CHRONIC WOUND CARE:

A Clinical Source Book for Healthcare Professionals

Second Edition

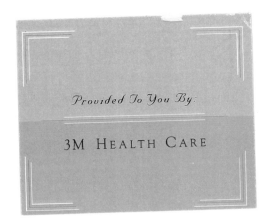

Provided To You By:

3M HEALTH CARE

CHRONIC WOUND CARE:

A Clinical Source Book for Healthcare Professionals

Second Edition

Edited by

Diane Krasner, MS, RN, CETN
Dean Kane, MD, FACS

Health Management Publications, Inc.
Wayne, PA

Managing Editor: Elizabeth G. Woytovich
Editorial Director: Harry J. Hurley
Publisher: Patrick D. Scullin

Chronic Wound Care: A Clinical Source Book for Healthcare Professionals, Second Edition

Copyright © 1997
Health Management Publications, Inc.
950 West Valley Road
Suite 2800
Wayne, PA 19087

ISBN 096280844X

Accurate indications, adverse reactions, and dosage schedules for wound care products and drugs are provided in this book, but it is possible that they may change. The reader is urged to review the package information data of the manufacturers of the products mentioned.

Printed in the United States of America

Dedication

To those persons who suffer
with chronic wounds,
whose plight inspires us
to envision and to provide
the best in Advanced Wound Caring.

Contents

Section I

Fundamentals

Section II

Management

Section III

The Cutting Edge

Contributors

Sue Bale, BA, RGN, NDN, RHV, DipN
Director of Nursing Research
Wound Healing Research Unit
Department of Surgery
University of Wales College of Medicine
Cardiff, UK

Sharon Baranoski, MSN, RN, CETN
Director of Nursing Education and Quality
Systems
Silver Cross Hospital and
President of Private Consulting Service
Wound Care Dynamics, Inc.
Shorewood, IL

Jane Ellen Barr, MSN, RN, CETN
Clinical Nurse Specialist
Mercy Medical Center
Rockville Centre, NY

Barbara Bates–Jensen, MN, CETN
Assistant Professor of Clinical Nursing
University of Southern California
Los Angeles, CA

Anne E. Belcher, RN, PhD, FAAN
Chairperson and Associate Professor
University of Maryland at Baltimore
School of Nursing
Baltimore, MD

Laura Bolton, PhD
Director of Scientific Affairs
ConvaTec, a Bristol–Myers Squibb Company
Skillman, NJ

Barbara J. Braden, PhD, RN, FAAN
Dean, Graduate School
Creighton University
Omaha, NE

Dale Buchbinder, MD, FACS
Chairman, Department of Surgery
Clinical Professor, Department of Surgery
University of Maryland and Chicago Medical
School
Greater Baltimore Medical Center
Baltimore, MD

Louise Colburn, RN, MS
Clinical Services Director
Johnson & Johnson Medical, Inc.
Arlington, TX

Philip D. Coleridge Smith, DM, FRCS
Senior Lecturer, Department of Surgery
UCL Medical School
London, UK

Janice C. Colwell, RN, MS, CETN
Clinical Specialist, Enterostomal Therapy
University of Chicago Hospitals
Chicago, IL

Sue Crow, RN, MSN
Nurse Epidemiologist
Associate Professor of Medical Administration
Louisiana State University Medical Center
Shreveport, LA

Jan Cuzzell, MA, RN, CNS
Director of Clinical Services
The Atlanta Consulting Group Healthcare
Practice, L.L.C.
Savannah, GA

Stephen C. Davis, BS
Instructor
University of Miami School of Medicine
Miami, FL

William H. Eaglstein, MD
Chairman and Harvey Blank Professor
University of Miami School of Medicine
Miami, FL

William J. Ennis, D.O.
Medical Director Wound Treatment Center
Columbia Olympia Fields Osteopathic
Medical Center
Olympia Fields, IL

Paula Erwin–Toth, MSN, RN, CETN
Manager, Enterostomal Therapy Nursing
Director, ET Nursing Education
Cleveland Clinic Foundation
Cleveland, OH

Vincent Falanga, MD, FACP
Professor of Medicine and Dermatology
University of Miami School of Medicine and
Miami VA Hospital
Miami, FL

Nancy A. Faller, RN, MSN, CETN
ET Nurse Clinical Specialist
Rutland Regional Medical Center
Rutland, VT

Carelyn P. Fylling, RN, MSN
Director of Educational Services
Curative Health Services
East Setauket, NY

Susan L. Garber, MA, OTR, FAOTA
Associate Professor, Department of Physical
Medicine and Rehabilitation
Baylor College of Medicine
Houston, TX

Judy L. Gates, RN, C
Wound Care Consultant
Olsten Kimberly Quality Care
Maricopa Medical Center
Adjunct Faculty at Arizona State University
Phoenix, AZ

Brian Gilchrist, BSc, MSc, RGN
Lecturer in Nursing Studies
King's College
London, England

Prem P. Gogia, PhD, PT
President
Wound Management Consultants, Inc.
Houston, TX

Julia E. Haimowitz, MD
Assistant Instructor of Dermatology
University of Pennsylvania School of Medicine
Philadelphia, PA

Keith Harding, MB, ChB, MRCGP
Director Wound Healing Research Unit
Senior Lecturer Rehabilitation, Wound Healing
University of Wales College of Medicine
Cardiff, Wales, UK

Ann H. Harris, MSN, RN, CS
Independent Practice
Spring Lake, MI

Cathy Thomas Hess, BSN, RN, CETN
President
Wound Care Strategies, Inc.
Harrisburg, PA

Mary Mayes Hilton, RN, BSN, CDE
Program Director
Greater Baltimore Wound Care Center
Baltimore, MD

G. Allen Holloway, Jr., MD, RVT
Director, Vascular Laboratory
Director, Medical Research
Maricopa Medical Center
Phoenix, AZ

Gloria J. Huber, RN
Clinical Manager
Greater Baltimore Wound Care Center
Baltimore, MD

Jeffrey P. Hurley, MD
Private Practive
Consulting Dermatologist
Fitzgerald Mercy Hospital
Darby, PA

Rick Jay, BA, MBA
President
RIK Medical
Boulder, CO

Dean P. Kane, MD, FACS
Plastic and Reconstructive Surgeon
Solo Practice
Assistant Clinical Professor
Division of Plastic Surgery
Johns Hopkins Hospital
Baltimore, MD

Karen Lou Kennedy, FNP, RN, CS
Consultant in Wound and Skin Care
Fort Wayne, IN

Diane Krasner, MS, RN, CETN
ET Nurse Consultant
Executive Director
Association for the Advancement of Wound
Care
Baltimore, MD

Thomas A. Krouskop, PhD, PE
Professor, Department of Physical Medicine
and Rehabilitation
Baylor College of Medicine
Houston, TX

David J. Margolis, MD
Assistant Professor of Dermatology
University of Pennsylvania School of Medicine
Philadelphia, PA

Adrienne McNally
Manager of Regulatory Affairs
ConvaTec, A Bristol–Myers–Squibb Company
Skillman, NJ

Clifford F. Melick, PhD
Director, Surgical Research
Department of Surgery
Greater Baltimore Medical Center
Baltimore, MD

Patricio Meneses, PhD
Assistant Director Magnetic Resonance Lab
Midwestern University
Chicago, IL

Patricia M. Mertz, BA
Dermatology Professor
University of Miami School of Medicine
Miami, FL

Glenda J. Motta, RN, BSN, MPH, ET
President
GM Associates, Inc.
Mitchellville, MD

Gerit D. Mulder, DPM, MS
University of California, San Diego
Wound Center, Department of Surgery
University of Colorado
Healthy Sciences Center
Department of Aging
Denver, CO

Diane K. Newman, RNC, MSN, FAAN
Adult Nurse Practitioner
Access to Continence Care & Treatment
DKN & Associates
Philadelphia, PA

Maria Oliveira–Gandia, DVM
Technical Specialist
University of Miami School of Medicine
Miami, FL

Nancy L. Parenteau, PhD
Senior Vice President
Chief Scientific Officer
Organogenesis Inc.
Canton, MA

Tania J. Phillips, MD
Associate Professor of Dermatology
Boston University School of Medicine
Boston, MA

Gayle Pinchcofsky–Devin, RD, FACN, L.D.
Vice President/Co–Owner
Stat Home Care, Inc.
Elmhurst, IL

Jay Portnow, MD, PhD
President
J. P. Healthcare Consulting and Management
Editor/Publisher
Norwell, MA

Lia van Rijswijk, RN, ET
Nurse Consultant
Newtown, PA

George T. Rodeheaver, PhD
Professor and Director of Plastic Surgery
Research
University of Virginia Medical Center
Charlottesville, VA

Bonnie Sue Rolstad, RN, BA, CETN
Director and ET Nurse Specialist
Healtheast
St. Paul, MN

Amy Roma, RN, CETN
Enterostomal Therapy Nurse
Columbia Hospital at Medical City Dallas
Dallas, TX

David T. Rovee, PhD
President and Chief Operating Officer
Organogenesis Inc.
Canton, MA

Cecilia Rund, RN, CETN
Clinical Nurse Consultant
Smith & Nephew United, Inc.
Largo, FL

Michael L. Sabolinski, MD
Senior Vice President
Corporate Development and Medical Affairs
Organogenesis Inc.
Canton, MA

Janice M. Stanfield, RN, BS, CETN
President and CEO
Stanfield Associates
Santa Clarita, CA

David L. Steed, MD
Professor of Surgery
University of Pittsburgh
Pittsburgh, PA

Brenda P. Stenger, MEd, RN, CETN
Faculty, ET Nursing Education
Cleveland Clinic Foundation
Cleveland, OH

Nancy A. Stotts, RN, EdD
Professor
Department Physiological Nursing
University of California San Francisco
San Francisco, CA

Thomas Taddonio, MT (ASCP), CTBS
Director, University of Michigan Skin Bank
and Trauma Burn Laboratory
University of Michigan Medical Center
Ann Arbor, MI

Robert Tallon, MD, MBA
President
Strategic Healthcare Analysts
Ormond Beach, FL

Philip D. Thomson, PhD
Associate Director, Technology Planning
Mallinckrodt Inc.
St. Louis, MO

Daniel L. Tritch, MD
Clinical Professor in Medicine
University of Chicago Hospitals and Clinics
Chicago, IL

Terence D. Turner, OBE, FRPharmS, MPharm, M.C.P.P.
Director, Surgical Dressings Research Unit
Welsh School of Pharmacy
University of Wales, Cardiff
Wales, UK

Keith Van Meter, MD
Section Chief, Emergency Medicine at LSU
School of Medicine
Charity Hospital of New Orleans
Louisiana State University School of Medicine
New Orleans, LA

Donald W. Wallace, Jr., MD
Investigator
Clinical Pharmacology Research Unit
Allegheny University of the Health Sciences
Medical Director
Clinical Services for Access to Continence Care
and Treatment
Philadelphia, PA

Joyce Wallace, RNC, MSN, CRNP
Clinical Preceptor and Lecturer
University of Pennsylvania
Philadelphia, PA

Laurel A. Wiersema–Bryant, MSN, RN, CS, ANP
Clinical Nurse Specialist
Barnes Jewish Hospital
Washington University Medical Center
St. Louis, MO

Deidre D. Wipke–Tevis, RNC, CVN, PhD
Assistant Professor of Nursing
University of Missouri–Columbia
Columbia, MO

Foreword

George T. Rodeheaver, PhD
Professor and Director of Plastic Surgery Research
University of Virginia Medical Center
Charlottesville, VA

Wound management has become a serious concern for healthcare professionals. With the restructuring of healthcare, financial demands require rapid resolution of complex problems such as chronic wounds. Unfortunately, the education that our healthcare professionals receive contains very little emphasis on the details of wound care. Practitioners interested in wound care usually have to educate themselves.

In this time of technological advancement, education is a continuous lifelong process. Even those practitioners and researchers who have dedicated their careers to wound care have difficulty keeping pace with the rapidly expanding information on the subject. This wealth of new information is manageable only if there is a well–organized, basic foundation upon which to correctly add and interpret the importance of these new bricks of information. Without the basic foundation, the dedicated practitioner is buried in a random pile of facts and figures.

Diane Krasner, a nurse specialist in the care of chronic wounds, and Dean Kane, a plastic surgeon with special focus on repairing wounded tissue, have provided practitioners with the components for building a strong foundation in wound care. This second edition of *Chronic Wound Care* is even more informative than the first edition. All seventy–one contributors provide state–of–the–art presentations on their special focus in wound care. Each one of these chapters is an essential brick for building the foundation of knowledge required of each wound care specialist. Whether you are a beginning practitioner or an experienced professional, this book will educate or re–educate you on the optimal ways to manage chronic wounds.

Preface

Diane Krasner, MS, RN, CETN
ET Nurse Consultant
Executive Director
Association for the
Advancement of Wound Care
Baltimore, MD

Dean P. Kane, MD, FACS
Plastic and Reconstructive Surgeon
Solo Practice
Assistant Clinical Professor
Division of Plastic Surgery
Johns Hopkins Hospital
Baltimore, MD

Stagnant or deteriorating chronic wounds and chronic diseases stand in sharp contrast to the advancing and dynamic nature of modern society. The care requirements of individuals with chronic wounds call for focused interventions and continuity of care. Optimal chronic wound care is holistic and individualized, demanding the most skilled, expert practices of interdisciplinary healthcare professionals with an eye toward prevention and a heart toward healing the mind, body and soul.

We term the optimal care requirements for chronic wound patients "Advanced Wound Caring." The nature and scope of advanced wound caring are detailed in the fifty–three chapters of this source book. Seventy–one contributors share their insights and make their predictions about advanced wound caring at the dawn of the new millennium.

Section 1, entitled Fundamentals, addresses the basics of wound healing, terminology, prevention, assessment, documentation, nutrition, infection and infection control. Section 2, entitled Management, reviews current management strategies, everything from wound cleansing to care in alternative settings. Section 3, entitled The Cutting Edge, introduces a number of advanced wound care concerns, such as practice issues, new technologies, palliative care, pain management, economic, regulatory, and research issues.

We hope that this source book will inspire you to:
- hone your wound caring skills and mentor your colleagues,
- embrace the challenge of life–long learning,
- be critical consumers of wound care practice and research,
- protect the rights and entitlements of persons who suffer,
  with chronic wounds worldwide.

Here's to Advanced Wound Caring!

Acknowledgements

In Appreciation:

To the contributors to this source book
who by sharing their expertise and insights
also serve as role models
for interdisciplinary collaboration
and wound care excellence.

To the publisher and editors
at Health Management Publications
for their technical expertise, encouragement,
and unwavering support of this source book.

To those healthcare professionals
whose untiring benevolence
fosters improved quality of life
for persons with chronic wounds.

Section I

FUNDAMENTALS

1

Wound Healing and Wound Management

Dean P. Kane, MD, FACS and Diane Krasner, MS, RN, CETN

Kane D, Krasner D. Wound healing and wound management. In: Krasner D, Kane D. *Chronic Wound Care, Second Edition*. Wayne, PA, Health Management Publications, Inc., 1997, pp 1–4.

Advanced Wound Caring

Wound healing is a complex process influenced by the host (the patient), the environment, and the healthcare professional. Despite the tenacity of many slow–to–heal, chronic wounds and the resultant frustration felt by patients, caregivers and healthcare professionals alike, with perseverance, many of these wounds can be healed. For patients where healing is not anticipated, expert palliative wound management can prevent deterioration and provide comfort.

This chapter will present an overview of wound healing and wound management from a broad, clinically focused perspective. The aim is to integrate state–of–the–science knowledge with state–of–the–art caring: into advanced wound caring. The objective of advanced wound caring is to improve the outcomes and the quality of life for all individuals who have sustained chronic wounds.

Extent of the Problem

The most common chronic wounds include lower extremity ulcers, diabetic ulcers and pressure ulcers. Other types of chronic wounds include non–healing surgical wounds, infected wounds and fistulae. As opposed to acute wounds that usually heal in a matter of days or weeks, chronic wounds can persist for months or even years (Plates 3 to 10).

The dimension of the worldwide chronic wound care problem is epidemic, although exact figures continue to be elusive. Lower extremity ulcerations are the most frequently occurring chronic wounds. Venous ulcers account for eighty to ninety percent of lower extremity ulcers. The incidence in Europe is documented to range from 0.12 percent for patients with an active venous ulcer at the time of study to approximately 1.0 percent when patients with a history of venous ulceration are included in the statistical analysis.[1] As many as ten to fifteen percent of diabetic patients will develop foot ulcers,[2] with 50,000 to 60,000 amputations performed on diabetics annually in the United States.[3]

In 1990 over 2.1 million pressure ulcers were reported in the United States alone at a yearly cost of greater than 1.3 billion dollars.[4] Certain groups, including elderly patients admitted to the hospital for femoral fracture (66 percent incidence of pressure ulcers) and critical care patients (33 percent incidence), are at particularly high risk for pressure ulcers.[4] Older adults are more likely to develop chronic wounds and since the global population is aging, the number of chronic wounds worldwide is expected to rise dramatically in the future. In the United States alone there are currently 35 million adults over the age of 65 and 4 million over the age of 85.

Acute Versus Chronic Wounds

When injury occurs to the skin, its normal barrier function is destroyed. A series of events and cascades initiate homeostasis and protection of all internal organs.[5–7] Traumatic abrasions, lacerations and superficial skin and soft tissue injuries generally heal without complications, sealing the offending external environment from the internal bodily environment within a short period. In the healthy, uncompromised host, acute wounds heal spontaneously without complications through the three normal phases

Table 1
The Wound Healing Trajectory

Phase	Goal	Duration	Principle Cells
I	Inflammatory Response	Injury to day 4 post injury	Platelets Neutrophils Lymphocytes Macrophages Epithelial cells
II	Granulation Tissue Formation	Day 4 to day 21 post injury	Fibroblasts
III	Remodeling	Day 21 to 2 years post injury	Fibroblasts

of the wound healing trajectory: inflammation, proliferation and remodeling (Table 1). Near normal tensile strength of the scar is achieved over time, with 30 percent tensile strength in 3 weeks, 60 percent in 6 weeks and 90 percent in 6 months.

If the natural healing progression is delayed, a chronic wound results. In 1992, Lazarus, et al. of the Wound Healing Society defined chronic wounds as those that "fail to progress through a normal, orderly and timely sequence of repair or wounds that pass through the repair process without restoring anatomic and functional results."[8] Many wound complications can result including infection; increased length of healing, length of stay or cost of healing; pain; disability; loss of work productivity; catabolism; deformity; disuse atrophy; reduced self esteem; and potential loss of limb or loss of life. Clinically, our experience has been that those wounds that do not heal within six weeks (with adequate tensile strength and stable barriers against re–injury or infection) will need wound specialist intervention and chronic wound management.

Chronic Wound Management

As each of us ages, many of us will acquire systemic chronic ailments. These conditions will force upon us less tolerance for maintaining a normal homeostatic environment and for achieving a well healed wound. The "plasticity" of healing as a newborn and infant is contrasted with the frailty and compromised healing of the aged.

Chronic wound care involves a series of distinct wound management goals (Table 2). The primary goal for any patient with a wound, whether it is caused by trauma or complicated by infection, is to save the patient's life. Patients with diabetes, vasculitis and peripheral vascular disease (including arterial or venous insufficiencies) have a high risk of limb threat which should be minimized if possible in order to achieve greater rehabilitative potential.

A healed wound in the shortest period of time with the least amount of energy and healthcare expenditure is the overall goal. Traditionally, it has been the only goal. A more holistic view of wound healing is necessary to meet patients' requirements for perfusion, nutritional support, mobility enhancement, incontinence management, pain control and self–esteem with that of their wound(s). In order to achieve improved outcomes with greater efficacy in healing, both function and aesthetic appearance of the final wound should also be considered at the time of the initial assessment. Certainly by adopting this holistic appreciation for form and function, the wound care specialist will be best able to address the unique requirements of the wounded patient. This will also reduce the number of staged procedures necessary to achieve the goal of a healed wound.

Each wound is unique in that its host is an individual with unique chronic ailments and potential for healing. Many times patient comfort and quality of life supersede aggressive intervention, despite the attendant risks of limb loss, pain and death. Careful consideration of wound care versus wound repair (taking into consideration unique social, economic and medical factors) is warranted if we are to return patients to their greatest functional state.

Delayed Wound Healing

As noted previously, each wound is influenced by many internal and external co–factors. Common

KANE AND KRASNER

co–factors that disrupt or delay wound healing include compromised perfusion, malnutrition, and infection. Without control of these variables wound healing cannot be optimized. See Chapter 9 in this source book for further information on co–factors that impair wound healing.

All wounds are colonized by bacteria, most of which are not virulent and cause no invasion, multiplication or inflammatory response. Virulent and invasive bacteria, such as *pseudomonas aeruginosa* and *staphylococcus aureus*, can cause infection, morbidity, limb loss, and mortality. Infection control is critical: if you do not control the infection, the infection will control the host. For further information on wound infection, refer to Chapters 8, 11, 12, and 14 in this source book.

Wound Healing from a Builder's Perspective

Many of us have difficulty understanding the complexities of the wound healing process. The following model is proposed as a way to facilitate understanding without oversimplification. Placed into the context of building a house, one can begin to appreciate the intricacies of the interactive phases of the wound healing trajectory, commonly referred to as inflammation, proliferation and remodeling. Multiple delays can occur with every step of the process. Wounding destroys the various layers of the skin and underlying soft tissues, just as a hurricane, tornado or bombing can destroy a house and the land site around it (Plate 2). Imagine . . . just like damaged water and electrical conduits, the arteries, veins and nerves become exposed during wounding. Just as utility workers must cap conduits to prevent further destruction and losses, platelets and fibrin cap damaged vessels at the site of injury. During the inflammatory phase, the polymorphonucleocytes or non–specific laborers initiate the clean–up process to remove debris and tidy up the area of wounding. Communication occurs during the entire reconstructive process much like that in building a house. Chemotaxins will signal for the next set of laborers to begin their work. Without the proper stimulation of wound healing events, the various phases would not occur.

To build a house various steps must be organized and synchronized (running conduits, laying foundations, framing the walls, siding the habitat and finishing the roof). It is the same for wound regeneration and repair. Without the proper signals at the right time, the macrophage or "contractor" cell, whose job it is to further organize the entire wound healing process, will not show up for work. In certain disease processes, such as diabetes and autoimmune diseases, and in immunocompromise due to

certain medications, the absence of a full inflammatory response delays the wound healing process.

Without the building materials or adequate nutrition to provide sustenance, including protein, carbohydrate, fat, fluid, vitamins and minerals, wound healing delays occur. Granulation tissue, the foundation of the house, is dependent on angiogenesis and neurogenesis. Without the foundation, the house cannot be built. Without growth factors or cytokines to stimulate granulation tissue formation, the wound will not heal.

Continued anabolism of the host must be maintained in order to achieve healing during the fibroblastic and fibrocyte stages of collagen formation, which is the scaffolding for repair of the wound site. Fibroblasts and fibrocytes are like sub–contractors in the building process, providing the scaffolding for myoblasts and myocytes. Other sub–contractors of the wound healing phase pull together and provide strength for the walls of the wound. As these last subcontractors leave the building or the wound site, the finishers or epithelial cells, provide the siding and the roofing, the barriers against the external environment.

If the epithelium is injured as in a burn, a deep sloughing injury, or a venous ulcer, such as happened with the loss of roofs in Florida during hurricane Andrew, then one would only repair or replace the roof, i.e. skin graft the epithelial surface lost. If deeper structures are lost, such as skin and subcutaneous tissue during wide excision of skin cancers, superficial ulcers, or traumatic injury, then approximating the wound edges or carrying adjacent tissues from redundant areas still attached to their random blood supply can hasten healing by primary intention. Perfusion and the cells needed for wound healing are more readily available, so healing is more rapidly achieved than with healing by secondary intention. This is much like building a split trailer house and riveting the edges with collagen rivets.

Certainly if the entire trailer house can be brought to the building site, much like that of an adjacent

---

<table>
<tr><td>
Table 2
Chronic Wound Management Goals

1. Saving life
2. Saving limb
3. Infection control
4. Pain management
5. Complete and durably healed wound
6. Optimal function or a stable chronic wound
7. Aesthetic result
</td></tr>
</table>

random flap into the wound, healing can be hastened. In wounds greater than 2 to 2.5 cm in diameter, even with adequate granulation tissue and contracture, wound epithelialization may remain unstable in the center and constantly bleed and crack if re–injured. For this reason, reconstructive surgical repair should be considered in these wounds. If larger amounts of healthy tissue are carried into the wound the repair will be more permanent. This is much like the total destruction of a landsite and placement of a new portable facility, such as a trailer house with conduits, foundation, frame and siding, at the repaired landsite.

Large amounts of energy, resources, time and money are necessary to reconstruct tissue that has been lost. Reconstructive surgery may be a cost–effective and efficient option for selected patients. The reader is referred to Chapter 30 on Surgical Repair in this source book for further information.

Differential Diagnoses for Chronic Wounds

Each wound or ulcer is created by unique physiologic events. Accurate assessment and diagnosis of each wound is therefore essential in order to achieve optimal healing. Common differential diagnoses for chronic wounds are listed in Table 3. Detailed discussions on the assessment, classification and management of pressure ulcers, arterial ulcers, venous ulcers and diabetic wounds can be found in Chapters 18 to 21 of this source book.

Wound Management from an Interior Decorator's Perspective

If wound healing is like building a house, than wound management is like interior decorating to make the house a home. Careful selection of wound products and devices to optimize the wound environment is like choosing the carpeting, furniture and accessories that make a house habitable. Attention to patient pain and comfort can be equated to selecting the color schemes and styles that turn a generic house into a comfortable, personalized living space. Decisions about wound care and/or wound repair should be made by the entire healthcare team, including the patient whenever feasible. After evaluating the patient's overall health, the severity of the wound, the repair options and the potential for optimal outcomes, the management plan can be developed. Wound management strategies vary widely and are both an art and a science. The reader is referred to Section II of this source book for detailed discussions on the interdisciplinary management of chronic wounds.

The Challenge of Advanced Wound Caring

Each wound and each patient is unique. Optimal wound care involves customizing standard approaches based on the latest recommendations for each chronic wound patient. This process is always challenging and often rewarding. Special attention must be given to the changing healthcare environment, to cost–effectiveness, to measurable outcomes and to quality of life. Such holistic care requires an interdisciplinary approach. The better we healthcare professionals are able to integrate our efforts across the continuum of care, the more likely we will be to deliver positive outcomes for our chronic wound patients, thereby providing advanced wound caring.

References

1. Burton C. Venous ulcers. *Am J Surg* 1994;167(1A):37S–41S.
2. Levin ME. Diabetic foot ulcers: pathogenesis and management. *JET Nurs* 1993;20:191–198.
3. Miller OF. Essentials of pressure ulcer treatment, the diabetic experience. *J Dermatol Surg* Oncol 1993;19:759–63.
4. Bergstrom N, Bennett MA, Carlson CE, et al. *Treatment of Pressure Ulcers*. Clinical Practice Guideline, No. 15. Rockville, MD: U.S. Department of Health and Human Services, Public Health Service, Agency for Health Care Policy and Research, AHCPR Pub. No. 95–0622, December 1994.
5. Cooper, D. The physiology of wound healing: An overview. In: Krasner D. *Chronic Wound Care: A Clinical Source Book for Healthcare Professionals*. King of Prussia, PA, Health Management Publications, 1990, pp 1–11.
6. Cohen IK, Diegelmann RF, Linblad WJ. *Wound Healing: Biochemical & Clinical Aspects*. Philadelphia, PA, W.B. Saunders, 1992.
7. Bryant R.(Ed.). (1992). *Acute and Chronic Wounds: Nursing Management*. St. Louis, MO, Mosby, 1992.
8. Lazarus G, Cooper D, Knighton D, Margolis D, Pecoraro R, Rodeheaver G, Robson M. Definitions and guidelines for assessment of wounds and evaluation of healing. *Archives of Dermatology* 1994;130:489–493.

2

The Language of Wounds

Lia van Rijswijk, RN, ET

van Rijswijk L. The language of wounds. In: Krasner D, Kane D. *Chronic Wound Care, Second Edition*. Wayne, PA, Health Management Publications, Inc., 1997, pp 5–8.

Language is not simply a reporting device for experience but a defining framework for it.
(Benjamin Whorf, 1897–1941)

Introduction

What is the framework of wound care and dressing changes? Most importantly, how can an understanding of the words we use contribute to improving patient care? If you have ever spent time explaining why you do wound care and what it is, you know the language we use is not well–understood outside the circle of "wound care" practitioners. This chapter may help you understand why and may help you communicate more effectively with patients, caregivers and others who do not have the same language framework as healthcare professionals.

Wound

Historically neither the word nor the meaning of the word "wound" has undergone much evolution. The skin has many functions, but its ability to protect and provide a permanent armor (Figure 1) against the elements has had a profound impact on our culture and our attitudes toward wounds. Definitions and expressions common hundreds of years ago are still used today. The word "wound" describes a separation of the tissues of the body, defines an injury due to external violence, or describes an imperfection.[1] Specifically, the word "wound" often can be found in the context of physical or emotional violence and is used to represent serious damage that may be difficult to repair. Historically, individuals with wounds would succumb to their injuries, be scarred for the rest of

their lives or be banned from society because "A wound though cur'd, yet leaves behind a scar" (Oldham, Sat Jesuits III, 1681).

Today, when the word "wounded" is used to describe what happened to a social system or the emotional well–being of a person (e.g. the political party was wounded, his pride was wounded) it still means that restoring complete function will probably be difficult and certainly take time. Wounds are not to be taken lightly!

Vulnerability

A separation of the tissues of the body may cause complications (e.g. infection), hence, a wounded person is vulnerable. Similarly, when using the word "wound" as a figure of speech, a psychologically or emotionally wounded person is more vulnerable than an intact person. Indeed, "vulnerable" is derived from the Latin word "vulnus," meaning wound, and the word "woundless" is defined as "that which cannot be wounded or invulnerable."[1] The vulnerability of wounded individuals increases when they have to depend on others for care since they often have little control over caregiver ability, sensitivity or availability. Finally, cultural and socio–economic circumstances can create in someone a sense of vulnerability and defenselessness and a loss of self–esteem. For example, for those who believe that physical "completeness" extends into an afterlife or later lives, any type of disfigurement can cause deep depression.[2] Similarly, for hundreds of years the lives of people suspected of having leprosy were affected by, among others, Old Testament Laws dictating that the person who was found to be unclean had to "dwell apart, making his abode outside the camp." (Leviticus 13)

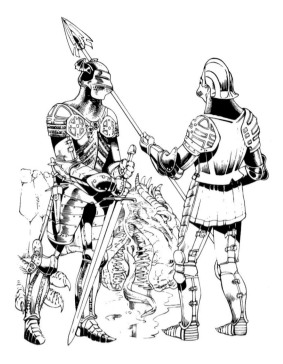

Figure 1. Advanced Dungeons & Dragons, Arms and Equipment Guide. Artwork courtesy of and © 1991, TSR, Inc.

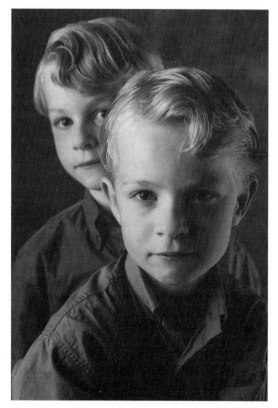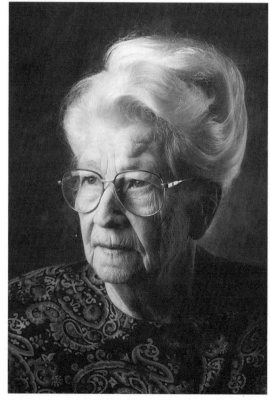

Figures 2 and 3. Photographs courtesy of and © 1994 Peter Dellenbag.

VAN RIJSWIJK

Perfection and Punishment

A wound is also defined as an imperfection. Wounded tissue not only limits function, but once healed the original perfection will never return. The latter may have profound psychological and social implications. Consider one's "natural" inclination to look at perfection and touch the unblemished skin of children. Conversely, blemishes, open wounds and disfigurement tend to cause people to "look the other way," repelling physical contact" (Figures 2 and 3).

Furthermore, the belief that skin disorders in general are a visible mark of sin (or punishment) has persisted over the years. Even today patients with unexplained skin disease tend to attribute their disorder to "poor lifestyle choices" (e.g. diet, drinking).[3] This view may, in part, explain why leg ulcer patients report depression, anxiety, anger, a negative self–image and social isolation.[4] Similarly, the idea that pressure ulcers are a result of poor patient care, i.e. "a visible mark of caregiver sin," has been around for a long time.[5,6]

Dressing

For thousands of years, people have applied almost every naturally occurring substance as well as a plethora of "specially developed" concoctions in an attempt to help wounds heal and lessen the burden of the wounded. Even today, many wound care practices are ritualistic instead of science–based. There are two explanations. First, healthcare professionals are reluctant to let go of wound care rituals, perhaps because of the level of comfort they provide. They can make events, such as caring for large malodorous wounds, socially manageable.[7] Second, history may provide us with an explanation because to dress a wound does not mean that it is simply covered up. Derived from the old French "drecier" (to arrange), "to dress" literally means to make straight, to make right, to tend or to put in proper order .[1] The term "dress" was also often used in the military; "the batallion dressed its rank with precision" (Kinglake, Crimea, 1877). Dressing wounds was such an important ritual that surgeons in 18th Century England employed assistants called dressers to care for the wounds. Thus, while the word "wound" may invoke images of serious harm and vulnerability, the word "dress" implies that "everything is going to be all–right."

Chronic Wounds

A chronic wound can be defined as a wound that has "failed to proceed through an orderly and timely process to produce anatomic and functional integrity, or proceeded through the repair process without establishing a sustained anatomic and functional result." [8] Literally, the word "chronic" as it pertains to disease means lasting a long time, lingering, inveterate, continuous or constant. For hundreds of years, the word "chronic" was also commonly used as a synonym for the word "invalid".[1] Individuals with chronic wounds not only have to deal with being wounded, but they also have to face the unfulfilled expectation of healing. They have to come to terms with their (seemingly) failing body.[9] The "failing body" may, in turn, cause a loss or negative alteration of body image which can be extremely traumatic and stressful. The need to be physically whole is strongly associated with remaining mentally and emotionally intact.[10]

Chronic Wound Care

Wound care professionals are usually called to care when it has been determined that the wound in question is not healing the way it should. Care in the context of "to care for" is defined as "take thought for, provide for, look after." In general, the word "care" means to grieve, feel concern or trouble oneself for someone or something.[1] Why do people in general, and healthcare professionals in particular, care? Louis Berman gives eight meanings of being called to care including these four: entering into a relationship with the other, suffering with the other, responding to the needs of, and hoping with another person.[11] When we perform wound care, we not only physically manage and cover the wound, we respond to a need and bring hope for healing. We dress the wound; we are supposed to "make it all better." We care. However, caring, being open to experiencing another's pain, inevitably leads to vulnerability and being "prone

> *The need to be physically whole is strongly associated with remaining mentally and emotionally intact.*[10]

to injury."[11] Thus, the feelings of vulnerability that may accompany the wounded person can be similar to the feelings experienced by those who care. For example, when asked to reflect on pressure ulcer patients' pain, one nurse said, "I get upset when someone is in pain due to something I am doing. I felt very helpless in this situation"[12]

Failing to acknowledge that there is a problem or "accepting" that one cannot respond to the call, are common strategies to avoid the call to care and thus vulnerability. Finding limited social support while caring for her elderly husband with pressure ulcers, a woman explained that her son "can't even look at his father, he is unable to cope."[13] Caring can wound, and wounded persons are vulnerable.

References

1. *Oxford English Dictionary, Twenty–Sixth Edition*. Oxford, UK, University Press, 1987.
2. Ryan TJ. Wound healing in the developing world. *Dermatology Clinics* 1993;11(4):791–800.
3. Kligman AM. Psychologic aspects of skin disorders in the elderly. *J Geriatric Dermatol* 1993;1(1):15–21
4. Phillips T, Stanton B, Provan A, Lew R. A study of the impact of leg ulcers on quality of life: Financial, social, and psychologic implications. *J Am Acad Dermatol* 1994;31:49–53.
5. Dealy C. Pressure sores: The result of bad nursing? *Br J Nurs* 1992;15(1):748.
6. Parish LC, Witkowski JA, Millikan LE. Cutaneous torsion stress alias the decubitus ulcer: a felony. *Int J Dermatol* 1988;27(6):375.
7. Wolff ZR. Nurses' work: the sacred and the profane. *Holistic Nurs Practice* 1986;1(1):29–35.

Caring can wound, and wounded persons are vulnerable.

The Language of Wounds

The rituals of wound care as well as the language we use are steeped in tradition. As a result, almost everyone has a frame of reference when talking about wounds and wound care. That does not mean, however, that we all speak the same language. Defining a "universal" framework for the language of wounds may be difficult, but being aware of the different interpretations of the words we use can make our life easier. What healthcare professionals call a "nicely healing" wound may be viewed as a disfigurement by others. Some may consider pressure ulcers "a normal occurrence among bedbound" whereas others view them as the "mark of caregiver sin." Dressing change procedures, interpreted as "standard procedure" by many healthcare professionals may invoke images of "making it all better" in patients or caregivers.

Knowing that the patient's frame of reference is based on his/her experience with an aunt or uncle who also "had a sore" or the neigbor who lost his foot because his wounds didn't heal, will help us communicate more effectively.

Asking patients how they feel about their wounds and what they expect does require getting involved. Understanding the patients' and caregivers' language of wounds requires caring. Caring may not always be easy but it has rich rewards. When we care for a wounded, vulnerable individual, we respond to, practice, and nurture the human potential to care. We explore the common grounds of meaning in human existence. In so doing, we can call ourselves wound care professionals.

8. Lazarus GS, Cooper DM, Knighton DR et.al. Definitions and guidelines for assessment of wounds and evaluation of healing. *Arch Dermatol* 1994;130:489–493.
9. Krasner D. Preface. In: Krasner D (ed). *Chronic Wound Care: A Clinical Source Book for Healthcare Professionals*. King of Prussia, PA, Health Management Publications, 1990.
10. Drench ME. Changes in Body image secondary to disease and injury. *Rehab Nurs* 1994;19(1):31–36.
11. Lashley ME, Neal MT, Slunt ET, Berman LM, Hultgren FH (eds). *Being Called to Care*. Albany, NY, State University of New York Press, 1994.
12. Krasner D. Using a gentler hand: reflections on patients with pressure ulcers who experience pain. *Ostomy Wound Management* 1996;42(3):20–2.
13. Baharestani MM. The lived experience of wives caring for their frail, homebound, elderly husbands with pressure ulcers. *Advances in Wound Care* 1994;7(3):40–52.

VAN RIJSWIJK

3

Prevention of Chronic Wounds

Louise Colburn, RN, MS

Colburn L. Prevention of chronic wounds. In: Krasner D, Kane D. *Chronic Wound Care, Second Edition.* Wayne, PA, Health Management Publications, Inc., 1997, pp 9–15.

Introduction

It is well known that chronic wounds can cause immense problems including pain, suffering, financial burden, work loss and psychosocial stressors. Whenever possible, prevention of wounding is the most obvious and sensible course to take. While it is often said and written that "most pressure ulcers are preventable," information related to the efficacy of prevention programs and associated costs is scarce. For example, there is very little research and documentation regarding outcomes associated with specific preventive activities. Most of the literature that does exist on wound prevention addresses pressure ulcers. Data on prevention of other chronic wounds such as venous and arterial ulcers is sparse. Prevention of wounds poses a huge challenge for providers in all healthcare settings. Development of wounds, especially pressure ulcers, is increasingly identified as an indicator of less–than–quality care, yet there has been no universally agreed upon approach to prevention.

The AHCPR Guideline

The greatest advance in pressure ulcer prevention was the development and publication of the Agency For Health Care Policy and Research (AHCPR) Clinical Guideline, "Pressure Ulcers in Adults: Prediction and Prevention."[1] This report describes a research–based approach to pressure ulcer prevention. Although many of the recommendations are reflective of minimally conclusive research, the guideline does offer the benefit of a complete literature search and ranking of evidence. Where the data are inconclusive or lacking, the recommendations reflect the opinion of the expert multidisciplinary panel.

The AHCPR Guideline first recommends identifying at–risk individuals and the specific factors placing them at risk. The document then groups preventive care into three categories: Skin Care and Early Treatment, Mechanical Loading and Support Surfaces, and Education:

Skin Care and Early Treatment

Goal: To maintain and improve tissue tolerance to pressure in order to prevent injury

• Inspect the skin daily, paying particular attention to bony prominences. Results of the inspection should be documented.

• Individualize bathing frequency based on need and/or patient preference. Bathing an elderly person daily may cause further drying of the skin leading to increased risk for breakdown. Use a mild cleansing agent. Avoid hot water and excessive friction.

• Minimize environmental factors leading to dry skin including low humidity (less than 40 percent) and exposure to cold. Treat dry skin with moisturizers.

• Avoid massages over bony prominences as they may cause trauma.

• Assess and treat incontinence. When incontinence cannot be controlled, cleanse the skin at the time of soiling and apply a topical moisture barrier. Select underpads or briefs that are absorbent and that provide a drying surface to the skin.

• Utilize proper positioning, transferring, and turning techniques to minimize skin injury due to friction and shear forces.

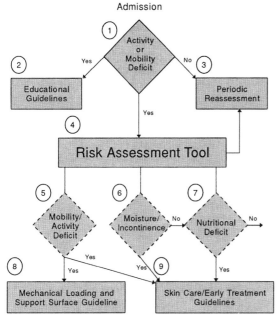

Figure 1. *"Management of Pressure Ulcers Overview" from AHCPR Clinical Practice Guideline Number 3: Pressure Ulcers in Adults: Preduction and Prevention*

• Use dry lubricants (e.g., cornstarch) or protective coverings (e.g., transparent films) to reduce friction injury.

• Identify and correct factors compromising protein/calorie intake. Consider nutritional supplementation/support for nutritionally compromised persons if such support is consistent with overall treatment goals.

• Institute a rehabilitation program consistent with the goals of care, to maintain or improve mobility/activity status.

• Monitor and document interventions and outcomes.

Mechanical Loading and Support Surfaces

Goal: To protect against the adverse forces of external mechanical forces: pressure, friction and shear.

• Reposition chair bound persons hourly and bedfast persons at least every two hours. Use a written repositioning schedule to ensure consistency and continuity.

• Place at-risk persons on a pressure reducing mattress and chair cushion. Do not use donut type devices.

• Teach chair bound persons, who are able, to shift weight every 15 minutes.

• Use lifting devices (e.g., trapeze or bed linen) to move rather than drag persons during transfers and position changes.

• Use pillows or foam wedges to keep bony prominences such as knees and ankles from direct contact with each other.

• Use devices that totally relieve pressure on the heels (i.e., place pillows under the calf to raise the heels off the bed).

• Avoid positioning directly on the trochanter when using the side–lying lateral position (i.e., use the 30° lateral inclined position).

• Maintain head of bed elevation at 30° or less if consistent with the person's overall medical condition.

Education

Goal: To reduce the incidence of pressure ulcers through educational programs

• Implement structured, organized, and comprehensive educational programs for the prevention of pressure ulcers. Direct these programs to patients, family and caregivers at all levels of healthcare providers.

• Include information on etiology, risk factors, risk assessment tools and their application, skin assessment, selection and use of support surfaces, individualized skin care programs, and demonstration of positioning to decrease risk of tissue breakdown. Also include information on accurate documentation of pertinent data.

• Use principles of adult learning with built in mechanisms, such as quality assurance standards and audits, for evaluating educational programs.

Figure 1 depicts the algorithm from the AHCPR Guideline, illustrating the process of managing persons at risk.

Guideline Implementation

Publication of the guideline is, of course, only the first step toward decreasing the incidence of pressure ulcers. The challenge for clinicians in all settings is to successfully implement these guidelines into clinical practice and to evaluate the effect.

Implementation is complex as it requires changing existing protocols and procedures, a daunting task at any time, but especially challenging in today's rapidly changing healthcare environment.[2]

Many authors have described and recommended that a multidisciplinary committee provide the leadership for a pressure ulcer prevention program. In a collaborative benchmarking study conducted in a large hospital group, a list of best practices identified included multidisciplinary involvement and protocols based on the AHCPR Guideline. In fact, all of the benchmarks met these criteria.[3]

Many programs based on this model have reported "success." While it is true that this "shared vision" often ensures continuity and consistency of care, most programs require a "champion" to keep the program on track.

In 1992, Barr suggested that guideline implementation requires an innovative approach by a change agent, a wound care specialist or educator with problem solving skills.[4] She also suggested that new tactics, such as utilizing a risk assessment tool, developing documentation forms, revising standards, policies and procedures and educating staff and patients, may be needed. After implementation, the expected outcomes must be evaluated for success. This approach should result in identification of new patients at risk and should demonstrate a decreased incidence of nosocomial pressure ulcers.

Bergstrom (1992) reported that the desired outcome for any pressure ulcer research is absence of pressure ulcers at the end of the course of care for a high risk group of patients. Intermediate outcomes such as interface pressure do not help clinicians determine if an intervention such as a support surface actually prevents pressure ulcers from forming in debilitated patients. Studies demonstrating the relationship between intermediate outcomes (e.g., interface pressure or dietary intake) and the desired outcome (pressure ulcer status at the end of the study) are needed to establish the validity of these intermediate outcomes.[5]

There are many reports of prevention programs in the literature, but most describe a plan or a program that was implemented and presumed to decrease pressure ulcers. Few describe the actual clinical outcomes of the program. There are, however, some examples of evaluation of specific interventions.

Cheney describes implementation of a program to reduce the incidence of heel ulcers in post–operative hip replacement patients. After the introduction of patient education, elevation of the heels off the mattress and the use of heel protectors, no post–operative heel wounds were found in 30 patients.[6]

In one study of a pressure ulcer prevention program modeled on the AHCPR Guideline, the incidence of pressure ulcers in a 125 bed long term care facility decreased significantly at each of the four initial post–program follow–ups and at an 11 month follow–up.[7]

The Cost of Prevention

Cost issues have not been well addressed in the literature. One research group examined the cost of implementing the AHCPR Guideline and found that the cost was no greater than the cost of current practice. The authors suggest that there is a cost saving for prevention vs. treatment cost, but more information is needed.[8]

A study performed in a 600 bed long term care facility examined the cost of four preventive measures including turning, pressure reducing mattresses, chair cushions, and miscellaneous devices. The facility's total 3 month cost of prevention was $132,114. Of this amount, turning was the most expensive intervention.[9]

In a study at a long term care facility, cost analysis revealed savings of more than $230,000 for an eight month time period. The authors point out that the cost in terms of human suffering also decreased.[7]

It is curious that saving patients from pain and suffering does not provide adequate rationale for preventive actions. Healthcare providers have traditionally dedicated themselves to relieving pain and suffering without expecting a cost saving. However, in today's managed care and outcome oriented environment, it is expected that definitive clinical and cost efficacy data will be provided. This expectation should be viewed as a positive development. The demand for outcome information will generate studies that provide more conclusive evidence than is currently available. Wound care clinicians would know which interventions and programs produce the desired outcomes, and the costs could be built into the systems and budgets. Precious resources including dollars would not be spent on ineffective or prohibitively high cost activities and products that produce negative or questionable results. Healthcare providers could make comparisons between interventions leading to informed decisions and programs that are clinically and economically effective.

Other Chronic Wounds

When the prevention of chronic wounds is discussed, the focus is most often on pressure ulcers.

However, there are preventive actions that can be put into place for other chronic wounds such as venous and arterial ulcers.

Arterial ulcers or "ischemic" ulcers are usually seen on the lower extremities and may be present in diabetics or non–diabetics with peripheral vascular disease. To prevent recurrences after surgical or medical interventions have assisted in healing the original ulcer, patient life–style changes are critical. Patients should be instructed to minimize situations that lead to vasoconstriction, for example, cold or constrictive clothing. It is important to facilitate blood flow through positioning. Patients must view control of risk factors including smoking, blood pressure, hyperlipedemia, and glucose as high priority. Depending on the individual, exercise may be recommended or curtailed. While there is no cure for the disease process that leads to ulcer formation, compliance with a prevention program can help to minimize the recurrence of wounds resulting from this condition.[10]

Neuropathic ulcers are pressure ulcers of the insensate foot and are associated with the vascular changes seen in diabetes. Primary goals are prevention of trauma that leads to wounding and relief of pressure. Orthotics and prescription shoes, specially fitted to re–distribute weight and prevent traumatic ulcers from forming, are used to achieve these goals. The primary focus of care is on prevention of foot injury through meticulous foot care and avoidance of trauma.

The large majority of leg ulcers are venous in origin. The mainstays of preventing recurrence are elevation of the extremity and compression. The most common cause of ulcer recurrence is failure to comply with compression therapy recommendations. The patient must be willing to wear prescription–grade stockings daily. Exercise is usually recommended as it may promote venous return. Educating at–risk patients in the management and prevention of venous ulcers can help prevent end–stage irreversible venous disease.[11]

Patient Education

Never before has patient and caregiver education been more important than it is in today's healthcare environment. Patients are discharged from acute care centers very early in the recovery process. The number of persons receiving home healthcare services is increasing exponentially. Healthcare professionals are responsible for giving patients and caregivers adequate information to assist them in prevention of pressure ulcers. Many persons not requiring an in–patient stay or receiving home care are seeking care for wounds at an ever increasing number of clinics. Prevention of re–wounding is key for these patients.

The primary goal of any patient education program is to provide patients and caregivers with information that will facilitate an understanding of the disease process. Hopefully, this knowledge will assist in recovery and in the prevention of future dysfunction. To whatever degree possible, the patient and family should be involved in prevention programs. Families or other caregivers may sincerely wish to give good care but may be unaware of the appropriate actions and the rationale for choosing them.

Spinal cord injured individuals play an integral role in their personal pressure ulcer prevention regimen since wounds are a life–long threat to this population. Compliance with prevention programs has been a challenge for healthcare providers working with these patients. Through education, effective teaching and monitoring, these patients may be motivated to become involved and responsible for their own care including wound prevention.

The AHCPR Guideline includes a consumer guide which details, in everyday terminology, the preventive recommendations of the clinical guideline for the health professional. There are diagrams to illustrate proper positioning and common sites for pressure ulcer development. In a critique, Ayello found this guide to meet many of the accepted criteria for patient teaching materials. There were some areas that could be improved including reading level (higher than recommended for the general population), small print size and clarification of illustrations.[12]

Fowler and Pelfrey describe a teaching plan to guide patients and families through the hospital to home transition.[13] The program includes a Patient Education Plan (PEP) incorporating outcomes and skills needed. This form outlines, tracks and evaluates achievement of these skills. The Teaching Guide provides step–by–step instructions based on the PEP (Figure 2).

There are many pamphlets and some videotapes available from skin and wound care manufacturers that are directed to patients and their caregivers. Videos have the advantage of providing visual demonstrations of positioning techniques and other interventions and are preferable if the required video equipment is available.

Healthcare professionals today must make every effort to offer patients and their caregivers adequate education in pressure ulcer or re–wounding prevention. It may be the deciding factor between maximizing health status and coping with debilitating wounds.

I. EDUCATIONAL PATHWAY

TEACHING STEPS	Give Handout	Discuss A-B-C	Show Video D-E-F-G & H	Discuss E-F-G Home	Home Care Products/Equipment	Discuss Home Care
TARGET DATE(S)	Day 1	Day 1	Day 2	Day 3	Day 4	Upon D/C

II. EDUCATIONAL TOPIC AND CONTENT OUTLINE

CONTENT	TEACHING METHOD	TEACHING RESOURCE
A. Definition of a Pressure Ulcer 1. A pressure ulcer is an area of skin where blood flow has been blocked by unrelieved pressure and has caused the skin cells to die. 2. Ask patient/S.O. to define pressure ulcers in their own terms.	Discussion Anatomy/ Physiology of the skin	Patient Guide Booklet the Pressures Off pg. 1
B. Causes of Pressure Ulcers 1. Anyone who is unable, unwilling, restricted or prevented from changing his own position and for whom repositioning supervision or assistance must be provided. 2. Other factors that may increase risk for developing skin irritation/breakdown include pressure OVER time, friction/shear and moisture, poor nutrition. 3. Help patient/S.O. identify risk factors that make patient at risk.	Discuss hazards of immobility friction & moisture	
C. Skin Assessment 1. Pressure ulcers usually occur observe a bony area; tailbone, hip, buttocks, ankle, heels. 2. Observe skin for signs and symptoms (s/s) of redness, irritation breakdown.	Illustration in handout.	Booklet pg. 1

Figure 2. Teaching Guide for a patient at high risk to develop a pressure ulcer (page 1 of 2). Reprinted with permission from Ostomy/Wound Management 1993;39(8):22–23. © 1993, Medical Center Education, Kaiser Permanente, Bellflower, CA.

CONTENT	TEACHING METHOD	TEACHING RESOURCE
D. Movement/Activity/Support Surface 1. To prevent soft tissue damage, an appropriate bed/chair surface used to evenly distribute/reduce/relieve/pressure. 2. Help patient/S.O. choose appropriate type of bed/chair surface. 3. To exercise joints, relieve pressure and prevent contracture. 4. Teach range of motion to all joints as tolerated at least 2 times a day. 5. Teaching positioning, bridging techniques to relieve pressure.	Show Video	Pressure Ulcer Prevention Video

E. Skin Care
 	
1. Healthy skin is soft, clean and supple.
2. Inspect skin daily for color changes, signs of redness.
3. Bathe regularly and after each episode of incontinence. Use skin cream/ointments to protect skin from drying, cracking and moisture.
  • Cleanse the affected area with soap/water or skin cleanser.
  • Dry area thoroughly.
  • Apply a thin layer of cream/ointment and rub gently over area, or
  • Apply Barrier Film over area and dry thoroughly (approximately 40 seconds).
  • Build 2-3 layers of Barrier Film.
  • Layers must be completely dry between layers.
	Demonstrate with mirror skin areas of high risk
	
	Demonstrate with skin care products
		Instruction Sheet

F. Nutrition 1. To provide sufficient intake to meet the body's needs. body's needs. 2. Help patient/s.o. understand the need for a well balanced diet, fluid intake to 2000 cc/D (unless contraindicated, and increased protein & calories.		Dietician

Figure 2 Continued. Teaching Guide for a patient at high risk to develop a pressure ulcer (page 2 of 2). Reprinted with permission from Ostomy/Wound Management 1993;39(8):22–23. © 1993, Medical Center Education, Kaiser Permanente, Bellflower, CA.

Summary

Whenever possible, prevention of chronic wounds is the optimal course to take in wound management. The AHCPR Guideline provides a research–based approach to preventing pressure ulcers. Much work needs to be done to evaluate the clinical outcomes and efficacy of each of the preventive interventions and associated costs. At this time, there are no AHCPR or other nationally recognized guidelines for other chronic wounds such as venous and arterial ulcers. With all chronic wounds, patient and/or caregiver knowledge and compliance with recommendations is critical. In this "revolutionary" time of a healthcare system moving rapidly toward managed care, it has never been more important to document clinical and cost benefits and to involve patients in their own care. Only through vigilant pursuit of these goals will wound prevention become a reality.

References

1. Panel for the Prediction and Prevention of Pressure Ulcers in Adults.(1992). *Pressure Ulcers in Adults: Preduction and Prevention. Clinical Practice Guideline, Number 3.* AHCPR Publication No. 92–0047, Rockville,MD. Agency for Health Care Policy and Research, Public Health Service, US Department of Health and Human Services.

2. Colburn L.*Wound Caring: A Guide to Wound Management Protocol Development.* Johnson & Johnson Medical,Inc., 1995.

3. Bankert K, et al. The application of collaborative benchmarking to the prevention and treatment of pressure ulcers. *Advances in Wound Care* 1996;9(3):21–29.

4. Barr JE. *Sound Advice on Implementing New AHCPR Guideline for Pressure Ulcers.* Convatec, A Bristol Myers Squibb Company. Sound Advice No.4., 1992.

5. Bergstrom N. A research agenda for pressure ulcer prevention. *Decubitus* 1992;5(5):22–30.

6. Cheney A. Portrait of Practice: A successful approach to preventing heel pressure ulcers after surgery. *Decubitus* 1993;6(4):39–40.

7. Regan MB, et al. Efficacy of a comprehensive pressure ulcer prevention program in an extended care facility. *Advances in Wound Care* 1995;8(3):49–54.

8. Hu T, et al. (1993). Cost analysis for guideline implementation in prevention and early treatment of pressure ulcers. *Decubitus* 1993;6(2):42–46.

9. Xakellis G, et al. Cost of pressure ulcer prevention in long term care. *Journal of the American Geriatric Society* 1995;43(5):496–500.

10. Bryant R.(ed). *Acute and Chronic Wounds: Nursing Management.* St. Louis, MO, Mosby, 1992.

11. Elder, DM, Greer KE. Venous disease: How to heal and prevent chronic leg ulcers. *Geriatrics* 1995;50(8).

12. Ayello E. A critique of the AHCPR's "Preventing Pressure Ulcers— A Patient's Guide" as a written instructional tool. *Decubitus* 1993;6(3):44–50.

13. Fowler E, Pelfrey M. Survival skills: A patient teaching model for the prevention of pressure ulcers. *Ostomy/Wound Management* 1993;39(8):18–24.

4

Wound Assessment and Documentation

Lia van Rijswijk, RN, ET

van Rijswijk L. Wound assessment and documentation. In: Krasner D, Kane D. *Chronic Wound Care, Second Edition*. Wayne, PA, Health Management Publications, Inc., 1997, 16–28.

Introduction

Appreciation of the wound healing process, factors that may affect it, and the number of devices available to manage wounds have increased dramatically during recent years. However, a significant portion of our wound healing knowledge is based on laboratory data, and the clinical effectiveness of most wound care devices has not been studied extensively.[1] One of the many reasons for this relatively slow clinical progress is the challenge of wound assessment. Questions such as: "Which indices of wound healing are most appropriate to evaluate?"remain unanswered.[2] In addition, wound assessment validity and reliability studies are often conducted from a research rather than a clinical perspective. However, with respect to clinical practice there is agreement about one wound assessment issue: it is better to regularly assess using the same, possibly less–than–perfect, tool than not to assess at all.[3] Every plan of care and intervention as well as the clinician's ability to determine the effectiveness of care is based on a complete patient history, assessment, and regular follow–up assessments.[4] This publication will focus on the practical application of available research as it pertains to the clinical assessment of non–sutured wounds and on the practical implications of documentation. The assessment of pressure ulcers and the use of a computerized pressure ulcer assessment tool will be reviewed in Chapter 6 of the source book.

Assessment: What it is and What it is Not

Verbs commonly used to describe the process of follow–up care include *assessing, monitoring, evaluating or inspecting*. It is important not to use them interchangeably because their use affects the level of knowledge required to implement the process. To *monitor* or *inspect* means to watch, to keep track of, check, or closely view a person or condition.[5] To *evaluate*, to determine the significance of an observation through appraisal and study, requires specific skills and knowledge. Similarly, collecting, verifying and organizing data, e.g. to *assess*, is impossible without specific skills and an understanding of the condition involved.[4] For example, the plan of care for a home–bound patient may include two visits per week; once a week the home health aide will change the dressing and monitor the patient and wound for signs of infection or deterioration, and once a week the registered nurse will change the dressing and complete a wound assessment to quantify healing.

Clinical Wound Assessment Rationale

Goal of Care. The patient history and wound assessment findings are the foundation for developing the goal of care and patient care plan; e.g. it will help the clinician determine if a wound is infected, whether it can be surgically closed, and which dressing should be used. If pressure redistribution is needed, a patient history and assessment will determine if frequent turning is appropriate

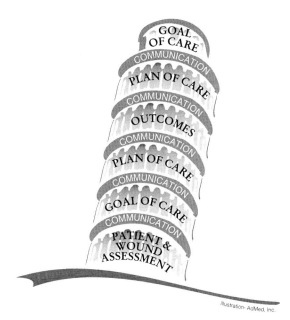

Figure 1. Clearly defined and realistic goals of care, as well as assessment tools which improve communication among healthcare professionals, may help achieve the desired outcome by stabilizing the seemingly unstable pattern of chronic wounds.

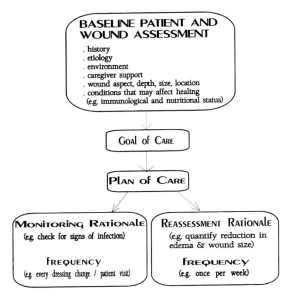

Figure 2. Wound reassessment and monitoring frequency/ rationale are affected by the overall patient condition, wound severity, patient care environment, goal of care and plan of care.

and feasible. Subsequent follow–up assessments, designed to monitor outcome(s), will determine whether the wound is moving in the direction of the "ultimate" outcome, the goal of care.[4]

Developing a realistic and clearly defined goal of care is particularly important when managing patients with chronic wounds because they often have a number of concomitant conditions that may affect the healing process or the plan of care. A chronic wound presents a considerable burden to patients, caregivers and healthcare professionals.[6] If the goals of care are not realistic or clearly defined, patients and caregivers may become discouraged and lose sight of the goal of care; the wound has turned into a "frustrating" problem that "challenges" our resources. Defining short–term as well as long–term goals of care may help. The overall goal of care for a full–thickness wound with necrotic tissue may be complete healing, but the short–term goal of care could be to reduce pain and to obtain a granulating wound bed. In addition to developing realistic long–term and short–term goals of care, it helps to remember that even seemingly unstable patterns may result in a desired outcome, providing one does not lose sight of it (Figure 1).

Outcome and Treatment Effectiveness. To determine whether a condition is moving in the direction of the goal of care or desired outcome,

regular reassessments are imperative. The effectiveness of interventions, their ability to produce the "decided, decisive, or desired effect," cannot be ascertained unless baseline assessment data are compared to follow–up data. In addition to monitoring the effectiveness of the plan of care, regular reassessments may help motivate patients and caregivers. Systematically gathered assessment and reassessment data will also help clinicians to develop a treatment outcome data base. The gathered data can be reviewed, analyzed, and compared to outcomes reported in the literature which will help the development or modification of general wound care policies and procedures as well as individual patient care plans. In summary, wound assessment and reassessment policies and procedures are a necessary and integral part of the individual patient's plan of care as well as a tool to accumulate much needed outcome data on chronic wound care.[7]

Clinical Wound Assessment Frequency

After gathering the baseline or admission assessment data, clinicians have to decide how often the wound should be reassessed and why. The reassessment and monitoring frequency and rationale is affected by the overall patient condition, wound severity, the patient care environment

Wound Classification Algorithm

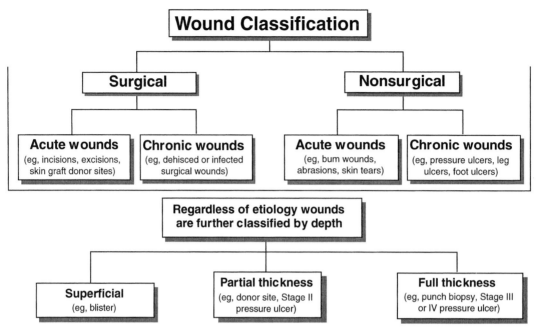

©1994 Diane Krasner, Lia van Rijswijk

Figure 3. Wounds are classified by cause and depth.

and the goal and plan of care (Figure 2). For example, when a patient has a systemic condition that has been shown to increase the risk of infection, the wound may require more frequent monitoring and assessments. Dressing/treatment selection may also be affected by the reassessment frequency, e.g. a wound that needs to be reassessed daily should not be covered with a dressing that is designed to remain in place for a number of days.

The Panel for the Prediction and Prevention of Pressure Ulcers in Adults recommends daily monitoring of patients with Stage I pressure ulcers.[8] The uses of risk assessment tools for patients with Stage I pressure ulcers are discussed in Chapter 5 of this source book. The AHCPR Clinical Practice Guideline on the Treatment of Stage II, III and IV pressure ulcers includes recommendations for a baseline assessment, regular monitoring and weekly reassessments. A reassessment rationale for Stage I through IV pressure ulcers has been reviewed elsewhere.[4]

Since the reassessment frequency depends on the reassessment rationale, it is not uncommon for the frequency interval to change over time. During the first few weeks of home care, for instance, more frequent skilled nursing visits may be needed for teaching purposes and to ensure that caregiver monitoring procedures are understood and followed. Similarly, a weekly or once–every–two–week assessment of venous ulcers is usually sufficient, but initially more frequent assessments may be needed to evaluate the effectiveness of interventions, e.g. a reduction in edema should be observed during this time.[10] Also, after initiating wound care treatments, allergic reactions to the dressing(s) or bandages used may become evident. These reactions usually present as irritation of the surrounding skin.

Assessing the Wound

General Wound Classification. The first step in the patient and wound assessment process is to classify the wound. For this purpose, two general categories are commonly used. The first category is related to the cause (surgical or non–surgical) and whether the wound is chronic or acute (Figure 3). A chronic wound can be defined as "a wound that has failed to proceed through an orderly and timely process to produce anatomic and functional

VAN RIJSWIJK

Table 1
Staging and Describing the Extent of Tissue Damage

Structures involved	Examples of wounds, commonly used wound descriptions, classification, or staging system
• Epidermis *(stratum corneum, granulosum, spinosum and germinativum)*	Superficial wound Stage I pressure ulcer* Grade 0 diabetic foot ulcer** First degree burn
• Epidermis • Dermis *(hair follicles, apocrine and sebaceous glands, blood and lymph vessels, nerve endings)*	Partial thickness wound Shave biopsy Abrasion Skin graft donor site Stage II pressure ulcer* Grade 1 diabetic foot ulcer** Venous disease: clinical classification Class 6*** Second degree burn
• Epidermis • Dermis • Subcutaneous tissue/Superficial fascia *(fat, fibrous and elastic tissue, deeper blood vessels)*	Full thickness wound Punch biopsy Penetrating wound Stage III pressure ulcer* Grade 2 diabetic foot ulcer** Venous disease: clinical classification Class 6*** Third degree burn
• Epidermis • Dermis • Subcutaneous tissue • Deep fascia/underlying structures *(muscle, tendon, bone)*	Full thickness wound Dehisced surgical wound Stage IV pressure ulcer* Grade 3 diabetic foot ulcer (if osteitis, abscess or osteomyelitis is present)** Venous disease: clinical classification Class 6*** Third degree (sometimes called fourth degree) burn

* National Pressure Ulcer Advisory Panel: Pressure ulcer prevalence, cost and risk assessment. Consensus Development Conference Statement. *Decubitus* 1989;2:24.

** Wagner FW. The dysvascular foot: A system for diagnosis and treatment. *Foot and Ankle* 1981;2:64–122.

*** Beebe HG, Bergan JJ, Bergqvist D, et al. Classification and grading of chronic venous disease in the lower limbs. A consensus statement of the North American Society of Phlebology. *Dermatol Surg* 1995;21:642–647.

integrity, or proceeded through the repair process without establishing a sustained anatomic and functional result."[11] Even though few (if any) differences exist in the actual processes of healing chronic and acute wounds, clinically it is important to distinguish them. For example, appropriate goals of care for acute versus chronic wounds are different since, as a rule, acute wounds heal more expediently than chronic wounds.[1] Similarly, because superficial and partial–thickness wounds usually take less time to heal than full–thickness wounds, the second general category is based on initial wound depth.[12]

With respect to classifying and grading chronic venous disease of the lower limbs, a recently published consensus statement includes classification and grading of clinical signs, etiologic classification, anatomic distribution and pathophysiologic dysfunction.[13] Using this classification, patients presenting with lower leg skin changes (e.g. pigmentation, venous eczema, lipodermatosclerosis) and active ulceration of any depth would receive a Clinical Classification (C0–6) of Class 6.

Choosing a wound assessment method. Wound assessment is not an exact science. It is primarily rooted in clinical observation, a skill that has lost value compared to the use of instruments and machines.[2] When it comes to skillful observation, available instruments and machines may enhance the process, but they cannot replace the adept examination of the clinician nor integrate and evaluate the significance of all the patient and wound information obtained during the assessment. In other words, the assessment process, defined as collecting, verifying and organizing data, will always require the talents of a skilled professional. Before reviewing the various wound assessment methods that can be used, it is important to understand one of the reasons for healthcare professionals' increased reliance on the use of equipment and tests. Many provide easy to understand numbers which communicate the same message to everyone involved in the care of that patient. Because communication, including communicating wound assessment data, is such an integral part of achieving the goal of care, standardization of the terminology and techniques used is crucial (Figure 1).

Reliability and validity. Reliability and validity are not just research concerns. Clinical assessments should also be reliable, that is, when two or more people make the same assessment the findings should be similar. For example, with respect to wound measurements, specifying which position the patient should be in when the wound is measured and which tape measure or tracing to use will greatly increase reliability. The validity of an assessment, i.e. it assesses what it is supposed to, can be increased by choosing the appropriate method, e.g. assessing wound depth by looking at a regular photograph would significantly reduce assessment validity. To simplify the process of determining which methods are valid to assess a specific aspect of the wound, those discussed are reviewed in the context of what they are supposed to measure.

Qualitative and Quantitative Methods. A wound assessment method can be descriptive, qualitative, or quantitative. Descriptive and qualitative methods are often used in clinical practice; e.g. the wound has improved, it is red, smaller than last week, the surrounding skin is healthy and the patient does not complain of pain. For the person who made the assessment, this chart entry makes perfect sense and provides an accurate description of the observations. However, it does not provide a complete "picture" for someone who has not seen the wound. This entry will not facilitate continuity of care. If the same wound assessment is made using a combination of standardized descriptive and quantitative methods, e.g. it includes pain and wound measurements and standardized descriptions of the surrounding skin condition, the findings are easier to understand by someone who has not seen the wound, thus facilitating communication and continuity of care.

Assessing wound depth. Neither wound depth nor the appearance of the wound bed can be accurately assessed if the wound contains loose debris, particulate matter or dressing residue. Therefore, wound cleansing is the first step in the wound assessment process. For assessment purposes, rinsing the wound with saline will usually suffice. However, when particulate matter is adherent to the wound bed, higher pressures (e.g. between 4 and 15 pounds per square inch) may be needed.[9]

Assessing wound depth is not always possible. If a wound is covered with eschar, depth cannot be ascertained. In these instances, document "unable to stage," or "unable to assess wound depth" and explain why wound depth cannot be established.[9] Also, the exact depth of wounds with sinus tracts or tunnels may be difficult to assess because the "bottom" of the tunnel cannot be seen. These wounds can be classified as full thickness (Table 1) and the amount of wound care product needed to fill the tract or tunnel can be used as a gauge for determining the extent of tissues involved.

Many wounds do not fit into "simple" depth categories and contain areas of partial and full thickness dermal involvement.[14] When using a pressure ulcer or foot ulcer staging system, the stage corresponding with the deepest area of the wound is documented. Similarly, a wound containing areas of partial and full–thickness dermal involvement is classified as a full–thickness wound.

Staging. Wound depth is a very important assessment variable since it has a direct effect on how long the wound may take to heal. Hence, most descriptive wound assessment methods or systems are based on depth. The work of Shea, with subsequent modifications by the International Association of Enterostomal Therapy and the National Pressure Ulcer Advisory Panel, has resulted in the Pressure Ulcer Staging System.[15–17] Other pressure ulcer staging systems, such as the Yarkony–Kirk scale and the UK consensus classification of pressure sores, are also based on the level of tissue involved.[18,19] The Pressure Sore Status Tool includes, among others, 5 parameters related to depth, including the variable "obscured by necrosis."[20]

Burn wounds are classified based on depth and area. For example, partial thickness wounds are classified as superficial or deep second degree burns, and wound area is defined as Total Body Surface Area involved. Classification systems for diabetic foot ulcers, e.g. the Wagner scale, are based on wound depth and the presence or absence of infection.[21]

These classification systems all have one major advantage; they standardize the terminology used, thus facilitating communication. However, they all rely on the clinician's ability to assess wound depth which may not always be easy to do. Assessing the extent of dermal involvement can be particularly difficult because dermal thickness varies with age (thin at birth and after the fifth decade of life), sex (thicker in men than in women) and anatomical location, e.g. it ranges from < 1 mm on the eyelids to > 4 mm on the back.[22] Indeed, the results of one pilot study indicate that, for most nurses, it is difficult to distinguish a Stage II from a Stage III pressure ulcer.[23] Only a few chronic wound classification systems have been tested for reliability and validity.[18,20]

Finally, staging systems were not designed to capture changes that occur during the healing process and they should be used to facilitate admission diagnostic procedures only.[3] We do not change the admission assessment of a deep second degree burn to a superficial second degree burn when it is healing, and we should not "downstage" pressure ulcers when they heal. The only time a wound stage can change is if it was incorrect on admission, e.g. when all necrotic tissue was debrided/removed, the wound was found to be less deep or deeper than originally thought.

The use of staging systems based on depth can help healthcare professionals because many clinicians are familiar with them and, as such, they facilitate communication. However, baseline and follow–up depth assessments should include a description of the tissues involved, and/or actual depth or volume measurements.

Describing the extent of tissue damage. The staging difficulties described earlier also apply to describing the extent of tissue damage. First, clinicians can try to find "markers" of wound depth. For example, islands of epithelium in the wound bed may be indicative of a superficial or partial thickness wound (Table 1). When underlying structures such as fascia or tendon are visible, the wound extends down through the dermis and can be classified as "full thickness." Second, it helps to remember that dermal thickness ranges from approximately 1 to 4 mm; thus, most wounds that are deeper than 4 mm involve subcutaneous tissue and can be classified as full thickness wounds.[22] Finally, document if the wound bed is irregular. For example "lateral aspect of wound extends through subcutaneous tissue, proximal aspect of the wound contains dermis."

Measuring wound depth, undermining and tunneling. Wound depth is most commonly measured and quantified by gently inserting a sterile swab into the wound. Find the deepest point and put a gloved forefinger on the swab at skin level. Remove the swab and place it next to a measuring guide, calibrated in centimeters.[24] This wound assessment method is not very useful for partial thickness or superficial wounds but can provide valuable information for deeper wounds. The presence or absence of undermining, a space between the surrounding skin and wound bed, and tunneling can also be determined in this manner. The depth of a tunnel or pocket of undermining can be measured using the same technique as described for wound depth. The accuracy of this method depends on the skill of the clinician and documentation.

First, determine if you need assistance to help the patient remain in the position required to perform the assessment and make sure that you have all the equipment needed. For example, the ruler and a pen to record the assessment should be close to the wound on a flat surface. If you are measuring different aspects of the wound, do not try to memorize every observation until you are finished.

Second, the value of the measurement for evaluating change (reliability) also depends on documenting how (patient position), and where (most lateral area) in the wound it was obtained. If tunneling or undermining is present, record the percentage of the wound margin involved and the location.

Table 2
Commonly used methods to measure wounds in the clinic

Method	Description	Advantages	Disadvantages	Comments
Tape measure or ruler	• *Length* (longest area of tissue breakdown or head–to–toe measurement) and *width* (narrowest area of tissue breakdown or side– to–side measurement) are measured using a disposable measuring guide/ruler calibrated in centimeters. • *Record* length, width, method of measurement (e.g. head–to–toe), patient position at time of assessment.	• Easy • Inexpensive • Fast • Good interrater and intrarater reliability	• Difficult to decide which dimension to measure if wound is irregular • Overestimates actual wound size • Reliability decreases with increasing wound size	• Good correlation between ruler measurements and tracings
Tracing	• Disposable acetate sheet, measuring guide, or plastic bag is held over the wound while tracing the edges with a permanent, fine tip marker. Add location markers (e.g. head, toes), date, patient number. • Clean the sheet or remove contaminated side of plastic bag/ measuring guide. • Attach tracing to chart and/or calculate area using 1.0 or 0.5 cm grid paper.* • *Record* area, method of obtaining and calculating measurement, patient position at time of measurement.	• Easy • Expense is determined by materials used • Fast • Excellent interrater and intrarater reliability • Reliability increases with increasing wound size	• May be difficult to see wound margins • Reliability decreases with decreasing wound size • If transparency does not contain grid, tracing has to be copied to grid paper to calculate area.	• Tracings can be a valuable part of patient records and changes in wound area can easily be compared.

* Some measuring guides incorporate a 1.0 or 0.5 cm grid or 0.5 cm grid. See Figure 4.

If it is difficult to describe where the measurement was obtained, draw a picture of the wound and mark the area or use a "clock" system. For example, for all assessment findings the area of the wound closest to the patient's head is 12 o'clock.

There are no limitations on how many depth measurements can be made and it may be helpful to take two or three different measurements in different areas to get a clear "picture" of the wound dimensions. Taking multiple measurements close together and recording the average may improve accuracy. Insertion of any object into the wound may cause trauma, and if cotton swabs are used particles can remain in the wound bed. These concerns have led some experts to recommend assessing depth by gently inserting a gloved finger instead of a swab.[25]

Regardless of how depth is measured, once a method has been chosen for a particular wound, standardizing the procedure is crucial in order to evaluate whether the wound is moving in the direction of the goal of care.

Assessing Wound Area/Size. Measuring and recording the size of a wound upon admission will help the clinician develop the goal of care and patient care plan. First, initial wound size may affect time to healing as studies of acute wounds have shown that large deep wounds take more time to heal than small deep wounds.[26] Clinical studies of deep chronic wounds have also shown that initial wound size affects healing time, but the importance of these findings is often overshadowed by the powerful effect of other patient and wound variables on healing chronic wounds.[27–31] However, all else being equal, the size of a patient's wound provides information about what can and cannot be expected during the course of treatment.

The second important reason for regularly measuring wounds relates to quantifying change in wound area/size. Change in wound size cannot be assessed by just "looking" at it because it is virtually impossible to remember its size one week ago. Also, a reduction in pressure ulcer area within the first 2 to 4 weeks of treatment may prove to be the best predictor of subsequent healing.[32] Specifically, clinical studies on full thickness pressure as well as on leg ulcers have shown that ulcers which decrease 20 to 40 percent in area after 2 to 4 weeks of treatment will heal significantly faster and are more likely to heal than ulcers that do not exhibit a considerable reduction in area at that time.[27,29,31]

When developing a patient's plan of care and reassessment rationale, it is important to remember the goal of assessing wound size. For example, if the goal of care is healing, the size of Stage II as well as Stage III and IV pressure ulcers should be determined at baseline and at weekly intervals thereafter.

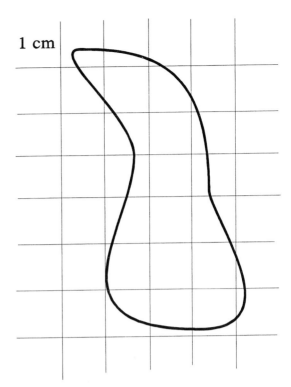

Figure 4. *Using a 1.0 cm grid to determine wound size, count the crosspoints that fall completely within the ulcer. This ulcer measures 13 cm². When using a 0.5 cm grid, count the crosspoints and divide the number by 4.*

However, the rationale for obtaining the measurements may vary because the latter usually take more time to heal.[4]

The most commonly used techniques for measuring wound area/size include tape measurements or tracings (Table 2) (Figure 4). Color photographs can also be used to measure wound area/size. Photographs can be taken using a 35 mm camera with a linear measurement scale next to the wound and/or at a "standard" distance. The slide can be projected and the wound size calculated. Clinicians who possess the expertise and skill to take quality photographs and calculate wound area following projection will find that this method correlates strongly with obtaining tracings.[33] In addition, photographs can be a very useful addition to the patient chart (see documentation). When using specialty cameras with a grid film, clinicians can simply calculate the number of squares that fall within the wound margins. The reliability and validity of using this type of specialty camera for measuring wound size has not been determined. Regardless of the type of camera used, wound size cannot be accurately assessed from two–dimensional photographs when the wound is on a curved surface.[34]

Wound Assessment Model

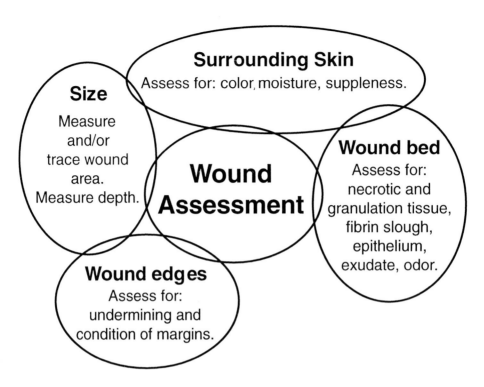

Figure 5. *Wound assessment model*

All measurement methods have advantages and disadvantages (Table 2) and their accuracy depends to a large extent on the ability of the clinician to precisely find the wound edge. For example, it may take practice to see newly formed epithelium at the wound margins. From a research perspective, measurement accuracy is very important and clinicians should also strive for accuracy. However, in the clinic, small variations are unlikely to effect the goal of re–assessment; to quantify change in wound area over time. As with other assessments, patient position at the time of measurement and recording how the measurements were obtained (see measuring wound depth) are important. At this time, measurement of wound surface is considered sufficient for the routine clinical documentation of pressure ulcer healing.[35] Finally, it is encouraging to note that assessing wound size does not involve a significant amount of time. When feasibility was evaluated, researchers found that using paper tape or a grid transparency takes approximately 1 minute.[36]

Volume. Wound volume can be calculated as follows: area x depth x 0.327; however, this method is not very exact. Indeed, variations of up to 40 percent of volume have been found when this method is used.[37] Other methods of measuring volume, e.g. using dental impression materials or filling a lesion with saline, are more precise but also more expensive and difficult to perform. Concerns about cast materials being used in wounds have also been voiced. In deep wounds, excellent correlations between wound volume and wound circumference, and wound area and circumference have been found.[38,39] In summary, obtaining area measurements has been found to provide clinically useful and valid information, whereas the need to measure wound volume will probably remain a subject of discussion in the foreseeable future.

Assessing the wound bed. After measuring the size of the wound, the appearance of the wound bed needs to be assessed and documented (Figure 5). Traditionally, clinical wound assessment systems include "yes" or "no" options to indicate the presence or absence of granulation tissue, necrotic tissue, fibrin slough, etc. Unfortunately, "yes" or "no" options will only capture changes when they are complete, e.g. if a wound contains necrotic tissue the "yes" option for necrotic tissue will be marked until the wound is completely free of eschar. Similarly, the red, yellow, black system, which translates granulation tissue into red, fibrin slough into yellow and dried debris (eschar) into black, will only capture present or absent changes. Even though this system is easy to teach and use, it has not been tested for reliability and validity and other limitations have to be kept in mind, e.g. bone and tendon are also yellow, topical treatments may discolor a wound, sutures may be black, and the presence of foreign bodies has to be documented separately.[40]

Many wounds contain a combination of granulation and necrotic tissue or fibrin slough. When trying to document the effect of treatments on wound debridement, investigators have used rating scales, e.g. no necrotic tissue, some necrotic tissue, some fibrin slough, etc., or have quantified the amount of necrotic tissue by estimating the percentage of tissue involved. No validity or reliability studies on the use of rating scales or quantifying the percentage of tissue involved (e.g. ± 50 percent of wound bed contains necrotic tissue, ± 25 percent contains granulation tissue and ± 25 percent contains fibrin slough) have been conducted; however, it is evident that these methods are more precise than "yes"/"no" options. Specifically, they will facilitate the assessment and documentation of changes in the wound bed related to debridement.

Estimating a range, e.g. < 25 percent necrotic tissue or 25 to 50 percent necrotic tissue has been studied as part of the Pressure Sore Status Tool. See Chapter 6 of the source book. The authors of the Pressure Sore Status Tool recommend using a transparent metric measuring guide with concentric circles divided into four (25 percent) pie–shaped quadrants to help clinicians assess the wound bed.[20] In another study, drawings of venous ulcers were used to compare the results of visually quantifying wound bed appearance to using a digital image analysis system for this purpose.[41] In this small study, considerable inter– and intra–observer variations were found in the visual estimation of the percentage of tissues involved. However, the average did not differ significantly from the average obtained using the equipment. Based on the limited research available, visual estimations may be considered too unreliable for research purposes. However, from a clinical perspective, they are more precise than commonly used "present" or "absent" ratings and more likely to meet the goal of reassessment; to quantify and document change in the wound bed over time.

Assessing the wound edges and surrounding skin. In addition to assessing the extent and depth of undermining, the condition of the wound edges should be also noted. Assessment of the wound edges includes distinctness, degree of attachment to the wound base, color, and thickness.[42] For example, if it is difficult to see where the wound ends and the surrounding skin starts, reepithelialization may be taking place and this observation should be charted. Chronic wounds may also present with thick ("rolled") wound margins. They are usually an indication that the wound has been present for some time and that the newly formed epithelial cells have migrated "down and around" the wound edge because they did not "find" moist, healthy, granulation tissue in the wound bed.

The condition of the surrounding skin provides very important information about the status of the wound as well as the result of treatment. Surrounding skin assessment includes evaluating color, induration, edema and suppleness (Figure 5). Redness of the surrounding skin can be indicative of less–than–optimal patient and wound care, i.e. unrelieved pressure or prolonged inflammation.[14] Irritation of the surrounding skin, which may also impair wound healing, can result from contact with feces or urine, from a reaction to the dressing or tape used, or from a reaction to frequent or inappropriate dressing/tape removal. In patients with darkly pigmented skin, skin color changes (e.g. a difference between the patient's usual skin color and the color of the skin surrounding the wound) should be noted.[43] Furthermore, inflammation/ vasodilation will cause an increase in skin temperature. A temperature difference between the skin immediately surrounding, and a little distance from, the wound can be assessed using the back of the hand or finger.[44] Also, redness, tenderness, warmth, and swelling of the surrounding skin are the classic clinical signs of infection.[45] When the surrounding skin has been exposed to moisture for a prolonged period of time, signs of maceration (pale, white or grey) may be observed. In leg ulcer patients the surrounding skin may exhibit signs of capillary leakage (hemosiderin pigmentation, lipodermatosclerosis) or ischemia (absence of hair growth, cool, clammy skin). Assessing and documenting suppleness of the surrounding skin is important because overly moist as well as overly dry skin (commonly seen in patients with impaired peripheral perfusion) is more prone to injury. Induration (an abnormal firmness of the tissues) and edema are assessed by gently pressing the skin within approximately 4 cm of the wound. Document the location and the extent (in centimeters) of induration and edema as well as pitting or nonpitting characteristics. The percentage of wound and area involved can be estimated using a transparent metric measuring guide with concentric circles divided into four (25 percent) pie–shaped quadrants.[20]

Assessing exudate and odor. Wound exudate characteristics, e.g. type and amount, should be assessed because they provide important information about the status of the wound and the most appropriate treatment. However, at this time no reliable and valid wound exudate assessment tool exists. One proposed definition includes a combination of qualitative descriptions and quantifying the amount of exudate when using gauze.[46] In this definition minimal exudate (< 5 cc/24 hrs) equates to no more than one (gauze) dressing change per day, moderate exudate (5 to 10 cc/ 24hrs) will result in two to three dressing changes per day, whereas wounds with high amounts of exudate (> 10 cc/day) require three or more dressing changes per day. Unfortunately, quantifying exudate in this manner is not possible when using modern absorptive or moisture–retentive dressings, but the proposed descriptions may facilitate the development of a universally applicable assessment tool.

Another commonly used method involves assessing the amount of moisture in the wound bed and the condition of the surrounding skin.[20,47] In the clinic, rating the amount of wound exudate will be useful only if a description of each rating is provided. For example, when the wound is dry there is no exudate, whereas a moist wound is indicative of scant or small amounts of exudate. When the tissues are wet/saturated and there is exudate in the wound bed, the amount of exudate could be rated as moderate, and when the tissues are saturated (sometimes including maceration of the surrounding skin) and the wound is bathing in fluid, the amount of exudate could be considered large. In addition to amount, the type of exudate should be described. Most commonly, exudate type is recorded as serous (clear fluid without blood, pus or debris), serosanguineous (thin, watery pale red to pink fluid), sanguineous or bloody (bloody, bright red) or purulent (thick, cloudy, yellow or tan).[20,46]

Traditionally, the presence of wound odor (and pus) was used to diagnose infection. Hence, when moisture–retentive dressings were first used, the odor that inevitably accompanies their removal was sometimes mistaken for infection. All wounds, particularly after they have been occluded, will emit an odor. Necrotic wounds tend to have a more "repulsive" odor than clean wounds, and wounds infected with anaerobic bacteria tend to produce a distinct acrid or putrid smell.[48] Because odor is a subjective assessment it cannot be quantified. However, a descriptive odor assessment can provide important information because a change in the type or amount of odor may be indicative of a change in wound status. As with all assessment parameters, standardizing what to assess, how to assess, and how to document it, will increase their usefulness. Odor assessments can include a description of the odor (e.g. sweet, like fresh blood, putrid, etc.) as well as a description of the "amount" of odor (e.g. filled the room, could only smell it immediately following dressing removal, disappeared when dressing was discarded).

When caring for patients with fungating wounds, the goal of odor assessment may be to evaluate the effectiveness of odor control measures. To assess odor with the dressing in place the following scale can be used: no odor at close range, faint odor at close range, moderate odor in room, or strong odor in room.[49]

Clinical assessment of infection. The classic clinical signs of infection, defined as "the invasion and multiplication of microorganisms in body tissues that result in local cellular injury," include redness, tenderness, warmth, swelling of the surrounding skin and the presence of pus.[45] One or more of these signs of infection are usually readily recognizable in acute wounds. In chronic wounds, however, unrelieved pressure, chronic inflammation and allergic reactions to dressings can also cause redness, tenderness, warmth and swelling of the surrounding skin. As a result, infections in chronic wounds, particularly pressure ulcers, can easily be overdiagnosed or underdiagnosed. For example, the presence of a yellowish coating is usually not indicative of an infection, rather, it is a fibrinous film that will dissolve when a moisture–retentive dressing regimen is instituted.

It has been suggested that traditional definitions of wound infection may be too narrow for all granulating wounds.[48] When looking for signs of infection, other assessment criteria that should be considered are delayed healing, discoloration, friable granulation tissue which bleeds easily, unexpected pain/tenderness, pocketing at base of wound, bridging (with epithelium) at base of wound, abnormal smell and wound breakdown. For example, when assessing the wound bed, clinicians should routinely look for the green or blue "hue" of pseudomonas, the "dull" appearance of wounds infected with anaerobes, as well as granulation tissue that bleeds easily and has a gelatinous texture. Also, it has been found that if a diabetic foot ulcer extends down to bone, osteomyelitis and/or joint infection may be present.[50] If, based on the clinical assessment findings, a wound infection or osteomyelitis is suspected, a quantitative or semiquantitative culture, roentgenogram(x–ray), bone scan, magnetic resonance imaging or indium 111 scan may be ordered to confirm the diagnosis.[11,51]

Finally, when baseline patient and wound assessment findings (Figure 2) indicate that the patient has an increased risk of infection, consider increasing the wound assessment frequency and obtaining a culture if the wound fails to improve one to two weeks after appropriate therapy has been instituted; delayed wound healing may be the only indicator of cutaneous candidiasis or carcinoma.[52]

Documentation. In addition to documenting all assessment findings in a standardized manner, color photographs can serve as a permanent record of the status of the wound at baseline and at regular intervals thereafter. Photographs may also facilitate reimbursement and patient/caregiver teaching and can serve as motivational tools.[53]

Regardless of the type of camera used, it is helpful to remember the definition of a medical photograph: "a photograph that accurately maximizes clinical information while minimizing irrelevant data."[54] Focus on the wound and try to eliminate clutter around the area to be photographed. Always include a measuring tape next to the wound to increase perspective. To maximize clinical information it may also be helpful to take a picture showing the location of the wound, e.g. the entire back or leg. Obtain informed consent and label the photographs by writing the patient's initials and date on the measuring tape or on the edge of the photograph/slide. To prevent problems, it is advisable to appoint one or two people who are "in charge" of camera storage and maintenance and to establish procedures for releasing photographs to third parties.

Conclusion

Wound assessments provide the foundation of the plan of care and are the only means of determining the effectiveness of the interventions. Regular reassessments may motivate patients and caregivers and will help clinicians develop a treatment outcome data base. While research will continue to try to answer remaining questions related to the appropriateness, validity and reliability of commonly used methods, existing knowledge can be applied in the clinic. In so doing, health care professionals will not only provide optimal patient care, but can also contribute to the accumulation of much needed outcome data on wound care.

References

1. van Rijswijk L. General principles of wound management. In: Gogia P (ed). *Clinical Wound Management.* Thorofare, NJ, Slack Inc., 1995, pp 31–52.
2. Cooper DM. Wound assessment and evaluation. In: Bryant R (ed). *Acute and Chronic Wounds; Nursing Management.* St.Louis, MO. Mosby Year Book, 1992, pp 69–90.
3. Maklebust JA, Margolis D. Pressure ulcers: Definition and assessment parameters. *Adv in Wnd Care* 1995;8(4)Suppl:6–7.
4. van Rijswijk L. Frequency of reassessment of pressure ulcers. *Adv in Wound Care* 1995;8(4)Suppl:19–24.
5. *Merriam–Webster's Collegiate Dictionary, Tenth Edition.* Springfield, Mass. Merriam–Webster, Inc., 1994.
6. Fowler E. Chronic wounds: An overview. In: Krasner D (ed). *Chronic Wound Care, A Clinical Source Book for Healthcare Professionals, First Edition.* King of Prussia, PA, Health Management Publications, Inc., 1990, pp 12–18.
7. Polansky M, van Rijswijk L. Utilizing survival analysis techniques in chronic wound healing studies. *WOUNDS* 1994;6:150–158.
8. Panel for the Prediction and Prevention of Pressure Ulcers in Adults. *Pressure Ulcers in Adults: Prediction and Prevention.* Clinical Practice Guideline, Number 3. AHCPR Publication No.92–0047. Rockville, MD: Agency for healthcare Policy and Research, Public Health Service, US Department of Health and Human Services, May 1992.
9. Bergstrom N, Bennett MA, Carlson CE et al. *Treatment of Pressure Ulcers.* Clinical Practice Guideline, No 15. Rockville, MD. US Department of Health and Human Services. Public Health Service, Agency for Health Care Policy and Research. AHCPR Publication No.95–0652. December, 1994.
10. Burton C. Venous ulcers. *Am J Surg* 1994;167:37S–41S.
11. Lazarus GS, Cooper DM, Knighton DR et al. Definitions and guidelines for assessment of wounds and evaluation of healing. *Arch Dermatol* 1994;130:489–493.
12. Clark RAF. Cutaneous tissue repair: basic biological considerations, I. *J Am Acad Dermatol* 1985;13:705–725.
13. Beebe HG, Bergan JJ, Bergqvist D, et al. Classification and grading of chronic venous disease in the lower limbs. A consensus statement of the North American Society of Phlebology. *Dermatol Surg* 1995;21:642–647.
14. Bolton L, van Rijswijk L. Wound dressings: Meeting clinical and biological needs. *Derm Nurs* 1991;3:146–161.
15. Shea JD. Pressure sores: Classification and management. *Clin Orthop* 1975;112:89–100.
16. International Association for Enterostomal Therapy. *Standards of Care for Dermal Wounds: Pressure Ulcers.* Irvine, California, 1987.
17. National Pressure Ulcer Advisory Panel. Pressure ulcers prevalence, cost, and risk assessment. Consensus development conference statement. *Decubitus* 1989;2:24.
18. Yarkony GM, Kirk PM, Carlson C, et al. Classification of pressure ulcers. *Arch Dermatol* 1990;126:1218–1219.
19. Reid J, Morison M. Classification of pressure sore severity. *Nurs Times* 1994;90:46–50.
20. Bates–Jensen BM, Vredevoe DL, Brecht ML. Validity and reliability of the pressure sore status tool. *Decubitus* 1992;5:20–28.
21. Wagner FW. The dysvascular foot: A system for diagnosis and treatment. *Foot and Ankle* 1981;2:64–122.
22. Odland GF, Short JM. Structure of the skin. In: Fitzpatrick TB, et al. (eds). *Dermatology in General Medicine.* New York, NY, McGraw–Hill Book Co., 1971.
23. Arnold N, Watterworth B. Wound staging: can nurses apply classroom education to the clinical setting? *Ostomy/Wound Management* 1995;41(5):40–44.
24. Krasner D. Wound measurement: Some tools of the trade. *Am J Nurs* 1992;May:89–90.
25. Maklebust JA, Sieggreen M. *Pressure Ulcers: Guidelines for Prevention and Nursing Management, Second Edition.* Springhouse , PA, Springhouse Publications, 1995.
26. Marks J, Hughes LE, Harding KG, Campbell H, Ribeiro CD. Prediction of healing time as an aid to the management of open granulating wounds. *World J Surg* 1983;7:641–645.
27. van Rijswijk L, Polanksy M. Predictors of time to healing deep pressure ulcers. *WOUNDS* 1994;6(5):159–165.
28. Skene AI, Smith JM, Dore CJ et.al. Venous leg ulcers: A prognostic index to predict time to healing. *Brit Med J* 1992;305:1119–1121.

29. van Rijswijk L and the Multi–Center Leg Ulcer Study Group. Full–thickness leg ulcers: Patient demographics and predictors of healing. *J Fam Pract* 1993;36:625–632.

30. Robson MC, Phillips LG, Lawrence WT, et al. The safety and effect of topically applied recombinant basic fibroblast growth factor on the healing of chronic pressure sores. *Ann Surg* 1992;216:401–406.

31. Arnold TE, Stanley JC, Fellow EP et al. Prospective, multicenter study of managing lower extremity venous ulcers. *Ann Vasc Surg* 1994;8:356–362.

32. Allman RM. Outcomes in prospective studies and clinical trials. *Adv in Wnd Care* 1995;8(4)Suppl:61–64.

33. Brown–Etris M, Pribble J, LaBrecque J. Evaluation of two wound measurement methods in a multi–center, controlled study. *Ostomy/Wound Management* 1994;40(7):44–48.

34. Harding KG. Methods for assessing change in ulcer status. *Adv in Wnd Care* 1995;8(4)Suppl:37–42.

35. Rodeheaver GT, Stotts NA. Methods for assessing change in pressure ulcer status. *Adv in Wnd Care* 1995;8(4)Suppl:34–36.

36. Liskay AM, Mion LC, Davis BR. Comparison of two devices for wound measurement. *Derm Nurs* 1993;5:437–441,434.

37. Plassman P, Melhuish JM, Harding KG. Methods of measuring wound size: a comparative study. *WOUNDS* 1994;6(2):54–61.

38. Melhuish JM, Plassman P, Harding KG. Circumference, area and volume of the healing wound. *J Wound Care* 1994;3(8):380–396.

39. Hayward PG, Hillman GR, Quast MJ, Robson MC. Surface area measurement of pressure sores using wound molds and computerized imaging. *J Am Ger Soc* 1993;41:238–240.

40. Krasner D. Wound care: How to use the Red–Yellow–Black system. *Am J Nurs* 1995;5:44–47.

41. Mekkes JR, Westehof W. Image Processing in the study of wound healing. *Clin Dermatol* 1995;13:401–407.

42. Stotts NA. Impaired wound healing. In: Carrieri–Kohlman VK, Lindsay AM, West CM (eds). Pathophysiological phenomenon in nursing. Philadelphia, PA, WB Saunders Co., 1993, pp 343–366.

43. Bennett MA. Report of the task force on the implications for darkly pigmented intact skin in the prediction and prevention of pressure ulcers. *Adv in Wnd Care* 1995;8(6):34–35.

44. Lowthian P.Pressure sores: A search for definition. *Nurs Stand* 1994;9(11):30–32.

45. Altemeier W, Burkerts F, Pruitt B, Sandusky W. *Manual on Control of Infection in Surgical Patients, Second Edition.* Philadelphia, PA, JB Lippincot, 1984.

46. Mulder GD. Quantifying wound fluids for the clinician and researcher. *Ostomy/Wound Management* 1994;40(8):66–69.

47. Baranoski S. Wound assessment and dressing selection. *Ostomy/Wound Management* 1995;41:7A:7S–12S.

48. Cutting KF, Harding KG. Criteria for identifying wound infection. *J Wnd Care* 1994;3(4):198–201.

49. Faller NA, Lawrence KG. (Modified Baker–Haig) odor scale.© 1992 Faller & Lawrence.

50. Newman LG, Waller J, Palestro CJ et.al. Unsuspected osteomyelitis in diabetic foot ulcers: diagnosis and monitoring by leukocyte scanning with indium in 111 oxyquinoline. *JAMA* 1991;266:1246–1251.

51. Stotts NA. Determination of bacterial burden in wounds. *Adv in Wnd Care* 1995;8(4)Suppl:46–52.

52. Giandoni MB, Grabski WJ. Cutaneous candidiasis as a cause of delayed surgical wound healing. *J Am Acad Dermatol* 1994;30:981–984.

53. Faller NA, Lawrence KG, Frank S, Barnard A. Wound photography: An alternate use. *Ostomy/Wound Management* 1994;40(4):10–11.

54. Gilbert G. *The Complete Photography Careers Handbook, Second Edition.* New York, NY, The Photographic Arts Center, 1992.

5

Risk Assessment in Pressure Ulcer Prevention

Barbara J. Braden, PhD, RN, FAAN

Braden BJ. Risk assessment in pressure ulcer prevention. In: Krasner D, Kane D. *Chronic Wound Care, Second Edition*. Wayne, PA, Health Management Publications, Inc., 1997, pp 29–36.

Introduction

In recent years a consensus has developed that the incidence of pressure ulcers in a facility or agency is an important indicator of quality of care. Unfortunately, as healthcare providers adjust to the increasing acuity of patients being cared for in every setting, they are suffering a sort of "sensory overload." As more problems compete for their attention and less time is available to analyze the implications of all the data they collect, certain basic assessments and interventions are sometimes overlooked. There is evidence that pressure ulcer risk assessment and prevention have been among these overlooked problems.[1,2]

There is also evidence that a program of prevention guided by risk assessment can simultaneously reduce the institutional incidence of pressure ulcers by as much as 60 percent and bring down the costs of prevention at the same time.[3] This chapter is, therefore, devoted to an exploration of issues in implementing a research–based program of pressure ulcer risk prediction and prevention.

Choosing a Risk Assessment Tool

Risk assessment is not confined to the problem of pressure ulcers. It is part of prevention of many diseases. Risk assessment tools are analogous to screening tests which are used to detect incipient disease in persons who are asymptomatic. An assortment of screening tools have been used or proposed to determine whether patients are at risk for pressure ulcer development. These tools vary from simple (rating scales, serum albumin, serum transferrin) to complex (thermography, laser doppler flowometry, ultrasound).

The U.S. Preventive Services Task Force recommends certain criteria in qualitatively evaluating the appropriateness of screening tests.[4] The first criterion is related to the effectiveness of the treatment for the condition predicted; namely, does the treatment do more good than harm, is it more effective in asymptomatic than symptomatic patients and is there good evidence of that effectiveness? The second criterion relates to the burden of suffering in terms of mortality, morbidity, discomfort, dissatisfaction, or destitution should the disease be contracted. The third criterion relates to quality of the test in terms of reliability, validity, acceptability, safety, simplicity and cost. It is clear that risk assessment for pressure ulcer prevention is appropriate, given the first two criteria. The third criterion as it relates to risk for pressure ulcer development requires further exploration.

In looking at the various screening tools available, the paper and pencil rating scales possess the best balance of characteristics (reliability, validity, acceptability, safety, simplicity and cost). Indices such as serum albumin or serum transferrin, while somewhat lower in patients who develop pressure ulcers, are not valid predictors of pressure ulcer development.[5] The more complex tools, such as laser doppler flowometry and ultrasound, have higher cost, lack simplicity and practicality of use and are less accurate as predictors than the paper and pencil rating scales.

		Physical condition		Mental condition		Activity		Mobility		Incontinent		Total Score
		Good	4	Alert	4	Ambulant	4	Full	4	Not	4	
		Fair	3	Apathetic	3	Walk/help	3	Slightly limited	3	Occasional	3	
		Poor	2	Confused	2	Chairbound	2	Very limited	2	Usually/urine	2	
		Very bad	1	Stupor	1	Bed	1	Immobile	1	Doubly	1	
Name	Date											

Figure 1. The Norton Scale.

BRADEN SCALE
For Predicting Pressure Sore Risk

Patient's Name _____   _____   Evaluator's Name_____   Date of Assessment

SENSORY PERCEPTION — ability to respond meaningfully to pressure-related discomfort	1. Completely Limited Unresponsive (does not moan, flinch, or grasp) to painful stimuli, due to diminished level of consciousness or sedation. OR limited ability to feel pain over most of body	2. Very Limited Responds only to painful stimuli. Cannot communicate discomfort except by moaning or restlessness OR has a sensory impairment which limits the ability to feel pain or discomfort over ½ of body.	3. Slightly Limited Responds to verbal commands, but cannot always communicate discomfort or the need to be turned. OR has some sensory impairment which limits ability to feel pain or discomfort in 1 or 2 extremities.	4. No Impairment Responds to verbal commands. Has no sensory deficit which would limit ability to feel or voice pain or discomfort..				
MOISTURE — degree to which skin is exposed to moisture	1. Constantly Moist Skin is kept moist almost constantly by perspiration, urine, etc. Dampness is detected every time patient is moved or turned.	2. Very Moist Skin is often, but not always moist. Linen must be changed at least once a shift.	3. Occasionally Moist: Skin is occasionally moist, requiring an extra linen change approximately once a day.	4. Walks Frequently Walks outside the room at least twice a day and inside room at least once every 2 hours during waking hours.				
ACTIVITY — degree of physical activity	1. Bedfast Confined to bed.	2. Chairfast Ability to walk severely limited or non-existent. Cannot bear own weight and/or must be assisted into chair or wheelchair.	3. Walks Occasionally Walks occasionally during day, but for very short distances, with or without assistance. Spends majority of each shift in bed or chair	4. Walks Frequently Walks outside room at least twice a day and inside room at least once every two hours during waking hours				
MOBILITY — ability to change and control body position	1. Completely Immobile Does not make even slight changes in body or extremity position without assistance	2. Very Limited Makes occasional slight changes in body or extremity position but unable to make frequent or significant changes independently.	3. Slightly Limited Makes frequent though slight changes in body or extremity position independently.	4. No Limitation Makes major and frequent changes in position without assistance.				
NUTRITION — usual food intake pattern	1. Very Poor Never east a complete meal. Rarely eats more than ⅓ of any food offered. Eats 2 servings or less of protein (meat or dairy products) per day. Takes fluids poorly. Does not take a liquid dietary supplement OR is NPO and/or maintained on clear liquids or IV's for more than 5 days.	2. Probably Inadequate Rarely eats a complete meal and generally eats only about ½ of any food offered. Protein intake includes only 3 servings of meat or dairy products per day. Occasionally will take a dietary supplement. OR receives less than optimum amount of liquid diet or tube feeding	3. Adequate Eats over half of most meals. Eats a total of 4 servings of protein (meat, dairy products per day. Occasionally will refuse a meal, but will usually take a supplement when offered OR is on a tube feeding or TPN regimen which probably meets most of nutritional needs	4. Excellent Eats most of every meal. Never refuses a meal. Usually eats a total of 4 or more servings of meat and dairy products. Occasionally eats between meals. Does not require supplementation.				
FRICTION & SHEAR	1. Problem Requires moderate to maximum assistance in moving. Complete lifting without sliding against sheets is impossible. Frequently slides down in bed or chair, requiring frequent repositioning with maximum assistance. Spasticity, contractures or agitation leads to almost constant friction	2. Potential Problem Moves feebly or requires minimum assistance. During a move skin probably slides to some extent against sheets, chair, restraints or other devices. Maintains relatively good position in chair or bed most of the time but occasionally slides down.	3. No Apparent Problem Moves in bed and in chair independently and has sufficient muscle strength to lift up completely during move. Maintains good position in bed or chair.					

© Copyright Barbara Braden and Nancy Bergstrom, 1988

Total Score

Figure 2. The Braden Scale.

Two rating scales recommended by the AHCPR Panel in the Pressure Ulcer Prevention Guidelines,[6] the Norton Scale[7] (Figure 1) and the Braden Scale[8] (Figure 2), were judged to have undergone sufficient testing to justify their use in making clinical judgements.

The parameters examined to establish the validity of this type of screening tool are sensitivity (ability to identify true positives while minimizing false negatives) and specificity (ability to identify true negatives while minimizing false positives). The Norton Scale has been reported to have good sensitivity but low to moderate specificity at a score of 14.[9,10] No tests of interrater reliability have been reported. The Braden Scale [8,11–13] has demonstrated good sensitivity and specificity in a variety of settings at cutoff scores that range from 16 to 18. The Braden Scale has also been demonstrated to have excellent interrater reliability when used by RNs, but a much lower level of reliability when used by licensed practical nurses or nursing assistants.[8,11]

These risk assessment tools measure broad categories of factors that most commonly put patients at risk and can be committed to interval ratings, e.g. 1 to 4. Other factors enter into pressure ulcer risk, however. Some of the risk factors that have been found to predict who develops pressure ulcers and who does not are advanced age, low diastolic blood pressure, elevated body temperature, and inadequate current intake of protein.[5] Other factors are also thought to contribute to risk but have not been adequately studied (smoking, vasoactive drugs, elevated cortisol levels due to either exogenous or endogenous corticosteroids).

Clinicians should keep in mind that risk assessment tools are intended to supplement nursing judgement, not to replace it. These additional factors should be considered when patients are assessed for risk of pressure ulcer development. Providers should also keep in mind that patients who are rapidly improving (e.g. young persons recovering from surgery) are probably at lower risk though their scores at the time may indicate otherwise. Likewise, persons with declining levels of function or health may be at higher risk than their scores would indicate.

Using Risk Assessment in Prevention Programs

At risk patients should be identified on admission to healthcare facilities and home care services. The activity subscales of either the Norton Scale or the Braden Scale can be used to determine whether patients require a full assessment for pressure ulcer risk. Reassessment should take place 48 hours after the admission assessment, at periodic intervals depending on the rapidity with which the condition changes, and whenever a major change occurs in the condition.

Special vigilance is required during acute illness and during the first two weeks following admission to long term care as these are times of high risk for pressure ulcer development. In one prospective study of nursing home residents,

---

Table 1
Protocols by level of risk

Mild Risk (15–16)*

Turning Schedule
Maximal Remobilization
Protect Heels
Manage Moisture, Nutrition, Friction and Shear
Pressure Reduction support surface if bed– or
    chair–bound
(* If other major risk factors present, advance to next
    level of risk)

Moderate Risk(12–14)

Turning schedule with 30° rule
Plus all interventions for mild risk

Severe Risk (< 11)

Increased frequency of turning
Facilitate 30° lateral turns with foam wedges
Supplement turning with small shifts
Plus all interventions for mild risk

Low Air–Loss Beds and Prevention*

Uncontrolled pain or
Severe pain exacerbated by turning or
Braden Scale Score < 9
Additional risk factors ameliorated by low
    air–loss beds

(** Low air–loss beds do not substitute for turning
    schedules.)

---

investigators followed new admissions for three months and found that 80 percent of those who developed a pressure ulcer did so within two weeks of admission and 96 percent did so within three weeks of admission.[5] Thus, an appropriate schedule for reassessment of pressure ulcer risk in nursing homes might be every week for four weeks with routine quarterly assessments thereafter.

In hospital settings, reassessments are commonly done in ICU and every other day in general medical–surgical units. If this schedule is burdensome, it may be sufficient to assess on admission and 48 hours later. In home care, screening should probably be done with every RN visit as

Table 2
Turning Schedules

These turning schedules may be used to organize care on nursing units with large numbers of patients who are at risk for pressure ulcers. Patients on a team or unit can be assigned to one of three schedules in a balanced manner, e.g., if six patients are at risk, two would be assigned to each of the three schedules. These schedules may have to be adjusted to each day, depending on other components of the patient's schedule.

Direction of Turn	Schedule 1	Schedule 2	Schedule 3
1. Back (breakfast and bath)	7:00 to 9:00	7:30 to 9:30	8:00 to 10:00
2. Right side	9:00 to 11:00	9:30 to 11:30	10:00 to 12:00
3. Back (lunch)	11:00 to 1:00	11:30 to 1:30	12:00 to 2:00
4. Right side	1:00 to 3:00	1:30 to 3:30	2:00 to 4:00
5. Left side	3:00 to 5:00	3:30 to 5:30	4:00 to 6:00
6. Back (dinner)	5:00 to 7:00	5:30 to 7:30	6:00 to 8:00
7. Left side	7:00 to 9:00	7:30 to 9:30	8:00 to 10:00
8. Right side	9:00 to 11:00	9:30 to 11:30	10:00 to 12:00
9. Left side	11:00 to 1:00	11:30 to 1:30	12:00 to 2:00
10. Back	1:00 to 3:00	1:30 to 3:30	2:00 to 4:00
11. Right side	3:00 to 5:00	3:30 to 5:30	4:00 to 6:00
12. Left side	5:00 to 7:00	5:30 to 7:30	6:00 to 8:00

the frequency of these visits is generally predicated on the severity of illness or the ability of the condition of the patient.

Preventive Protocols Based on Level of Risk

Preventive interventions should become more frequent and/or intense as risk increases. Braden and Bergstrom have made specific recommendations based on level of risk (Table 1).[12] Risk assessment, however, not only allows the healthcare provider to identify the level of risk, but also to identify specific problems or factors that contribute to that level of risk. In some cases the problems are amenable to intervention and other times they are not. It may be possible, for example, to restore mobility to some persons and not to others. In instances where mobility, activity or sensory perception cannot be restored, the potential consequences (exposure to prolonged, intense pressure) can be addressed.

Reducing the Exposure to Pressure

Turning schedules. Close attention should be paid to individualized turning schedules. Sample turning schedules that account for periods when the patient must be on his/her back, such as during meals and morning care can be seen in Table 2. These schedules can be further altered to meet individual patient needs. Repositioning should be done with assistance and with attention to good body mechanics, using pillows and pads to protect bony prominences.

To protect the heels when the patient is in the supine position, pillows should be used to support the entire length of the legs, ending at the ankles and suspending the heels above the mattress. The heels must be checked frequently to assure that, as the pillows compress, they remain free of pressure. If use of the pillows is not effective in protecting the heels, consult a physical therapist or occupational therapist to construct devices that adequately protect the heels from excessive pressure.

For emaciated patients or those at higher levels of risk, turning schedules should include either increased frequency of turns or assisted frequent, small shifts in body weight. Lateral turns should not exceed 30 degrees[14] and, if at all possible, the head of the bed should not be elevated beyond 30 degrees. Foam wedges are helpful in lateral positioning and should be pulled out slightly every thirty minutes to an hour to increase the frequency of repositioning. If narcotics or sedatives are being used, extra attention should be paid to turning during times of heavy sedation.

When a patient can tolerate the prone position, it should be added to the turning schedule as it allows the most common sites of pressure ulcer formation (sacrum, trochanters, heels) to be totally relieved of pressure while also preventing flexion contractures of the hips. Careful padding and positioning are required if the prone position is to be employed.

difficult to evaluate, but findings converge on these areas: 1) almost any surface tested reduced interface pressure below those seen with a standard hospital mattress;[15–17] 2) foam overlays that were 2 to 3 inches thick did not compare favorably to other pressure–reduction surfaces[18] including thicker foam surfaces;[19] 3) gel filled overlays and mattresses reduced pressure better

---

If the patient is bed–bound or chairbound, an overlay or replacement support surface is recommended to decrease interface pressure over bony prominences.[6]

Remobilization of the immobile. When a patient is found to have deficits in activity or mobility, the healthcare provider should always be alert to the patient's potential to become remobilized. It is very easy during an episode of illness for an elderly person to be less active than warranted and to enter into a spiral of deconditioning and gradual decline. This process leads to a myriad of complications besides increased pressure ulcer risk. A physical therapy consult may be helpful in determining the degree to which remobilization is possible and to begin the process. The physical therapist, the nurse and, if possible, the patient should collaborate in developing a plan that is clear about the responsibilities that each one holds in the process of remobilization.

In cases where the return to full mobility is not possible, the patient can be taught to make small shifts in body position, such as moving the legs and shifting weight from one buttock to another. If the patient is wheelchair–bound, he/she needs to be taught to lift his/her buttocks off the seating surface every 20 minutes. Teaching the patient to use some external cue (like television commercials) to remember to "lift–off" may be helpful. If the patient is incapable of performing "lift–offs" or making shifts in their seating position, an hourly schedule for repositioning must be implemented by the provider or caregiver.[6]

Use of special support surfaces. Support surfaces include overlays (mattress or wheelchair seating), mattress replacements and specialty beds. Mattress overlays and mattress replacements may be classified as either static (i.e. foam, gels) or dynamic (i.e. alternating pressure surfaces). Specialty beds are classified as either low air loss or air–fluidized.

The comparative effectiveness of mattress overlays, mattress replacements, and specialty beds is

than most foam overlays;[19,20] and 4) the air–fluidized bed and low air loss beds offered substantial pressure reduction and appeared to be beneficial in healing pressure ulcers though results were not always dramatic.[21–24]

If the patient is bed–bound or chairbound, an overlay or replacement support surface is recommended to decrease interface pressure over bony prominences.[6] If the Braden Score is below 9 or the patient has intractable or severe pain exacerbated by turning, use of a low air–loss bed may be indicated. It is important to remember that (in spite of pressure relief) turning will still be necessary to prevent pressure ulcers and other complications of immobility. However, all team members must be clear about the goal of care for these patients. If the patient is terminally ill and the goal of care is provision of comfort, a rigorous schedule of turning is not appropriate.

Managing moisture. Exposure of the skin to excessive moisture from any source can weaken the outer layers and increase the opportunity for skin injury. Incontinence is a common cause of skin maceration and breakdown. A variety of interventions aimed at reducing or eliminating incontinent episodes are available to clinicians, including use of bladder training, prompted voiding or other behavioral methods.[25] After each incontinent episode, the nurse or caregiver should use a very mild soap to cleanse the skin, rinse thoroughly, pat the skin dry and apply a commercial moisture barrier. Absorbent underpads or briefs should be used, checked frequently and changed as needed. The use of thin, plastic backed underpads should be avoided as these keep the mattress dry while the patient sits in a pool of urine or liquid stool.

Diarrhea is very caustic to the skin and can lead quickly to skin breakdown. An attempt should be made to determine the cause of the diarrhea and to eliminate that cause. Such diarrhea may be related to hyperosmolar tube feedings or impaction. If intervention to stop the diarrhea does not bring quick results, a fecal incontinence collector should be used while further attempts at control are made.

Perspiration can be problematic when it is constant, trapped between skin folds or held close to the skin by an unbreathing support surface. Absorbent materials should be used beneath the patient and next to the patient's skin. Use of absorbent powders are generally not advisable as they may collect in skin folds and become a source of injury. If perspiration is the result of a non-breathing support surface, an alternative surface should be sought.

Friction and shear. Friction and shear are very harmful to the skin and make it particularly susceptible to the effects of pressure. Dinsdale used swine to investigate the effects of friction.[26] He found that in the absence of friction a pressure of 290 mm Hg was required to produce ulceration while a pressure of only 45 mm Hg wound produce ulceration in skin pretreated with friction.

Several interventions may be used to prevent or ameliorate exposure of the skin to friction and shear. A trapeze or turning sheet may be used to assist movement in bed. Ankle and heel protectors, while doing nothing to relieve pressure, may be very helpful in protecting these areas from friction. In some instances, hydrocolloid dressings may be used over a particular prominence that is being exposed to friction.

Shearing can occur in the sacral area when the head of the bed is elevated. Maintaining the elevation of the head of the bed at or below 30 degrees will prevent shearing as well as excess pressure at the sacrum. This may not be possible at all times but the duration of higher elevations should be minimized in patients at higher levels of risk.

Nutritional repletion. Both long-term and short-term problems with nutrition make patients more prone to pressure ulcer development. It appears that even slightly lower than optimal current dietary intake of protein is an especially strong risk factor.[5] It is possible that immediate nutritional repletion, particularly for protein intake, may provide some protection. If the patient has good liver and renal function, it may be helpful to increase protein intake beyond 100 percent of the RDA and to increase general caloric intake so as to spare the protein from being used for energy. Though there is no direct evidence that vitamin and mineral deficiencies increase the risk for developing pressure ulcers, it is known that certain vitamins and minerals such as A, C and zinc are important in building new tissue and healing injured tissue. Nutritional supplementation with these vitamins and minerals may be helpful.

When there are problems with nutrition, a consultation with a registered dietician should be considered. This is particularly important when the patient is being fed enterally to assure adequacy of the feeding for individual patient needs. If the patient develops diarrhea, a change to a feeding with a lower osmolality, higher fiber content and/or lack of artificial coloring may be sufficient to take care of the diarrhea. Bacterial contamination from the feeding equipment should be considered as a potential contributing factor. Occasionally, anti-diarrheal medication may be necessary.

Evaluating a Program of Prevention

Developing an evaluation plan for a program of prevention is important for a variety of reasons. One important but seldom recognized reason is that the act of periodically evaluating progress and giving feedback to the healthcare providers has been shown to enhance the effectiveness of the overall program. For example, one Midwestern tertiary care hospital, using a continuous quality improvement strategy that allowed for this periodic feedback, cut the incidence of pressure ulcers from 18.7 percent to 6.4 percent over a 3 year period of time.[3]

Baseline data is important to accurate measurement of the impact of the program of prevention. While many clinical facilities/agencies have sophisticated management information systems which enable them to determine how many pressure ulcers had been documented in a given previous time period, a point prevalence study is a better method of obtaining an accurate baseline. This is because, prior to implementation of a formal program of prevention, the staff may not be attentive to certain pressure ulcers, particularly partial thickness lesions. This inattentiveness leads to underdocumentation and therefore underestimation of the problem. A point prevalence study will provide more accurate information.

The purpose of a point prevalence study is to determine the percentage of persons with pressure ulcers in the facility or agency at one point in time (usually one day). Conducting such a study requires a team of healthcare providers who have been trained to stage and measure pressure ulcers. All nursing units that will participate in the program

Table 3			
Formulas for Program Evaluation			

Prevalence:
$$\frac{\text{\# with pressure ulcers}}{\text{\# surveyed during study}}$$

Incidence:
$$\frac{\text{\# with ulcer during study - \# with ulcers on admission}}{\text{\# of patients surveyed during study}}$$

Severity Index:
$$([\text{length} + \text{width}]\ /2)\ \text{x stage}$$

Severity Index for Hospital:
$$\frac{\text{total severity index for all pressure ulcers}}{\text{total \# with pressure ulcers}}$$

of prevention should be part of the point prevalence study. If possible, every patient currently in the facility should be examined for the presence or absence of pressure ulcers on that day. If the facility is too large to inspect the skin of every patient, a good size random sample should be selected for study.

If a patient is found to have one or more pressure ulcer, the stage, size (length and width) and location of each should be recorded on the data collection sheet. From these data, a severity index may be calculated for each ulcer and for the facility (Table 3). The researcher should also note whether any of the admissions assessments indicated the presence of any of these ulcers, as this information will allow one to estimate the incidence or the percent of nosocomial ulcers found (Table 3).

A chart review should be conducted at the same time as the point prevalence study. The chart review usually consists of calculating the percentage of times that the risk assessment score is charted on admission notes. Evidence of implementation of preventive interventions are present on the care plan and in the charting. The results of both should be reported to nursing staff on various units. In most facilities, the association between the point prevalence study and the chart review will be obvious; nursing units with the lowest prevalence, incidence and severity indexes are usually the units on which the staff are most diligent in performing risk assessment and implementing preventive measures. Unitswhich have high incidence rates and low compliance with

protocols are usually targeted for additional education or assistance in strengthening their care procedures.

The baseline point prevalence study should be conducted as close to the time of start–up as possible. In other words, the study should be conducted a few weeks before the facility–wide educational programs are begun. After the staff has been educated, the point prevalence study should be conducted at specific intervals, such as every six months.

Conclusion

While not all pressure ulcers are preventable, many are. The cost and human suffering associated with treatment of pressure ulcers is tremendous and, for the most part, unnecessary. Prevention of pressure ulcers requires a systematic approach that begins with risk assessment and ends with appropriate preventive measures being delivered in a timely manner to those who are in need. A careful reading of this chapter should supply healthcare providers with the necessary information to initiate formal, research–based programs of prevention in their facilities.

References

1. Xakellis GC, Frantz RA, Arteaga M, Nguyen M, Lewis A. A comparison of patient risk for pressure ulcer development with nursing use of preventive interventions. *J Am Geriatr Soc* 1992;40(12):1250–4.
2. Bergstrom N, Braden BJ, Kemp M, Champagne M, Ruby E. Multi–site study of the incidence of pressure ulcers and the relationship between risk level, demographic characteristics,

diagnoses and prescription of preventive interventions. *J Am Geriatr Soc* 1996;44(1):1–10.

3. Bergstrom N, Braden BJ, Boynton P, Bruch S. Using a research–based assessment scale in clinical practice. *Nurs Clin North Am* 1995;30(3):539–551.

4. O'Malley MS, Fletcher SW. Screening for breast cancer with breast self–examination. *JAMA* 1987;257(16):2196–203.

5. Bergstrom N, Braden B. A prospective study of pressure sore risk among institutionalized elderly. *J Am Geriatr Soc* 1992;40:747–58.

6. Panel for the Prediction and Prevention of Pressure Ulcers in Adults. *Pressure Ulcers in Adults: Prediction and Prevention.* Clinical Practice Guideline, Number 3. AHCPR Publication No. 92–0047. Rockville, MD: Agency for Health Care Policy and Research, Public Health Service, U.S. Department of Health and Human Services. May 1992.

7. Norton D, McLaren R, Exton–Smith AN. *An Investigation of Geriatric Nursing Problems in Hospitals.* London, England, National Corporation for the Care of Old People, 1962.

8. Bergstrom N, Braden BJ, Laguzza A, Holman B. The Braden Scale for Predicting Pressure Sore Risk. *Nurs Res* 1987;36(4):205–10.

9. Goldstone LA, Roberts BV. A preliminary discriminant function analysis of elderly orthopaedic patients who will or will not contract a pressure sore. *Int J Nurs Stud* 1980;17(1):17–23.

10. Goldstone LA, Goldstone J. The Norton score: an early warning of pressure sores? *J Adv Nurs* 1982;7(5):419–26.

11. Braden BJ, Bergstrom N. Predictive validity of the Braden Scale for Pressure Sore Risk in a nursing home population. *Research in Nursing & Health* 1994;17:459–470.

12. Braden BJ, Bergstrom N. Pressure reduction. In: Bulechek GM, McCloskey JC (eds). *Nursing Interventions, Essential Nursing Treatments, Second Edition.* Orlando, FL, W.B. Saunders Co., 1992, pp. 94–108.

13. Braden BJ, Bergstrom N. Clinical utility of the Braden Scale for Predicting Pressure Sore Risk. *Decubitus* 1989;2(3):44–51.

14. Seiler WO, Stahelin HB. Decubitus ulcers: preventive techniques for the elderly patient. *Geriatrics* 1985;40(7):53–8,60.

15. Bliss MR, McLaren R, Exton–Smith AN. Preventing pressure sores in hospital: controlled trial of a large–celled ripple mattress. *Br Med J* 1967;1(537):394–7.

16. Goldstone LA, Norris M, O'Reilly M, White J. A clinical trial of a bead bed system for the prevention of pressure sores in elderly orthopaedic patients. *J Adv Nurs* 1982;7(6):545–8.

17. Jacobs MA. Comparison of capillary blood flow using a regular hospital bed mattress, ROHO mattress, and Mediscus bed. *Rehabil Nurs* 1989;14(5):270–2.

18. Stapleton M. Preventing pressure sores—an evaluation of three products. *Geriatr Nur London* 1986;6(2):23–5.

19. Krouskop TA. The effect of surface geometry on interface pressures generated by polyurethane foam mattress overlays. A compilation of reports by The Rehabilitation Engineering Center at the Institute for Rehabilitation & Research. Houston, TX, 1986.

20. Berjian RA, Douglass HO Jr., Holyoke ED, Goodwin PM, Priore RL. Skin pressure measurements on various mattress surfaces in cancer patients. *Am J Phys Med* 1983;62(5):217–26.

21. Allman RM, Walker JM, Hart MK, Laprade CA, Noel LB, Smith CR. Air–fluidized beds or conventional therapy for pressure sores. A randomized trial. *Ann Intern Med* 1987;107(5):641–8.

22. Bennett RG, Bellantoni MF, Ouslander JG. Air–fluidized bed treatment of nursing home patients with pressure sores. *J Am Geriatr Soc* 1989;37(3):235–42.

23. Jackson BS, Chagares R, Nee N, Freeman K. The effects of a therapeutic bed on pressure sores: an experimental study. *J Enterostomal Ther* 1988;15(6):220–6.

24. Ferrell BA, Osterweil D, Christenson P. A randomized trial of low–air–loss beds for treatment of pressure ulcers. *JAMA* 1993;269(4):494–7.

25. Panel for Urinary Incontinence in Adults. *Urinary Incontinence in Adults*: Clinical Practice Guideline. AHCPR Publication No. 92–0038. Agency for Health Care Policy and Research, Public Health Service, U.S. Department of Health and Human Services. March, 1992.

26. Dinsdale SM. Decubitus ulcers: role of pressure and friction in causation. *Arch Phys Med Rehabil* 1974;55(4):147–52.

6

Pressure Ulcer Assessment and Documentation: The Pressure Sore Status Tool

Barbara M. Bates–Jensen, MN, CETN

Bates–Jensen BM. Pressure ulcer assessment and documentation: The Pressure Sore Status Tool. In: Krasner D, Kane D. *Chronic Wound Care, Second Edition.* Wayne, PA, Health Management Publications, Inc., 1997, pp 37–48.

Introduction

A pressure ulcer is defined as an area of local tissue necrosis usually developing where soft tissues are compressed between bony prominences and any external surface for prolonged periods.[1,2] Pressure ulcers are the result of mechanical injury to the skin and tissues causing hypoxia and ischemia. The Wound Healing Society, in 1992, commissioned a panel of experts to define language related to chronic wounds and chronic wound healing. This group of experts defined chronic in relation to wounds, as wounds that fail to progress through a normal, orderly and timely sequence of repair or wounds that pass through the repair process without restoring anatomic and functional results.[3] Margolis suggests that as pressure ulcers have traditionally been classified as "chronic wounds" and based on the work of the Wound Healing Society, including failure to progress through the repair process in a timely and orderly manner might also be appropriate in defining pressure ulcers.[4]

Pressure ulcer assessment forms the foundation for treatment and evaluation. The initial assessment provides baseline data, and follow up assessments at regular intervals allow for comparison to the baseline data to monitor progress or deterioration of the ulcer. In this manner the therapeutic plan can be evaluated for effectiveness. Indices for pressure ulcer assessment should provide data for two purposes, examining the severity of the lesion

and monitoring changes in the lesion over time. The assessment data enables clinicians to communicate clearly about a patient's pressure ulcer, to provide for continuity in the plan of care, and to allow evaluation of treatment modalities. This chapter focuses on pressure ulcer assessment, reviews pertinent research in pressure ulcer assessment, discusses assessment and documentation issues related to pressure ulcers and reports on the use of the Pressure Sore Status Tool (PSST) and the Wound Intelligent System (WIS) for pressure ulcer assessment. Although the principles used for assessing pressure ulcers apply in general to other wound types, the clinician is referred to Chapter 4 for a more general approach to all wound assessment.

Overview

Pressure ulcer assessment must encompass evaluation of the total patient. The clinician must remember the importance general patient assessment has for evaluating wound healing in pressure ulcers. The patient should be evaluated for nutritional status, presence of risk factors for pressure ulcer development, pressure ulcer pain, and adherence to the therapy plan since all of these factors may influence the healing of pressure ulcers. The primary focus of this chapter is on assessment of the pressure ulcer wound itself.

A composite of wound characteristics is necessary for accurate documentation of the wound's status and overall health.[5–7] A single wound characteristic does not provide information essential in determining the adequacy of the therapy nor does it allow for monitoring progress or deterioration of the wound. The indices for pressure ulcer assessment include all of the following: location, size of the ulcer, stage of the ulcer, depth of tissue involvement, condition of the wound edges and presence of undermining or tunneling, necrotic tissue characteristics, exudate characteristics, surrounding tissue conditions and wound healing parameters of granulation tissue and epithelialization.[2,3,6,8,9]

assessment of the dark skinned patient with a pressure ulcer. Some general guidelines for assessment in dark skinned individuals can assist in more accurate and meaningful communication regarding pressure ulcers in these patients.

Another assessment issue for pressure ulcers is the use of a staging classification system to document healing, termed "downstaging" or "back–staging." Downstaging is using the staging system (a system which evaluates the wound based on clinical observation of tissue layers involved) as a dynamic continuum to show healing in pressure

---

Methods of documenting assessment data should allow for tracking of individual assessment characteristics and promote quantification of observations for easy examination of changes in the ulcer status.

Surprisingly, there are few tools for assessing pressure ulcer characteristics and healing. The Sessing Scale[10] and the Pressure Sore Status Tool (PSST)[11] are reviewed here as examples of research–based instruments for assessment. Once the pressure ulcer is evaluated, the information must be recorded in a manner that allows for monitoring changes in individual wound characteristics as the wound heals or deteriorates.

Methods of documenting assessment data should allow for tracking of individual assessment characteristics and promote quantification of observations for easy examination of changes in the ulcer status. The PSST, a research–based instrument for assessment and documentation of pressure ulcers, incorporates the necessary indices for pressure ulcer assessment, provides for quantification of observations and allows for tracking the condition of the ulcer over time.[6] The automated PSST, the Wound Intelligence System (WIS), involves total patient and wound assessment with convenient documentation abilities and without some of the problems associated with manual recording systems for monitoring changes over time.[12] Use of an organized method of pressure ulcer assessment is a beginning in addressing several issues related to pressure ulcer assessment and documentation.

The issues surrounding pressure ulcer assessment and documentation include use of staging and size as stand–alone assessment criteria to demonstrate healing, assessment of the dark skinned individual, and documentation for reimbursement of therapy. One of the most pressing issues for clinicians and researchers alike is the

ulcers (documenting a pressure ulcer initially as a Stage IV and as it heals as a Stage III, Stage II, Stage I, healed). Generally downstaging has been used to document healing in pressure ulcers and has been used as criteria for determining reimbursement for treatments. Downstaging has been used, in particular, in long term care facilities where there is a mandate to demonstrate wound healing, where facilities' documentation of pressure ulcer status is regulated, and where facilities are routinely surveyed for compliance with documentation regulations. Documentation of pressure ulcers may be more of an issue in different healthcare settings as third party reimbursement is often based on written records of pressure ulcer status and healing. This dependency may present issues related to documentation and assessment.

The most commonly used assessment indicators of pressure ulcer status are size and staging systems. There are problems associated with both of these measures. The most frequently used methods for assessment of size and stage and the disadvantages associated with use of these two measures in isolation are presented. Each of the other major indicators included in pressure ulcer assessment are also discussed. The major issues related to assessment and documentation of pressure ulcers are discussed and finally, the WIS is described as a useful automated tool for assessing pressure ulcers.

Assessment Issues

One of the reasons for limited studies and limited usefulness of previous work on wound healing in pressure ulcers is related to the difficulties in assessment of healing in pressure ulcers. These difficulties relate to terminology definitions, tools available for measurement and lack of specificity for dark skinned patients. The major tools used by clinicians to determine pressure ulcer status have been staging classification systems and measurement of the size of the ulcer. The issue of assessment of dark skinned patients with pressure ulcers is a special assessment issue.

Assessment of the dark skinned patient. Dark skin does not show the erythematous skin color changes so evident in lighter skinned persons. In assessing the dark skinned patient, be aware that dark skin exhibits early pressure tissue trauma with different observable tissue changes. The tissues over the bony prominence may become taut and shiny with evidence of induration or firmness of the tissues present. The tissues may have an orange peel appearance where visually the pores are more prominent in the skin.[13]

The skin may feel warmer with localized increase in temperature in the early stages of tissue inflammation. The tissues later exhibit a decrease in temperature as the tissue trauma progresses. Assessment of skin temperature changes can be performed using the skin thermometers available in most drug stores. Apply the skin thermometer to an area of intact, undamaged skin for a baseline skin temperature reading and then apply the skin thermometer over the bony prominence of concern. Compare the skin temperature over the bony prominence to that of the healthy tissues to evaluate for localized heat.

Skin color does change in dark skinned individuals. It may be observed as a deepening of normal ethnic tone or a bluish, purple hue to the skin.[14] In some cases, a greyness to the skin may be determined. Use of adequate and consistent lighting sources for evaluating dark skin are essential for evaluation of the tissue changes.[13]

Staging systems. Prior to 1989, the primary tool used to assess pressure ulcer status was staging classification systems. Pressure ulcers are commonly classified according to grading or staging systems based on the depth of tissue destruction. Historically, one problem in assessment was the lack of a universal staging system for classifying the severity of pressure ulcers. A variety of systems existed with little uniformity between systems. These staging systems were generally clinical descriptions that focused on a single variable, usually depth of tissue loss, and were not comprehensive in scope. Although staging pressure ulcers was a commonly accepted practice it was an area with little or no agreement on the number of stages or specific criteria for each stage. This general lack of

congruence between systems made comparison difficult. Additionally, several classification systems combined physiological development descriptors with clinical manifestations, which made using the systems confusing and ambiguous. Maklebust discussed the major concern that existed in using a staging system as the assessment model of skin breakdown,[15] i.e. that no system was universally accepted.

Cooper points out that use of a staging system (any system) requires a degree of skill and knowledge in recognition of tissue layers not necessarily taught to most healthcare professionals.[16] Identification of specific wound characteristics requires a certain amount of time to develop and healthcare providers using staging systems may be at various levels of ability in using the system. Accurate, meaningful communication is difficult as clinicians may not have the experience necessary to recognize the various tissue layers that identify the stage or grade. In addition, clinicians may use the same system but interpret the stage criteria differently.

The best known and most widely used of the staging systems was the system introduced by Shea in 1975. Shea's four stage system formed the basis for most of the systems in use.[17] Shea did not report on reliability of the system nor was any specific validity testing reported. Shea analyzed tissue biopsies for determination of the histopathologic trauma within the tissues. More recently, Witkowski and Parish reviewed the histopathology and documented tissue damage at the cellular level for each of Shea's stages.[18]

The First National Consensus Development Conference on Pressure Ulcers sponsored by the National Pressure Ulcer Advisory Panel (NPUAP) in 1989 recommended adoption of a uniform staging system to assist with communication and research in the field.[1] This system was later recommended for universal use by the Agency for Health Care Policy and Research (AHCPR) panel.[2,19] The recommended staging system follows:

Stage I—Non–blanchable erythema of intact skin; the heralding lesion of skin ulceration. In individuals with darker skin, discoloration of the skin, warmth, edema, induration, or hardness may also be indicators.

Stage II—Partial–thickness skin loss involving epidermis or dermis, or both. The ulcer is superficial and presents clinically as an abrasion, blister or shallow crater.

Stage III—Full–thickness skin loss involving damage or necrosis of subcutaneous tissue, which may extend down to but not through underlying fascia. The ulcer presents clinically as a deep crater with or without undermining of adjacent tissue.

Stage IV—Full–thickness skin loss with extensive destruction, tissue necrosis, or damage to muscle bone or supporting structures (such as tendon, joint capsule).

many cases there is greater tissue damage in the Stage I lesion (the non–blanchable erythema may be the early manifestation of trauma at the bony tissue interface involving deeper tissue layers).

There are other validity problems. Stage I lesions vary in presentation and pose questions regarding

---

The staging system is best used as a diagnostic tool to determine the depth of the tissue insult and should remain static over time even as the wound itself heals and recovers.

Staging systems only measure one characteristic of the wound and should not be viewed as a complete assessment independent of other indicators. Staging classification systems do not assess for criteria in the healing process and hinder tracking of progress because of the inability of the staging system to demonstrate change over time. This is especially true if one considers pressure ulcer development as a continuum that begins as a reversible superficial injury that may progress to a significant problem. The staging system does not allow for movement within or between stages.[20,21] Many clinicians attempt to use the staging system as a dynamic continuum, despite the difficulties associated with back–staging or downstaging. Use of the pressure ulcer stages in reverse order to demonstrate healing suggests that the tissues replaced during the normal repair process are structurally similar to the lost soft tissue layers.

Questions regarding the validity of the staging system relate to the Stage II lesion, characteristics of the Stage I lesion and use of the system on wounds of various etiology. Theoretically, pressure ulcer trauma starts at the bony tissue interface and works outward to the top layer of the skin. Stage II lesions are usually caused by friction or shearing of the tissues causing superficial, partial thickness damage to the epidermis. The use of the term "pressure" in the label pressure ulcer, implies the cause of the lesion. Maklebust points out the difficulty in applying this label to the Stage II lesion.[22] Stage II pressure ulcers are partial thickness wounds most commonly caused by friction or shearing forces, not necessarily pressure forces. Maklebust poses the question, is the Stage II pressure ulcer a true pressure ulcer?[22] Another concern with the pressure ulcer staging system is the use of numbers to identify the stages. The use of numbers implies that pressure ulcers develop in a specific sequence and order.[22] This underlying implication would suggest that the Stage II lesion is more severe than Stage I lesions. In

the validity of the system. Some Stage I lesions may be the indicator of deep tissue damage just beginning to manifest on the skin, and others may indicate only superficial insult where damage is somewhat reversible and not indicative of underlying tissue death. Identification of Stage I lesions is difficult in dark skinned patients and important tissue changes may be overlooked due to inexperience in examining dark skin.

Often wounds caused by factors other than pressure (for example, vascular, neurotrophic, traumatic, incontinence) are classified using the same staging system which further confuses the issue.

The disadvantages of staging as a single indicator of pressure ulcer status include the need for past experience/education in tissue layer identification, reliability of the system, validity of the staging system, inability to measure change, and the inability to account for wound recovery. These problems are not easily overcome and make staging of pressure ulcers an ineffective assessment when used alone. The staging system is best used as a diagnostic tool to determine the depth of the tissue insult and should remain static over time even as the wound itself heals and recovers.

Measurement of size. Verhonick in her early study of decubitus ulcer observations noted the first obvious measurable aspect of pressure ulcer healing is wound size.[23] Today, assessment of size of the ulcer remains a critical characteristic for evaluating pressure ulcer status and healing. Measurement of wound size has received much attention in the literature. Measurement generally involves either two–dimensional or three–dimensional measurements. Two–dimensional measurements are the most widely used approach to measure wound healing in the clinical area.

Linear measurements, wound tracings with or without planimetry and photographs with or without planimetry are examples of tools used for two–dimensional measurement. Bohannon and Pfaller evaluated wound tracings and planimetry as techniques to determine the area of wound perimeter tracings and concluded that most difficulties were encountered with the irregularly shaped wound and the ability to obtain the wound tracing itself.[24] Serial photographs can provide information on both wound assessment and measurement.

Rigorous technique should be used with all three methods to ensure validity and accuracy (reliability) of results. The photo should be taken from the same distance, with the patient in the same position. Linear measurements must be taken from the same point of reference and wound tracings must be carefully obtained. Wound tracings and photographs can also be used with planimetry methods to estimate surface area measurements. Either manual or computer–assisted planimetry may be used, but the approach may be time intensive for the bedside clinician.

The usual methods of obtaining area measurements involve measuring the length and width (and/or depth) of the wound in centimeters and recording area measurement on a flow sheet for tracking purposes. Area measurement of the ulcer is considered an index of wound healing by most clinicians.[25] Consistent documentation of area measurements allows determination of whether the ulcer has decreased in size over a period of time.[26]

The following suggestions may improve the results obtained. Measurements should be taken in a consistent manner; always measure the longest and widest aspect of the wound or measure from head to toe and side to side of the wound to increase the reliability of the results.[27] Calculating the surface area estimates from the length and width (length x width) allows for tracking of a single number which will improve the ability to monitor for changes in size over time. Use of caution in concluding that minute changes in size are evidence of healing (more likely they are evidence of the unreliable nature of the measure). Assessing for overall gross changes in size as the indicator of wound healing is also important.

Three dimensional measurements have some of the same difficulties discussed in relation to two–dimensional measurements. Three dimensional measurements can be obtained by linear measurements, wound molds, foam dressings or fluid instillations. Linear measurements for length, width and depth can be obtained in two ways. The clinician can use any measuring device and simply measure as requested or there is a device developed by Kundin[28] available to measure depth as well as length and width. Thomas and Wysocki compared three clinically useful methods of measurement: the Kundin gauge, photographs, and acetate tracings.[25] They found the three measures highly correlated, although the Kundin gauge had a tendency to underestimate wound area on larger, irregularly shaped wounds. The acetate tracings and photos had the highest correlation.

There are several problems with area measurement reliability. When used alone, area measurements may not accurately indicate the rate of wound healing.[29] One common problem with using size as the only indicator of wound healing is the case of the debrided pressure ulcer. When an ulcer is debrided, the size generally increases although the wound has usually improved. Variations in clinicians' abilities to define the wound edge and approach measurement with rigor may influence reliability of findings. Wounds with irregular shapes and depth present additional problems with validity of linear measurements of size. Irregularly shaped wounds pose the problem of where along an uneven wound edge to place the measuring device to obtain the measurement reading. Ulcers with depth may make two–dimensional measurements meaningless, and three–dimensional measurements are difficult. Depth may be measured linearly as part of the determination of size by inserting a cotton–tipped applicator into the wound, marking the level of the skin, and measuring the applicator to the mark in centimeters. The difficulty in measuring depth with linear measurements is discussed by Cooper[7] and relates to the imprecise nature of the measure. Where to insert the cotton–tipped applicator on the uneven wound base is problematic and raises questions about the reliability and validity of the measure.

Wound volume is an additional approach to measurement of wound size. Wound molds have been used to assess the volume of the wound. Resch, Kerner and Robson used this technique to measure wound status in pressure ulcers.[30] The placement of the mold medium does not affect the granulating tissues nor does it cause discomfort to the patient. It does provide a visual record of the wound's progress, but does not lend itself to the clinical area. Cooper reported on a new foam elastomer dressing that also provides information like the molds on wound volume.[27] To date, these products have not been approved for use in the United States. The last method of three–dimensional measurement is fluid instillation. A transparent film dressing is applied over the wound and fluid is instilled via syringe and needle into the wound cavity until the dressing approaches normal body contours. The amount of fluid instilled is then recorded. Problems arise with maintaining the patient in the same position for each measurement, or because of the position of the wound on the body various amounts of the fluid are retained. A major difficulty with methods to measure three–dimensions is the inability to determine whether the volume is related to healthy, healing tissues or a necrotic debris–filled wound. Gentzkow questions the necessity of obtaining wound volume measurements for clinical studies on pressure ulcer wound healing and suggests that wound volume measurements do not provide any advantage for assessing wound healing over simple area measurements of the wound.[31] Until further research demonstrates the importance of wound volume measurements, it is not likely to become part of the standard assessment for pressure ulcer status.[31] Size is an important indicator for pressure ulcer assessment. As wounds heal, wound surface area and volume must decrease. Recent studies suggest that the rate of decrease in the size of the wound may be a predictor to ultimate healing. Van Rijswijk and Polansky studied predictors of time to healing deep Stage III and IV pressure ulcers.[32] Time to healing analysis methods (Kaplan–Meier time until healing curves) were used to evaluate healing time in Stages III to IV ulcers as a function of patient and wound characteristics at baseline and after two weeks of therapy. Results demonstrated that pressure ulcers in patients who were 60 to 70 years old, who had good nutritional status at baseline, and whose ulcers reduced at least 39 percent in size after two weeks, healed more quickly. However, size is only one characteristic of the wound and should not be the only index to status of the ulcer.

Assessment of Pressure Ulcer Status

Assessment of pressure ulcer status is perhaps the most useful method in evaluation of pressure ulcers. Assessment of status evaluates macroscopic indices of healing. The NPUAP concurred with the need for better assessment and evaluation of healing and focused the 1995 NPUAP Consensus Development Conference on assessment. The conference reached consensus on several issues: first, assessment must encompass a composite of characteristics; second, pressure ulcer staging is useful but is a static tool used for diagnosis purposes only—not as a continuum; and finally, size and stage are insufficient measures of healing and an inappropriate assessment data base when used in isolation of other wound characteristics.[33] The AHCPR guidelines for treatment of pressure ulcers views assessment as the starting point in preparing to treat or manage a person with a pressure ulcer, and the panel acknowledges that assessment forms the basis for planning and evaluating therapy.[2] The panel further recommends assessment of a composite of characteristics associated with pressure ulcers.

The indices for pressure ulcer assessment include all of the following: location and size of the ulcer, stage or depth of tissue involvement, condition of the wound edges and presence of undermining or tunneling, necrotic tissue characteristics, exudate characteristics, surrounding tissue conditions and wound healing characteristics of granulation tissue and epithelialization.[2,3,6,8,9] There are few tools available to help the clinician evaluate the overall wound status: the early work by Verhonick on Decubitus Ulcer Observations,[23] the Pressure Sore Status Tool[11] and the Sessing Scale[10] are the available instruments for pressure ulcers. The PSST developed in 1990 by this author, Barbara Bates–Jensen[11] evaluates 13 characteristics and rates them on a modified Likert scale with 1 being the best of the characteristic and 5 being the worst possible for the characteristic. The Sessing scale[10] is a modified classification system that evaluates wound characteristics in addition to stage of the ulcer.

Verhonick addressed decubitus ulcer observations with the use of criterion–measures.[23] Verhonick in 1961 designed decubitus ulcer criterion–measures to meet four specifications: relevance or validity, freedom from bias, reliability or precision, and convenience or availability.

The Criterion Measure for Decubitus Observations includes eight categories: size, color, skin tone, skin condition, drainage, sensation, infectious process and other factors. The size of induration, excoriation, necrosis, scar and depth were all measured. Size of the ulcer was determined by actual tracings and circumference in square centimeters. Color of the lesion was assessed using a color scale consisting of 25 shades of red, 22 shades of purple and blue, 21 shades of yellow and 19 shades of gray to black. The color samples were encased in a plastic cover and placed next to the ulcer; the code number corresponding to the color was then recorded. Verhonick cited difficulties in using this measure: the paper colors were flat compared to tissue color, the range of colors was not wide enough to be inclusive of patients with different skin color, subtle changes in color were difficult to determine and variables such as race, general complexion, skin thickness, and location distorted observer selection of colors.[23] These difficulties in assessing color remain problems for assessment today.

Skin tone was defined as loose to pinch, moderate to pinch or hard and taut. Skin condition was measured using the characteristics of dehydration, edema, erythema, pallor, purple, hot and dry, perspiration, rash and mottling. These characteristics were rated on a scale of negative (0), slight (1), moderate (3), marked (5), or profuse (7). Drainage was measured with serous, serosanguineous and purulent being measured as scanty, moderate or profuse. Sensation characteristics observed were recorded as no complaint, numbness, tingle, itching, irritated, mild pain, moderate pain, or severe pain.

Verhonick reported that experience with the tool and the accompanying nursing diagnosis checklist, in 45 patients over a two–year period, met the four specifications stated earlier, although no statistics were presented.[23] No information was available on use of the tool since its development. The strength of the instrument is that it was one of the first attempts to quantify wound observations. The major weakness in the tool is the lack of uniformity in scaling and the lack of current use of the tool.

necrotic tissue type, necrotic tissue amount, exudate type, exudate amount, surrounding skin color, peripheral tissue edema, peripheral tissue induration, granulation tissue, and epithelialization. Two items are non–scored items: location and shape. The remaining 13 are scored items and each appears with characteristic descriptors rated on a modified Likert scale (1 = best for that characteristic and 5 = worst attribute of the characteristic). The individual items can be summed and the total score may be an index of overall wound status. Total scores range from 13 to 65.[34] The goal of the PSST is to enhance meaningful communication between healthcare professionals involved in pressure ulcer care by providing a framework for assessment and documentation with an attempt at quantification. An objective method of assessing pressure ulcers and monitoring changes over time

An objective method of assessing pressure ulcers and monitoring changes over time allows for evaluation of the therapeutic plan of care and may be used to guide and direct therapy.

More recently, Ferrell and colleagues reported use of the Sessing Scale.[10] This tool combines specific wound descriptors into six categories and places a numerical value on each category. Test–retest reliability was determined on two consecutive days, using ten pressure ulcer patients in long term care facilities with wounds on the trunk or trochanter. Agreement was evaluated using a weighted kappa statistic and resulted in a kappa = 0.90. Inter–rater reliability was evaluated on the same 10 patients with two nurse observers and resulted in a weighted kappa = 0.80. The Sessing scale demonstrated concurrent validity with both the Shea scale[17] and surface area measurements with moderately strong relationships between the Sessing scale and Shea, Spearman's r = 0.52, p < 0.0001; and the Sessing scale and surface area, Spearman's r = 0.35, p < 0.001. The strengths of this newer tool are the concurrent validity tests with Shea's classification staging system[17] and surface area measurements. The major disadvantages of the tool include that it is an additional classification system with several additional stages added; no attempt is made to quantify individual wound characteristics; and the tool has only been tested on a small sample with educated and experienced clinicians as observers.

The Pressure Sore Status Tool (PSST) is a pencil and paper instrument comprised of 15 items: location, shape, size, depth, edges, undermining,

allows for evaluation of the therapeutic plan of care and may be used to guide and direct therapy. The purpose of the tool is to provide a framework for objective assessment of pressure ulcers for clinicians and researchers. The tool is research–based and was developed using a modified Delphi technique with 20 multi–disciplinary experts on wound healing and pressure ulcers.[11] Content validity was established for each individual item on the tool and for the total tool with a nine member judge panel of nurse experts.[11] Concurrent validity was evaluated in a long term care setting and involved comparing medical record documentation of pressure ulcer Stage II with the PSST depth item for a correlation coefficient of 0.90.[12]

Pilot reliability with two ET nurses (with experience and education in wound care) in an acute care setting has been reported with inter–rater agreement as r = 0.91 (p = 0.0001) and mean intra–rater reliability was r = 0.975 (p = 0.0001).[11] Reliability in a long term care setting with licensed practical nurses, one physical therapist, and registered nurses with no additional wound care training resulted in acceptable reliability. Item by item inter–rater reliability yielded a coefficient of 0.78, lower than that previously reported for ET nurses but above a pre–set agreement criterion of 0.75. Intra–rater agreement was higher, r = 0.89 and the agreement with the expert resulted in a coefficient of 0.82.[12]

Since the PSST involves a Likert–type ordinal scale and the probability of chance agreement between two raters is 0.20 for any item, the data were also subjected to analyses using kappa statistics and each item on the scale yielded coefficients above 0.60.[12]

The PSST allows for temporal tracking of individual characteristics as well as of the total tool. Each characteristic is assessed and given a value from the Likert scale, thus the scores can be monitored for improvement or deterioration in each characteristic. Additionally, the 13 item scores can be summed and the total plotted on a continuum to allow for overall tracking of the wound status. This quantification of observations allows for monitoring not only individual items and total score but also groups of characteristics. For example, the characteristics of necrotic tissue type and amount and exudate type and amount may be tracked to evaluate debridement or infection management.[12]

Another benefit associated with the assignment of numerical values to items on the tool is the ability to set realistic goals. Clinical experience shows that not all pressure ulcers heal and certainly not always in the same setting. The goal may not always be that "the wound will heal." The PSST allows for more realistic goal setting as appropriate to the healthcare setting and the individual patient and pressure ulcer. For example, the patient with a large necrotic full–thickness ulcer in acute care will probably not be in the facility long enough for the wound to actually heal; however, the tool would enable clinicians to make smaller goals, such as, the wound will decrease in type and amount of necrotic tissue. In some instances a pressure ulcer may never heal because of host factors or other contextual circumstances, so the goal might be to maintain the total wound score between 20 and 22.

Appropriate assessment requires documentation of findings. The PSST incorporates the necessary indices for pressure ulcer assessment, provides for quantification of observations and allows for tracking the condition of the ulcer over time.[6]

Assessment of Pressure Ulcer Characteristics

Wound edges. Wound edges are a composite of characteristics that include distinctness, degree of attachment to the wound base, color and thickness.[21] As tissues degenerate, broad indistinct areas, where any edge is difficult to discern, become shallow lesions with more distinct, thin, separate edges. As tissue trauma progresses, the reaction intensifies with a thickening and rolling inward of the epidermis, so the edge is well–defined and sharply outlines the ulcer with little or no evidence of new tissue growth.

Finally, fibrosis and scarring result from repeated injury and repair. The edges become indurated and firm[17] with possible impairment in migratory ability of epithelial cells.[35]

Partial–thickness wounds heal by regeneration and the edges provide a supply of intact epithelial cells to proliferate, and assist in re–surfacing the wound by lateral migration.[8,36,37] For full–thickness wounds, healing must occur via repair and scar formation. The wound fills with scar tissue, contraction occurs and the edges assist with either epithelialization or proliferation and migration of epithelial cells to re–surface the wound.[8,36,37]

Edges may be assessed at regular intervals by measuring the distance the edge extends into the wound base or by tracing the perimeter of the wound on acetate or plastic.[38]

Undermining. Pressure ulcers with undermining have more aerobic and anaerobic bacteria present than wounds in the process of healing with no undermining.[39] The degree and amount of undermining indicates the severity of the tissue necrosis. As subcutaneous fat necroses, the skin undermines. Initially, deep fascia limits the depth of penetration, encouraging more internal undermining spread. Once the fascia is penetrated, undermining of deeper tissues may proceed rapidly.[17] Undermining may be thought of as involving a significant proportion of the wound edges whereas tunneling may only involve a small edge of the wound and extend for a significant length in that one direction. Internal wound dimensions are commonly measured by using cotton tipped applicators and gently probing the wound.[8]

Necrotic tissue type and amount. Necrotic tissue characteristics, such as color, consistency, adherence and amount present in the wound, must be incorporated into the pressure ulcer assessment. As tissues die during pressure ulcer development, they change in color, consistency and adherence to the wound bed. The level and type of tissue death influences the clinical appearance of the necrotic tissue. For example, as subcutaneous fat tissues die, a collection of stringy, yellow slough is formed. As muscle tissues degenerate, the dead tissue may be more thick or tenacious. Histologic studies of human skin during pressure ulcer development demonstrate that as the insult to the tissue progresses, the level of necrosis deepens.[18] Hard black eschar represents full thickness destruction possibly occurring from prolonged ischemia and anoxemia, or a sudden large vessel disruption from shearing forces.[40] Fat and dermal necrosis and the formation of a slough may be compounded by infection from previous contamination by normal skin flora.[41,42] The debris may appear as yellow slough or a mucoid substance.

The characteristic "necrotic tissue type" is a qualitative variable; most clinicians use descriptions of clinical observations of a composite of factors as a method of assessment. The characteristics of color, consistency and adherence are most often used to describe the type of necrosis. As necrosis worsens, color varies from white/grey non–viable tissue to yellow slough and finally to black eschar. Consistency refers to the cohesiveness of debris (i.e. is it thin or thick? stringy or clumpy?). Consistency also varies on a continuum as necrosis deepens and becomes more dehydrated.

The terms "slough" and "eschar" refer to different levels of necrosis and are described according to color and consistency. The term "slough" is defined as yellow (or tan) and either thin, mucinous or stringy, whereas, "eschar" is described as black, soft or hard and representing full thickness tissue destruction.[17] Adherence refers to the adhesiveness of the debris to the wound bed and the ease with which the two are separated. Necrotic tissue tends to become more adherent to the wound bed as the level of damage increases. Clinically, eschar is more firmly adherent than yellow slough.

The amount of necrotic tissue retards wound healing because it is a medium for bacterial growth and a physical impediment to epithelialization, contraction or granulation.[43,44] The more necrotic tissue present in the wound bed, the more severe the insult to the tissue and the longer the time required to heal the wound.[17] In the process of treating the necrotic wound, the amount of necrotic tissue present leads to modification of treatment and debridement techniques. The stage of the pressure ulcer can not be assessed in the presence of necrosis, which obscures visualization of the total wound.

Exudate type and amount. Exudate should be assessed for the amount and type of drainage that occurs. The type and color of wound exudate varies depending on the degree of moisture in the wound and the organisms present. For example, when a wound becomes dry, the exudate darkens. Also, the presence of *pseudomonas* produces a thick, malodorous, green drainage.[21] Wounds with foul smelling drainage are generally infected and healing time is prolonged as tissue destruction progresses.[39] Characteristics used to examine exudate are color, consistency, adherence and distribution in the wound, and presence of odor.[8]

Excess exudate uses substrates and energy that could be used for the wound healing process.[21] Estimating the amount of exudate in the wound is difficult due to wound size variability and topical dressing types. Cooper suggests estimating the percentage of exudate in the wound by clinical observation.[8] Estimation of wound drainage can also be determined by noting the number of dressings saturated during a period of time. One problem with assessment of exudate amount is the size of the wound. What might be considered a large amount of drainage for the smaller wound may be considered a small amount for the larger wound, making clinically meaningful assessment of exudate difficult to obtain. Mulder advocates using standardized terminology for describing amount and type of wound exudate.[45]

Surrounding tissue condition. The tissues surrounding the wound should be assessed for color, induration and edema. These characteristics are indicators for further tissue damage and possible impairment in the wound healing process. Cellulitis or infection may be suspected, based on the presence of redness and tenderness around the wound.[46] Further tissue trauma due to pressure may appear as blanchable to non–blanchable erythema around the wound. Blanchable erythema may be red, dark red or purple discoloration of the skin. As the condition becomes more chronic the area can remain blue–brown with no blanching.[47] Erythema can be evaluated by testing for blanching in light skinned patients. Skin color is a qualitative variable with no simple, objective assessment method. Tissue induration and edema may be an indication of additional tissue damage or infection.[18,46] Edema is assessed by location and pitting or non–pitting characteristics. Induration may be assessed using linear measurements. Edema impedes neoangiogenesis and prolongs the healing process. Induration signals further tissue ischemia and damage.

Granulation tissue and epithelialization. Granulation tissue provides the scaffolding for scar tissue in full–thickness wounds and consists of new blood vessels and an immature collagen matrix.[8] The color of granulation tissue is a reflection of the health of the wound. For example, impaired arterial circulation to the wound site results in pale pink tissue, while venous circulation impairment results in a dusky, ruby color.[21] The color of the granulation tissue may also indicate the length of time it has been present in the wound with fresh granulation tissue appearing pink and progressing to beefy red as the depth builds. Harding suggests that a red friable appearance may signify infection rather than wound health.[26] The percent of the wound filled with granulation tissue and the color of the tissue are characteristics indicative of the health of the wound.[6]

Partial thickness wounds heal by epidermal resurfacing and regeneration. Epithelialization happens from lateral migration at the wound edges and the base of hair follicles, as epithelial cells proliferate and resurface the wound.[8,36,37] Full–thickness wounds heal using scar formation: the tissue defect fills with new blood vessels and collagen, edges contract and the wound is resurfaced by epithelialization. So the process of epithelialization may occur throughout the wound bed in partial thickness wounds but only occurs from wound edges in full thickness wounds.

Assessment of epithelialization can occur by evaluating the amount of the wound that is surrounded by new tissue and the distance new tissue extends into the wound base.[8,21]

Once assessment data are collected they must be recorded for monitoring purposes. The key to assessment of pressure ulcer status is what is accomplished once the information is obtained. Monitoring the data routinely allows easy identification of trends and evaluation of outcomes of interventions. Methods of monitoring the data should be relatively simple and efficient to ensure compliance and use of the information obtained during the assessment.

Documentation and the Wound Intelligence System. Documentation of pressure ulcer status is notoriously poor.[48] Documentation may be required for reimbursement of specific therapies in use to support the healing of the wound. Using the pencil and paper PSST as a form for assessment of the pressure ulcer wound has the advantage of providing a means for documentation that is simple and time effective. The paper assessment form is simply entered into the patient's medical record. Paper forms such as skin care flow sheets in long term care facilities provide other examples of documentation formats. Long narrative notes are rarely kept together in an organized manner for easy retrieval of ulcer information. Monitoring data using narrative notes or skin care flow sheets is problematic. It is often difficult and time consuming to analyze the information and determine quickly whether or not the interventions in use are effective. The PSST has the advantage of including a scale at the bottom of the paper form for entering the total wound score to see at a glance the health or degeneration of the wound. All paper forms have disadvantages.

Manual tools like the PSST provide formidable information regarding pressure ulcer characteristics as well as a method of documenting findings. Yet, as data accumulate over time the pencil and paper PSST is susceptible to the same conditions that plague most temporally based documentation systems; the available information soon overcomes the clinician's ability to interpret and use the findings. Automation of tools such as the PSST, should be the next logical step. Development of a database that is reliable and valid requires identification of the essential nursing elements, development of definitions for each element and standard procedures for data collection.[49] The Wound Intelligence System (WIS) incorporates the criteria for a valid and reliable database system. The automated version of the PSST tool increases the clinician's ability to synthesize and act on large volumes of wound assessment data. The purposes of the WIS are clinical assessment, management, and documentation, providing feedback based on aggregate data within the system and monitoring progress. Data are collected routinely (usually weekly) on standardized forms and then transferred to the computerized file by the nurse or designated clerk. Patient files consist of demographic and clinical data, type and cost of treatment, and agency/facility and staff data. Methods to insure validity of data include the following strategies: 1) all data are entered into the system through a fixed format screen, 2) out of range values and certain illogical entries are not permitted, and 3) data that have odd or unrealistic patterns are trapped in an outlier file for individual evaluation.

Three clinical assessment items appear on the WIS that were not part of the original PSST, they are ulcer pain, nutritional status, and functional ability. These three items are not calculated with the total score of the PSST wound parameters and are examined individually. The automated system has several additional features that will help ensure valid data. For example, the automated version does not allow users to enter incompatible data on the PSST, whereas the pencil and paper version has no control for incompatible data.

Relational data bases archive facility, patient, treatment, background and assessment data. The system allows for easy data input and a variety of graphic and reporting capabilities. Users enter the relevant characteristics of the patient including demographic data, risk factor and nutritional data, medical and nursing diagnoses and support surface and topical treatment data. Initial and follow up wound assessment data are entered and from these data the computer automatically tracks and graphically displays changes in the PSST total and individual scores over time. The system also tracks and monitors the pattern in the scores for the 13 items on the assessment tool. The ability to visually determine general and specific changes in wound status over time and relate these changes to interventions has been greatly aided by the data base system. The system allows users to relate pressure ulcers with specific chronic wound healing patterns, with specific demographic and medical characteristics to specific interventions and to evaluate resulting changes in pressure ulcer status based on those interventions. It allows for differentiation of success of treatment strategies as applied in various practice settings. The WIS is an integrated relational set of data bases and essentially "learns" from all the data entered. Given a sufficient amount of data in the system it should be possible to make discriminations about the relative efficacy of various interventions on pressure ulcer healing. The system is connected to a network system which allows for aggregate data analysis based on all users of the system. This analysis will enable users to evaluate individual practices with the collective experience of all users of the system.

Summary

A composite of wound characteristics is necessary for accurate documentation of the wound's status and overall health of the wound. A single wound characteristic does not provide information essential in determining the adequacy of the therapy nor allow for monitoring progress or deterioration of the wound. The indices for pressure ulcer assessment include all of the following: location, size of the ulcer, stage of the ulcer, depth of tissue involvement, condition of the wound edges and presence of undermining or tunneling, necrotic tissue characteristics, exudate characteristics, surrounding tissue conditions and wound healing parameters of granulation tissue and epithelialization.

Tools for assessing pressure ulcer characteristics and healing are minimal. The Sessing Scale and the Pressure Sore Status Tool were discussed as examples of research based instruments for assessment. Once the pressure ulcer is evaluated, the information must be recorded in a manner that allows for monitoring changes in individual wound characteristics as the wound heals or deteriorates.

Methods of documenting assessment data should allow for tracking of individual assessment characteristics and should promote quantification of observations for easy examination of changes in the ulcer status. The PSST, a research-based instrument for assessment and documentation of pressure ulcers, incorporates the necessary indices for pressure ulcer assessment, provides for quantification of observations and allows for tracking the condition of the ulcer over time. The automated PSST, the Wound Intelligence System (WIS), involves total patient and wound assessment with convenient documentation abilities and without some of the problems associated with manual recording systems for monitoring changes over time. Use of an organized method of pressure ulcer assessment is a beginning in addressing several issues related to pressure ulcer assessment and documentation.

Development of a national data base on chronic wounds is still in the beginning stages. The advent of an artificial intelligence system which analyzes large volumes of data and provides feedback based on the aggregate data will change wound care practices and enhance assessment and documentation.

References

1. National Pressure Ulcer Advisory Panel. Pressure ulcers: Incidence, economics, risk assessment. Consensus Development Conference Statement, West Dundee, Illinois, S–N Publications, Inc., 1989, pp 3–4.
2. Bergstrom N, Bennett MA, Carlson CE, et al. *Treatment of Pressure Ulcers.* Clinical Practice Guideline, Number 15. Rockville, Md.: U.S. Department of Health and Human Services, Agency for Health Care Policy and Research. AHCPR Publication No. 95–0653, December 1994.
3. Lazarus G, Cooper D, Knighton D, Margolis D, Pecoraro R, Rodeheaver G, Robson M. Definitions and guidelines for assessment of wounds and evaluation of healing. *Archives of Dermatology* 1994;489–493.
4. Margolis DJ. Definition of a pressure ulcer. *Advances in Wound Care* 1995;8(4):28(8)–28(10).
5. Ayello E. Teaching assessment of patients with pressure ulcers. *Decubitus* 1992;5(7):53–54.
6. Bates–Jensen B. The Pressure Sore Status Tool: An outcome measure for pressure sores. Topics in Geriatric Rehabilitation 1994;9(4):17–34.
7. Cooper DM. (1995). Indices to include in wound assessment. *Advances in Wound Care* 1995;8(4): 28(15)–28(18).
8. Cooper DM. Human wound assessment: Status report and implications for clinicians. *American Association of Critical Care Nursing Clinical Issues* 1990;1:553–565.
9. Yarkony GM, Kirk PM, Carlson C, Roth EJ, Lovell L, Heinemann A, King R, Lee MY, Betts HB. Classification of pressure ulcers. *Archives of Dermatology* 1990;126:1218–1219.
10. Ferrell BA, Artinian BM, Sessing D. The Sessing scale for assessment of pressure ulcer healing. *Journal of the American Geriatric Society* 1995;43:37–40.
11. Bates–Jensen BM, Vredevoe DL, Brecht ML. Validity and reliability of the Pressure Sore Status Tool. *Decubitus* 1992;5(6):20–28.
12. Bates–Jensen B, McNees MP. Toward an intelligent wound assessment system. *Ostomy/Wound Management* 1995;41(Supplement 7a): 80–88.
13. Bennett MA. *Skin Assessment: Implications for Darkly Pigmented Intact Skin in the Prediction and Prevention of Pressure Ulcers* 1995.
14. Graves DJ. Stage I in ebony complexion (letter). *Decubitus* 1995;3(4):4.
15. Maklebust J. Pressure ulcers: Etiology and prevention. *Nursing Clinics of North America* 1987;22(2): 359–377.
16. Cooper DM. Wound assessment and evaluation of healing. In: Bryant RA (ed). *Acute and Chronic Wound Care: Nursing Management.* St. Louis, MO, Mosby Year Book, 1992, pp 69–90.
17. Shea JD (1975). Pressure sores: Classification and management. *Clinical Orthopaedics and Related Research* 1975;112: 89–100.

18. Witkowski JA, Parish LC. Histopathology of the decubitus ulcer. *Journal of the American Academy of Dermatology* 1982;6(6):1014–1021.

19. Panel for the Prediction and Prevention of Pressure Ulcers in Adults. *Pressure Ulcers in Adults: Prediction and Prevention.* Clinical Practice Guideline, Number 3. AHCPR Publication No. 92–0047. Rockville, Md.: Agency for Health Care Policy and Research, Public Health Service, U.S. Department of Health and Human Services. May 1992.

20. Maklebust J, Sieggreen M. *Pressure Ulcers: Guidelines for Prevention and Nursing Management.* West Dundee, Illinois, S–N Publications, 1991, pp 14–30.

21. Stotts NA. Impaired wound healing. In: VK Carrieri–Kohlman VK, Lindsay AM, West CM. (eds). *Pathophysiological Phenomenon in Nursing, Second Edition.* 1993, pp. 343–366. Philadelphia, PA, W.B. Saunders Company.

22. Maklebust J. Pressure ulcer staging systems. Advances in Wound Care,1995; 8(4):28(11)–28(14).

23. Verhonick J. Decubitus ulcer observations measured objectively. *Nursing Research* 1961;10(4):211–214.

24. Bohannon RW, Pfaller BA. Documentation of wound surface area from tracings of wound perimeters. *Physical Therapy* 1983;63:1622–1624.

25. Thomas AC, Wysocki AB. The healing wound: A comparison of three clinically useful methods of measurement. *Decubitus* 1990;3(1):18–25.

26. Harding KG. Wound care: Putting theory into clinical practice. *WOUNDS* 1990;2(1):21–32.

27. Cooper DM. Challenge of open–wound assessment in the home setting. *Progressions* 1990;2(3):11–18.

28. Kundin J. A new way to size up a wound. *American Journal of Nursing* 1989;89(1):206–207.

29. Gilman TH. Parameter for measurement of wound closure. *WOUNDS* 19902(3):95–101.

30. Resch CS, Kerner E, Robson MC, Heggers JP, Scherer M, Boertman JA, Schileru R. Pressure sore volume measurement. *Journal of the American Geriatrics Society* 1988;36(5):444–446.

31. Gentzkow GD. Methods for measuring size in pressure ulcers. *Advances in Wound Care* 1995;8(4):28(34)–28(45).

32. Van Rijswijk L, Polansky M. Predictors of time to healing deep pressure ulcers. *WOUNDS* 1994;6:159–165.

33. National Pressure Ulcer Advisory Panel. Pressure ulcer healing: Controversy to consensus Assessment methods and outcomes, Consensus Conference. Washington DC, 1995.

34. Bates–Jensen B. New pressure ulcer status tool. *Decubitus* 1990;3(3):14–15.

35. Seiler WO, Stahelin HB. Identification of factors that impair wound healing: A possible approach to wound healing research. *WOUNDS* 1994;6(3): 101–106.

36. Jackson D, Rovee D. Current concepts in wound healing: Research and theory. *The Journal of Enterostomal Therapy* 1988;15:133–137.

37. Winter G. Epidermal regeneration studied in the domestic pig. In: Hunt, TK, Dunphy JE (eds). *Fundamentals of Wound Management.* New York, NY, Appleton–Century–Crofts, 1979, pp. 71–111.

38. Sussman CA. The role of physical therapy in wound care. In: Krasner D (ed). *Chronic Wound Care.* King of Prussia, PA, Health Management Publications, Inc., 1990, pp.327–366.

39. Sapico FL, Ginunas VJ, Thornhill–Hoynes M, Canawati HN, Capen DA, Klein NE, Khawam S, Montgomerie JZ. Quantitative microbiology of pressure sores in different stages of healing. *Diagnostic Biology and Infectious Disease* 1986;5(1):31–38.

40. Black J, Black S. Surgical management of pressure ulcers. *Nursing Clinics of North America* 1987;22(2):429–438.

41. Haury B, Rodeheaver G. Debridement: An essential component of traumatic wound care. *American Journal of Surgery* 1978;135(2):238–242.

42. Nichter L, Williams J. Ultrasonic wound debridement. *Journal of Hand Surgery* 1988;13:142–145.

43. Alterescu V, Alterescu K. Etiology and treatment of pressure ulcers. *Decubitus* 1988;1(1):28–35.

44. Rodeheaver G, Baharestani M, Brabec ME, Byrd J, Salzberg A, Scherer P, Vogelpohl T. Focus on debridement. *Advances in Wound Care* 1994;7(1):22–36.

45. Mulder G. Quantifying wound fluids for the clinician and researcher. *Ostomy/Wound Management* 1994;40(8):66–69.

46. Alvarez OH, Mertz PM, Eaglstein WH. The effect of occlusive dressings on collagen synthesis and epithelialization in superficial wounds. *Journal of Surgical Research* 1983;35:142–148.

47. Seiler WD, Stahelin HB. Recent findings on decubitus ulcer pathology: Implications for care. *Geriatrics* 1986;41(1):47–60.

48. Pieper B, Mikols C, Mance B, Adams N. Nurse's documentation about pressure ulcers. *Decubitus* 1990;3(1):32–34.

49. Jacobson, T. Standardized ET nursing database: Imagine the possibilities. *Journal of Wound, Ostomy, Continence Nursing* 1996;23(1):5–9.

BATES–JENSEN

7

Moist Wound Healing

Julia E. Haimowitz, MD and David J. Margolis, MD

Haimowitz JE, Margolis DM. Moist wound healing. In: Krasner D, Kane D. *Chronic Wound Care, Second Edition*. Wayne, PA, Health Management Publications, Inc., 1997, pp 49–56.

Introduction

Chronic wounds are a major cause of morbidity as well as a source of frustration for both the patient and the clinician. For the patient, much of the frustration of wound care involves the time for healing. For the clinician, however, much of the frustration is related to confusion regarding wound care. The aim of this chapter is to provide a better understanding of moist wound healing and its impact on the treatment of chronic wounds. Included in this section is a review of normal wound healing followed by a discussion of the advantages and disadvantages of occlusive dressings. This chapter is designed to assist the clinician in the fundamentals of occlusive wound dressings so that he/she can make a rational treatment plan, rather than choosing arbitrarily amongst the many wound care products now available.

Acute vs. Chronic Wounds

A wound is a disruption of normal anatomic structure and function. The designation of a wound as "acute" versus "chronic" is academic, based on both the wound and the patient.[1–4] An acute wound which is the result of surgery or trauma in a healthy individual is expected to heal quickly. Chronic wounds occur in individuals with underlying local or systemic ailments. The majority of chronic wounds are associated with a limited number of ailments including venous disease, arterial disease, diabetes mellitus and local pressure. These wounds do not heal in a reasonable period of time.

Since chronic wounds are usually associated with a local or systemic disease, recognizing this association is essential. Therefore, before initiating therapy, it is imperative to perform a complete patient evaluation. A careful history, including both a patient and wound history, should be taken. A psychosocial assessment should be carried out to determine whether the patient comprehends the treatment plan and has motivation to adhere to this regimen. The clinician must also assess the impact of this chronic condition on the patient's life.[1,5,6]

When deemed necessary, laboratory tests to diagnose or confirm the diagnosis of the chronic wound should be performed.[1,5,6] Tests may be invasive or non–invasive. Unusual chronic wounds or wounds that fail to heal after adequate therapy may require a biopsy to help in the detection of infection or malignancy. After establishing the cause of the chronic wound, as well as identifying underlying and/or contributory medical conditions, specific treatment can be instituted.

Fundamentals of Wound Healing

After an injury occurs, a complex series of events is set in motion by the body in order to heal the defect.[1,7] The process of wound healing is continuous, but is usually divided into three overlapping phases: the inflammatory phase, the proliferative phase and the remodeling phase. In uncomplicated cases, this process proceeds in an orderly and predictable fashion. The inflammatory phase, which lasts several days, begins immediately after injury and is marked by the processes of blood clotting and platelet degranulation. Cellular components of this stage include platelets, polymorphonuclear leukocytes and macrophages.

The next phase is the proliferative phase which can last for several weeks. The dominant cellular components of this phase include fibroblasts,

Table 1
Advantages and Disadvantages of Moist Wound Healing

Advantages
—prevention of wound desiccation
—increased re–epithelialization rate
—prevention of eschar formation
—increased dermal repair
—decreased inflammation and better
      cosmetic results
—enhanced autolytic debridement
—bacterial barrier and decreased rate
      of infection
—cost effective
—maintenance of normal voltage gradient
—functioning neutrophil and complement
      activity maintained
—decreased pain
—psychosocial benefits
—ease of use

Disadvantages
—bacterial colonization
—hematoma
—seroma
—folliculitis
—need for healthy ulcer borders
—trauma to peri–ulcer skin
—allergy to dressing material

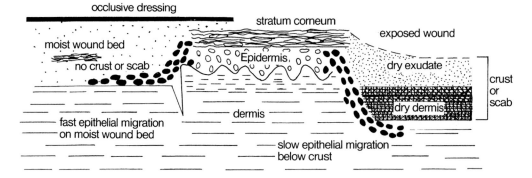

Figure 1. Diagrammatic representation of epidermal migration in moist vs. dry environment. (Reprinted with permission from Chronic Wound Care, First Edition, © Health Management Publications, Inc., 1990.

epithelial cells and endothelial cells. All of these cell types secrete growth factors that allow for cellular communication which is critical for the formation of granulation tissue, epithelialization, and angiogenesis.

The final phase is tissue remodeling which may occur over several months to years. During this phase the dermis responds to the injury with the production of collagen and matrix, thus attempting to restore the tensile strength of the wound to its pre–injury state.

This model is well established for acute wounds in non–human species, but it has not been fully replicated in humans. More importantly, the cellular and molecular events which ultimately lead to

non–healing or healing are poorly documented in human chronic wounds. No established animal model truly replicates the human chronic wound experience.

Methods of Moist Wound Healing or Occlusion

Moist wound healing can be achieved in several ways. The most popular methods involve covering the wound with wet gauze or covering the wound with an occlusive dressing. Occlusive dressings are wound coverings that isolate the wound from the external environment. The occlusiveness of a dressing is often measured by the evaporation of fluids

HAIMOWITZ AND MARGOLIS

from the surface of the wound through the dressing or by the passage of oxygen from the external environment into the wound. The benefits of moist wound healing and occlusion are based on a combination of factors working synergistically. Some of the more important effects of moist wound healing will be discussed briefly (Table 1).

Effects of moist wound healing on epidermal and dermal repair

Increase rate of re–epithelialization. Epidermal cells require a supply of blood and nutrients as they spread over a wound bed. Occluded wounds are kept moist, thereby preventing crust formation, so that the epithelium may spread more rapidly across the wound surface (Figure 1). [8,9,10]

Dermal repair and inflammation[10,11] demonstrate increased collagen synthesis in the dermis of occluded wounds. This increase has been noted under both oxygen–permeable and oxygen–impermeable dressings. In these studies, the exact relationship, if any, between increased dermal collagen synthesis and increased re–epithelialization awaits determination. Other reports suggest that occlusion is responsible for enhanced angiogenesis and granulation tissue formation.[12,13] Linski, et al.[14] and others[15] reported less clinical inflammation and finer, less pigmented, and more attractive scars in human wounds treated with occlusive dressings.

Choices for Occlusion

In the past decade, many products which provide a moist healing environment have been introduced,[7] each product having its own chemical composition, adhesive properties, effect on wound hydration, and effects on gas permeability. In developing a treatment plan, the healthcare provider must consider the patient and his/her environment, the wound and its etiology and the dressing(s). The following sections will provide brief descriptions of the major categories of occlusive dressings. However, the selection of the proper dressing should never detract from the appropriate attention to nutritional support, pressure relief in patients with pressure ulcers, compression for those with venous insufficiency, and other support.[5,16,17] For more detailed discussions of dressings, see Chapters 16 and 17.

General Principles

There are some general principles that apply for the proper use of occlusive dressings. The first is to become familiar with each class of wound dressing and know a number of examples from each class.[7] When treatment is implemented, there may be a rather alarming accumulation of exudate from the wound.[3] Maximally, most occlusive dressings have been approved for use for up to seven days; however, there is no set rule for how long an occlusive dressing should stay on a wound in a particular patient. Rather, it is recommended that the dressing stay in place until it starts leaking fluid from the sides, and then it should be gently removed. In some patients, after the exudative phase has resolved, dressings may remain in place for several days. Following are some general rules that apply when choosing a dressing:
• Use a dressing that will keep the ulcer bed continuously moist.
• Use clinical judgment to select the type of moist wound dressing suitable for the ulcer.
• Choose a dressing that keeps the surrounding intact skin dry.
• Choose a dressing that controls exudate but does not desiccate the ulcer bed.
• Consider caregiver time when selecting a dressing.[5]

Saline/gauze dressings. Gauze dressings are among the most popular dressings currently in use. They are frequently used as wet–to–dry dressings. Wet–to–dry dressings adhere to the wound and frequently injure granulation tissue and epidermis on removal. This injury occurs despite resoaking the dressings.[10,11] As such, they are useful dressings for wound debridement and cleansing, but should not be considered to be occlusive dressings.

Wet–to–damp saline dressings are made continuously wet with solutions. Careful attention by the patient or caregiver is required to keep these dressings wet. These treatments need to be changed two to three times a day and can be neither too dry nor too damp. If these dressings are allowed to dry, they will in effect become wet–to–dry dressings.[17]

One–hundred percent cotton open weave gauze is traditional gauze as described here. Due to cost constraints, availability of traditional gauze has diminished and patients are using rayon/silk tight weave paper dressings on "infected" wounds without the expected results of traditional gauze. Wet dressings are also damaging to peripheal wound edges causing maceration and breakdown. Please consider describing these dressing/packaging changes as moist–to–moist saline dressings.

Films. Film dressings are composed of thin, transparent, adherent polyurethane. They transmit water vapor, oxygen and carbon dioxide.[3,18] They are not absorbent and are useful for abrasions, skin tears, and selected nonhealing wounds with minimal drainage.[17] Polyurethane films are used most commonly to dress intravenous and other catheter sites.[19] With most films, the adherent material comes in direct contact with the wound. Initially, this contact poses no problem, since they adhere only to dry, unwounded tissue. However, once epithelialization begins, the potential exists for stripping away newly formed skin.[6,10,11,19] Alternatively, the adhesive portion of the film may be blocked with petrolatum impregnated gauze, but this obstacle alters the dressing's ability to transmit moisture vapor. Films, especially when used on highly exudative wounds, are prone to wrinkling and forming crevices which may permit entrance of microbes into the wound. When used in moderately exudative wounds, the dressing should extend 2 to 3 cm beyond the wound edge so that an adequate seal may be maintained.[7,18,19]

Wounds and the surrounding tissue covered by films may have a yellow, dark beige, or brown liquid that accumulates after time. This appearance is often similar to pus. Unless the wound is clinically infected, this liquid reflects healthy autolytic debridement that is easily cleansed from the wound. Examples of films include Acu–derm® (Acme United Corporation, Fairfield, CT) Bioclusive* (Johnson & Johnson Medical, Inc. (Arlington, TX), Blisterfilm® (Sherwood Medical, St. Louis, MO), Op–Site* (Smith & Nephew United, Inc., Largo, FL), Polyskin® II (Kendall Healthcare Products Co., Mansfield, MA), Pro–Clude® transparent wound dressing (ConvaTec®, Princeton, NJ), and Tegaderm™ (3M Health Care, St. Paul, MN).

Foams. Foam dressings, composed of polyurethane, are highly conformable and permeable and are easy–to–apply nonadherent dressings. The amount of wound fluid absorbed tends to be minimal. Moisture is absorbed into the foam layer and decreases maceration. A moist wound environment is maintained, and removal of the dressings does not result in reinjury to the wound.[3,7,17,18] As they are nonadherent, foams require additional dressings to be secured in place.[19] Included in the list of foams are Allevyn* Cavity Dressing (Smith & Nephew United, Inc., Largo, FL), Cutinova® Plus (Beiersdorf–Jobst, Inc., Charlotte, NC), Hydrasorb® (ConvaTec®, Princeton, NJ) and Lyofoam® (Acme United Corporation, Fairfield, CT).

Hydrocolloids. Hydrocolloids consist of a water–impermeable, polyurethane outer covering separated from the wound by a hydrocolloid material.[3,11] Hydrocolloid dressings are adherent and non–permeable to water vapor and oxygen, hence, moisture is absorbed into the dressing over normal skin. As hydrocolloids dissolve over the wound, softening and discoloration of the dressing occurs. This phenomenon allows removal of the dressing without injury to the wound.[10,11,19] One of the major disadvantages of these dressings is that most are opaque, making wound inspection difficult. Additionally, the gelatinous melt–down product is brownish red and can be falsely alarming to untrained providers and patients.

Hydrocolloids have been extensively used since their introduction in 1982. Their efficacy has been well–established and they assist in rapid autolysis of necrotic debris, improved tissue repair, and pain relief. Hydrocolloids, which are available in sheets and gels, are quite easy to use and, because most may be left in place for up to seven days, there is less maintenance required. A brief list of products includes Comfeel® Ulcer Care Dressing (Coloplast Sween Corp., Marietta, GA), DuoDerm®, ConvaTec®, Princeton, NJ), and Tegasorb™ (3M Health Care, St. Paul, MN).[7,18] These dressings are available in sheets or gels.

Hydrogels. Hydrogels are polymers with a water content often between 90 and 95 percent. They are semitransparent and nonadherent.[7,17] They are available as sheets or gels. The sheets are highly conformable and permeable and absorb wound exudate without losing their initial sheet form. They absorb varying amounts of drainage, but generally should be used in moist granulating wounds with little or no exudate. Because they are nonadherent, additional dressings must be placed to ensure immobilization.[19] Examples of hydrogels include Biolex™ wound gel (Bard Medical Division, Covington, GA), Carrasyn™ Hydrogel Wound Dressing (Carrington Laboratories, Inc., Irving, TX), Elasto–Gel™ (Southwest Technologies, Inc., Kansas City, MO), Hypergel® (SCA Mölnlycke, Eddystone, PA), Nu–Gel™ (Johnson & Johnson Medical, Inc., Arlington, TX) and Vigilon® (Bard Medical Division, Covington, GA).

Absorptive dressings. Absorptive, starch–based copolymer dressings are able to absorb fluid amounts many times their own weight. The dressings may be purchased pre–mixed and packaged or can be mixed by the care provider. Mixing the dressing oneself allows the provider to adjust the consistency of the slurry (either slightly wetter or drier) to accommodate the varying amounts of exudate for a given wound as it heals. Confinement of the dressing slurry to the wound cavity can be difficult, thus resulting in maceration of surrounding skin as the dressing oozes onto surrounding skin.[17] Exudate absorbers include Bard® Absorption Dressing (Bard Medical Division, Covington, GA), Dermanet® Wound Contact Layer (DeRoyal Wound Care, Powell, TN) and Multidex® Hydrophilic Powder Wound Dressing (DeRoyal Wound Care, Powell, TN).[7]

of keratinocytes and fibroblasts and the release of growth factors by tissue macrophages.[20,22,23]

Altered wound microenvironment. Wound fluid is thought to contain a variety of factors that can modulate both connective tissue production and epithelial cell migration. With moist wound

---

A fine balance needs to be established to prevent dehydration of the wound leading to eschar formation versus maceration of peri–wound skin due to excessive moisture.

Calcium alginates. Calcium alginates, derived from seaweed, can be used as sheets, mats or "ropes" of absorbent material. They are nonantigenic, hemostatic and bioabsorbable. As the calcium alginate mixes with wound fluid, a viscous hydrogel is produced. Calcium alginates are useful in exudative wounds of the lower extremities, pressure ulcers and surgical wounds. They are contraindicated in dry wounds, as a small amount of fluid is needed to transform the fibers into a moist gel.[17] There is evidence that calcium alginates may have hemostatic properties[19] and limited antibacterial actions.[4] Examples of alginates include Curasorb® (Kendall Healthcare Products Company), DermaSorb™ (ConvaTec®, Princeton, NJ), Kaltostat® (ConvaTec®, Princeton, NJ) and Sorbsan™ wound dressings (Dow Hickam Pharmaceuticals Inc., Sugar Land, TX).

Conditions of Moist Wound Healing

Moist wound healing—alterations of wound environment

Gas exchange and oxygen permeability. Comparisons of oxygen–permeable and oxygen–impermeable dressings suggest that atmospheric oxygen permeability through a dressing may be of little importance in wound healing.[10,20,21] Epidermal resurfacing is enhanced under both types of dressings.[21] It seems that regardless of the type of dressing used, the normal repair of wounds takes place in a low–oxygen environment and the oxygen needed for wound repair is provided through the local blood supply.[3,11] A low pO2 enhances the healing process. As mentioned above, this hypoxic environment may stimulate angiogenesis as well as promote the growth

healing, the wound exudate is not lost via absorption by gauze, but rather kept in contact with the wound bed. This persistent contact between acute wound fluid and the wound may explain some of the beneficial effects of occlusive dressings on epidermal repair.[3,6] This same benefit may not be achieved with occlusion of chronic wounds. Several studies suggest possible detrimental effects of chronic wound fluid on the local wound environment.[24–26]

Occlusion maintains a normal voltage gradient across the wound. Transcutaneous potential differences are decreased by wounding, and dry wounds effectively maintain no electrical gradients. Evidence suggests that maintenance of such electrical fields may be important to epidermal cell migration.[3,18]

Moist wound healing, by occluding the wound bed, decreases transepidermal water loss from the wound. Most investigators agree that an appropriately moist wound bed maintained by occlusion is responsible for the increased rate of re–epithelialization seen in covered wounds.[20,27] However, the optimal water permeability of the ideal dressing is not known.[28] A fine balance needs to be established to prevent dehydration of the wound leading to eschar formation versus maceration of peri–wound skin due to excessive moisture.

Effects of Moist Wound Healing

During the past three decades there has been increasing interest in wound dressings to enhance the healing of cutaneous wounds. In a landmark article in 1962, Winter demonstrated that an occlusive dressing nearly doubles the rate of wound re–epithelialization when compared with an air exposed wound on the domestic pig.[8] In the following year, Hinman and Maibach reported parallel

Table 2
Signs of infection

—purulent drainage or exudate
—induration
—erythema and warmth
—edema
—pain
—lymphadenitis
—elevation of peripheral neutrophil count
—uncharacteristic odor
—fever

studies, with similar results, performed in human volunteers.[9] Since these observations, a host of studies have been performed to better understand the effects of "moist wound healing."

As mentioned earlier, there is no adequate animal model of chronic wounds that mimics the human experience. The majority of animal studies on moist wound healing have used an acute wound model. Unfortunately, few studies on chronic wounds have used human subjects.

Neutrophils and other inflammatory cells play a major role in wound repair. In addition to phagocytosis of bacteria and other debris, neutrophils are responsible for the release of biologically active mediators that stimulate cellular proliferation. Adequate numbers of viable and functionally active neutrophils have been recovered from wound fluid under occlusive dressings.[13,20] Available evidence indicates that more neutrophils are able to infiltrate an occluded wound than one that can dry out.[16] In addition to functional neutrophils, the compliment system functions normally under occlusive dressings.[13]

Benefits of Moist Wound Healing

Enhanced autolytic debridement. Moist wound healing can assist in the painless debridement of chronic wounds. This debridement may be due to proteolytic enzymes released by neutrophils which reach the wound surface under occlusion.[3]

Bacterial barrier. As long as an edge seal is maintained, occlusive dressings can act as excellent barriers from microorganisms in the environment external to the wound. Additionally, many occlusive dressings maintain an acidic pH that is found to retard bacterial growth.[20,27,28]

Increased quality of life. The cost of chronic wounds in terms of loss of productivity and personal suffering including decreased self–esteem cannot

be estimated. Phillips, et al. demonstrated that leg ulcers have a significant impact on a patient's quality of life, having financial, social and psychological implications.[29] As occlusive dressings hasten wound healing, their benefits cannot be underestimated.

Decreased pain. Local wound pain is significantly reduced in occluded wounds due to hydration of the wound by the dressing which insulates and protects nerve endings.[12] There is also a reduction in pain because less oxygen is available for wound macrophages to metabolize arachidonic acid whose metabolites are believed to play a role in modulating pain.[18]

Cost. Currently, the projected cost of caring for chronic wounds has been estimated at over seven billion dollars worldwide.[2] As concerns regarding healthcare costs increase, it is likely that there will be further studies on the cost–benefits of wound occlusion. Many authors suggest that a delay in healing as well as the need for fewer dressing materials and dressing changes support the use of moist wound healing.[5,16,30]

Microbiology of Occlusion

A common fear of wound occlusion is that of infection. Distinguishing wound colonization from wound infection is important. A wound is colonized with microorganisms when there is no invasion of bacteria into viable tissue and a minimal host immune response. Wound infection pertains to organisms binding host tissues, invading, multiplying and eliciting a strong host immune response.[4] While colonization may not delay wound healing, infection may. Evidence for infection includes purulent drainage or exudate, induration, erythema, edema, pain, lymphadenitis, elevation of neutrophil count, uncharacteristic odor, or fever[4,13,16] (Table 2).

The effect of bacterial contamination on chronic wound healing often depends on wound type. A quantitative wound culture may help differentiate colonization from infection. There are a number of ways of obtaining quantitative wound cultures, including the swab and scrub technique, and biopsy.[31] Unfortunately, quantitative cultures are not available from all microbiology labs.

Obtaining a sterile wound environment is nearly impossible; wounds are readily contaminated from the normal surrounding skin. Wound fluid, necrotic tissue and the cracks and crevices of chronic wounds provide a supportive environment for microorganisms. The exact relationship between healing and bacterial count is not known. Robson, et al. defined wound infection as the presence of greater than 10^5 colony forming units of a specific pathogen per gram of tissue.[32] Lookingbill, et al. supported this definition by reporting that chronic leg wounds with more than 10^5 organisms per square centimeter failed to heal or healed more slowly than those with fewer organisms.[33] In contrast, Alper, et al. found large numbers of organisms in occluded chronic wounds shortly before clinical healing took place.[34] Others have suggested that the presence of bacteria might even be beneficial to wound healing by aiding in desloughing and stimulating inflammation.[13]

Moist wound healing has several effects on wound microbiology. The moist environment provided by occlusive wound dressings is conducive to increased bacterial growth. However, wound re–epithelialization occurs more rapidly in occluded wounds compared to those left exposed to the air despite this increase in bacterial counts.[4,17,27,31,35,36] Most studies have demonstrated that occlusive dressings are not associated with an increased rate of wound infections.[16] The main caveat is that occlusive dressings are contraindicated in wounds that clinically appear to be grossly contaminated or that may contain certain gram negative or anaerobic organisms, especially *B. fragilis*, *P. aeruginosa* and *Proteus mirabilis*.[4,13,36]

Complications of Occlusive Dressings

Eaglstein described a number of other concerns with occlusion,[8] including hematoma or seroma formation, folliculitis, need for healthy borders, trauma to adjacent skin and possible allergy to the dressing material.

Conclusion

Over the past several decades, great progress has been made in understanding wound healing and wound repair. As the pathophysiology of wounds has become better understood, the care of wounds, both acute and chronic, has also improved. One major step has been the institution of moist wound healing. The benefits of moist wound healing are many and varied, including faster epidermal and dermal repair as well as decreased pain and inflammation. Additionally, moist wound dressings are potentially cost–effective. Infection, the fear of which has been a deterrent to using moist wound dressings, has not been shown to be a complication. Several classes of wound dressings are now available. Researchers aspire to achieve a greater understanding of wounds and wound care in order to lead to better patient care.

References

1. Kirsner RS, Eaglstein WH. The wound healing process. *Dermatol Clinics* 1993;11(4):629–640.
2. Lazarus GS, Cooper DM, Knighton DR, Margolis DJ, Pecoraro RE, Rodeheaver G, Robson MC. Definitions and guidelines for assessment of wounds and evaluation of healing. *Arch Derm* 1994;130:489–93.
3. Falanga V. Occlusive wound dressings: Why, when, which? *Arch Derm* 1988;124:872–7.
4. Mertz PM, Ovington LG. Wound healing microbiology. *Dermatol Clinics* 1993;11(4):739–47.
5. U.S. Department of Health and Human Services: Clinical Practice Guideline No. 15: *Treatment of Pressure Ulcers*. Rockville, MD, 1994.
6. Phillips TJ, Dover JS. Leg ulcers. *J Amer Acad Dermatol* 1991;25:965–87.
7. Hess CT. N*urse's Clinical Guide: Wound Care*. Springhouse, PA, Springhouse Corporation, 1995.
8. Winter GD. Formation of the scab and the rate of epithelialization of superficial wounds in the skin of the young domestic pig. *Nature* 1962;193:293–4.
9. Hinman CD, Maibach H. Effect of air exposure and occlusion on experimental human skin wounds. *Nature* 1963;200:377–8.
10. Alvarez OM, Hefton JM, Eaglstein WH. Healing wounds: Occlusion or exposure. *Infection in Surg* 1984;3:173–81.
11. Alvarez OM, Mertz PM, Eaglstein WH. The effect of occlusive dressings on collagen synthesis and re–epithelialization in superficial wounds. *J Surg Res* 1983;35:142–8.
12. Friedman SJ, Su WPD. Management of leg ulcers with hydrocolloid occlusive dressings. *Arch Dermatol* 1984;120:1329–36.
13. Hutchinson JJ, Lawrence JC. Wound infection under occlusive dressings. *J Hosp Infect* 1991;17:83–94.
14. Linsky CB, Rovee DT, Dow T. Effects of dressings on wound inflammation and scar tissue. In: Hildick–Smith G (ed). *The Surgical Wound*. Philadelphia, PA, Lea & Febiger, 1981, pp. 191–205.
15. Eaton AC. A controlled trial to evaluate and compare a sutureless skin closure technique (Op– Site skin closure) with conventional skin suturing and clipping in abdominal surgery. *Br J Surg* 1980;67:857–60.
16. Hutchinson JJ, McGuckin M. Occlusive dressings: A microbiologic and clinical review. *Amer J of Infect Control* 1990;18(4):257–68.
17. Jeter KF, Tintle TE. Wound dressing of the nineties: indications and contraindications. *Clinic Pod Med Surg* 1991;8(4):799–816.
18. Eaglstein WH, Mertz PM, Falanga V. Occlusive dressings. *Am Fam Phys* 1987;35(3):211–6.
19. Kannon GA, Garrett AB. Moist wound healing with occlusive dressings: A clinical review. *Dermatol Surg* 1995;21:583–590.
20. Varghese MC, Balin AK, Carter M, Caldwell D. Local environment of chronic wounds under synthetic dressings. *Arch Derm* 1986;122:52–7.
21. Eaglstein WH. Experiences with biosynthetic dressings. *J Am Acad Dermatol* 1985;12:434–40.
22. Berardesca E, Vignoli GP, Fideli D, Maibach H. Effect of occlusive dressings on the stratum corneum water holding capacity. *Am J Med Sci* 1992;304(1):25–8.
23. Knighton DR, Hunt TK, Scheuenstuhl H, Halliday BJ, Werb Z, Banda MJ. Oxygen tension regulates the expression of angiogenesis factor by macrophages. *Science* 1983;221:1283–5.
24. Falanga V. Growth factors and chronic wounds: The need to understand the microenvironment. *J Dermatol* 1992;19:667–72.
25. Wysocki AB, Staiano–Coico L, Grinnel F. Wound fluid from chronic leg ulcers contains elevated levels of metalloproteinases MMP–2 and MMP–9. *J Invest Dermatol* 1993;101:64–8.
26. Wysocki AB, Grinnell F. Fibronectin profiles in normal and chronic wound fluid. *Lab Invest* 1990;63(6):825–31.

27. Aly R, Shirley C, Cunico B, Maibach HI. Effect of prolonged occlusion on the microbial flora, pH, carbon dioxide and transepidermal water loss on human skin. *J Invest Dermatol* 1978;71:378–381.

28. Agren MS, Wijesinghe C. Occlusivity and effects of two occlusive dressings on normal human skin. *Acta Derm Venereol* (Stockh) 1994;74:12–4.

29. Phillips T, Stanton B, Provan A, Lew R. A study of the impact of leg ulcers on quality of life: Financial, social, and psychologic implications. *J Amer Acad Dermatol* 1994;31:49–53.

30. Xakellis GC, Chrischilles EA. Hydrocolloid versus saline–gauze dressings in treating pressure ulcers: A cost effectiveness analysis. *Arch Phys Med Rehabil* 1992;73:463–9.

31. Mertz PM, Eaglstein WH. The effect of a semiocclusive dressing on the microbial population in superficial wounds. *Arch Surg* 1984;119:287–9.

32. Robson MC, Heggers JP. Quantitative bacteriology and inflammatory mediators in soft tissues. In: Hunt TK, Heppenstall RB, Pines E, Rovee D (eds). *Soft and Hard Tissue Repair: Biological and Clinical Aspects.* Praeger, New York, NY, 1984, pp 483–507.

33. Lookingbill DP, Miller SH, Knowles RC. Bacteriology of chronic leg ulcers. *Arch Dermatol* 1978;114:1765–8.

34. Alper JC, Welch EA, Maguire P. Use of the vapor permeable membrane for cutaneous ulcers: Details of application and side effects. *J Am Acad Dermatol* 1984;11:858–66.

35. Katz S, McGinley K, Leyden JL. Semipermeable occlusive dressings: Effects on growth of pathogenic bacteria and reepithelialization of superficial wounds. *Arch Dermatol* 1986;122:58–62.

36. Marshall DA, Mertz PM, Eaglstein WH. Occlusive dressings: Does dressing type influence the growth of common bacterial pathogens? *Arch Surg* 1990;125:1136–9.

8

The Wound Environment: Implications from Research Studies for Healing and Infection

Patricia M. Mertz, BA; Stephen C. Davis, BS; Maria Oliveira–Gandia, DVM and William H. Eaglstein, MD

Mertz PM, Davis SC, Oliveira–Gandia M, Eaglstein WH. The wound environment: Implications from research studies for healing and infection. In: Krasner D, Kane D. *Chronic Wound Care, Second Edition.* Wayne, PA, Health Management Publications, Inc., 1997, pp 57–63.

Introduction

A basic understanding by healthcare practitioners of research data gathered from animal and human models can lead to improved patient care. Although human clinical trials remain the gold standards, studies on animal models in a controlled environment with a limited number of variables allow the examination of selected features and may be extrapolated to the clinical situation. We hope that the data generated from our animal studies will heighten our understanding of the mechanisms and potential therapies for various types of wounds, including non–healing chronic wounds. Recently the following studies have been done at the University of Miami.

Growth Factors

We have a particular interest in IL–1, a polypeptide growth factor which possesses a wide spectrum of inflammatory, metabolic, physiologic, and immunologic properties. IL–1α is the predominant form produced by keratinocytes.

In 1990 we reported that the addition of exogenous IL–1α enhanced wound epithelization in our partial thickness wound model.[1] The enhancement of epithelization was comparable to the effects of an occlusive film dressing (Figure 1). Studies by Mizutani demonstrated that human keratinocytes

do not process IL–1ß receptors *in vitro*.[2] IL–1α and IL–1ß are both expressed by keratinocytes; however, only IL–1α is indeed active upon release.[2] The addition of IL–1ß in a swine second degree burn model for epithelization did not demonstrate a stimulatory effect on epithelization, again suggesting that IL–1α is the Interleukin which plays a significant role in epithelization (non–published data). To further investigate this hypothesis we used ultraviolet radiation (UVR), which is known to stimulate keratinocyte IL–1α production.[3] Non–wounded skin was irradiated with a UVR source that contained mostly UVB, the portion of light which is responsible for sunburn. The radiated skin–sites received three times as much UVR as was needed to develop a slightly visible redness [3 MED]. Partial thickness wounds were then made on the radiated site using an electrokeratome according to the model of Eaglstein and Mertz.[4] Three treatment groups were studied: 1) no additional UV radiation, 2) additional treatment with UVR after wounding (to the wounds), and 3) the control consisting of wounds and sites which never were exposed to UVR.

The results showed that UVR exposure both prior to wounding and after wounding stimulated epidermal repair. The control wounds healed at the usual rate suggesting that UVR has a local not a systemic effect.[3] We hypothesized that the increased healing was related to IL–1α.

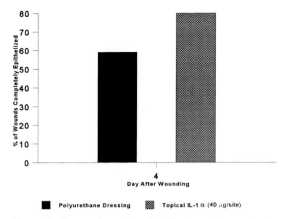

Figure 1. *Comparison of topical IL–1α and an occlusive dressing on the rate of epithelization of partial thickness wounds*

The control of epithelization continued to fascinate us. Since occlusive dressings speed epithelization as do some growth factors we wanted to study the possibility that occlusive dressings stimulate epithelization by their effect on growth factors, IL–1α in particular. Toward that end, we conducted two sets of experiments. We first used a polyanionic drug, suramin, which had been shown to block receptors for growth factors which are considered important to epithelization of wounds. Suramin in a topical suspension of 0.4 M concentration was placed into wounds which were then covered with an occlusive dressing. The occlusive dressing–suramin treated wounds were compared to occlusive dressing–saline treated wounds. Suramin decreased the relative rate of healing of occluded wounds by 19 percent.[5] Although this is not direct proof of the role of occlusive dressings and growth factors, these data do suggest that occlusive dressings work at least in part by way of growth factors.

Our second experiment, designed to detect growth factor activity under an occlusive dressing, was directed at IL–1α. We used an IL–1α receptor antagonist (IL–1α R) applied topically under occlusion to see if this application would block the stimulatory effect of occlusion on epithelization. Using the excision wound healing model, wounds treated with the IL–1α R antagonist under an occlusive dressing healed at the same rate as wounds left open to the air (a relative healing rate of -20 percent). These data supply further support for the vital role of IL–1α in wound repair and suggest that IL–1α is one of the factors associated with the occlusive dressing effect on epithelization.[6]

Electrical Effects

Another hypothesis put forth regarding the mechanism by which occlusive dressings enhance epithelization is the maintenance of the naturally occurring electrical potential that occurs in moist wounds after injury. This "current–of–injury" is shut–off when a wound dries out.[7] The presence of this current of injury may also be related to growth factor receptors since skin cells placed in electrical fields have been shown to have more receptor–sites for certain growth factors.[8]

Dr. Kang Cheng, who recently completed his Biomedical Engineering thesis work in our department on the role of pulsed electrical stimulation, measured the electrical potentials in wounds treated with occlusive dressings. He devised a system using tiny silver–chloride electrodes connected to voltmeter (Keithley™). One of the electrodes contacted the center of a wound and another contacted the normal skin when the dressing was removed. These electrodes measured the electrical potential in partial thickness wounds that were occluded or air exposed. He found that the electrical potential was identical between occluded and air exposed wounds for day 0, day of wounding (35 to 38 mvs). However, the occluded wounds maintained a high mean potential of 29.6 mv for the 4 days needed for epithelization. By comparison, in the air exposed wounds the potential fell to mean 5.2 mv. The mean electrical potential of the occluded wounds returned to a similar potential to that of air exposed after 4 days. Dr. Cheng's work is consistent with the hypothesis that occlusive dressings may work by way of their electrical potential.[9] Further experiments need to be carried out to delineate how this electrical potential influences growth factors and their receptor sites *in vivo*.

Experiences with Skin Substitutes

Cultured keratinocyte wound dressing. During the past ten years, biotechnology has begun to make substantial advances in the development of biological useful cells, tissues, and organs. Phrases such as "cell therapy" and "tissue engineering" have emerged to describe this biotechnologic development. Among the materials tested for use in wounds are cultured keratinocyte dressings, dermal substitutes, and skin (epidermal/dermal) substitutes.

To study the role of a wound dressing containing cultured keratinocytes, we used a surgically debrided second degree burn model in pigs.[10] This model creates an environment which can support a keratinocyte wound dressing (Acticel™) because a viable burn wound bed is made by excising the eschar until punctate bleeding occurs in the burned area. Second degree burn wounds were made on the backs of young domestic pigs with a heated brass rod of 0.8 mm in diameter. The burn wounds were debrided (excised) 48 hours after burning at a depth of 0.4 mm. Bleeding was stopped with direct pressure, and the keratinocyte dressing and its overlying backing were stapled in place directly on the debrided burn wounds. The control burn wounds on the same animal were covered with the backing used for the keratinocyte sheet.

The results of the keratinocyte dressing treatment compared to backing treatment for epithelization are seen in Figure 2. These findings show that a keratinocyte wound dressing stimulates epithelization.[11] The optimum dressing backing has not been identified and work continues toward understanding what the role of the addition of keratinocytes to a dressing contributes to the healing process. The theory proposed as to the method of action is that the keratinocyte sheet contributes growth factors that stimulate epithelization or that the host keratinocytes in the wound are somehow stimulated by the mere presence of the cells in the expanded keratinocyte dressing.

Epidermal/Dermal (composite) skin substitute. To evaluate a recipient's response to a skin substitute, a bioengineered skin equivalent was placed on acute surgical wounds. The skin equivalent known as Graftskin™ (Organogenesis, Canton, MA) has been characterized as a living skin equivalent (LSE). It is made of a bovine collagen matrix containing human fibroblasts and an overlying sheet of stratified human epithelium. This composite was grafted onto the site of cancer removal in 14 of 15 patients. In one patient, a fast growing benign lesion had been removed. Overall, Graftskin™ proved easy to handle and a typical clinical appearance of the skin substitute during "take" was detected. Blood and cell studies for allergy were negative. Compared with expectations, improved healing occurred. Twelve of the fifteen patients had 10 percent initial clinical take while at three months eleven of the fifteen appeared to have 75 percent or greater clinical take. We conclude that Graftskin™ was not clinically rejected and was not toxic. It often appeared to take and produce better–than–expected healing.

Burn Wound Debridement

One of the chief goals of wound care is to close the wound in a timely fashion in order to help prevent burn infection and other morbidity and mor-

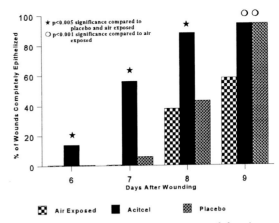

Figure 2. *The effect of a keratinocyte wound dressing on the rate of epithelization of partial thickness wounds.*

tality. In burn wounds it is important to remove as much devitalized tissue as possible prior to adjunct treatment. The current clinical protocol in many burn centers is to surgically debride deep second degree burn wounds within five to seven days after burning.

We have recently studied the effect of early debridement of deep second degree burn wounds using our already existing burn wound model.[12] The burn wounds were created on the anterior two–thirds of white domestic pigs. Burn wounds were randomly assigned to one of the following treatment groups: 1) control, no debridement; 2) early debridement at 24 hours post–burning; or 3) late debridement at 96 hours post–burning. Wounds from each treatment group were harvested, incubated to allow separation of the dermis and epidermis, then examined macroscopically for complete epithelization. On day seven after burning, the percent of burn wounds completely epithelized was as follows: 41 percent non–debrided, 75 percent of 24 hour early debrided, and 22 percent of 96 hour late debrided (Table 1). We hypothesize that debridement of the burn wound accelerates healing by creating a bleeding injury which allows the introduction of platelet factors. Early introduction of these platelet factors is more beneficial to the healing process. Additionally early debridement may intervene in the depth progression of the burn wound itself. (These burn wounds have been shown to progress in depth over a 48 hour time period.)

These data supported the importance of debridement in stimulating healing in chronic wounds. Steed, et al. found that debrided diabetic foot ulcers had the same response rate as diabetic foot ulcers treated with a platelet derived growth

Table 1
The effect of early debridement on second–degree burn wounds

Treatment	Days after burning			
	6	7	8	9
Non–debrided	0/31[†] (0%)[°]	13/32 (41%)	26/32 (81%)	32/32 (100%)
24 hour early debridement	2/32 (6%)	24/32* (75%)	29/32 (91%)	32/32 (100%)
96 hour late debridement	0/31 (0%)	7/32 (22%)	30/32 (94%)	32/32 (100%)

[†] Data is presented as the number of burn wounds epithelized over the number of burns assessed.
[°] Percent of burn wounds completely epithelized.
* $p < 0.02$ significance to non–debrided and 96 hour debridement.

factor. He concluded that debridement was a vital adjunct to healing chronic wounds.[13]

Infection Control

Wound infection is defined as the adherence and the penetration of bacteria into viable tissue. A simple equation for infection is as follows: infection = dose x virulence /host resistance.

Potential sources of bacterial wound contamination include the following: person to person (direct) contact, direct contact with contaminated foreign matter, animal vectors, and the patient's own endogenous micro flora.

Chronic wounds offer a distinct environment for micro flora that often features copious wound fluid, necrotic tissue and deep cracks and crevices on the wound surface. In addition, individuals with chronic wounds often have underlying pathology and a weakened host defense mechanism. The environment of a chronic wound offers a suitable habitat for a great variety of colonizing micro flora. These micro flora are in greater numbers and types than in acute wounds because of the presence of non–viable tissue which serves as a banquet of nutrients for the micro flora's growth. The role of the colonizing micro flora in the chronicity of chronic wounds is controversial.

Chronic wounds often have a characteristically offensive odor which can be attributed to both gram–negative and anaerobic micro flora colonization.[14] Ulcers may be a potent source of such gram–negative bacilli such as Pseudomonas species, including *P. aeruginosa*. Examination of a chronic ulcer with a woods light in a darkened room can give a clinician evidence of *P. aeruginosa* colonization. Areas heavily colonized by *P. aeruginosa* will have a characteristic blue–green fluorescence made by water soluble fluorescence pigments. Other frequently isolated gram–negative species include *Proteus sp.* and *Acinetobacter calcoaceticus*. Teng, et al. collected routine cultures from 75 leg ulcer patients and 48 infected dermatoses patients.[15] Leg ulcers yielded a greater proportion of cultures which contained mixed flora (56 percent) than the cultures from infected dermatoses (18.8 percent). The most frequently isolated organisms from chronic leg ulcers were *P. aeruginosa* and *Staphylococcus aureus*. When Bacteroides species are isolated from chronic wounds, clinicians should be alerted to the possibility of septicemia since the isolation of bacteroides from chronic wounds has been associated with septicemia.

Lookinghill, et al. reported that chronic ulcers with greater than 10^5 organisms per square centimeter either healed more slowly or failed to heal.[16] In contrast, Alper, et al. found large numbers of organisms present in chronic ulcers shortly before healing.[17] These ulcers were treated with a polyurethane film dressing. These findings in

MERTZ, ET AL.

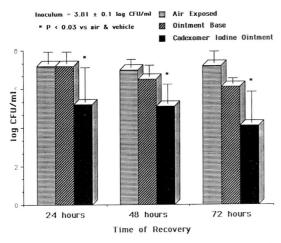

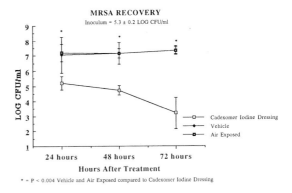

Figure 3. The effect of a cadexomer iodine ointment on the multiplication of Staphylococcus aureus in partial thickness wounds

Figure 4. The effect of a cadexomer iodine dressing on the multiplication of methicillin resistant Staphylococcus aureus (MRSA) in partial thickness wounds

chronic wounds are supported by our animal studies of acute wounds, which demonstrate that polyurethane dressing enhances the growth of micro flora while still promoting healing.[18] The enhancement of micro flora growth was shown to be unrelated to a greater number of reported wound infections as supported by a literature review by Hutchinson and Laurence.[19]

We have developed and used an animal model with acute wounds that are inoculated with known amounts of pathogens to predict the efficacy of antimicrobial agents.[20] Since *Pseudomonas aeruginosa* and *Staphylococcus aureus* are the most prevalent pathogens causing wound infection, strains of these bacteria are the most commonly used in our laboratory. We have also used the multi–drug resistant *S. aureus*, better known as methicillin–resistant *S. aureus* (MRSA). MRSA has a recognized importance as a wound pathogen due to its difficult eradication and increased incidence in the past decade.

A known quantity of pathogens is inoculated into the wound bed and scrubbed for 10 seconds with a Teflon spatula, favoring the adequate colonization of the tissue by the microorganism. The inoculum is allowed to dry on the wound before the application of the treatment. The wounds are assessed 24, 48, and 72 hours after wounding and treatment. The bacteria are recovered using the modified scrub technique. This technique consists of scrubbing the wound with a Teflon spatula for 30 seconds using 1 mL of a neutralizer solution. The neutralizer solution inactivates the active ingredient of the treatment preventing its further

action against the microorganism present during the quantification process. The bacteria are plated using a Spiral Plater which allows bacterial quantification.

In one of our studies we evaluated the antimicrobial activity of a cadexomer iodine ointment (Iodosorb®) against *P. aeruginosa* and *S. aureus* and its effect on wound healing.[21] Our study determined that the cadexomer iodine ointment does not have a detrimental effect on wound healing and has a substantial antimicrobial activity against *S. aureus* (Figure 3). *P. aeruginosa* was not significantly reduced by the use of this ointment.

Based on the effectiveness of the cadexomer iodine ointment against *S. aureus* we decided to evaluate the microbial activity of a cadexomer iodine dressing (Iodoflex™) against MRSA. Epithelization was not evaluated in this study. The cadexomer iodine dressing demonstrated to be highly effective against the MRSA challenge strain (Figure 4). This is an exciting finding since the treatment of infections with drug–resistant bacteria is calculated to cost over $4 billion annually in the USA (ASM).[22] By effectively treating the wound sites, the spread of the bacteria can be prevented and the morbidity reduced, with enhanced health and decreased cost of treatment as final outcomes.

Control of *Pseudomonas aeruginosa* multiplication with topical application of silver sulfadiazine has been demonstrated in a similar model of non–debrided and debrided burn wounds. Silver sulfadiazine significantly reduced the number of *P. aeruginosa* in the burn wounds at each time point

Table 2
The effect of silver sulfadiazine (SSD) on the multiplication of *Pseudomonas aeruginosa* in debrided and non–debrided burn wounds

Treatment	Time after Treatment (hours)		
	24	48	72
SSD cream (non–debrided)	3.9 ± 0.6	3.9 ± 0.5	3.4 ± 0.0
SSD cream (debrided)	3.0 ± 0.6	2.8 ± 0.5	3.8 ± 0.1
Occlusive dressing (non–debrided)	5.2 ± 0.8	6.9 ± 0.2	6.9 ± 0.2
Occlusive dressing (debrided)	4.7 ± 0.9	7.4 ± 0.1	6.8 ± 1.3

Inoculum
- non–debrided = 4.24 log CFU/ml
- debrided = 4.13 log CFU/ml
- wounds inoculated immediately after debridement

Debridement
- 24 hours after burning

Wound treatment
- applied immediately after inoculation (SSD cream covered with occlusive dressing)
- all treatments were applied once per day.

evaluated (Table 2). These data suggest that silver sulfadiazine used topically in chronic wounds colonized with *Pseudomonas aeruginosa* would reduce the wound's bacteria burden.

Conclusion

The "ideal" animal model to study chronic wounds does not exist. Since it is difficult to obtain appropriate controls for human studies and many patients are either elderly or have co–existing disorders, the use of controlled animal models to elucidate wound healing mechanisms and treatment modalities is of great importance.

Although strict extrapolation cannot be made between animal and human studies or acute, burn and chronic wounds, it is advantageous to obtain much knowledge on all wound types. A particular therapy for one type of wound may be determined to also be useful for another.

Current therapies such as cadexomer iodine, electrical stimulation, UV light therapy, and wound debridement are being used to stimulate the healing of chronic wounds. Although electrical stimulation is being used by many practitioners, no device has been approved by the FDA at this time. Debridement is routinely used for chronic wounds; however, state laws vary as to who can perform these procedures. The addition of various exogenous growth factors to chronic wounds has been studied; however, a definitive growth factor regimen to stimulate repair has not been identified. Additional studies, both pre–clinical and clinical, need to be performed to help identify optimum therapies.

References

1. Sauder DN, Kilian PL, McLane JA, Quick TW, Jakubovic H, Davis SC, Eaglstein WH, Mertz PM. Interleukin–1 enhances epidermal wound healing. *Lymphokine Res* 1990;9(4):465–473.
2. Mizutani H, Black R, Kupper TS. Human keratinocytes produce but do not process pro–Interleukin–1 (IL–1) beta. Different strategies of IL1 production and processing in monocytes and keratinocytes. *J Clin Invest* 1991;87:1066–1071.
3. Kaiser ME, Davis SC, Mertz PM. The effect of ultraviolet irradiation–induced inflammation on epidermal wound healing. *Wound Repair and Regeneration* (in press).
4. Eaglstein WH, Mertz PM. New method for assessing epidermal wound healing: The effect of triamcinolone acetonide and polyethylene film occlusion. *J Invest Dermatol* 1978;71(6):382–4.
5. Rotman DA, Cazzaniga A, Helfman R, Falanga V, Mertz PM. Suramin application to porcine partial thickness wounds delays epithelization. *J Invest Dermatol* 1992;98:610.
6. Mertz PM, Wu D, Oliveira–Gandia MF, Davis SC, Dinarello C, Sauder DN. Evidence for the role of IL–1 in the healing process: An IL–1 antagonist decreased the healing time of occluded partial thickness wounds. *J Invest Dermatol* 1995; 104(4):631.
7. Jaffe LF, Vanable JW. Electrical fields and wound healing. *Clin Dermatol* 1984;2(3):34–44.

MERTZ, ET AL.

8. Falanga V, Bourguignon GJ, Bourguignon LY. Electrical stimulation increases the expression of fibroblast receptors for transforming growth factor–beta. *J Invest Dermatol* 1987;88:488.

9. Cheng K, Tarjan PP, Oliveira–Gandia MF, Davis SC, Mertz PM, Eaglstein WH. An occlusive dressing can sustain natural electrical potential of wounds. *J Invest Dermatology* 1995;104(4):662.

10. Davis SC, Bilevich ES, Cazzaniga AL, Mertz PM. Early debridement of second–degree burn wounds enhances the rate of epithelization: An animal model to evaluate burn wound therapies. *J Burn Care & Rehabil*, (in press).

11. Mertz PM. Preclinical research finding in wound healing: Cultured human keratinocytes xenografts stimulate the healing of second degree burn wound in the pig. (Abstract) Symposium on Advanced Wound Care, April 1994, Miami Beach, FL.

12. Davis SC, Mertz PM, Eaglstein WH. Second degree burn healing: The effect of occlusive dressings and a cream. *J Surg Res* 1990;48:245–248.

13. Steed D, Donohoe D, Webster M, Lindsley L. Extensive debridement of human diabetic foot ulcers is a vital adjunct to healing. PDGF study group. (Abstract) European Tissue Repair Society, August 30, 1995.

14. Academiluyi SA, Rotime VO, Coker AO, et al. The anaerobic and bacterial flora of leg ulcers in patients with sickle–cell disease. *J Infect* 1988;18:115–120.

15. Teng P, Falanga V, Kerdel FA. The microbiological evaluation of leg ulcers and infected dermatoses in patients requiring hospitalization. *WOUNDS* 1993;5:133–136.

16. Lookinghill DP, Miller SM, Knowles RC. Bacteriology of chronic leg ulcers. *Arch Dermatol* 1978;114:1765–1768.

17. Alper JC, Welch EA, Maguire P. Use of the vapor permeable membrane for cutaneous ulcers: Details of application and side effects. *J Am Acad Dermatol* 1984;11:858–866.

18. Mertz PM, Eaglstein WH. The effect of a semiocclusive dressing on the microbial population in superficial wounds. *Arch Surg* 1984;119:287–289.

19. Hutchinson JJ, Lawrence JC. Wound infection under occlusive dressings. *J Hosp Infect* 1991;17:83–94.

20. Mertz PM, Alvarez OM, Smerbeck RV, Eaglstein WH. A new in vivo model for the evaluation of topical antiseptics on superficial wounds: The effect of 70% alcohol and povidone–iodine solution. *Arch Dermatol* 1984;120(January):58–62.

21. Mertz PM, Davis SC, Brewer LD, Franzén L. Can antimicrobials be effective without impairing wound healing? The evaluation of a cadexomer iodine ointment. *WOUNDS* 1994;6(6):184–193.

22. Report of the ASM task force on antibiotic resistance. Antimicrob agent and chemo. *Am Soc Microbiol* 1973;23 (Suppl):244–52.

9

Co–Factors in Impaired Wound Healing

Nancy A. Stotts, RN, EdD and Deidre Wipke–Tevis, RNC, PhD

Stotts NA, Wipke–Tevis D. Co–factors in impaired wound healing. In: Krasner D, Kane D. *Chronic Wound Care, Second Edition.* Wayne, PA, Health Management Publications, Inc., 1997, pp 64–72.

Introduction

Healing chronic wounds is a complex biological process that requires the interaction of many co–factors for normal repair. Impairment in healing is manifest as a delay in the rate of healing, the development of complications, or abnormal bio–chemical responses of factors associated with healing.

This chapter describes the major co–factors in impaired healing of chronic wounds and the mechanism by which each co–factor contributes to impairment. Types of wounds considered are chronic surgical wounds, pressure ulcers, and vascular ulcers. Co–factors addressed are age, insufficient oxygenation/perfusion, malnutrition, bioburden, excess pressure, psychophysiological stress, concomitant conditions, and adverse effects of treatment (Table 1). Understanding the co–factors that contribute to impaired healing allows the practitioner to identify high risk patients and treat persons at high risk proactivity so the disruption in healing can be mitigated.

Age

Age has been associated with impairment in healing, perhaps because there are differences in healing in the fetus, child, adult, and elderly. Fetal wound healing is virtually scarless. Although the mechanism is not entirely understood, it is thought to be the consequence of a reduced inflammatory response and lower concentration of cytokines.[1] In childhood, wound contraction occurs more rapidly than in adulthood. Beginning in adulthood and continuing into advanced age, cellular changes occur in wound healing. There is a decrease in the density of collagen, fewer fibroblasts are present, there is fragmentation of elastin fibers, and the number of mast cells diminishes with age.[2]

Advanced age has long been viewed as a co–factor in impaired healing. Yet when elderly persons do not have concomitant diseases, their rate of healing is only slightly slower or within the normal range and it is primarily re–epithelialization which is delayed.[2–4] The elderly have plagued many chronic illnesses that are associated with impaired healing (e.g. vascular disease). Because of the frequent occurrence of these conditions in the elderly, age is often noted as a co–factor in impaired healing.

Insufficient Oxygen and Perfusion

Insufficient oxygenation and perfusion are often related to impaired healing. Lack of molecular oxygen results in slowed deposition of collagen. At tissue levels below 20 mm Hg, collagen synthesis stops. Collagen lysis, however, continues and wounds may actually break down in a hypoxic environment.[5] Hypoxia also inhibits phagocytic activity. When neutrophils or macrophages ingest foreign material and microorganisms, there is a respiratory burst. Lack of sufficient oxygen slows the activity of the leukocytes and may lead to overgrowth of micro–organisms.[6] On the other hand, hypoxia stimulates fibroblast replication, macrophage secretion of angiogenic substances as well as release of transforming growth factor beta, endothelin–1, and vascular endothelial growth factor. It is important, however, to recognize that providing adequate oxygenation will not inhibit these processes[7,8] and oxygen is needed to have a functional healed product.

Normally oxygen is carried in the blood dissolved in plasma and bound to hemoglobin. Hemoglobin is carried by red blood cells. The oxygen used for healing is dissolved in plasma and comprises only a small portion of the oxygen in the blood. The majority of oxygen in the blood is carried bound to hemoglobin (Figure 1).

To appreciate the role of insufficient oxygen in impaired healing, it is important to distinguish between hypoxemia and hypoxia. Hypoxemia is present when oxygen levels are decreased in the blood and it may or may not impair healing. Hypoxia is decreased tissue oxygen; it usually results in impaired healing.

To evaluate the amount of oxygen in the vasculature, both dissolved oxygen and that bound to hemoglobin are measured in the blood vessels; the dissolved oxygen is measured using an arterial blood gas. The amount of oxygen carried by the hemoglobin is measured by assessing the hemoglobin saturation. In the tissues, only dissolved oxygen is present. Measurement of oxygen in the tissues is done directly with a subcutaneous optode[9] or more indirectly at the capillary level with a transcutaneous oxygen sensor.[10] The optode is used primarily in research while transcutaneous oxygen is measured more often in the diagnostic vascular laboratory.

As most of the oxygen content in the blood is carried by hemoglobin, theoretically anemia should be an important factor in reduced tissue oxygen and impaired healing. Data, however, suggest that anemia does not result in impaired healing. Early research shows that oxygen tension is not decreased when subjects are anemic, as long as the subjects have adequate circulating volume.[11] Recent research confirms these early findings and shows that the hydroxyproline level, a major component of collagen, is not decreased in subjects with anemia.[12,13] Thus, data suggest that anemia is not a co–factor in impaired healing when perfusion is sufficient.

Smoking tobacco may produce both hypoxemia and hypoxia. The triad of nicotine, carbon monoxide, and hydrogen cyanide interact to produce deleterious effects.[14] Nicotine acts as a potent vasoconstrictor, increases platelet adhesiveness and enhances the risk of microvascular thrombosis and ischemia. Carbon monoxide aggravates the situation by binding with hemoglobin, reducing the available sites for oxygen carrying and lowering oxygen saturation. Hydrogen cyanide inhibits the enzyme systems necessary for oxidative metabolism and the cellular transport of oxygen.

Table 1
Co–factors in impaired healing

Age
  Fetus
  Child
  Adult

Insufficient oxygenation/perfusion
  Hypoxemia
  Hypoxia
  Anemia
  Hypovolemia

Malnutrition
  Protein–calorie
  Vitamins
  Minerals

Bioburden
  Contamination
  Infection

Excess pressure
  Pressure
  Shear
  Friction

Psychophysiological stress
  Stress
  Pain
  Noise

Concomitant conditions
  Peripheral vascular disease
  Diabetes
  Uremia
  Immunocompromise

Adverse effects of treatment
  Radiation
  Chemotherapy
  Steroid therapy
  Anti–inflammatory drugs
  Local anesthetics

Hypovolemia, lack of adequate intravascular volume, also has been shown to be associated with impaired healing.[7,8,14] With hypovolemia there is an insufficient circulating volume to take oxygen and nutrients to the tissues; if this state is prolonged, collagen production and leukocyte activity are diminished.

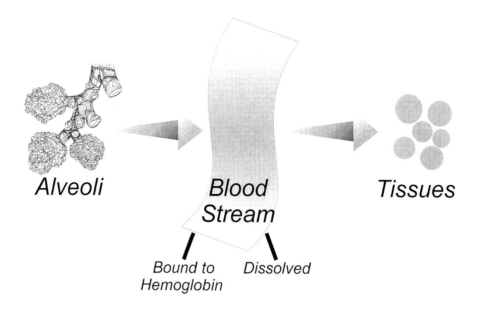

Figure 1. *Oxygen transport.*

When there are overt clinical signs of hypovolemia, it is treated. A more difficult situation occurs when subclinical hypovolemia is present. Subclinical hypovolemia by definition means there are no overt clinical signs and symptoms. Currently the only method available for measuring subclinical hypovolemia is the measurement of subcutanoeus tissue oxygenation using an optode. In a study examining the effects of increasing the fraction of inspired oxygen on subcutaneous tissue and wound oxygen levels in surgical patients, Chang, et al. found that a portion of their sample had tissue hypoxia in the presence of increasing ambient oxygen.[15] A bolus of fluid was given that resolved the hypoxia and they concluded that subclinical hypovolemia was present in this subset of patients. It is important to note that no signs or symptoms were present that would have allowed the clinician to diagnose the hypovolemia. Follow–up studies were performed and showed that low tissue oxygen levels in surgical patients in the early post–operative period were normalized with supplemental fluid.[12,16] In the chronic wound population, subclinical hypovolemia has not been studied. However, it may occur in several situations, e.g. diuretics, renal dialysis, blood loss.

Fluid administration for hypovolemia, however, is not without iatrogenic effects. Using an animal model, Heughen, Ninikoski, and Hunt showed that large volumes of saline provided to rats resulted in a decrease in oxygenation due to excess fluid administration. The fluid overload in the rat was equal to less than a liter of extra fluid in a normal human.[17] Thus, when enhancing perfusion, care must be taken to maximize intravascular volume without causing fluid overload.

In considering oxygenation and perfusion, the issue of edema should be addressed. It is commonly found in individuals with venous leg ulcers. Traditional therapy for these ulcers is leg elevation and compression to reduce lower extremity edema. Theoretically, the increased interstitial fluid present with edema results in reduced oxygenation because of slowed diffusion. There are limited data on this issue. However, available data do indicate that edema reduction using a pneumatic compression device does not improve oxygenation in patients with lower extremity ulcers. The authors conclude that removal of edema fluid is unlikely to be related to improved tissue oxygenation[18] and thus, the mechanism by which reduction in edema improves healing remains unclear. However, it should be noted that this study is limited by its small sample size (n = 8) and further work is needed to confirm these findings.

Malnutrition

Protein–calorie malnutrition, manifest as a weight loss of 20 percent of the body weight, slows

STOTTS AND WIPKE–TEVIS

the gain of tensile strength in wound healing.[5,6,19,20] Usually wound healing abnormalities are associated with protein–calorie malnutrition rather than depletion of a single nutrient.[5,20]

Studies provide data on how the absence of adequate quantities of specific nutrients affect healing. Deficiencies of protein result in decreased fibroblast proliferation, reduced proteoglycan and collagen synthesis, decreased angiogenesis, and disrupted collagen remodeling.[19–22] With insufficient carbohydrate intake, catabolism of body protein is initiated. Protein is then diverted from repair to provide the glucose needed for cellular maintenance. Cellular maintenance is especially important in fighting infection as leukocytes require glucose for phagocytosis. Fat inadequacy is seen only in prolonged starvation or severe hypercatabolic states and deficiencies of the fat soluble vitamins (A, D, E, and K) may be seen at those times.[5]

A relationship means that two events occur at the same time and are thus correlated. Cause and effect means that a prospective clinical trial has demonstrated that "A" causes "B." In the nutrition literature, there are many studies that show the relationship between nutritional deficiencies and the development of ulcers. Although there are well designed clinical trials based on surgical patients with acute wounds that demonstrate a cause and effect relationship between nutritional supplementation and healing,[29,30] limited data exists in the chronic wound population. Feeding with a normal diet, either orally or by tube, has not been shown to result in increased healing. Several relevant studies suggest that protein is important in the diet of persons with pressure ulcers. Bergstrom and Braden show a correlation between the development of pressure ulcers and decreased nutritional intake, particularly of protein.[31] Work by Breslow, et al. supports the importance of a high

---

Lack of Vitamin A can result in inadequate inflammatory response, while an excess of it may cause an excessive inflammatory response; both impair healing.

Lack of Vitamin A can result in inadequate inflammatory response, while an excess of it may cause an excessive inflammatory response; both impair healing. Thiamine (B1) deficiency results in decreased collagen formation while pantothenic acid (B5) deficiency results in decreased tensile strength and fibroblasts.[23,24] Insufficient quantities of Vitamin C may result in lysis of collagen exceeding synthesis so new wounds may have delayed collagen formation and old wounds may come apart. Vitamin E in levels in excess of the recommended 100 IU daily retards healing and fibrosis.[5]

Zinc, iron, copper and manganese are needed in small quantities for normal collagen formation. Of these elements, zinc is the best studied and data, although inconclusive, strongly suggest that zinc deficiencies impair healing and repletion in states of deficiency returns healing to its normal rate.[25,26] Zinc deficiencies are seen in the elderly, those with chronic metabolic stress, and those with persistent diarrhea. Iron deficiency is primarily a problem in infants and in that situation will impair collagen formation.[5]

The majority of studies in nutrition and chronic wounds address the pressure ulcer population.[27,28] Research has not demonstrated a cause and effect relationship between nutritional status or intake and the development or healing of pressure ulcers. Here it is critical to understand the difference between showing a relationship and demonstrating cause and effect.

protein supplement in healing of patients with pressure ulcers; however, limitations in the research methods dictate cautious interpretations of the findings.[32]

Limited data are available related to overall nutritional status and intake in persons with vascular ulcers. Burton, in a review article on management of chronic lower extremity wounds, does not mention nutritional status.[33] Pecoraro and associates, in their conceptual model of pathways to amputation, do not identify nutrition as a factor to consider.[34] Falanga, on the other hand, does note that nutrition probably plays a role in the overall pathogenesis of chronic wounds (decubitus, venous and diabetic); details of the mechanism are not elucidated.[35] Preliminary work by Wipke–Tevis and Stotts supports this assertion. In their research, nutritional deficiencies are present in a large proportion of vascular ulcer patients.[36] Additional work is needed to confirm these early findings.

Bioburden

Bioburden, the metabolic load imposed by bacteria in tissue, is often a co–factor in impaired repair. Bacteria compete with normal cells for oxygen and nutrients, and their by–products are toxic to normal cells.[37] It is important to differentiate between contamination and infection.

Contamination refers to colonization found on the surface of the wound. Contamination normally involves less than 10^5 organisms per gram of tissue. Surface contamination occurs in all wounds but rarely are the organisms on the surface of the wounds those that cause infection.[38] Nonetheless, contamination is important because the organisms compete with the new tissue for nutrients and oxygen. Furthermore, the by–products of the organisms are deleterious to the normal physiological balance of the healing wound. Overall, contamination predisposes the patient to delayed healing and may progress to infection.

Excess Pressure

Pressure, shear, and friction are co–factors in all types of chronic wounds. They are most often associated with pressure ulcers,[44] but in fact, they are significant factors in the majority of chronic wounds. Little documentation exists to support this triad as contributing to chronic wounds, but clinical experience supports these as important factors in impaired healing. In the venous ulcer population, this problem is seen in the shear and friction that occur when compression stockings and/or bandages are applied. Often co–existing arterial

---

Environmental factors that contribute to bacterial proliferation and the development of impaired healing include the presence of devitalized tissue, dirt in the wound, an abscess remote from the site of the injury, and a hematoma or large wound space.[37]

Infection is present when there is an invasion of the tissue by a microorganism. Diagnosis is usually made with clinical signs, i.e., the presence of pus, warmth, pain, erythema, induration. In immuno-compromised persons and those with neuropathy, often the only sign of infection is a change in the sensation around the wound. Also, poorly granulating tissue may be a sign of infection in chronic wounds.[39] Confirmation of the diagnosis and identification of the specific organism is done with wound culture. A culture that shows 10^5 or greater organisms per gram of tissue confirms the diagnosis of infection.[40,41] The exception to this quantitative criterion is with *beta hemolytic streptococci* where fewer organisms (10^3 per gram of tissue) are required to produce infection.[37]

Host resistance and the local environment are important in determining whether a wound that is contaminated becomes infected.[8] Normal tissue is resistant to microorganisms. In fact, tissue contamination of 10^2 organisms per gram of tissue or less actually activates leukocytes and so has been seen as a factor that supports healing, rather than impairing it.[42] Host resistance refers primarily to immunocompetence, which is discussed later in this chapter.

Environmental factors that contribute to bacterial proliferation and the development of impaired healing include the presence of devitalized tissue, dirt in the wound, an abscess remote from the site of the injury, and a hematoma or large wound space.[37] Fecal incontinence with its large bacterial load is also associated with delayed healing.[43]

disease is present in the patient with venous ulcers. Inappropriate application of compression stockings and/or bandages may result in additional tissue damage due to ischemia.[45] Similarly, friable epithelial tissue may be disrupted under the stocking or bandage, especially along the previously intact skin of the shin, over the bony prominences of the ankle, and around the edge of the ulcer. Shear and friction occur most often with ambulation or during stocking application or removal. Clinically, this problem is most often seen in the elderly who have limited strength and manual dexterity.[46]

Neuropathic ulcers occur in persons with decreased sensation. Excess pressure which is not sensed and which continues beyond tissue tolerance causes damage and prevents repair.

In the pressure ulcer population, it is believed that low pressures for long periods of time or high pressures for short periods produce pressure ulcers.[43] There is controversy over what level of pressure causes vessel occlusion that leads to ischemia and necrosis. For purposes here, it is important to recognize that at–risk persons are immobile, bed–bound, chair– bound and those with impaired sensory capacity or insufficient cognitive ability to interpret excess pressure.[43,48]

Psychophysiological Stress

Stress has been identified as a potential co–factor in impaired healing. The proposed mechanism is through stimulation of the sympathetic nervous system, with the outflow of vasoactive substances,

STOTTS AND WIPKE–TEVIS

Table 2
Effects of radiation therapy on tissue over time

Phase	Time after treatment	Latent effects
Acute	0–6 months	Clinically silent organ damage.
Subacute	7–12 months	Clinically silent vascular deterioration, especially fibrosis.
Chronic	2–6 years	Hypoperfusion of irradiated tissue with atrophy and fibrosis of area. Radiation cancer.
Late	6+ years	Tissue deterioration with parenchymal deterioration.

and subsequent vasoconstriction. The major stressors in this category are psychological stress, pain, and noise.

Braden explored the effect of stress associated with the development of pressure ulcers in persons transferred from acute care hospital to long term care. Cortisol was used as an objective measure of stress and although the numbers are small, data show that subjects with higher cortisol levels developed ulcers; subjects with lower cortisol levels did not develop pressure ulcers.[49] Similarly, work by Holden–Lund explored the effect of relaxation and guided imagery on stress and healing in persons with wounds.[50] Stress, measured with cortisol levels, as well as inflammation were reduced with this intervention. These data suggest that available therapies might be used to decrease the sympathetic nervous system response to stress and thus support healing in persons with wounds.

While intuitively pain is thought to be an important issue in healing chronic wounds, data does not indicate if it is a co–factor in impairment of healing. Transcutaneous electrical nerve stimulation (TENS)[51] and music[52] have been shown to reduce pain in persons with open wounds. Unfortunately, healing was not an outcome measured when evaluating these treatments. It would seem logical that a reduction in pain would mitigate vasoconstriction, thus increasing wound perfusion. Whether or not it does remains to be established.

Noise is another stressor that results in a dynamic cardiovascular response that may affect repair. Noise has been shown to increase epinephrine levels[53] and later *in vitro* leukocyte function.[54] In addition, intermittent noise has been shown to decrease healing in an animal model.[55] Studies have not specifically addressed this issue in the chronic wound population.

Concomitant Conditions

The presence of concomitant conditions often is a co–factor in impaired healing. Peripheral vascular disease, diabetes mellitus, uremia, and immunocompromise are all associated with impaired healing.

Persons with vascular disease are at risk for impaired healing. In arterial disease the cause is accepted as hypoxia due to arteriosclerotic disease. In venous disease, various hypotheses exist to explain the impaired healing. One hypothesis suggests that fibrin cuffs around dermal vessels lead to impaired skin nutrition and eventually to local ischemia and ulcers.[56] Other scientists suggest that neutrophil adherence to damaged tissues releases free radicals that result in tissue damage and eventually ulcers.[57] A recent hypothesis suggests that macromolecules that leak into the dermis lead to trapping of growth factors, making normal constituents of healing unavailable for the process.[35] Only time and additional research will resolve the issue of which theory is correct; what is important is that both arterial and venous disease are co–factors in impaired healing.

Persons with diabetes are at high risk for impaired healing. Glucose control is essential for normal healing and high glucose levels often are seen in diabetics during periods of physiological stress and repair. The high glucose levels result in altered leukocyte functioning and risk of infection. In the more advanced stages of diabetes where Charcot foot and neuropathy occur, lack of sensation is a serious problem. When persons lack normal protective sensation, initial damage may occur to the foot without the person being aware of it. In addition, existing wounds may be exacerbated by excess pressure and mechanical or thermal damage in persons who lack sensation.[34]

Uremia also has been implicated as a co–factor in impaired healing. The exact cause of the impairment is not known although it is recognized that collagen deposition is disrupted and the amount of granulation tissue in the wound is decreased.[58]

signs of inflammation are suppressed. If steroids are administered at the time of injury, their impact is greater than if they are administered several days after injury because they suppress the inflammatory response that accompanied initial injury.

...treatment for one condition may be a co–factor in impairment of healing. Examples of such treatments are radiation therapy, chemotherapy, steriod therapy, anti–inflammatory drugs, and possibly the use of local anesthetics for debridement.

Immunocompromised patients include persons who are HIV–positive, those with cancer, the malnourished, those receiving immunosuppressive agents, and the aged. Persons who are immunocompromised are either unable to mount an adequate inflammatory response or the response is delayed. With immunocompromise, all phases of healing are delayed and patients may be at risk for infection or wound disruption.

Adverse Effects of Treatment

Iatrogenic effects of many therapies may result in impaired healing. Thus, treatment for one condition may be a co–factor in impairment of healing. Examples of such treatments are radiation therapy, chemotherapy, steriod therapy, anti–inflammatory drugs, and possibly the use of local anesthetics for debridement.

Radiation disrupts cell mitosis at the time of the treatment and has on–going effects for the individual's life. The dose and dose–rate determine the extent of damage and the rate at which it occurs[59,60] (Table 2). Bone marrow is the organ most sensitive to radiation exposure and its effects are felt immediately in terms of numbers of various types of circulating cells. Recovery depends on the dose of radiation and the half–life of the various cells.[59,60]

Chemotherapy is designed to interrupt the cell cycle. It affects cells while they are dividing. Chemotherapy is accomplished in most anticancer drugs by damaging DNA or preventing DNA repair. Hormonal anticancer agents prevent binding of hormones while others antagonize receptors to inhibit tumor growth.[58] The primary effects of chemotherapy on healing are experienced during the treatment period and immediately after it.

Steroids impair all phases of healing. They suppress the inflammatory response, reduce immunocompetent lymphocytes, decrease antibody production, and diminish antigen processing. Clinically

When the initial inflammatory response is decreased, all subsequent phases of healing are delayed and the risk of infection is increased.[56]

Other medications such as the non–steroidal anti–inflammatory agents, phenylbutazone, and Vitamin E disrupt the normal healing process. Their effects are primarily anti–inflammatory and thus are seen early after injury.[6]

Local anesthetics have been shown to have deleterious effects at the cellular level in some wounds. They produce decreased leukocyte activity as well as opsonization,[61] inhibit host defenses, and support bacterial proliferation.[62] Interestingly, however, there is no difference in infection or necrosis between subjects injected with lidocaine and those treated with topical EMLA cream (Lidocaine 2.5 percent/ Prilocaine 2.5 percent).[63] Also, when EMLA is compared with placebo, it has been shown to decrease pain intensity and frequency without adversely affecting healing.[64] These data suggest that some cellular impairment occurs with the use of local anesthetic, but data suggest that pain relief is achieved with no clinically significant impairment in the rate of healing. Further research is needed to clarify this issue.

Conclusion

Caring for individuals with chronic wounds is a complex process and requires a multi–disciplinary approach. One cannot simply dress the wound and expect healing to occur. It is important to assess the individual for the presence of each of the potential co–factors described in this chapter (Table 1). Typically, evaluation of co–factors for impairment is integrated into the initial history and physical and should be an integral part of the ongoing assessment. Early identification of co–factors for impaired healing allows the clinician to make a differential diagnosis, initiate appropriate referrals, and develop a comprehensive plan of care.

STOTTS AND WIPKE–TEVIS

Management of local and systemic co–factors that impact repair will mitigate their adverse effects and facilitate healing of chronic wounds.

References

1. Adzick N, Larynx HP. Cells, matrix, growth factors, and the surgeon. *Ann Surg* 1994;220(1):10–18.
2. van de Kerkhoff PCM, van Bergen B, Spruijt K, Kuiper JP. Age–related changes in wound healing. *Clin & Experi Derm* 1994;19:369–374.
3. Holt DR, Kirk SJ, Regan MC, et al. Effect of age on wound healing in healthy human beings. *Surg* 1992;112(2):293–297.
4. Olerud JE, Odland GF, Burgess EM, et al. A model for the study of wounds in normal and elderly adults and patients with peripheral vascular disease or diabetes mellitus. *J Surg Res* 1995;59(3):349– 360.
5. Goodson WH and Hunt TK: Wound healing. In: Kinney JM, Jeejeebhoy KN, et al. (eds). *Nutrition and Metabolism in Patient Care.* Philadelphia, PA, WB Saunders Company, 1988, pp 635– 642.
6. Stotts NA. Impaired wound healing. In: Carrieri–Kohlman V, Lindsey AM, West C (eds). *Pathophysiological Phenomena in Nursing: Human Responses to Illness, Second Edition.* Philadelphia, PA, WB Saunders Company, 1993, pp 443– 469.
7. Falanga V, Grinnel F, Gilcrest B, et al. Experimental approaches to chronic wounds. *Wound Rep Reg* 1995;3:132–140.
8. LaVan FB and Hunt TK. Oxygen and wound healing. *Clin Plas Surg* 1990;17(3):463–472.
9. Wipke–Tevis DD. Subcutaneous tissue oximetry: Implications for wound healing and monitoring critically ill patients. *Crit Care Clin N Am* 1995;7(2):275–285.
10. Rooke TA. The use of transcutaneous oximetry in the noninvasive vascular laboratory. *Intl Angiology* 1992;11(1):36–40.
11. Heughen C, Grislis G, Hunt TK. The effect of anemia on wound healing. *Ann Surg* 1974;179(2):163–167.
12. Jonsson K, Jensen JA, Goodson WH, et al. Tissue oxygenation, anemia, and perfusion in relation to wound healing in surgical patients. *Ann Surg* 1991;214(5):605–613.
13. Jensen JA, Goodson WH, Vasconez LO, Hunt TK. Wound healing in anemia. *West J Med* 1986;144(4):465–467.
14. Silverstein P. Smoking and wound healing. *Am J Med* 1992;93(Suppl 1A):22S–24S.
15. Chang N, Goodson WH, Gottrup F, Hunt TK. Direct measurement of wound and tissue oxygen tension in postoperative patients. *Ann Surg* 1983;197(4):470–478.
16. Hartmann M, Jonsson K, Zederfeldt B. Effect of tissue perfusion and oxygenation on accumulation of collagen in healing wounds. *Eur J Surg* 1992;158:521– 526.
17. Heughan C, Ninikoski J, Hunt TK. Effect of excessive infusion of saline solution on tissue oxygen transport. *Surg Gynec Obst* 1972;135:257–260.
18. Nemeth A, Phalange V, Alstadt S, Eaglstein W. Ulcerated edematous limbs: Effect of edema removal on transcutaneous oxygen measurements. *Am Acad Derm* 1989;20(2, Part I):191–196.
19. Irvin TT. Effects of malnutrition on wound healing. *Surg Gynec Obst* 1978;146:33–37.
20. Daly JM, Vars HM, Dudrick SJ. Effects of protein depletion on strength of colonic anastomoses. *Surg Gynec Obst* 1972;134:15–21.
21. Albina JE. Nutrition in wound healing. *JPEN* 1994;18(4)367:376.
22. Fitzpatrick DW, Fisher H. Carnosine, histidine and wound healing. *Surg* 1982;91:56–60.
23. Alvarez OM, Gilbreath RL. Thiamine influence on collagen during the granulation of skin wounds. *J Surg Res* 1982;32:24–31.
24. Grenier JF, Aprahamian M, Genot C, et al. Pantothenic acid (vitamin B5) efficiency on wound healing. *Acta Vitaminol Enzymonol* 1982;4:81–85.
25. Sandstead HH, Henriksen LK, Greger JL, et al. Zinc nutriture in the elderly in relation to taste acuity, immune response, and wound healing. *Am J Clin Nutri* 1982;36(Suppl 5):1046–1059.
26. Pories WJ, Henzel JH, Robb CG, Strain WH. Acceleration of healing with zinc sulfate. *Ann Surg* 1967;165(3):432–436.
27. Breslow R. Nutritional status and dietary intake of patients with pressure ulcers: Review of research literature 1943–1989. *Decubitus* 1991;4(1):16–21.
28. Finucane TE. Malnutrition, tube feeding and pressure sores: Data are incomplete. *JAGS* 1995;43:447– 452.
29. Haydock DA, Hill GL. Improved wound healing response in surgical patients receiving intravenous nutrition. *Br J Surg* 1987;74:320–323.
30. Daly JM, Lieberman MD, Goldfine J, et al. Enteral nutrition with supplemental arginine, rna, and omega–3 fatty acids in patients after operation: Immunologic, metabolic, and clinical outcome. *Surg* 1992;112:56–67.
31. Bergstrom N, Braden BJ. Nutritional status during the development and resolution of pressure sores. In: Funk SG, Tournquist EM, Champagne MT, et al. (eds). *Key Aspects of Recovery: Improving Nutrition, Rest, and Mobility.* New York, NY, Springer Publishing, 1990, pp 183–187.
32. Breslow RA, Hallfrisch J, Guy DG, et al. The importance of dietary protein in healing pressure ulcers. *JAGS* 1993;41:357–362.
33. Burton CS. Management of chronic and problem lower extremity wounds. *Derm Clin* 1993;11(4):767–773.
34. Pecoraro RE, Reiber GE, Burgess EM. Pathways to diabetic limb amputation: Basis for prevention. *J Diab Care* 1990;13(5): 513–521.
35. Falanga V. Chronic wounds: Pathophysiologic and experimental considerations. *J Invest Derm* 1993;100(5):722–725.
36. Wipke–Tevis DD, Stotts NA. Nutritional risk, status and intake of individuals with venous ulcers: A pilot study. *J Vasc N* 1996;XIV(2):127–33.
37. Robson MC, Stenberg BD, Hegger J. Wound healing alterations caused by infection. *Clin Plas Surg* 1990;17(3)485–492.
38. Rudensky B, Lipshits M, Isaacsohn M, Sonnenblick M. Infected pressure sores: Comparison of methods for bacterial identification. *S Med J* 1992;85(9):901– 903.
39. Harding KG. Wound care: Putting theory into clinical practice. *WOUNDS* 1990;2(1):21–32.
40. Horan TC, Gaynes RP, Martone WJ, et al. CDC definition of nosocomial surgical site infections, 1992: A modification of CDC definitions of surgical wound infections. *AJIC* 1992;20(5):271–274.
41. Stotts NA. Determination of bacterial burden in wounds. *Adv Wound Care* 1995;8(4)suppl: 46–52.
42. Laato M, Lehtonen OP, Ninikoski J. Granulation tissue formation in experimental wounds inoculated with staphylocccus aureus. *Acta Chir Scand* 1985;151:313–318.
43. Allman RM, Laprade CA, Noel LB, et al. Pressure sores among hospitalized patients. *Ann Intern Med* 1986;107(5):641–648.
44. Bergstrom N, Bennett MA, Carlson CE, et al. Pressure ulcer treatment. Clinical practice guideline. *Quick Reference Guide for Clinicians.* No. 15, 1994.
45. Callam MJ, Ruckley CV, Dale JJ, Harper DR. Hazards of compression treatment of the leg: An estimate from Scottish surgeons. *Br J Med* 1987;295:1382.
46. Morison M,Moffatt C. Treatment options. In: *A Color Guide to the Assessment and Management of Leg Ulcers, Second Edition.* London, England, Mosby Year Book, 1994, pp 55–94.
47. Koziak M. Etiology and pathology of ischemic ulcers. *Arch Phys Med Rehabil* 1959;40(2):62–69.
48. Breslow RA, Bergstrom N. Nutritional prediction of pressure ulcers. *J Am Dietet Assoc* 1994;94(11):1301–1304.
49. Braden BJ. The relationship between emotional stress and pressure sore formation among the elderly recently relocated to a nursing home. In: Funk SG, Tournquist EM, Champagne MT, et al. (eds). *Key Aspects of Recovery: Improving Nutrition,*

Rest, and Mobility. New York, NY, Springer Publishing, 1990, pp 188–196.

50. Holden–Lund C. Effects of relaxation with guided imagery on surgical stress and wound healing. *Res Nurs Health* 1988;11:235–244.

51. Hargreaves A, Lander J. Use of transcutaneous electrical nerve stimulation for postoperative pain. *Nurs Res* 1989;38:159–161.

52. Angus JE, Faux S. The effect of music on adult postoperative patients' pain during a nursing procedure. In: Funk SG, Tournquist EM, Champagne MT, et al. (eds). *Key aspects of recovery: Management of pain, fatigue and nausea.* New York, NY, Springer Publishing, 1989, pp 166–172.

53. Schmid P, Horejsi RC, Miekusch W, Paletta B. The influence of noise stress on plasma epinephrine and its binding to plasma protein in the rat. *Biomed Miochim Acta* 1989;48:453–456.

54. McCarthy DO, Quimet ME, Daun JM. The effect of noise stress on leukocyte function in rats. *Res Nurs & Health* 1992;15(2):131–137.

55. Wysocki AB. The effect of intermittent noise exposure on wound healing. *Adv Wound Care* 1996;9(1):35–39.

56. Burnand KG, Whimster I, Naidoo A, Browse NL. Pericapillary fibrin in the ulcer–bearing skin of the leg: The cause of lipodermatosclerosis and venous ulceration. *Br J Med* 1982;285:1071–1072.

57. Coleridge–Smith PD, Thomas P, Scurr JM, Dormany JA. Causes of venous ulceration: A new hypothesis. *Br J Med* 1988;296:1726–1727.

58. Hunt TK. Disorders of repair and their management. In: Hunt TK, Dumphy JE (eds). *Fundamentals of Wound Management.* New York, NY, Appleton– Century–Crofts, 1979, pp 68–169.

59. Heimback RD. Radiation effects on tissue. In: Davis JC, Hunt TK (eds). *Problem Wounds: The Role of Oxygen.* New York, NY, Elsevier, 1993.

60. Mustoe TA, Porras–Reyes BH. Modulation of wound healing response in chronic irradiated tissues. *Clin Plast Surg* 1993;20(3):465–472.

61. Eriksson AS, Sinclair R, Cassuto J, Thomsen P. Influence of lidocaine on leukocyte function in the surgical wound. *Anesthesiology* 1992;77:74–78.

62. Powell DM, Rodeheaver GT, Foreman PA, et al. Damage to tissue defenses by EMLA cream. *J Emer Med* 1991;9:205–209.

63. Nykanen D, Kissoon N, Rieder M, Armstrong R. Comparison of a topical mixture of lidocaine and prilocaine (EMLA) versus 1% lidocaine infiltration on wound healing. *Ped Emerg Care* 1991;7(1):15–17.

64. Hansson O, Holm J, Lillieborg S, Syren A. Repeated treatment with Lidocaine/Prilocaine cream (EMLA®) as a topical anesthetic for the cleansing of venous leg ulcers. *Acta Derm Venereol* 1993; 73:231–233.

10

Nutritional Assessment and Intervention

Gayle Pinchcofsky–Devin, RD, FACN

Pinchcofsky–Devin G. Nutritional assessment and intervention. In: Krasner D, Kane D. *Chronic Wound Care, Second Edition*. Wayne, PA, Health Management Publications, Inc., 1997, pp 73–83.

Introduction

Surveys of hospital patients by nutritional assessment indicate that malnutrition may be a common problem. In 1974, Bistrian, Blackburn, Hallowell and Heddle showed that 50 percent of the patients in their hospital had evidence of protein calorie malnutrition and that 35 percent of the patients had at least one index less than 60 percent of standard, suggesting severe nutritional depletion.[1] These general findings were confirmed by Hill, et al. in 1977.[2]

Although the patients were not severely protein calorie malnourished, they had other nutritional abnormalities, which included anemia and vitamin and mineral deficiencies. Freed et al., using stricter nutritional assessment criteria, identified nutritional deficits that correlate with increased morbidity and mortality in patients on admission.[3]

Protein calorie malnutrition is associated with such clinical problems as poor wound healing, decreased strength of bowel anastomoses, impaired resistance to infection, and increased risk of morbidity and mortality.[4–6]

Nutritional Assessment

Despite the widespread occurrence of malnutrition and its associated consequences, there is no universally accepted definition of the malnourished state. Thus, nutritional assessment continues to consist of a vast array of anthropometric, immunologic, biochemical and body compositional parameters. The immediate goal of nutritional assessment is to identify patients at high risk of developing nutritionally based adverse clinical events. The ultimate goal is, of course, early identification to prevent the development of these poor clinical outcomes.[7]

There are three major components of a nutritional assessment: the visceral protein stores, the somatic protein stores, and the vitamin and mineral status of the patient. These three components comprise the patient's nutritional status. Combined with the patient's physiological status, these components form the building blocks for the patient's ability to deal with infection, heal wounds, fight trauma, and deal with cancer therapies (chemotherapy and radiation therapy).

Diet History

It is important to obtain a collection of the patient's social, medical and dietary intake information. Frequently, this information gives clues to the type of nutritional problems that may be encountered. The following questions should be used as a guide in obtaining a diet history.
– Is there recent significant weight gain or loss?
– Are there increased metabolic needs such as fever, infection, trauma or burns?
– Are there increased losses via draining fistulae, open wounds, draining abscesses, effusion, chronic blood loss or exudative enteropathies?
– Are there chronic diseases?
– Has there been recent major surgery or illness?
– Are there diseases of the GI tract?

Table 1
Somatic Proteins : Percent Deficit

Severe	≥ 30
Moderate	< 15 to 30
Mild	< 5 to 15

Assessment of The Somatic Compartment Weight and Height Indices

Body weight is the most commonly used and easily obtainable anthropometric measurement. However, it is subject to great error in interpretation, especially when used to compare one individual to another or to a group of individuals.[8] Such obvious factors as height and body frame size certainly influence body weight.[9,10] Even among patients of similar height and body build, however, great variation in weight measurements may result from additional factors such as the presence of anasarca, dehydration and any disease state or therapeutic regimen that may result in a significant alteration of body water. Nutritional deterioration and nutritional repletion have known influences on total body water and, thus, body weight.

An ideal weight/height table may provide a reasonable preliminary assessment of somatic protein status; however, as stated above, the disease state may distort the measurement. The change from the premarked weight to the present weight, together with the date of onset of illness, will provide a valuable index of nutritional assessment. A history of recent unintentional weight loss and/or a "weight for height" of less than 85 percent of standard has been related to functional consequences of malnutrition.[11] To determine a percent deficit of weight, the following calculation is used:

$$\text{percent deficit} = 100 - \frac{\text{actual weight}}{\text{ideal weight}} \times 100$$

Total Body Fat

Skinfold measurements, the mainstay of anthropometric techniques, are used to estimate the thickness of subcutaneous adipose tissue at various sites on the body. These sites include the triceps, biceps, subscapular, abdominal, suprailiac, medial calf, and anterior thigh locations.[12] The amount of subcutaneous adipose fat, as measured by skin foldcalipers, has been found to correlate well with determinations of adipose contents by densitometry, radiography, and autopsy techniques.[13,14] There is, however, great variability in skinfold thickness between individuals. This variability depends not only upon the site of the measurement and nutritional status, but also on the age, sex and race of the subjects.[15–17] Thus, one must be cautious in the interpretation of skinfold measurements, especially those obtained at a single site. Measurements of skinfold thickness at multiple sites may improve the reliability of this technique.[18]

Body Muscle Stores

The anthropometric evaluation of skeletal muscle has been predominantly restricted to assessment of the upper extremities. The commonly used anthropometric indicators of muscle mass include the middle upper arm circumference, the arm muscle circumference, and the arm muscle area. The mid–upper arm circumference is measured at the same level as the triceps skinfold thickness, that is, halfway between the acromial and olecranon process. Arm muscle circumference is obtained by the following formula: AMC = MAC – (TSF x 0.314) where AMC is arm muscle circumference in cm, MAC is mid–arm circumference in cm, and TSF is triceps skinfold thickness in mm.

Creatinine Height Index

The creatinine height index provides another estimate of skeletal muscle mass because urinary levels of creatinine are dependent primarily upon the extent of skeletal muscle catabolism, especially during protein depletion. Creatinine excretion remains relatively constant in direct proportion to defined amounts of muscle mass. With chronic wasting diseases, skeletal muscle mass and creatinine excretion decrease simultaneously. Lean body mass is depleted during malnutrition as muscle protein is catabolized for utilization as energy; creatinine excretion and the creatinine height index are lowered as a result.

The creatinine height index is expressed as a percentage and calculated as mg creatine excreted/24 hours by a normal subject of the same height and sex. A creatinine height index of less than 40 percent of standard is generally considered indicative of severe nutritional depletion; 40 to 60 percent of standard is interpreted as marginal depletion (Table 1).

Assessment of Visceral Proteins

The status of visceral proteins dictates the patient's ability to clinically respond to stress; i.e., mount an immune response, heal wounds, etc. The visceral proteins that should be included in a nutritional assessment are serum albumin, total protein, serum transferrin, and total lymphocyte count.

Serum Albumin

Albumin is a protein with a molecular weight of 65,000 daltons and a half life of approximately 20 days under normal conditions.[19] The normal serum albumin concentration is 3.5 to 5.0 gm/dl in the serum of the adult. This serum level is the equilibrium point between the production, distribution, and degradation of albumin. Forty percent of the albumin pool is intravascular and 60 percent is extravascular. The skin represents 30 to 40 percent of the extravascular albumin stores and large amounts are also stored in the muscle and viscera. Albumin is the major protein synthesized by the liver. This important protein serves to maintain plasma oncotic pressure and to function as a carrier for metabolites, enzymes, drugs, hormones, and metal in the bloodstream.[20,21]

Numerous studies have revealed increased morbidity and mortality in patients with decreased serum albumin levels. In 1955, Rhoads and Alexander documented an increased incidence of infection in post–operative patients with poor nutritional status and hypoalbuminemia.[22] Neumann, et al., in 1975, associated severe weight loss and low serum albumin concentrations with an increased rate of clinical sepsis.[23] Seltzer et al., in 1979, reported a four–fold increase in morbidity and six–fold increase in mortality in patients with serum albumin concentrations less than 2.5 gm/dl.[24] Additional studies have confirmed these observations and clearly demonstrate that the serum albumin concentration is a reliable indicator of patient prognosis.

Hypoalbuminemia results from inadequate synthesis, increased catabolism, or extraordinary corporal losses of albumin. Decreased albumin synthesis occurs in Kwashiorkor Malnutrition, such as feeding carbohydrate without protein, or Marasmus–Kwashiorkor Mix Malnutrition, liver disease, ethanol use, cancer cachexia,[25] and aging.[26]

Increased protein catabolism occurs during sepsis, wound healing, or any severe metabolic stress. Losses occur in severe burns, nephrotic syndrome, or severe diarrhea.

Within the intestine, the hypo–oncotic state from hypoproteinemia results in a marked shift of fluid into the interstitial space. This shift is associated with cells no longer being subjected to the normally net negative pressure but rather to a positive interstitial pressure.

In the hypo–oncotic state, the bowel becomes edematous and sausage–like and loses its ability to passively absorb water from the intraluminal space.

This hypo–oncotic state of the bowel is of vital importance when the patient is a candidate for abdominal surgery. Edematous tissues do not hold sutures. Edematous patients are at risk for anastomotic leaks, intra–abdominal sepsis, wound dehiscence, fistulization, and prolonged ileus.

Enteral feeding tolerance is decreased in the hypo–oncotic intestine. Under normal circumstances, water is absorbed from the gastrointestinal tract by passive diffusion at the mucosal epithelium. Absorption may occur anywhere along the GI tract, but the small intestine is the primary area of absorption due to its greater surface area. Water absorbed from the epithelium enters the intestinal space and subsequently enters the blood and lymph capillaries to be deposited into the systemic circulation.

The capillary colloid oncotic pressure in the intestine is approximately 28 mm Hg, while that in the interstitium of the intestine is between 4 and 9 mm Hg. The rates of filtration and absorption of water across the capillary beds of the intestine are equal in the healthy person. Thus, the total volumes shifted between the blood and the interstitial fluid are very small. A small amount of fluid escapes into the interstitial fluid, but it is returned via the lymphatics. The empty intestine behaves like an interstitial space, with respect to plasma, and fluid begins to leak into the lumen, resulting in diarrhea. Furthermore, the cells of the intestinal lumen can no longer optimally absorb nutrients.

There appears to be a direct correlation with gut function for all levels of hypoalbuminemia which tend toward sluggish GI function and bowel edema. This relationship clinically effects the length and severity of post–operative ileus as well as tolerance to enteral feedings.

Albumin and Wound Healing

Increased capillary permeability secondary to injury results in localization of some acute phase proteins around the injury site.[27–29] The increase in plasma protein availability very likely facilitates wound healing.[30] Albumin is the major plasma protein.

Albumin is an amino acid donor for extrahepatic tissue synthesis.[31] Decreased total plasma protein or albumin concentrations are associated with reduced wound tensile strength in a variety of clinical states such as Adult Kwashiorkor Malnutrition, wound infection, uremia and old age.

Albumin catabolism increases as a result of injury to the skin as does other plasma protein catabolism.[29,32] Albumin is made available to regeneration tissue in proportion to the extent of injury and inflammation. Changes in temperature and pH at the injury site denature the native albumin. Macrophages are then able to utilize the constituents of the albumin.[33]

Table 2
Rating Deficits of Visceral Proteins

	Severe	Moderate	Mild
Albumin	< 2.5	< 3.0 to 2.5	< 3.5 to 3.0
Transferrin	< 160	< 180 to 160	< 180 to 200
Total Protein	< 5.0	< 6.0 – 5.0	< 6.0 to 6.5
TLC	< 900	< 1500 to 900	< 1800 to 1500

Albumin synthesis decreases during trauma. If utilization of albumin increases at the wound site and albumin synthesis decreases, unless some attempt is made to support or increase synthesis, serum albumin in the wounded patient falls. If severe, such a decrease in serum albumin synthesis or increase in albumin utilization at a major wound site may impair wound healing in the patient with borderline visceral protein status. See Table 2 for rating deficits of visceral proteins.

Total Protein

The serum total protein level is determined primarily by the circulating albumin and globulin concentrations. Normal serum total protein levels in an adult are 6.5 to 8.6 gm/dl. Levels of 5.4 or below have been associated with decreased colloid osmotic pressure.

Transferrin

Transferrin is a glycoprotein with a molecular weight of approximately 76,000 daltons.[34] It is a Beta–globulin that is synthesized predominantly in the liver and transports iron in the plasma. Each molecule of transferrin has two specific iron binding sites. Under normal conditions, transferrin is present in the serum at a concentration of 180 to 260 mg/dl.[34]

Serum transferrin has a shorter half–life than albumin (7 days) and equilibrates rapidly because of its relatively small extravascular stores. Therefore, transferrin is more discriminating than serum albumin levels for assessing protein status.

Documentation of depressed serum transferrin concentrations in severe protein calorie malnutrition is inconclusive. Its usefulness in the diagnosis of subclinical malnutrition is somewhat controversial because serum transferrin concentrations vary over a wide range, even in clinically obvious malnutrition, and the response to treatment is often unpredictable.[19,35,36]

Total Lymphocyte Count

Malnutrition has repeatedly been associated with peripheral lymphocyte counts less than 2,000 cells/mm^3 and impaired cell–mediated immunity. The depressed total lymphocyte count has been associated with increased morbidity and mortality. The total lymphocyte count (TLC) is calculated as follows:

$$TLC = WBC \times \frac{Percent\ Lymphs}{100}$$

Significant lymphocytopenia has been defined as a total lymphocyte count of less than 1,000 to 2,000 cells/mm^3. A TLC of less than 2,000 cells/mm^3 indicates a need for further nutritional evaluation, since some defect in immune responsiveness may be present. Refer to Table 2 for rating deficits in TLC.

Classification of Types of Malnutrition

Kwashiorkor. Kwashiorkor or protein malnutrition is caused by consumption of adequate or more than adequate amounts of calories, in the form of carbohydrate and fat, and practically no protein. On nutritional assessment, the patient will have adequate or more than adequate somatic stores (fat reserves) but will have significant deficits in their visceral protein stores. The Kwashiorkor patient may appear well nourished or even obese. Without adequate nutritional assessment, the disease can go undetected.

Marasmus. Marasmus or protein calorie malnutrition is caused by a diet consisting of protein, fat and carbohydrate in limited amounts. On nutritional assessment, patients have deficits in their somatic stores, but on assessing their visceral stores, the parameters are normal. Visually, these patients look very thin and emaciated.

Kwashiorkor–Marasmus Mix. This type of malnutrition results from starvation. It presents with deficits in both the somatic and visceral protein stores. The patient will present with weight loss, fat, and muscle wasting as well as edema and the other complications caused by low visceral protein stores (Table 3).

Determining Calorie and Protein Requirements

There are numerous equations available to calculate calorie and protein requirements. One equation for calculating caloric requirements, which tends to be very accurate in meeting patient needs, is the Harris–Benedict Equation, which takes into account weight, height and age. The equation gives an estimate of the patient's resting energy expenditure (REE). Using various activity and stress factors, the equation can be further modified.

Harris–Benedict Equation

Male REE =
66.4230 + 13.7516W + 5.033H − 6.7750A
Female REE =
655.0955 + 9.6534W + 1.8496H − 4.6756A

W = Actual weight in kilograms
H = Height in centimeters
A = Age in years

Activity Factors:
Ambulatory 1.3
Bedridden 1.2

Stress Factors:
Minor surgery 1.2
Skeletal Trauma 1.35
Major sepsis 1.6
Severe Burns 2.1

(The large difference between the male REE and the female REE is due to differences in muscle mass metabolic rate.)

After calculating the REE by using the Harris–Benedict Equation, the result is multiplied by both an ambulation factor and a stress factor in order to calculate the patient's caloric requirement.

Another common method of determining the caloric requirement for the hospitalized patient is to estimate the protein requirement and then set caloric requirements based on an optimal calorie–nitrogen ratio. Estimates of the protein requirements for moderately malnourished patients vary but generally range between 1.0 and 1.5 gm protein per kilogram of body weight per day. Shizgal, for example, studied the moderately malnourished patient and found that 1.3 gm protein per kilogram of body weight per day was sufficient to maintain body cell mass.[37]

Table 3
Protein Calorie Malnutrition/ ICD9
International Classification

Kwashiorkor	267.0
Marasmus	268.0
Mix	269.9

Shizgal's data indicated that the restoration rate of a depleted body cell mass is related to caloric intake and the degree of malnutrition, but is not affected by increasing the protein intake from 1.3 to 2.4 gm/kg body weight per day.

According to Shizgal, there are no apparent advantages to increasing the daily protein intake to levels above 1.5 to 2 gm/kg body weight per day. Peters and Fisher found that 1.56 grams protein per kilogram of body weight per day was adequate to meet the needs of patients receiving TPN.[38] Long, et al. reported that the protein intake necessary to maintain a neutral nitrogen balance in the septic patient was approximately 1.5 gm/kg body weight per day when adequate nonprotein calories are provided.[39]

For the hospitalized patient, the optimal calorie to nitrogen ratio, defined as the non–protein calories administered per gram nitrogen (NPC per gm N) is a ratio of 120:1 to 180:1 when feeding a catabolic patient.

Using the figures of 1.5 gram protein per kilogram body weight per day and NPC per gm
N ratio of 150:1, the protein and calorie requirements of a patient can be determined. First, multiply the patient's weight in kilograms by a factor of 1.5:

Protein requirement = 1.5 x weight (kg)
= 1.5 x 52.3
= 78.43

The resulting protein requirement is 79 gm/day.
Next, determine the nitrogen equivalent of the protein requirement by dividing by a factor of 6.25 (6.25 gm of protein = 1 gm of nitrogen).

Nitrogen equivalent of protein requirement
= protein requirement (gm) divided by 6.25
= 79 divided by 6.25
= 12.6

The resulting figure is approximately 13 gm nitrogen. Finally, by utilizing the NPC per gm N ration of 150:1, the following is the result.

Table 4
Nitrogen Balance

Nitrogen In = $\dfrac{\text{Protein Intake (gm)} \times 24 \text{ hours}}{6.25}$

Nitrogen Out = gms urinary urea nitrogen/24 hrs + gms for other non–urea nitrogen losses

Nitrogen Balance = Nitrogen In – Nitrogen Out

Nitrogen intake is derived by dividing the patient's protein intake by a factor of 6.25.

Nitrogen In = Protein (gm)/6.25
Nitrogen Balance =
(gm protein intake/6.25) – UUN + 3

The correction factor of 3 accounts for non–urea urinary losses as well as for stool and cutaneous nitrogen losses.

Nonprotein calorie requirement = 150 x gm N
= 150 x 13
= 1950

A nonprotein calorie requirement for this particular patient would be 1950 kcal per day. Sufficient calories must be supplied for healing to occur while optimal nutritional status is preserved. When calories supplied are less than required, muscle and organ proteins breakdown to supply amino acids for gluconeogenesis.

A high calorie diet with 50 to 60 percent of calories as carbohydrates will help spare protein stores of vital tissue. Muscle and organ protein serves as an amino acid resource when dietary protein is inadequate.

It is essential to repeat nutritional assessments and monitor a patient's intake. Based on the results of the nutritional assessment, alter the calculation for determining caloric and protein requirements.

Nitrogen Balance

Nitrogen balance, defined as the difference between nitrogen intake and nitrogen excretion provides a quick and relatively effective means of evaluating the adequacy of the patient's nutritional intake or the efficacy of nutritional support therapy. When a subject's nitrogen intake exceeds his or her nitrogen excretion, the resultant "positive" nitrogen balance suggests the availability of protein for repair of nutritional deficits. In normal subjects, the rates of

anabolism and catabolism are in equilibrium, thereby preserving body protein mass and resulting in a nitrogen balance of zero. During trauma and infection, however, the turnover and loss of protein increases.

A nitrogen balance is simple to obtain and is based on a calculation using a 24–hour urine collection, which is assessed for its urine urea nitrogen (UUN) content. (Table 4).

Selection of Feeding Formulas

If a patient is severely hypo–oncotic and has dependent edema secondary to hypoproteinemia, the patient's total protein must first be repaired. As mentioned previously there are two circumstances that are associated with lowering total protein: 1) feeding non–protein calories, especially carbohydrates with no or inadequate amounts or protein fed and 2) infection.

If the patient is infected, the enteral feeding of a balanced diet will not result in an elevation of total protein. Where the patient is pitting in the peripheral tissue, he is also pitting in his intestine. The enteral feeding of severely hypoproteinemic patients is usually associated with severe loose and watery stools. This association is secondary to the inability of the vilus to absorb water from the intestine. Much of the water absorption is passive and is secondary to a total protein creating an oncotic pressure within the vilus capillary, drawing water from the intestine as it does from tissues from the interstitial space. This pressure can only be repaired by placing the patient on an IV maintenance solution of amino acids and then supplementing with 12.5 gm albumin per liter for a limited period of time. The clinician must be extremely careful when performing this procedure because as the total protein rises, the oncotic pressure rises and when it overcomes the hydrostatic pressure, there will be a translocation of the interstitial edema back into the circulating volume. At this point, the patient must be aggressively treated with diuretics. If not, the patient will develop fluid overload syndrome and acute respiratory distress.

Once the patient's oncotic pressure has been physiologically stabilized, then the old dictum "if the gut works – use it" comes into play. The formula used should be selected by a dietician. Its efficacy in repairing deficits should be reassessed on a weekly basis.

Sample Set of Enteral Orders

- Begin enteral hyperalimentation at 50 ml per hour.
- Check all voided specimens for glucosuria. If negative for two consecutive specimens and no loose stools are observed during that time, increase the rate to 75 ml/hr.

- If no glucosuria is observed for two more consecutive specimens (and no loose stools), increase the rate to 100 ml/hr.

When formulas are begun at half strength, the volume should be increased before increasing the concentration.

Complications of Enteral Feedings

Diarrhea. There should be no complications from enteral hyperalimentation. The most frequent complication is associated with loose bowel movements which can usually be addressed using the following technique. If a loose stool is observed, measures can be taken to control it with loperamid given immediately through the tube and added to the feeding solution for 7 days.

Diarrhea can also occur as a result of a reduction in the absorptive capacity and absorptive area associated with a loss of brush border enzymes, mucosal cells and microvilli. An elemental diet is used initially until visceral and structural proteins of the intestinal mucosa are restored. Severe hypoalbuminemia compromises absorption by reducing the intravascular osmotic force that draws fluid across the endothelium. The decreased absorptive power in the villi leads to malabsorption and eventually to diarrhea. If the patient is infected or severely stressed, raising the serum albumin by parenteral administration may be indicated.

Patients who have been hospitalized for extended periods of time and who have been on a series of antibiotics that alter bacterial flora may experience diarrhea due to an overgrowth of bacteria. The administration of Lacto–Bacillis, one packet via the tube three times a day for one day, will usually resolve this problem.

Frequent loose, foul–smelling stools are associated with failure or inadequate function of the exocrine pancreas. When an elemental diet is not used, a chemically defined diet and replacement of pancreatic enzymes will eliminate this problem.

Occasionally, administration of a fiber–containing formula is necessary to provide bulk and convert a watery stool to a more manageable semi–soft consistency.

Finally, lactose intolerance is so frequent that no feeding formula that contains lactose is suitable for the patient who is prone to diarrhea from multiple causes.

Glucosuria. Glucosuria produces an osmotic diuresis and is the cause of hyperosmolar hyperglycemic nonketotic dehydration. An increase in the rate of feeding is made only if there is no glucosuria.

If glucosuria persists, oral hypoglycemic agents can be added to the feeding. If the agent fails, insulin can be administered to match the feeding schedule and carbohydrate load.

Constipation. Many commercially available tube feeding formulas are low in residue; therefore, decreased frequency of bowel movements is to be expected. Magnesium oxide can be administered through the tube if constipation affects the patient's comfort. Due to the thickness of this medication, it is recommended that it be diluted with water prior to administration to avoid clogging the tube. This medication should be followed with irrigation of the feeding tube with 30 to 60 ml water. An agent to increase intestinal bulk can also be used or a fiber–containing enteral formula can be administered.

Nutrition and Wound Healing

Poor nutrition can contribute to the development of chronic wounds in several ways. A diet deficient in many nutrients, particularly those involved in protein synthesis, jeopardizes tissue integrity and contributes to skin breakdown. In addition, inadequate caloric intake causes weight loss and a reduction in subcutaneous tissue, allowing bony prominences to compress and restrict circulation to the skin. The resultant lessening of the nutrients supplied to that area also promotes tissue catabolism.

The wound healing response is a complex process following injury that optimally ends with complete restitution of tissue structure and function. However, delays in wound healing result in weak poor quality scars or indeed in complete failure to heal. An excessive healing response may determine keloids, contractions and other cosmetic functional alterations.

The classically described steps in the healing response involve and are dependent on nutritional substrates as follows:
1. Inflammation with recruitment of polymorphonuclear leukocytes, macrophages and lymphocytes;
2. Fibroblast proliferation and collagen production;
3. Collagen remodeling and re–epithelialization when appropriate.

The strength and integrity of tissue repair depend on collagen crosslinking and deposition.

Alterations in nutritional status or intake proceeding or during injury may clearly alter the normal wound healing response. The rebuilding of the body's immunologic defense system and the replacement of tissue destroyed by disease, surgery and problem wounds call for nutritional support. The best surgical and nursing care available will not heal the wound if there is inadequate nutritional substrates to make new tissue.

If the "fuel" for healing is not provided, the wound will not heal. Nutritional substrates are needed to make new tissue.

Role of Specific Macro–Nutrients

Wound healing is aided by adequate oxygenation, blood flow and nutrient supply. All of the steps involved in wound healing require numerous synthesis and other energy consuming reactions. It is possible that impaired healing may be a consequence of specific nutrient deficiencies. Proteins are the basic cellular component of all living organisms. Protein deficiency contributes to poor wound healing by prolonging the inflammatory response and impairing fibroplasia. When protein deprivation is prolonged, edema secondary to hypoalbuminemia occurs. This alteration may slow oxygen diffusion flow from the capillaries to the cell membrane and cause further insult to tissue.

Methionine, a precursor to cystine, is associated with collagen synthesis. Cystine's exact role is not completely defined, but it may be needed as a co–factor in enzyme systems responsible for collagen synthesis or it may contribute to the proper alignment and attachment to peptide chains in the formation of tropocollagen through disulfide bonds.[40]

A possible role for arginine as a promoting agent for wound healing has also been suggested.[41]

Carbohydrates and fats provide a source of cellular energy. The specific roles of carbohydrates and fat in wound healing are not well defined. Glucose, the simplest form of carbohydrate, is the primary fuel for cellular metabolism of many tissues, including leukocytes, fibroblasts and macrophages. When glucose is not available for cellular function, the body catabolizes protein and, to a lesser degree, fat to produce glucose to meet energy requirements. Glucose is needed to meet the metabolic demand for wound healing and preserve the body's structural and functional protein.[42]

Fats or lipids are the primary source of stored energy in the body. Energy from fat metabolism is used in all normal cell functions, and fat metabolism results in the formation of prostaglandins and other regulators of the immune and inflammatory process. Fat is an essential component of intracellular organelles, such as the mitochondria, and is an integral component of cell membranes.

Vitamins and Wound Healing

Vitamins play a role in wound healing.[43–48] The natural process of wound healing requires numerous energy consuming reactions and these energy consuming reactions all require increased amounts of vitamins, minerals and trace elements. Where specific vitamin deficiencies are diagnosed, individual supplements of up to 10 to 20 times the RDA may be needed.

Higher vitamin levels may be indicated because of increased excretion or decreased absorption as well as drug nutrient interaction. Supplementation is an extremely important component of the therapeutic nutrition care plan for the patient with a wound.

Ascorbic acid plays an important role in wound healing. Vitamin C functions as a cofactor in the hydroxylation of proline to hydroxyproline, an essential step in the synthesis of collagen. Hydroxyproline is needed to stabilize collagen. The role of ascorbic acid in epithelialization is less well defined; however, ascorbate is one of the stimulants for fibroblast mitosis and subsequent collagen synthesis.[49] Vitamin C deficiency markedly delays the wound healing process and causes capillary fragility. In Vitamin C deficiency states, old wounds may reopen due to loss of tensile strength and degeneration of the extracellular matrix.

Ascorbic acid has also been shown to enhance the cellular and humoral responses to stress. *In vitro* studies suggest there is an increased utilization of Vitamin C during phagocytosis and ascorbic acid may increase the activation of leukocytes and macrophages to the injured site.[50,51] The reducing property of Vitamin C may assist in preventing the oxidation of the membranes of chemotactic proteins allowing for rapid response during inflammation.[51]

There appears to be a beneficial effect in the treatment of pressure ulcers with Vitamin C.[48] Other investigators have correlated delayed wound healing with decreased ascorbic acid levels in surgical patients.[52] Report of marginal Vitamin C levels in institutionalized persons may substantiate the rationale for supplementation during hospitalization, mainly where there is some evidence for its increased need during injury.[53]

Studies during deficiency states show that Vitamin A is important in maintaining the normal humoral defense mechanism and in limiting complications associated with wound infections either locally or systemically. Supplementation of retinoic acid has been shown to improve wound healing in patients receiving corticosteroid treatment.[54] Studies have shown that Vitamin A counteracts the catabolic effect that glucocorticosteroid exerts on wound healing.[54,55] *In vitro* studies by Demetrious, et al. suggest Vitamin A and retinoic acid enhance fibroplasia and collagen accumulation in wounds.[56]

Vitamin A, also known as retinol, is required for an adequate inflammatory response and is essential for the formation of mucopolysaccharides, which function as a protective sheath around collagen. It is essential for epithelial integrity and may also be a cofactor for collagen synthesis. Vitamin A stimulates cellular differentiation in fibroblasts and collagen synthesis, thus hastening the healing process and enhancing tensile strength. The supplementation of Vitamin A in steroid dependent patients prior to surgery may promote a rapid healing response and reduce the incidence of wound dehiscence.

Vitamin E, also known as tocopherol, is an antioxidant. It is essential for the stability of cell walls. Decreased levels of Vitamin E are associated with shortened survival of red and white blood cells. Vitamin E also enhances the immune response. Vitamin K plays an essential role in coagulation which is a prerequisite for healing.

Trace Elements and Wound Repair

Zinc acts as a cofactor in over 100 enzyme reactions. It is needed for the transcription of RNA in the promotion of protein synthesis, cellular replication, and collagen formation. Zinc is required for synthesizing and mobilizing plasma proteins such as retinol binding protein and albumin. Given its role in rapid tissue growth and protein synthesis, zinc is thought to be involved in wound healing. Zinc deficiency has an adverse influence on wound healing through its effect on reducing rates of epithelialization, decreasing of wound strength and collagen synthesis.

Iron is necessary for the hydroxylation of lysine and proline in the formation of collagen. Iron is necessary to transport oxygen in the body. Copper is a component of many enzyme systems including lysl oxidase. Copper is the enzyme necessary for collagen cross link formation. Together with iron, copper is essential to the production of erythrocytes.

Water

Providing adequate water should not be overlooked. Overhydration and dehydration must be avoided. Two formulas to calculate water requirements are 1) 1 cc of water per each calorie fed and 2) 30 cc of water per kilogram of body weight.

Wound Healing

Wound healing is a complex interaction of mechanical, physiologic and biochemical events.

An alteration in any facet of this intricate process will inevitably lead to prolonged or abnormal wound healing.[57] Malnutrition can adversely affect the normal healing process.

Evidence indicates that protein depletion or Vitamin C and Zinc deficiency can directly affect collagen synthesis. In addition, altered immunity accompanying malnutrition can have a major impact on wound strength and integrity.

Correlation of Pressure Ulcers and Nutritional Status

A study was performed on 232 nursing home patients from two metropolitan nursing homes.[58] The mean age of the patients was 72.9 years. Nutritional assessments were performed using the following parameters: percent ideal body weight, triceps skinfold, mid–arm circumference, arm muscle circumference, serum albumin, serum prealbumin, retinol binding protein and total lymphocyte count. The patients were examined by a physician noting mentation, hydration, presence, and degree of edema. Pressure points were checked for pressure ulcers.

Patients were divided into three groups based on their nutritional status. Severity of malnutrition was also graded as mild, moderate or severe. A patient was defined as having severe Kwashiorkor Malnutrition if two or more visceral proteins were severely low. Likewise, a patient was defined as having severe Marasmus if two or more of the somatic parameters were severely low. The same system was used to classify patients as mildly or moderately malnourished.

All patients with pressure ulcers (7.3 percent) were severely malnourished. The mean serum albumin level of this group was 2.3 gm/dl and the TLC was 1080.

Approximately 51.7 percent of the patients were mildly to moderately malnourished and did not have pressure ulcers. The mean serum albumin level of this group was 3.3 gm/dl and the TLC was 1220. It was found that 41 percent of the patients were well nourished, as judged by adequate visceral protein stores. The mean serum albumin was 4.0 and the TLC was 1942.

There was a significant difference between the mean serum albumin and the TLC in the severely malnourished group and the well–nourished group (p < 0.001). There was also a significant difference between the serum albumin and the TLC of the well–nourished and the mildly to moderately malnourished group (p < 0.05).

All patients with pressure ulcers were severely malnourished. The severity of malnutrition was correlated with the stage of the pressure ulcer; the more severe the malnutrition, the more severe the pressure ulcer (Table 5).

No well–nourished patients developed pressure ulcers. Nutritional assessments must be performed. From these data, one can infer that when the serum albumin level is below 3.3 gm/dl and the TLC is 1220 or lower, nutritional intervention should be implemented to prevent the nutritional consequences that will result in the development of pressure ulcers.

Table 5		
Malnutrition vs. Severity of Pressure Ulcer		
Ulcer stage	Number	Albumin (gm/dl)
I	1	x 3.4
II	1	x 2.6
III	9	x 2.4
IV	6	x 2.0

If the patient is able to eat, oral supplements are appropriate and should be used. A documentation of intake is necessary to see whether the patient is consuming the supplement, and a serial nutritional assessment should be performed twice a month for patients in a therapeutic phase.

The AHCPR guideline, *Pressure Ulcers in Adults: Prediction and Prevention*, states that nutritional risk should be periodically reassessed.[59] They recommend determining factors that are compromising oral intake and first offering the patient support with eating. If after this assistance, intake still remains inadequate, they recommend nutritional supplements or the use of more aggressive nutritional intervention such as enteral and parenteral support.

Summary

Early identification and monitoring of several nutrition risk factors may eliminate or reduce the complications associated with delayed wound healing. These nutrition risk factors include decreased serum albumin level below 3.5 gm/dl; low serum transferrin level below 180 mg/dl; low total lymphocyte count below 1800 cells/mm^3, anemia, hemoglobin below 12 mg/dl; and decreased oral intake.

The nutrition risk factors can be identified by performing a nutritional assessment. The immediate goal of a nutritional assessment is to identify patients at high risk of developing nutritionally based adverse clinical events. The ultimate goal is, of course, early identification to prevent the development of these poor clinical outcomes.

Malnutrition can contribute to delayed or impaired wound healing, and conversely delayed or impaired wound healing can be an indicator of malnutrition. Healing wounds are intensely anabolic, and malnutrition need not be severe to adversely affect the healing process. Additionally, overt symptoms or physical signs may not accompany specific nutritional or metabolic abnormalities. Early nutritional assessment and intervention

will help meet the protein, energy, vitamin and mineral requirements necessary to optimize healing.

Protein calorie malnutrition occurs in a significant number of hospitalized, home and institutionalized patients. It results in increases in morbidity and mortality, which are associated with increased length of stay and, therefore, increased cost of hospitalization.

Such malnutrition can be reversed and corrected by appropriate nutritional intervention, thereby reducing the severity of these complications. It is necessary to identify those patients with clinical and subclinical malnutrition. Protein–calorie malnutrition or patients at risk of developing malnutrition can be identified by performing a nutritional assessment as described in this chapter. After performing a nutritional assessment, nutritional intervention should be implemented and monitored for efficacy.

Outcome

The prevention and treatment of wounds depends heavily upon adequate nourishment and the correction of nutrient deficiencies. Sufficient calories, protein vitamins, minerals and water are fundamental to the optimal maintenance and repair of the body. Preventive nutrition is also an urgent necessity. Based on available references it seems reasonable to conclude that without the correction of nutritional deficiencies, concomitant with the correction of external factors, the application of proper wound care techniques alone cannot be expected to result in wound healing. Thus, nutrition assumes an equal footing with the other time honored pathogenic considerations in wound prevention and treatment.

References

1. Bistrian BR, Blackburn GL, Hallowell E, Heddle R. Protein status of general surgical patients. *JAMA* 1974;230:856–886.
2. Smith T, Corli A, et al. Hospital malnutrition. *Lancet* 1977;1:689–693.
3. Freed BA, Chase G, Kaminski MV. Initiation of admission nutritional screening program in an urban community. *Hospital Nutritional Support Services* 1982;2(8):19–23.
4. Bozzetti F, Terno G, Longoni. Parenteral hyperalimentation and wound healing. *Surg Gynecol Obstet* 1975;141:712–714.
5. Daley JM, Vars HM, Dudrick SJ. Effects of protein depletion on strength of colonic anastomes. *Surg Gynecol Obstet* 1971;134:15–22.
6. Law DK, Dudrick SJ, Abdou N. The effect of protein calorie malnutrition on immune competence of surgical patients. *Surg Gynecol Obstet* 1974;139:257–2656.
7. Mullen JM, Buzby G. Nutritional assessment of the hospitalized patient, Why bother? *Drug Therapy* 1984;10:220–227.
8. Morgan DB, Hill GL, Bukenshaw L. The assessment of weight loss from a single measurement of body weight: The problems and limitations. *Am J Clin Nutr* 198033:2101–2105.

9. Seonans N, Latham MC. Nutritional anthropometry in the identification of malnutrition in children. *J Trop Pediatr* 1971;17:98–104.

10. Metropolitan Life Insurance Company, Modified from data derived from the 1959 Build and Blood Pressure Study, Society of Actuaries.

11. Harvey KB, Ruggiero JA, Reagan CS, et al. Hospital morbidity–mortality risk factors using nutritional assessment. *JPEN* 1987;19:212–216.

12. Zenas AJ. Anthropometric field methods: General. In: Jelliffe DB, Jelliffe EF (eds). *Nutrition and Growth*. New York, NY, Plenum Press, 1979, pp 339–364.

13. Durnin JG, Womersley J. Body fat assessed from total body density and its estimation from skin fold thickness: Measurement on 481 men and women aged 16 to 72 years. *Research J Nutr* 1974;32:77–97.

14. Baker PT, Hunt E, Sen T. The growth and interrelations of skin folds and branchial tissues in man. *Am J Phys Anthropol* 1958;16:39–58.

15. Frisancho AR. Triceps skinfold in upper arm muscle size norms for assessment of nutritional status. *Am J Clin Nutr* 1978;27:1052–1058.

16. Himes JH, Roche AF, Sierwogel RM. Compressibility of skinfolds and the measurements of subcutaneous fatness. *Am J Clin Nutr* 1979;32:1134–1140.

17. Robson JR, Bazin M, Soderstrom R. Ethnic differences in skin fold thickness. *Am J Clin Nutr* 24:864–868, 1971.

18. Noppa H, Anderson M, Bengteson C, et al. Body composition in middle–age women with special reference to the correlation between body fat mass and anthropometric data. *Am J Clin Nutr* 1979;32:1388–1395.

19. Rothschild MA, Oratz M, Schreibers S. Albumin synthesis. *NEJM* 1982;286:745–757.

20. Rothschild MA, Oratz M, Schreiber S. Serum albumin. *Am J Dig Dis* 1969;14:711–744.

21. Peters T. Serum albumin. *Adv Clin Chem* 1970;13:37–111.

22. Rhoads JE, Alexander CE. Nutritional problems of surgical patients. *ANN NY Acad Sci* 1955;63:268–275.

23. Neumann CG, Lawlor ER, Steinham B, et al. Immunologic responses in malnourished children. *Am J Clin Nutr* 1975;28:89–104.

24. Seitzer MH, Bastidas JA, Cooper DM, et al. Instant nutritional assessment. *JPEN* 1979;3:157–159.

25. Tayek JA, Bistrian BR, Hehir DJ, et al. Improved protein kinetics and albumin synthesis by branch. Chain amino acid enriched TPN in cancer cachexia. *Cancer* 1986;58:147–157.

26. Gersovitz M, Munro HN, Udal J, et al. Albumin synthesis in young and elderly subjects using a neco stable isotope methodology. Response to level of protein intake. *Metabolism* 1980;29(11):320–329.

27. Fischer CL, Gill C, Forrester MC, et al. Quantitation of acute–phase proteins postoperatively. *Am J Clinical Pathol* 1976;66:840.

28. Agostoni A, Binagh BC, Radice F, et al. Acute phase proteins and healing of myocardial infarction. *J Mol Cell Cardiology* 1972;4:519.

29. Brown WL, Boker EG, Mason AP, et al. Protein metabolism and burned rats. *Am J Physiol* 1976;231:476.

30. Powanda MC, Moyer ED. Plasma proteins and wound healing. *Surg Gynecol Obstet* 1981;153:521–525.

31. Jeffay H. Metabolism of serum proteins–The kinetics of serum protein metabolism during growth. *J Bio Chem* 1960;235:2352.

32. Owen JA. Effect of injury on plasma proteins. *Adv Clin Chem* 1967;9:217–223.

33. Thakral KK, Goodson WH, Hunt TK. Stimulation of wound blood vessel growth by wound macrophages. *J Surg Res* 1979;26:430.

34. Morgan E. Transferrin and transferrin iron. In: Jacobs CA, Worwood M (eds). *Biochemistry and Medicine*. London, England, Academic Press, 1974, pp 29–71.

35. Young GA, Chem C, Hill GH. Assessment of protein–calorie malnutrition in surgical patients from plasma proteins and anthropometric measurements. *Am J Clin Nutr* 1978;31:429–435.

36. Shelty PS, Jungs RT, Watragewics KE, et al. Rapid turnover transport proteins: An indicator of subclinical protein energy malnutrition. *Lancet* 1979;23:230–232.

37. Shizgal HM. Body composition and nutritional support. *Surg Clin North Am* 1981;61(3):739–741.

38. Peters C, Fischer J. Studies on calorie nitrogen ration for total parenteral nutrition. *Surg Gynecol Obstet* 1980;151:1–8.

39. Long C, Crosby B, Geifer B, et al. Parenteral nutrition in the septic patient: Nitrogen balance. Limiting plasma amino acids and calories to nitrogen ration. *Am J Clin Nutr* 1976;29:380–391.

40. Ruberg RL. Role of nutrition in wound healing. *Surgical Clinics of North America* 1984;64:705.

41. Barbul A, Retture G, Levenson SM, et al. Arginine: A thymotropic and wound healing agent. *Surgical Forum* 1977;28:101.

42. Ruberg RL. Role of nutrition in wound healing. Surgical Clinics of North America 1984;67(705):526–530.

43. Alvarez OM, Gilbreath R. Thiamine influence of collagen during the granulation of skin wounds. *Journal of Surgical Residency* 1982;32:24–31.

44. Burr RG, Rajan KT. Leukocyte ascorbic acid and pressure sores in paraplegia. British *Journal of Nutrition* 1972;28(2):275–281.

45. Cohen C. Zinc sulfate and bed sores. *British Medical Journal* 1968;2(604):561.

46. Grenier J, Aprahamian M, Genot R, et al. Pantothenic acid (Vitamin B5) efficiency of wound healing. *Acta Vitamina* 1982;4(1,2):81–5.

47. Henken R. Zinc and wound healing. *New England Journal of Medicine* 1974;292(13):675–676.

48. Taylor TV, Rimmer S, Day B, et al. Ascorbic acid supplementation in the treatment of pressure sores. Lancet 1974;2(7880):544–6.

49. Orgill D, Denling RH. Current approaches to wound healing. *Critical Care Medicine* 1988;16:899.

50. Leibowitz B, Seigel BV. Ascorbic acid neutrophil function and the immune response. *International Journal Vitamin Nutrition Research* 1978;48:159.

51. Shilotry PG. Phagocytosis and leukocyte enzymes in ascorbic acid deficient guinea pigs. *Journal of Nutrition* 1977;107:1507.

52. Irvin TT. Challopadhyay DK, Smythe A. Ascorbic acid requirements in postoperative patients. *American Journal of Surgery* 1978;147:49.

53. Mason M, Matyk PW, Doolan SA. Urinary ascorbic acid excretion in postoperative patients. *American Journal of Surgery* 1978;147:49.

54. Ehrlich HP, Hunt TK. Effect of cortisone and Vitamin A on wound healing. *Annals of Surgery* 1968;167:324.

55. Hunt TK, Ehrlich HP, Garcia JA, et al. Effect of Vitamin A on reversing the inhibitor effect of cortisone on healing of wounds in animal and man. *Annals of Surgery* 1969;170:633.

56. Demetrious AA, Levenson SM, Retture G, et al. Vitamin A and retinoic acid–induced fibroblast differentiation in vitro. *Surgery* 1985;98:931.

57. Carrico TT, Riedrhof AT, Cohen IK. Biology of wound healing. *Surgical Clinic of North America* 1984;64:721.

58. Pinchcofsky–Devin G, Kaminski MV. Correlation of pressure sores and nutritional status. *JAGS* 1986;34:435–440.

59. AHCPR. *Pressure Ulcers in Adults: Prediction and Prevention.* U.S. Department of Health and Human Services. No. 92–0042.

11

Wound Infection

Philip D. Thomson, PhD and Thomas E. Taddonio, MA

Thomson PD, Taddonio TE. Wound infection. In: Krasner D, Kane D. *Chronic Wound Care, Second Edition.* Wayne, PA, Health Management Publications, Inc., 1997, pp 84–89.

Introduction

The medical dictionary definition of infection states that this process is the invasion and multiplication of microorganisms in body tissues which may be acute, subacute or chronic depending on the status of the body's defense mechanisms. This definition implies that the condition of the host may share equal importance with the microorganism in this process, and that the interaction between host and microorganism is the process known as infection. This host/microorganism interaction has been summarized by Mertz and Ovington[1] in an expression that considers dose and virulence of the organism as well as host resistance:

Infection = Number of Organisms x Virulence/Host Resistance

The condition of the host or host resistance may be the important factor in this equation and could tip the scale in favor of infection.

Wound infection has been based historically upon visual inspection with the findings of redness, swelling, heat and purulence. It is now accepted that these are visual signs of inflammation and of colonization of tissue by microorganisms or injury to tissue, and although each of these signs may be predictive of infection, each alone is not necessarily diagnostic for wound infection or sepsis.

Inflammation

Inflammation may play a pivotal role in the infectious process. Mechanisms of the inflammatory response are designed to be protective of host tissue, but when the inflammation process is out of control, the result may be host tissue auto destruction. This "vicious cycle" of tissue injury has been well described,[2,3] and as in the case of the severely burned patient who manifests a whole body inflammatory response to tissue insult, superimposing an infection may have devastating results.

The insult to tissue activates physiologic biochemical cascades that include the coagulation system, tissue enzyme system, white blood cell system and vascular microcirculation system.[4] Cytokine and complement activation feed the inflammatory process and result in the activation and production of oxygen metabolites, histamine and leukotrienes.[5] If these cascades are unchecked and are compounded by the effects of infectious toxins, collateral tissue damage occurs resulting in sepsis syndrome, organ system failure and death.

The early inflammatory response seen in acute wounds is initiated by the attraction of polymorphonuclear leukocytes (PMNs) to the site of injury. If microorganisms are encountered, degranulation of these white blood cells may lead to release of enzymes (proteases) and production of toxic oxygen radicals. If this inflammatory response is uncontrolled, local tissue destruction is compounded.

The wound milieu is an ideal growth medium for skin microflora, and if the organisms that colonize are not invasive, a chronic wound may develop. Chronic wound inflammation is generally characterized by the replacement of or addition to PMNs by macrophages. Macrophages are capable of extensive proinflammatory cytokine production[6] and, in the presence of persisting microbial flora, produce enzymes and oxygen free radicals that promote the inflammatory response and the continuation of the colonization processes. In general, the inflammatory response in acute and chronic wounds makes it difficult to determine wound infection visually, and therefore, some other means of diagnosis must be used.

Monitoring And Diagnosis

In the 1950's, Liedberg and his associates showed that when 10^5 bacteria per mL in solutions were delivered to skin graft beds, acceptance of skin grafts did not occur in a normal fashion.[7] In that same era, Elek showed that 10^6 staphylococci would form pustules in normal human skin, and that if an inflammatory response was initiated in the tissue by placement of a foreign body, the numbers of organisms required for pustule formation was significantly reduced.[8] Teplitz and colleagues in a series of landmark studies showed that *Pseudomonas aeruginosa* in numbers greater than 10^5 per gram of tissue in a burn wound was associated with invasion into undamaged, subjacent tissue and was associated with systemic sepsis.[9,10] Teplitz coined the term "burn wound sepsis" in relation to pseudomonas in the burn wound, but this term has been extrapolated, correctly or incorrectly, to encompass all wounds, organisms and patient populations. Robson and his associates, including Krizek and Heggers, have repeatedly reported over the past 20 years that successful wound closure may not be accomplished when wound microorganisms exceed 10^5 per gram of tissue.[11–13] Lookingbill, et al. showed an inverse relationship between wound healing and bacterial counts in chronic leg ulcers.[14] These studies signified the importance of quantifying wound flora and led to the preoccupation with new ways to monitor wounds more rapidly.

The following question remains: Where do these microorganisms come from? The origin of organisms in the wound may provide a clue as to where to monitor. There is evidence that some organisms invade from below the surface by surviving in skin appendages subjacent to the wound while others are delivered from the vasculature and/or lymphatics in acute wounds through translocation[15] from the gut. In other words, not all organisms reach the surface of the wound by aerosol or direct contact. Gut translocation of bacteria to chronic wounds has not been shown.

What is the best way to monitor wounds? When should one perform cultures? Is it more proper to biopsy or to swab a wound to determine the level of wound flora? This argument of swab versus biopsy has persisted for a long time, and the answer may be either or both, depending upon the level of information required and the type of wound being monitored.

Indications for wound culturing in either acute or chronic wounds are similar. Changes in the wound appearance or in the appearance of the surrounding tissue are good indicators. The visual indicators mentioned previously are useful, as are changes in wound color (black, green, etc.) and wound odor. In the acute setting, wound infection should be considered in instances where the systemic signs of sepsis are present without any other obvious cause. Chronic wound guidelines have been published[16] and are useful except that they state flatly that "no swab cultures" should be done. It seems contrary to good sense to biopsy a wound that has compromised perfusion and oxygenation when those biopsies only serve to enlarge such wounds. If performed properly, useful treatment information may be obtained by swab culture.

The following techniques are the most common methods used to monitor wound microbial flora and to determine soft tissue infection or colonization. It should be noted that chronic wounds, in some cases, may progress to affect underlying bone and cause osteomyelitis. It is beyond the scope of this chapter to review those diagnostic tests, such as roentgenogram MRI,[111] In labeled white blood cells or ^{99m}Tc bone scans. However, the biopsy techniques mentioned above can be applied to bone.[16,17]

The swab. The swab is one of the oldest techniques for wound monitoring and is attributed to Councilmen who used the technique to monitor diphtheria patients in 1893.[18] This technique may be divided into two types: the quantitative and the non–quantitative swab. For the purposes of quantifying wound flora, the swab must be moved over a known surface area of the wound and agitated in a known amount of growth media for a specified time period before a known amount of the diluting fluid is transferred to agar for culture.[19,20] The information is expressed as bacteria per square centimeter (cm^2) of surface area. Georgiade, et al. noted the importance of using a pre–moistened swab and demonstrated no statistically significant differences between the quantitative swab and other quantitative assessment techniques.[20] The informational, non–quantitative swab is merely rolled across the wound and then across the agar plate and streaked for isolation of individual colonies. This technique provides information as to types and distribution of microorganisms present.

In a survey of 60 burn centers, Taddonio, et al. reported that the majority continued to survey wounds using the swab technique,[21] although the literature suggested that the biopsy was the "gold standard." This same group also showed that there was a direct correlation between information obtained by swab and by biopsy in 150 burn wounds monitored by both techniques.[22] The swab, however, does not answer the question of colonization versus invasion into viable tissue, and there are those investigators who believe that if invasion does not occur, then numbers of organisms in tissue is immaterial. The swab, however, does provide a handle with which to grasp the information of bacterial type and burden in the wound, a means to anticipate problems in wound healing, and an aid to direct appropriate treatment regimens.

The quantitative biopsy. The quantitative wound biopsy culture became popular in the 1960's, and its use was stimulated by the work of Teplitz, et al.[10,11] Early use of this technique was limited to the evaluation of burn wounds, but it has since become a popular tool in a variety of surgical applications.[25–27] The procedure involves obtaining a tissue sample from a representative area(s) of the wound either by punch biopsy or by freehand excision with a scalpel. Prior to obtaining the biopsy, the wound should be cleaned with mild soap and water rinse, followed by 70 percent isopropyl alcohol and sterile saline rinse.[28] This cleaning procedure will minimize the number of surface microorganisms and eliminate any topical antimicrobial agents. The tissue is handled by

---

The finding of organisms within tissue may represent an active process of progressive infection which may require more aggressive treatments than those used for colonized wounds.

The capillary gauze. The capillary gauze technique described by Brentano and Gravens[23] is a more cumbersome technique than the swab but employs the same principle, namely, the direct physical contact of a moist, absorbent material (gauze) to a known area of wound for a specified time. Microorganisms from the wound are drawn into the gauze and can be extracted into sterile diluent and plated onto culture media for enumeration and identification. While this technique is reported to provide reproducible results,[24] it is limited to the evaluation of surface flora, and recent reports of its use have been scarce.

The contact plate. The contact plate technique involves the use of a special culture dish (RODAC plate) configured so that the sterile agar growth media protrudes above the rim of the plate. This configuration allows the growth media to be placed in direct contact with a known surface area of the wound and eliminates any intermediate dilution and transfer procedures. After incubation, the microbial colonies corresponding to individual organisms can be counted with the aid of the cm^2 grid etched into the bottom of each culture plate. Again, this technique will only provide information about the wound surface flora. It is impractical because any significant burden of organisms will cause a confluent blanket of growth over the entire surface of the plate, making isolation of individual colonies and quantification impossible. These contact plates may be more appropriately used to monitor environmental surfaces.

aseptic technique, and if a histology examination is to be performed, (see below) the specimen is divided approximately in half. The sample for quantification is weighed, placed in a sterile tissue grinder with a known volume of diluent and homogenized to free microorganisms from the tissue matrix. The homogenate is serially diluted, and a known quantity of each dilution is placed onto culture media. After incubation, colonies are enumerated and identified. Because the weight of the biopsy and dilution arithmetic is known, the determination of organisms/gram of tissue is easily calculated:

$$\text{Number of colonies} \times \text{Dilution} / \text{Biopsy weight (grams)} = \text{Organisms/gram tissue}$$

The advantage of the quantitative wound biopsy is that it evaluates for the presence of microorganisms within tissue as opposed to methods that evaluate surface colonization. The finding of organisms within tissue may represent an active process of progressive infection which may require more aggressive treatments than those used for colonized wounds. Investigators have shown a correlation between the quantitative biopsy technique and the quantitative swab;[22] however, there are some who question the validity of the quantitative wound biopsy to accurately assess the condition of the wound.[29] Volenec, et al. have performed a statistical analysis of the biopsy procedure and concluded that it is a reliable procedure to quantify wound organisms and that changes in sequential sampling give an indication of the dynamics of the infection process.[30] The quantitative wound biopsy continues to enjoy widespread use, but it should be noted that these punch wounds have been slow to heal in some chronic wound patient populations.[31] Chronic wound patients with underlying tissue or vascular deficiencies may require alternative monitoring methods. No chronic wound studies have been performed to determine if there is a correlation between the swab and biopsy techniques.

The rapid slide. The previously described wound monitoring techniques involve the growth and isolation of organisms on culture media over 24 to 48 hours. This delay from sample collection to reporting of results may impact patient care, especially when related to grafting or primary wound closure. Heggers[32,33] and Robson[13] described a rapid method to evaluate the microbial load in wounds using a quantitative gram stain technique. The technique was originally performed in conjunction with the quantitative biopsy described above. The rapid slide technique involves taking a known amount of ground biopsy homogenate and spreading it over a known area of a glass microscope slide. The sample is allowed to dry and is heat fixed, stained by the standard Gram method and evaluated by oil immersion light microscopy. The average number of organisms per field of view is determined after viewing multiple fields. In general, the presence of one or more organisms per field is prognostic of 10^5 or greater organisms per gram of tissue. The more organisms observed per field, the greater the precision to predict $> 10^5$ organisms per gram of tissue. The time from specimen collection to reporting can be as short as 10 to 15 minutes. Although organism identification cannot be made using this technique alone, organism morphology and staining characteristics can be discerned. It should be noted that gram–negative organisms are difficult to discern from the background tissue debris which tends to stain the same color. Nevertheless, this technique can be an effective tool and has been used to provide rapid clinical guidance for wound closure and treatment options.[34]

The histologic biopsy. The histologic biopsy involves the preparation and staining of thin sections of wound tissue biopsy samples. The sample may be half of the biopsy obtained for quantitative purposes or may be acquired solely for the purpose of histo-pathology. This technique has the advantage of microscopically assessing the invasion of microorganisms into viable tissue underlying the wound. In large wounds involving greater than 20 percent of the body surface area, or in the immuno-compromised host, the invasion of microorganisms into viable tissue can signify imminent systemic sepsis and its associated dire consequences. The value of the histologic biopsy for the management of burn wound infections has been described by several investigators.[35–38] The rapid technique used to make these permanent histologic specimens takes about four hours[38] and requires the services of a trained pathologist. Kim, et al. reported the development of a frozen tissue section technique that decreased the evaluation time to 30 minutes,[39] but it requires specialized equipment as well as a trained pathologist. These techniques will identify invasion if the appropriate wound area is chosen for monitoring. However, these techniques will not identify organism or determine susceptibility and, therefore, must be accompanied by one of the previously described culture techniques. The complexity and expense of this technique is not practical for most clinical settings where cost containment is a consideration.

Organisms

Chronic wounds generally harbor a mixed flora of aerobic and anaerobic, gram positive and gram negative origin. In a study of non–insulin–dependent diabetes mellitus (NIDDM) patients by Wheat, et al., *Staphylococcus aureus* accounted for approximately 64 percent of foot ulcer isolates. *Streptococcus* species were the next most prevalent organism (30 percent), followed by *Enterococcus* (26 percent).[40] *Peptococcus* species were the most common anaerobe (36 percent) in this study, followed by *Bacteroides* species (18 percent) and *Clostridium* (6 percent). Fifteen percent of all cultures contained anaerobic bacteria, and 60 percent contained more than one organism.

A recent multi–center study of 97 mixed chronic wounds from four centers found 63 different organisms (44 aerobic and 18 anaerobic) populating the tissue.[41] These swab cultures showed a mixture of normal skin flora with opportunistic pathogens such as *Staphylococcus aureus* (61 percent), *Enterococcus* (36 percent), *Streptococcus* (34 percent), *Proteus* (24 percent) and *Pseudomonas* (21 percent). Anaerobic bacteria were led by *Bacteroides* species (45 percent) and followed by *Peptostreptococcus* (24 percent).

Hutchinson reported heavy colonization as measured by quantitative swab cultures for a prospective study of leg ulcers (70 percent had $>10^5$ organisms per gram of wound fluid). However, he also reported an infection rate of only 5.38 percent under conventional dressings.[42] This rate compares favorably with his retrospective review showing ulcers to have an infection rate of 6.5 percent under conventional dressings.[43]

Outcome

In the aforementioned NIDDM study that spanned three years, 103 patients had 131 infections that included cellulitis, osteomyelitis, necrotizing cellulitis or fasciitis and abscess.[38] More than half of these patients required an amputation, and the average hospital length of stay was 22 days at a cost of $6,600 per patient. If one considers that there are at least 1.5 million pressure ulcers, 900,000 diabetic ulcers and 600,000 venous stasis ulcers to be treated in the United States alone,[44] and that approximately six percent will become infected with associated morbidity and mortality, then 180,000 infections would result in almost four million hospital days at a cost of approximately 1.2 billion dollars. As the population ages over the next 10 to 15 years, the numbers are expected to increase.

...it would serve us well to better understand the relationships between the chronic wound, the organisms they contain and the mechanisms to prevent infection and promote wound healing.

In light of these statistics, it would serve us well to better understand the relationships between the chronic wound, the organisms they contain and the mechanisms to prevent infection and promote wound healing. As time progresses, even a one or two percent chronic wound infection rate may not be affordable.

References

1. Mertz PM, Ovington LG. Wound healing microbiology. *Derm Clin* 1993;11:739–747.
2. Till GO, Guilds LS, Mahrougui M, et al. Role of xanthine oxidase in thermal injuruy of skin. *Am J Pathol* 1989;135:195–202.
3. Woolliscroft JO, Prasad JK, Thomson PD, et al. Metabolic alterations in burn patients: Detection of adenosine triphosphate degradation products and lipid peroxides. *Burns* 1990;16:92–96.
4. Thomson PD. Host defenses: basic physiology and management. In: Bartlett RH, Whitehouse WM, Turcotte JG (eds). *Life Support Systems in Intensive Care.* Chicago, IL, Yearbook Medical Publishers, 1984, p 179.
5. Baxter CR. Immunologic reactions in chronic wounds. *Am J Surg* 1994;167:12S–14S.
6. Schroder JM. Peptides and cytokines. *Arch Dermatol Res* 1992;284:S22–S26.
7. Liedberg NCF, Kuhn LR, Barnes BA, et al. Infection in burns. I. The problem and evaluation of therapy. *Surg Gynec Obstet* 1954;98:535–540.
8. Elek SD. Experimental staphylococcal infections in the skin of man. *Ann NY Acad Sci* 1956;65:85–90.
9. Teplitz C, Davis D, Mason AD, Moncrief JA. Pseudomonas burn wound sepsis. I. Pathogenesis of experimental burn wound sepsis. *J Surg Res* 1964;4:200–216.
10. Teplitz C, Davis D, Walker HL, et al. Pseudomonas burn wound sepsis. II. Hematogenous infection at the junction of the burn wound and unburned hypodermis. *J Surg Res* 1964;4:217–222.
11. Krizek TJ, Robson MC, Kho E. Bacterial growth and skin graft survival. *Surg Forum* 1967;XVIII:518.
12. Robson MC, Lea CE, Dalton JB, Heggers JP. Quantitative bacteriology and delayed wound closure. *Surg Forum* 1968;XIX:501–502.
13. Robson MC, Duke WF, Krizek TJ. Rapid bacterial screening in the treatment of civilian wounds. *J Surg Res* 1973;14:420–430.
14. Lookingbill DP, Miller SH, Knowles RC. Bacteriology of chronic leg ulcers. *Arch Dermatol* 1978;114:1765–1768.
15. Deitch EA, Specian RD, Berg RD. Endotoxin–induced bacterial translocation and mucosal permeability: role of xanthine oxidase, complement activation and macrophage products. *Crit Care Med* 1991;19:785–791.
16. U.S. Department of Health and Human Services. Quick Reference Guide for Clinicians – Number 15. Pressure Ulcer Treatment. AHCPR Publication No. 95–0653, 1994, p 18.
17. Ayton M. Infection control and chronic wounds. *Nursing Standard* 1991;5:30–33.
18. Levine NS, Lindberg RB, Mason AD, Pruitt BA. The quantitative swab culture and smear: A quick, simple method for determining the number of viable aerobic bacteria on open wounds. *J Trauma* 1976;16:89–94.
19. Georgiade NG, Lucas MC, O'Fallonn WM, Osterhout S. A comparison of methods for quantification in burn wounds. *Am J Clin Pathol* 1970;53:35–39.
20. Taddonio TE, Thomson PD, Smith DJ, Prasad JK. A survey of wound monitoring and topical antimicrobial therapy practices in the treatment of burn injury. *J Burn Care Rehabil* 1990;11:423–427.
21. Thomson PD, Taddonio TE, Tait MJ, et al. Correlation between swab and biopsy for the quantification of burn wound microflora. *Proc Int Cong Burn Inj* 1990;8:381.
22. Brentano L, Gravens DL. A method for the quantification of bacteria in burn wounds. *Appl Microbiol* 1967;15:670.
23. Edlich RF, Rodeheaver GT, Spengler M, et al. Practical monitoring of the burn victim. *Clin Plast Surg* 1977;4:561–569.
24. Robson MC, Shaw RC, Heggers JP. The reclosure of postoperative incisional abscesses based on bacterial quantification of the wound. *Ann Surg* 1970;171:279–282.
25. Marshall KA, Edgerton MT, Rodeheaver GT, et al. Quantitative microbiology: Its application to hand injuries. *Am J Surg* 1976;131:730–733.
26. Tobin GR. Closure of contaminated wounds. *Surg Clin N Am* 1984;64:639–652.
27. Woolfrey B, Fox J, Quall C. An evaluation of burn wound microbiology: I. Quantitative eschar cultures. *Am J Clin Pathol* 1981;75:532–537.
28. Lobel EC, Marvin JA, Heck EL, et al. The method of quantitative burn–wound biopsy cultures and its routine use in the treatment of burned patients. *Am J Clin Pathol* 1974;61:21–24.

THOMSON AND TADDONIO

29. Volenec FJ, Clark GM, Mani MM, et al. Burn wound biopsy bacterial quantitation: A statistical analysis. *Am J Surg* 1979;138:695.

30. Nemeth AJ, Eaglstein WH, Taylor JR, et al. Faster healing and less pain in skin biopsy sites treated with an occlusive dressing. *Arch Derm* 1991;127:1679–1683.

31. Heggers JP, Robson MC, Ristroph J. A rapid method of performing quantitative wound cultures. *Milit Med* 1969;63:666–667.

32. Heggers JP, Robson MC, Doran ET. Quantitative assessment of bacterial contamination of open wounds by a slide technique. *Trans Royal Soc Trop Med Hyg* 1969;63:532–534.

33. Taddonio TE, Thomson PD, Tait MJ, et al. Rapid quantification of bacterial and fungal growth in burn wounds: Biopsy homogenate gram stain versus microbial culture results. *Burns* 1988;14:180–184.

34. Pruitt BA, Foley DF. The use of biopsies in burn patient care. *Surgery* 1973;73:887–897.

35. Neal GD. Burn wound histologic cultures: A new technique for predicting burn wound sepsis. *J Burn Care Rehabil* 1981;2:35–39.

36. McManus WF, Goodwin CW, Mason AD, Pruitt BA. Burn wound infection. *J Trauma* 1981;21:753–756.

37. Parks DH, Linares HA, Thomson PD. Surgical management of burn wound sepsis. *Surg Gynecol Obstet* 1981;153:374–376.

38. Kim SH, Hubbard GB, McManus WF, et al. Frozen section technique to evaluate early burn wound biopsy: A comparison with the rapid section technique. *J Trauma* 1985;25:1134–1137.

39. Eckman MH, Greenfield S, Mackey WC, et al. Foot infections in diabetic patients. Decision and cost–effective analysis. *JAMA* 1995;273:712–720.

40. Wheat LJ, Stephen DA, Henry M, et al. Diabetic foot infections. Bacteriologic analysis. *Arch Int Med* 1986;146:1935–1940.

41. Thomson PD. Wound Microbiology. *WOUNDS* 1994;7:58–61.

42. Hutchinson JJ. A prospective clinical trial of wound dressings to investigate the rate of infection under occlusion. In: *Proceedings. Advances in Wound Management*. London, England, MacMillan, 1993, pp 93–96.

43. Hutchinson JJ, McGuckin M. Occlusive dressings: A microbiologic and clinical review. *Am J Infection Control* 1990;18:257–268.

44. The Genesis Report: The wound care market. September/October 1992, p 12.

12

Infection Control Perspectives

Sue Crow, RN, MSN

Crow S. Infection control perspectives. In: Krasner D, Kane D. *Chronic Wound Care, Second Edition*. Wayne, PA, Health Management Publications, Inc., 1997, pp 90–96.

Introduction

Mr. Johnathon White, an elderly male with diabetes, entered a community hospital for a removal of his gallbladder. While he was hospitalized he developed a nosocomial pneumonia and then a pressure ulcer. Treatment of the pneumonia consisted of several antibiotics. Soon after, his pressure ulcer became infected with a total resistant bacteria identified as *Enterococcus*. When his Medicare ran out, he was discharged with follow–up via home healthcare. In due time, with the appropriate medication, nutrition, and nursing care, he became free of the resistant microbe and his pressure ulcer eventually healed.

A similar scenario is occurring every day. It is important to recognize that patients and healthcare workers are at risk for infection in any healthcare environment which now includes the patient's home. The patient's skin is his number one defense against infection. When the skin is not intact this primary protection is shattered and he is at added risk for infection. Healthcare workers with broken skin, especially on their hands, are also at increased risk for infection. Methods of reducing cross-contamination for both the patient and healthcare worker will be reviewed in this chapter.

Colonization vs. Infection

Microbes are everywhere, they colonize the body and the environment. Colonization is defined as the presence of microbes without infection. The skin, especially body orifices are heavily colonized with microbes.[1] Fewer microbes are present deep within the body. For example, the heart, lungs, and bloodstream are sterile, while moist areas such as the mouth and nasal passages are colonized with many microbes.

The naso–pharynx is also colonized with many of the same microbes found in the nasal passages and mouth. At any given time, 20 to 40 percent of healthcare workers are colonized with *Staphylococcus aureus* in their noses. Fewer microbes are present farther into the respiratory tract. For example, the sinuses, trachea, bronchi, and lungs are considered sterile. Cultures from these normally sterile areas often are considered contaminated because they are retrieved through the heavily colonized mouth or nose. For example, even though the lungs are considered sterile, it is common to find microbes such as *staphylococci* in a sputum culture. This is because the specimen is contaminated as it passes through the mouth.

Infection occurs when the tissue is invaded and destruction of the cells occurs. Healthcare workers must understand the difference between colonization and infection because their actions will differ depending on the situation. Chapter 11 on wound infection by Philip D. Thomson and Thomas E. Taddonio further explores the concept of infection.

Some experts in pressure ulcer care[2] do not recommend culturing pressure ulcers via the traditional swab method because these ulcers will always be colonized but not necessarily infected. They recommend cultures be obtained by needle aspiration or biopsy only. While this is the preferred method to differentiate between colonization and infection, it may be impractical in some situations. For example, many nursing homes may not be successful in obtaining a physician's assessment of the patient much less having the physician perform this procedure. From a patient's perspective, the expense and pain involved in these procedures must also be considered. While culture of a pressure ulcer via a routine swab is not the most efficient method of collection, it may be helpful in an epidemiological workup where there is an outbreak investigation. If a swab culture is done, the wound is first cleaned, removing the purulent drainage and debris and swabbing the reddened area. Microbes are not found in purulent drainage since the drainage is the aftermath of the battle between the microbe and man. The battle continues in the indurated tissue and this is where the culture should be taken. Chapter 14 on infection and culturing by Brian Gilchrest discusses this issue in more detail. The transportation of the culture from the patient to the lab is also important and healthcare workers should be certain that they are in compliance with the individual laboratory's collection protocols.

Routine culturing of patients or the environment is unnecessary. Only when personnel know the difference in colonization can this information be useful. Routine culturing can cause unnecessary concern and be a waste of time and money.

Understanding Microbes

A microbe that is normal flora in one area of the body may become pathogenic (disease producing) when introduced into another area of the body. *Staphylococcus epidermidis*, for example, which is part of the skin's normal microbial flora, can be deadly when it enters the normally sterile bloodstream.

The pathogenicity of a microbe is a balance between the microbe and the susceptibility of its host. When patients are vulnerable, i.e., immunosuppressed, elderly, debilitated, having poor nutrition, chronically ill, their susceptibility to infection is increased regardless of the microbe's strength.

Microbes are becoming more and more resistant to antibiotics. Colonization/infections due to antibiotic–resistant *Klebsiella* pneumonia, multiple-resistant strains of *Serratia marcescens*, highly resistant *Staphylococcus epidermidis*, Methicillin–resistant *Staphylococcus aureus* (MRSA), Methicillin aminoglycocide–resistant *Staphylococcus aureus* (MARSA), and *Vancomycin* resistant *Enterococcus* (VRE) are only a few examples that now plague healthcare institutions.[3]

Recognition of plasmids inside microbes and their ability to cause resistance is important. Although initially weak, these enzyme–producing genes may grow stronger as antibiotics are continued. For example, plasmids containing penicillinase in MRSA existed long before the abuse of penicillin and sometimes even occur without antibiotic overuse.[4] However, many resistant microbes appear in healthcare institutions because of antibiotic over–use.[5,6]

Resistant microbes are often found on the patient or healthcare personnel in either the colonization or infection state. It is interesting that healthcare workers are a major reservoir of these microbes and that these microbes are often found on personnel's hands and in their nose.[7] The nose can become colonized from the common habit of touching the nose with contaminated hands. Studies indicate that nurses, doctors, physical therapists, and respiratory personnel carry resistant microbes more readily than other personnel. In fact, one study showed personnel without direct contact with patients, i.e., housekeeping personnel were colonized with MRSA less than 3 percent of the time.[8,9] Microbes are spread primarily by direct contact — touching the colonized patient and then failing to wash hands before going to the next patient.[10] Both gram–positive and gram–negative microbes are usually not spread by the airborne route.

Most microbes live on man; however, some have found a happy home in the environment.[10] Solutions such as normal saline, antiseptics, and disinfectants are often reservoirs for gram negative organisms, and they easily grow and multiply in these mediums. The significance of multiple–resistant microbes can be deadly in any healthcare institution. Each episode poses a serious threat to all patients and healthcare workers and should be stopped as quickly as possible.

It is difficult to keep current with developments in microbiology. New microbes, bacteria, and viruses are constantly being discovered. To provide a solid foundation for patient care, one must understand the microbial world and be able to interpret culture reports correctly. One must know which microbes are normal in various body sites.[1] This basic knowledge is crucial in making the correct patient–care decisions. Culture reports and sensitivities should be reviewed carefully. Booklets containing information about specific microbes are useful informational tools.[11]

There is usually an increase in the carrier status of microbes when patients are on cortisone or antibiotic therapy. Some people disseminate microbes more than others; however, most microbes fall out from the perineal area. Most resistant microbes colonize the skin for only minutes or hours; however, carrier status may be more lengthy. Application of a topical ointment such as mupirocin to the nose and systemic antibiotics may remove the resistant microbes for a short time.[12] Total bathing, including daily shampooing with an antiseptic, may also be helpful.

Table 1
Universal Aseptic Precautions

	Intervention	Handwashing	Gloves	Other Protective Attire / Gowns & Face Protection — Protecting Patient	Other Protective Attire / Gowns & Face Protection — Protecting Practitioner	Supplies (3x3s, pads etc)	Instruments
1.	Skin cleansing (intact skin and no contact with body fluids)	Yes	No	No	Yes, only if splashing occurs	*Sterile, Maintain as clean	Sterile
2.	Routine dressing change without debridement	Yes	No/Yes**	No	Yes, only if splashing occurs	*Sterile, Maintain as clean	Sterile
3.	Mechanical and/or chemical debridement	Yes	Clean	No	Yes, only if splashing may occur	*Sterile, Maintain as clean	Sterile
4.	Chemical debridement with peeling	Yes	Clean	No	Yes, only if splashing may occur	*Sterile, Maintain as clean	Sterile
5.	Intentional perforation of skin, i.e., surgical debridement	Yes	Sterile	No/Yes*** ***Sterile if needed	Yes, only if splashing may occur	*Sterile, Maintain as sterile	Sterile

*   Items are initially sterile, i.e., large container of 3 x 3s are sterile when opened but can be maintained as clean for future use.
**   Gloves are necessary if body fluids are encountered
***   Intervention determines if gown is necessary
****   Sterile gowns are necessary if debriding large area where possibility exists of contaminating patient's wound.

Aseptic Technique for Wound Intervention

There are several methods of caring for a wound that are addressed in other chapters in this book. The key is that care is indeed given and given conscientiously. It is the healthcare worker's responsibility to keep up–to–date with wound treatment methods and find the most effective one for each patient. Studies show that staff education on pressure ulcer development in elderly hospital patients can make a difference in decreasing pressure ulcers and can save money.[13] This chapter will focus primarily on the technique of wound care.

Chronic wounds are not sterile and can never be expected to be. Microbial colonization of the tissue is inevitable. When tissue is necrotic, it acts as an excellent culture medium for microbes to grow.[14]

One objective of pressure ulcer care is to assure that cross–contamination does not occur. To accomplish this objective, numerous attempts have been made to define the terms "clean technique" and "sterile technique." However, interpretations of these concepts have been confusing and filed with discrepancies, and have failed to define specific patient care practices. Questions persist. Should sterile or clean gloves be worn? Should gowns be worn? Should the supplies be clean or sterile? Instead of debating clean or sterile technique, adoption of a universal practice using the principles of aseptic technique may be more appropriate.

Aseptic technique provides the principles for assuring that cross–contamination does not occur. In fact, aseptic technique is, by definition, the purposeful prevention of the transfer of microbes. Another way to state this is that asepsis is doing what is necessary to assure the treated area does not become contaminated by the healthcare worker. As with clean and sterile techniques, aseptic technique requires that the practitioner know what is sterile, what is clean, and what is dirty. However, healthcare workers must also know what to do to keep these concepts apart and what to do if contamination does occur. The ability to keep these concepts apart and to remedy contamination are what distinguishes aseptic technique from clean and sterile technique. It also allows the healthcare worker a more holistic approach to wound care, which requires much more than simply making a distinction between clean and sterile conditions.

The principles of keeping clean, sterile, and dirty apart and of remedying contamination include technique and a conscientious attitude.[15] The cause of the nosocomial infections may well be attributed more to the attitude of the workers than to their materials. The development of the conscious–careful attitude is the last hope in the house

of healing. Discipline is an integral part of asepsis and the application of discipline depends on integrity.[16] In other words, prevention of cross–infection depends largely on attitude and practice. For example, a container of sterile 3 x 3s can be opened and used for other patients or future use if they are not contaminated by a negligent healthcare worker.

Aseptic practices have always been recognized as protective, for both the patient and the healthcare worker.[17] This is what the Centers for Disease Control and Prevention (CDC) had in mind when they introduced the concept of universal precautions.[18] Universal precautions require that the body fluids of all patients be treated as potentially infectious regardless of individual diagnosis. Aseptic technique is related to universal precautions in that, to be effective, it too must be applied to all wound care regardless of the patient diagnosis; hence, the term, universal aseptic precautions for wound care.[19] This term is thus defined as assuring that all pressure ulcers are handled in a manner so as not to promote contamination for the patient or the healthcare worker. Universal aseptic practices are cost–effective and practical, and provide consistency in the delivery of wound care.

The appropriate aseptic precautions are dictated by the activity and the situation. For example, a stage I ulcer may require only handwashing if no body fluids are encountered. In the framework of universal aseptic technique, pressure ulcer care is divided into five areas of intervention (Table 1). The assessment and the activity defines the aseptic practice.

The level of intervention with pressure ulcers also has implications for the degree of aseptic technique. The most basic level of intervention, skin cleansing, may or may not require other precautions depending on the body fluids encountered. The second level, basic dressing change without debridement, could be provided to Stage I or Stage II ulcers without gloves, if the wound is dry. When slough or eschar is being removed, gloves are indicated. The use of other protective attire is determined by the potential for splash.

Universal Aseptic Precautions

Handwashing. Handwashing is the single most important practice for preventing nosocomial infection; however, this simple practice is most difficult to achieve. Hands should be washed thoroughly for 10 to 15 seconds between each patient and when gloves are removed. An antiseptic soap such as chlorhexidine is used when bacteriostatic actions are needed.

Table 2
Universal Aseptic Precautions Philosophy

- The technique and attitude of the practitioner plays a key role in wound contamination.

- Aseptic technique assures that practitioners do not add more microbes to the wound than are already present.

- The type of intervention dictates the proper technique, reducing the sterile/clean confusion.

- Universal asepsis is appropriate for pressure ulcer care.

Gloves. In certain situations, gloves are worn to protect both the patient and the healthcare worker. Gloves are not necessary for contact with intact skin or if there is no contact with body fluids. Sterile gloves are used when invading the bloodstream; otherwise clean gloves are sufficient. Sterile gloves do not offer more protection than clean gloves. Gloves are removed carefully after each patient care activity is completed and hands are washed.

Gowns. Clean, splash–proof gowns are necessary if splashing may occur. Sterile barrier gowns are usually used only for surgical debridement of large wounds which risk contact with the practitioner.

Face protection. Face protection, such as goggles or a mask, is worn if splashing may occur. Masks are changed when they become moist. They are not left dangling around the neck to later be passed over the mouth.

Supplies. Sterile bulk supplies once opened may be kept in a clean controlled area for use in intervention categories 1 through 4. Sterile supplies must be used in intervention category 5 (Table 1).

Instruments. Instruments used for pressure ulcer care are cleaned thoroughly and sterilized between each patient use. Sterile technique mandates that instruments are kept sterile during use, whereas with clean technique, they are kept clean. Each procedure involves assessment and implementing appropriate nursing action.

Summary of Universal Aseptic Precautions

The level of asepsis should increase as the procedure becomes more invasive. For example, sterile technique is needed for surgical procedures. Clean technique is usually sufficient for local wound care. Whatever technique is used, it is the responsibility of the healthcare worker not to add any more microbes to the wound than are already present. This can be done using either clean or sterile technique. Universal aseptic precautions are summarized in Table 2. The person's skill and knowledge of asepsis are probably as important as the specific technique.

Healthcare Worker Protection

Healthcare workers who work directly with body fluids and where there is excessive splashing or direct exposure to body fluids continuously should be offered the Hepatitis B vaccine. The risk of developing Hepatitis B or Hepatitis C after a direct exposure, such as a needlestick, is increased and should be evaluated by an experienced employee health nurse or physician each time an exposure occurs. Each institution should establish protocols for Hepatitis vaccination, prevention, and exposure.

The influenza vaccine should be given each year to all healthcare workers and patients especially in long term healthcare facilities to avoid the illness and consequent pneumonia risk in the winter months.

Isolation

The CDC encourages healthcare institutions to develop and modify their isolation system to meet their individual needs. Treating all body fluids as potentially infected is the first principle of isolation. Besides using universal precautions, it may be wise to have a formal isolation system since there are diseases spread by methods other than the blood–borne route. The latest CDC recommendations for isolation standards should be reviewed and incorporated into each healthcare institution's specific policy.[20] Isolation must be directed toward the disease and not primarily at placing the patient in a private room.

Control Measures for an Outbreak of Resistant Microbes

When an outbreak of any infectious process occurs, the established protocols should be followed to protect patients and healthcare workers. The control measures will be determined by the microbe and the method of spread.

Isolation should be initiated immediately.[10] The type of isolation will depend on the institution's specific policy. Microbes usually do not travel further than five to six feet from the patient; therefore, a negative pressure room is not necessary. However, air turbulence should be avoided, i.e, making a bed, since the patient sheds microbes onto the sheets.

Sometimes a more strict isolation policy is needed to eliminate resistant microbes from the healthcare institution. In fact, in some outbreaks of MRSA and VRE, "strict" isolation has been necessary to rid the institution of the organism. Strict isolation includes private room, gowns, gloves, masks, handwashing when leaving the room, and strict adherence to technique. Isolation precautions should be continued until the patient is no longer on antibiotics and a minimum of three cultures reveal negative reports.[10]

In an outbreak situation, identification of the infected/colonized patients and personnel is necessary. Culturing patients and personnel may be indicated if there is an epidemiological investigation. The decision of culturing is made by an experienced infection control practitioner.

Disinfection/Sterilization

Instrument decontamination is cleaning an object to reduce the number of microbes.[1] This process is necessary before disinfection or sterilization because the processes cannot be effective unless the item is clean. Decontamination should be carried out in an area designated for cleaning. Personnel should wear gloves, gowns, and goggles to avoid splashing of debris into their eyes or mouth. Keep in mind the following points for appropriate decontamination:

- Decontamination is a dirty procedure and should be done in a controlled area by skilled and experienced personnel.
- An instrument cleaner should be used instead of routine soaps or antiseptics. These products may leave a fill on the item which will protect the microbe during disinfection or sterilization.

- The decontamination method should be the same for all items.

Decontamination is best achieved by washing an item in a washer–decontaminator, but can also be done using an instrument washer or an ultrasonic cleaner or by manually cleaning.

Whichever decontamination method is chosen, the item must indeed be clean before further processing. Decontamination is the first and perhaps the most important step in processing items.

Disinfection kills vegetative microbes, whereas sterilization removes all microorganisms, including spores. Sterility is critical for items that come into contact with normally sterile tissue. Sterility is preferred but not absolutely necessary for items that will come in contact with intact mucous membranes. At minimum, high level disinfection with a gluteraldehyde should be used for such items as laryngoscopes. When an item is used on patients whose mucous membranes are not intact, instruments should be sterile.[1]

Conclusion

More and more resistant microbes will infect the compromised patient population. Healthcare workers must have an understanding of the microbes found in the healthcare institution and how they are transmitted. Patients will suffer if healthcare workers do not exercise skill, common sense, and aseptic practice in all patient care activities. Cross–infection can be prevented by using knowledge of wound care, aseptic technique, and a conscious–careful attitude. The principles of containment and confinement are simple. When they are fully utilized, cross–infection can be eliminated.

References

1. Crow S. Asepsis: *The Right Touch, Something Old is now New*. Bossier City, LA, Everett Publishing Company, 1989.
2. U. S. Department of Health and Human Services, Public Health Service, Agency for Health Care Policy and Research, Treatment of Pressure Ulcers Guideline Panel, Nancy Bergstrom, PhD, RN, FAAN (Chair). *Treatment of Pressure Ulcers*. Clinical Practice Guideline, Number 15. Rockville, Maryland, US Dept of Health and Human Services, AHCPR Publication No. 95-0652, December 1994.
3. Berg R, Multiply-resistant gram negative bacilli: Methods for controlling intrahospital spread, Asepsis. *The Infection Control Forum* 1988:10(3);6-8.
4. Cohen ML. Epidemiology of drug resistant: Implications for a post-antimicrobial era. *Science* 1992;257:1050-1055.
5. Kunin CM, Lipton HL, Tupasi T, Sacks T, Scheckler WE, Jivani A, Goic A, Martin RR, Guerrant RL, Thamlikitkul V. Social, behavioral, and practical factors affecting antibiotic use worldwide. *Reviews of Infectious Diseases*. 1987;9(Suppl. 3):70-S285.
6. Kunin CM. Resistance to antimicroibal drugs - A worldwide calamity. *Annals of Internal Medicine* 1993;118(7):557-561.

7.	Brumfitt W, Hamilton-Miller J. Methicillin-resistant staphylococcus aureus. *New England Journal of Medicine* 1989:320(18):1188-1196.

8.	Ballou WR, Cross AS, Williams DY, Keiser J, Zierdt CH. Colonization of newly arrived house staff by virulent staphylococcal phage types endemic to a hospital environment. *J Clin Microbiol* 1986;23:1030-3.

9.	Casewell MW, Hill RL. The carrier state: methicillin-resistant staphylococcus aureus. *J Antimicrob Chemother* 1986;12(Suppl A):1-12.

10.	Centers for Disease Control and Prevention. Preventing the spread of vancomycin resistance - Report form the Hospital Infection Control Practices Advisory Committee. 59 Federal Register 25,757 (1994).

11.	Mikat DM, Mikat KW. *A Clinician's Dictionary Guide to Bacteria and Fungi*. Indianapolis, IN, Dista Products Company, 1981.

12.	American Health Consultants. Mupirocin lowers staph carriage but may lead to resistance. *Hospital Infection Control* 1992;19(3):35.

13.	Moody BL, Fanale JE, Thompson M, Vaillancourt D, Symonds G, Bonasoro C. Impact of staff education on pressure sore development in elderly hospitalized patients. *Archives of Internal Medicine* 1988;143:2241-3.

14.	Rudolph R, Noe JM, Sterile technique and wound infection: Sorting truth from fiction. In. Rudolph R, Noe JM (eds). *Chronic Problem Wounds*. Boston, MA, Little, Brown, and Company, 1983, pp 19–27.

15.	Brown, AF, Otterman JL. The coccus-conscious or the conscious-careful. *Infection Control* J 1987,8(1):34-35.

16.	Laufman H. Infection control: A moral issue. *Today's OR Nurse* 1983;6(9):38-45.

17.	Beck WC. Two-way asepsis. Complications in Surgery 1991;10(5):4–5.

18.	U.S. Department of Health and Human Services, Centers for Disease Control. Update: Universal precautions for prevention of transmission of human immunodeficiency virus, hepatitis B virus, and other bloodborne pathogens in health-care settings. *Morbidity and Mortality Weekly Report* 1988;37(24):377-384,387-388.

19.	Crow S. Universal aseptic precautions for pressure ulcers. *Nursing 95* 1995;volume?: pages?

20.	Department of Health and Human Services, Centers for Disease Control and Prevention. Draft Guideline for Isolation Precautions in Hospital; Notice. Federal Register. November 7, 1994;10(5):4-5.

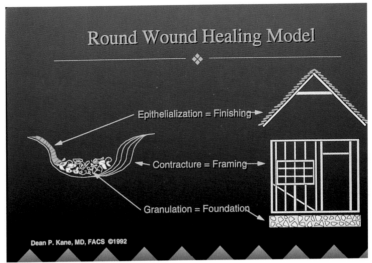

Plate 1. *Kane's Wound Healing Analogy. Chapters 1, 30. Courtesy of Dean Kane, MD, FACS.*

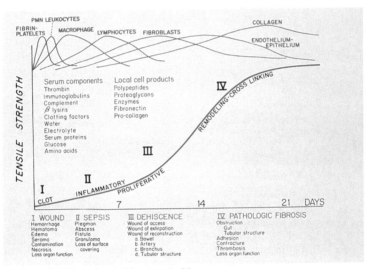

Plate 2. *Schilling chart. Chapters 1, 30. Courtesy of Dean Kane, MD, FACS.*

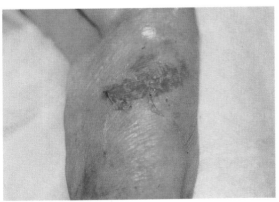

Plate 3. *Partial thickness skin tear. Chapter 1. Courtesy of Diane Krasner, MS, RN, CETN.*

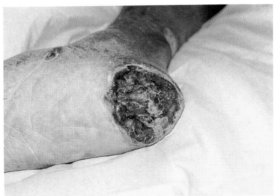

Plate 4. *Full thickness heel ulcer. Chapter 1. Courtesy of Diane Krasner, MS, RN, CETN.*

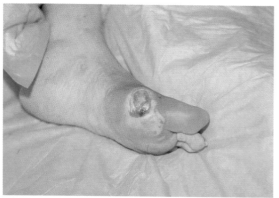

Plate 5. *Diabetic foot ulcer. Chapter 1.*
Courtesy of Diane Krasner, MS, RN, CETN.

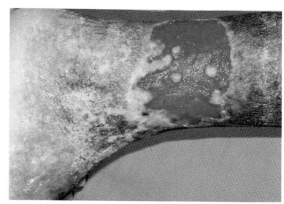

Plate 6. *Venous ulcer. Chapter 1.*
Courtesy of Dean Kane, MD, FACS.

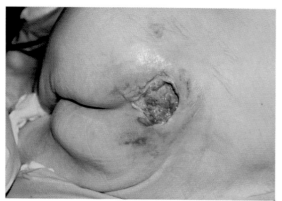

Plate 7. *Infected sacral pressure ulcer. Chapter 1.*
Courtesy of Diane Krasner, MS, RN, CETN.

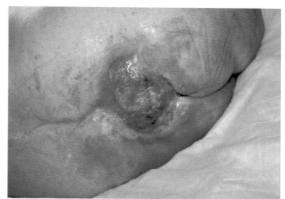

Plate 8. *Sacral pressure ulcer complicated by candidia-*
sis. See Plates 35, 36, 37 for reconstruction of this ulcer.
Chapter 1. Courtesy of Diane Krasner, MS, RN, CETN.

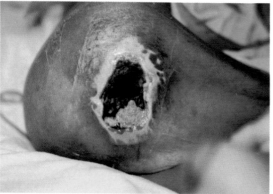

Plate 9. *Trochanteric pressure ulcer with eschar.*
Chapter 1. Courtesy of Diane Krasner, MS, RN, CETN.

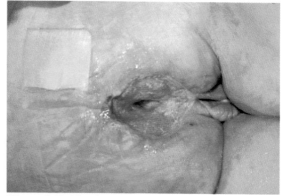

Plate 10. *Dehisced surgical wound following abdomi-*
no–perineal resection for cancer of the rectum.
Chapter 1. Courtesy of Diane Krasner, MS, RN, CETN.

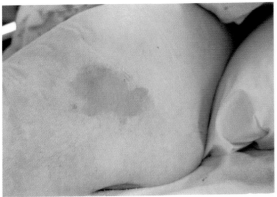

Plate 11. *Stage 1 trochanteric pressure ulcer. Chapter 18.*

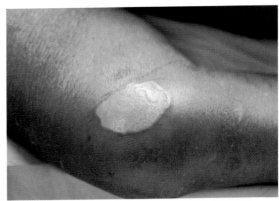

Plate 12. *Stage 2 pressure ulcer over knee. Chapter 18.*

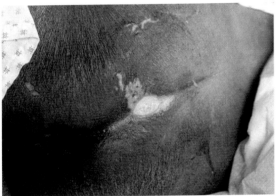

Plate 13. *Stage 3 sacral pressure ulcer. Chapter 18.*

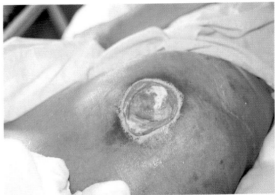

Plate 14. *Stage 4 trochanteric pressure ulcer. Chapter 18.*

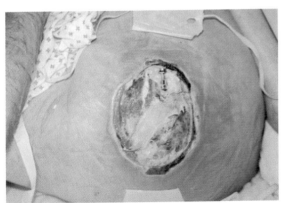

Plate 15. *Stage 4 trochanteric pressure ulcer with slough in the wound bed, and hip replacement hardware visible, prior to debridement. Chapter 18.*

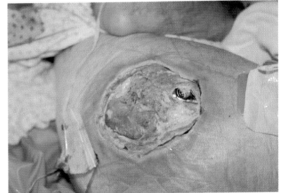

Plate 16. *Ulcer from Plate 16 following sharp debridement at the patient's bedside. Chapter 18.*

All photos on this page courtesy of Diane Krasner, MS, RN, CETN.

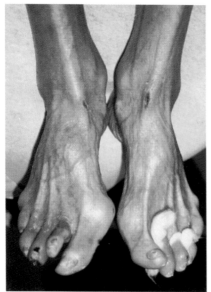

Plate 17. *Arterial feet. Chapter 19.*
Courtesy of G. Allen Holloway, MD.

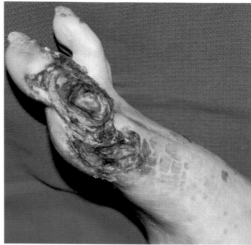

Plate 18. *Wound infection. Chapter 27.*
Courtesy of Bonnie Sue Rolstad, RN, BA, CETN
and Ann H. Harris, MSN, RN, CS

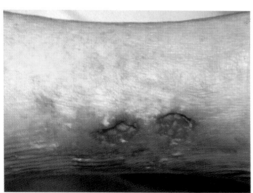

Plate 19. *Pain control. Chapter 27.*
Courtesy of Bonnie Sue Rolstad, RN, BA, CETN
and Ann H. Harris, MSN, RN, CS

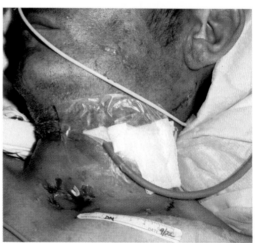

Plate 20. *Exudate management. Chapter 27.*
Courtesy of Bonnie Sue Rolstad, RN, BA, CETN
and Ann H. Harris, MSN, RN, CS

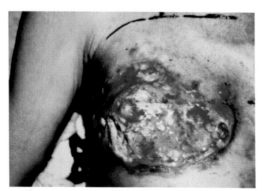

Plate 21. *Odor control. Chapter 27.*
Courtesy of Bonnie Sue Rolstad, RN, BA, CETN
and Ann H. Harris, MSN, RN, CS

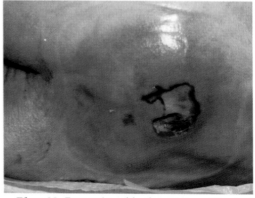

Plate 22. *Prevention of further reinjury. Chapter 27.*
Courtesy of Bonnie Sue Rolstad, RN, BA, CETN
and Ann H. Harris, MSN, RN, CS

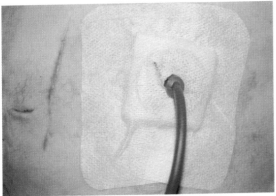

Plate 23. *Foam dressing and silicone disc with stretch tape stabilizing tube. Chapter 26.*

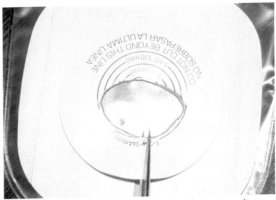

Plate 24. *Pouching over a tube with a large opposite or free end. Chapter 26.*

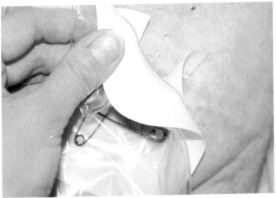

Plate 25. *Pouching over a tube with a drain with pins. Chapter 26.*

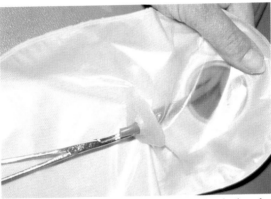

Plate 26. *Exiting tube through a pouch using hydrocolloid buttons. Chapter 26.*

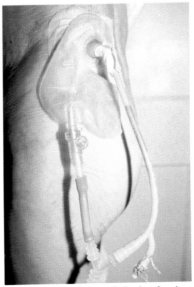

Plate 27. *Attaching a baby bottle nipple to a pouch with an upside down "convex flange" insert. Chapter 26.*

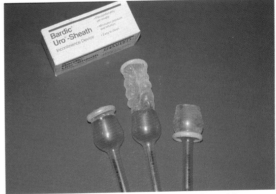

Plate 28. *Draining internal vaginal fistulae with a Bard® Uro–Sheath. Chapter 26.*

All photos on this page courtesy of Nancy Faller, RN, MSN, CETN.

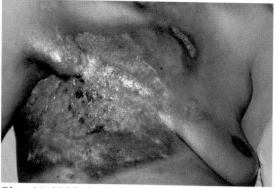

Plate 29. *STSG of radiation treated radical masectomy chest wall defect for breast cancer. Chapter 30.*

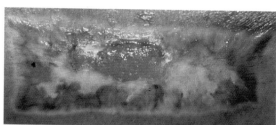

Plate 30. *Slow healing STSG thigh donor site with hypertrophic granulation tissue. Chapter 30.*

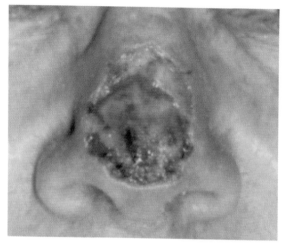

Plate 31. *Nasal defect from basal cell carcinoma excision. Chapter 30.*

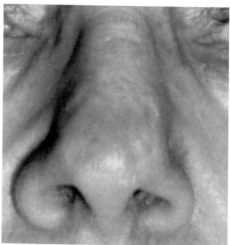

Plate 32. *FTSG reconstruction of nasal skin. Chapter 30.*

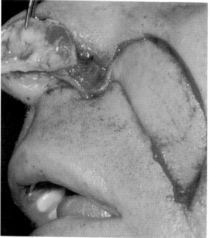

Plate 33. *(left) Nasal skin and cartilage defect following basal cell carcinoma excision. Chapter 30.*

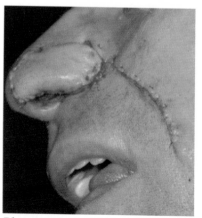

Plate 34. *Nasolabial flap and supporting cartilage reconstruction of nasal defect. Chapter 30.*

All photos on this page and the next page courtesy of Dean Kane, MD, FACS.

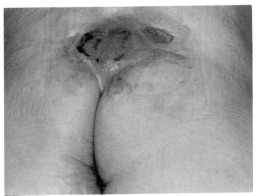

Plate 35. *Non–healing Stage 4 sacral pressure ulcer, cleared of candidasis (see Plate 8) and ready for reconstruction. Chapter 30.*

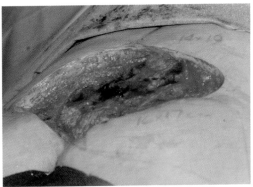

Plate 36. *Acute wound following ulcer excision and ostectomy. Chapter 30.*

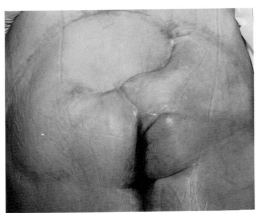

Plate 37. *Left gluteal rotation and right gluteal V–Y myocutaneous flap reconstruction. Chapter 30.*

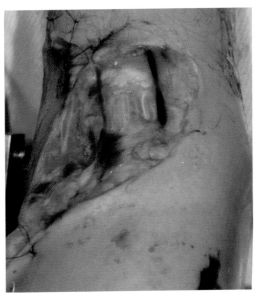

Plate 38. *Lawn mower injury to the right ankle. Chapter 30.*

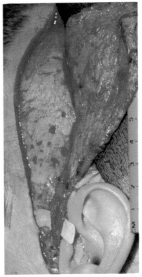

Plate 39. *Harvesting a temporalis fascia flap from the face for the ankle repair. Chapter 30.*

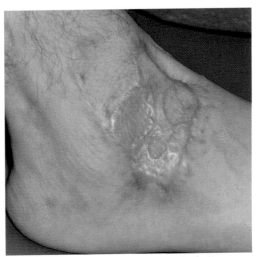

Plate 40. *Completed reconstruction, including STSG. Chapter 30.*

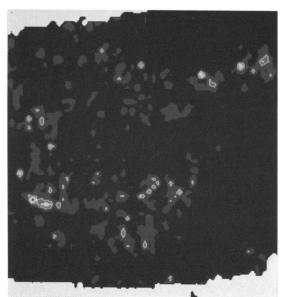

Plate 41. *Laser doppler imaging of patient #1 seen here at baseline. Chapter 41.*
Courtesy of William J. Ennis, DO.

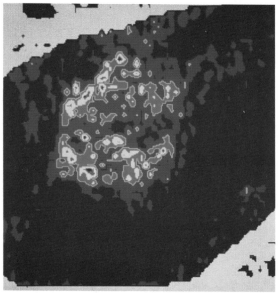

Plate 42. *Laser doppler imaging seen here 1 week after hydrocolloid therapy and compression in patient #1. Chapter 41.*
Courtesy of William J. Ennis, DO.

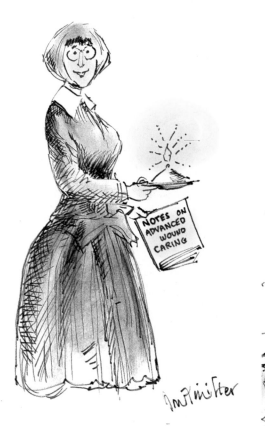

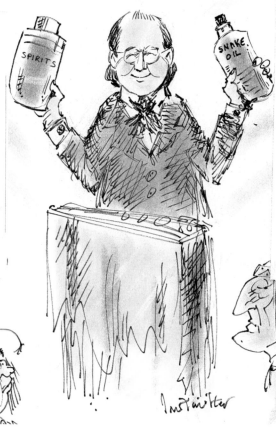

Section II

MANAGEMENT

13

Wound Cleansing, Wound Irrigation, Wound Disinfection

George T. Rodeheaver, PhD

Rodeheaver GT. Wound cleansing, wound irrigation, wound disinfection. In: Krasner D, Kane D. *Chronic Wound Care, Second Edition*. Wayne, PA, Health Management Publications, Inc., 1997, pp 97–108.

Introduction

Wound cleansing is one of the most important components of an effective wound management protocol. Optimal wound healing can not occur until all inflammatory foreign bodies have been removed from the wound. In its broadest sense, wound cleansing can encompass aggressive debridement of all devitalized tissue, extensive use of fluids for cleansing and selective use of topical antimicrobial agents to control bacterial contamination. Each of these steps is essential for obtaining a clean, vital wound that has the greatest potential for healing at an optimum rate. However, in its strictest meaning, wound cleansing is the use of fluids to gently remove loosely adherent contaminants and devitalized material from the wound surface. If the materials cannot be removed gently with fluids then more specific mechanical techniques are required. These mechanical techniques are termed "debridement." For further information on debridement refer to Chapter 29.

Wound cleansing is the process of using fluids to remove inflammatory contaminants from the wound surface. The benefits of obtaining a clean wound must be weighed against the trauma to the wound that results from the cleansing. Wound cleansing is a mechanical process that traumatizes the wound. The practitioner must always attempt to minimize wound trauma during wound cleansing. By definition, the wound is already a traumatic insult to the body's integrity, and any additional trauma inflicted in attempts to manage that wound will only delay the reparative process. If contaminants cannot be removed with gentle wound cleansing, then a more specific debridement technique should be employed.

Wound trauma incurred during wound cleansing can be chemical, mechanical or both. Mechanical trauma occurs when the mechanical forces of scrubbing and high pressure irrigation must be absorbed by the delicate wound tissue. Chemical trauma occurs when the fluids used to cleanse wounds contain chemicals that are toxic to the wound tissue. A philosophy to consider is: "Don't do to a wound what you wouldn't do to your own eye." Very few caregivers treat someone else's wound as sensitively as they would treat their own eye. Yet the sensitive care required for your eye is exactly the quality of care required for wounds to optimize their potential for rapid resolution.

Wound Cleansing

Cleansing Solutions. Definitive research on this topic has not yet been published, so the following recommendations are based on the best possible science to date and common sense.

Wound cleansing is the process of using fluids to gently remove inflammatory contaminants from the wound surface. In the majority of cases water or saline is sufficient for cleansing the wound surface; because of the limited contact time between the wound and the cleansing solution it is not essential for wound healing that the solution be isotonic (0.9 percent sodium chloride). For home care, an acceptable saline solution can be made by adding two teaspoons of salt to one liter of boiling water (eight teaspoons per gallon). Any water with

Table 1
Toxicity indexes for sixteen wound or skin cleansers

Cleanser	Intended Primary Use	Toxicity Index
Shur Clens® (ConvaTec®, Princeton, NJ)	Wound	10
Biolex™ (Bard Medical Division, Covington, GA)	Wound	
Saf Clens™ (ConvaTec®, Princeton, NJ)	Wound	100
Cara Klenz™ (Carrington Laboratories, Inc., Irving, TX)	Wound	
Ultra Klenz™ (Carrington Laboratories, Inc., Irving, TX)	Wound	
Clinical Care® (Carrington Laboratories, Inc., Irving, TX)	Wound	1,000
Uni Wash® (Smith & Nephew United, Inc., Largo, FL)	Skin	
Ivory Soap® (0.5%) (Procter & Gamble, Cincinnati, OH)	Skin	
Constant Clens™ (Sherwood – Davis & Geck, St. Louis, MO)	Wound	
Dermal Wound Cleanser (Smith & Nephew United, Inc., Largo, FL)	Wound	
Puri–Clens™ (Coloplast Sween Corp., Marietta, GA)	Wound	10,000
Hibiclens® (Stuart Pharmaceuticals, Wilmington, DE)	Skin	
Betadine® Surgical Scrub (Purdue Frederick, Norwalk, CT)	Skin	
Techni–Care™ Scrub (Care–Tech® Laboratories, St. Louis, MO)	Skin	
Bard Skin™ Cleanser (Bard Medical Division, Covington, GA)	Skin	100,000
Hollister™ Skin Cleanser (Hollister Incorporated, Libertyville, IL)	Skin	

known or suspected contaminants should not be used for this purpose.

When enhanced cleansing efficacy is needed, a commercial wound cleanser can be used. Commercial wound cleansers contain surface–active agents to improve removal of wound contaminants. Surface–active agents (surfactants), by the nature of their chemical structure and chemical charge, help break the bonds of the foreign bodies to the wound surface. The strength of their chemical reactivity is directly proportional to their cleansing capacity and toxicity to cells. Therefore cleansing capacity needs to be balanced against toxicity to wound healing cells.

Surfactants can be categorized according to their chemical charge in solution (cationic, anionic, or non–ionic). Most surfactants with charges and many non–ionic surfactants have been shown to be toxic to cells, delay wound healing, and inhibit the wound's defenses against infection.[1-5] Since the Food and Drug Administration (FDA) does not critically scrutinize the safety and efficacy of wound cleansers, it is the responsibility of the practitioner to select a wound cleansing solution that has been documented by independent testing to be safe for use in open wounds.

Documentation of safety is difficult since standardized tests for wound cleansers have not been established. However, tests that directly compare wound cleansers under controlled conditions can provide useful information on relative safety. One such study ranked the relative toxicity of several commercial wound cleansers based on their relative toxicity to white blood cells.[6] Polymorphonuclear leukocytes (PMNs) were isolated from rabbit blood, exposed for 30 minutes to increasing 1:10 dilutions of the test solutions, then assayed for viability (Trypan blue dye exclusion) and functionality (phagocytic efficiency). The extent of dilution required to provide viability and functionality similar to PMNs exposed to Hanks' Balanced Salt Solution alone was used as the basis of an index of toxicity. If a wound cleansing solution required a 1:1,000 dilution to eliminate its toxicity, then its toxicity index was 1,000. The results that were reported for both wound cleansers and skin cleansers are listed in Table 1.

Cleansers that are formulated to remove fecal contamination from intact skin (skin cleansers) are stronger, and thus more toxic than cleansers that are meant to be used in wounds. Skin cleansers should never be used in wounds. The relative toxicity values listed in Table 1 are based on the results of *in vitro* testing and their clinical relevance has not been determined. In addition, the values of relative toxicity should not be used as a guide for diluting the commercial wound cleanser. The commercial wound cleanser should be used at its recommended strength. The toxicity index is only a guide to help in the selection of a commercial wound cleansing agent.

A similar *in vitro* test of cleanser toxicity was conducted using fibroblasts.[7] Monolayers of cultured fibroblasts were exposed to dilutions of the various cleansers for 15 minutes and cell viability was determined by cell uptake of fluorescein diacetate. The results were very similar to those reported in Table 1.

A third study utilized human fibroblasts, red blood cells, and white blood cells as test cells for several wound cleansers.[8] This study involved Constant–Clens™, Shur–Clens®, Saf–Clens™, Cara–Klenz™, and Ultra–Klenz™. The relative results were somewhat different than those shown in Table 1. Constant–Clens was found to be the most biocompatible cleanser tested and Shur–Clens to be the worst. Analysis of the Shur–Clens tested indicated that it did not meet the manufacturer's specification on pH which accounted for its unexpected toxicity. The relative results for the other cleansers were similar to those reported in Table 1.

Many wound cleansers contain an antimicrobial agent such as benzethonium chloride (0.1 percent) or benzalkonuim chloride (0.1 percent). Preliminary studies, using the previously described model,[6] have indicated that the presence of these antiseptic agents in the wound cleanser result in a relative toxicity index of 10,000. The benefit of adding the antiseptic agent to the wound cleanser has not been documented.

Scrubbing Devices. The efficacy of wound cleansing solutions can be enhanced by using a scrubbing device such as a cloth, sponge, or brush. Whenever these devices are used, the user must realize that mechanical trauma is being imparted to the wound. It is essential to minimize this trauma by using nonabrasive devices and as little force as necessary to achieve appropriate cleansing. If the desired cleansing is not achieved with moderate force, then other means of wound cleansing should be considered. One should not try to cleanse the wound by increasing the force applied to the scrubbing device.

Saline has a minimal ability to reduce the frictional forces encountered by the wound tissue from a scrubbing device. The surfactant properties of commercial wound cleansers significantly reduce the coefficient of friction between a scrubbing device and the wound tissue.[9]

The coarseness of the scrubbing device should be as low as possible while still providing cleansing action. Wounds scrubbed with coarse sponges were shown to be significantly more susceptible to infection than less traumatized wounds scrubbed with a smoother sponge.[9]

Wound Irrigation

Wound cleansing can also be accomplished by irrigating the wound with fluid. The hydraulic forces generated by the stream of fluid act on the debris on the wound surface and try to flush it from the wound. In order to remove the wound debris, the force of the irrigation stream has to be greater than the adhesion forces holding the debris to the wound surface. Therefore, it would be logical to assume that increasing the pressure of the irrigation stream would increase the cleansing efficiency of the irrigation process.

Several studies have documented that increasing the pressure of the irrigating stream enhances removal of bacteria and soil from wounds.[10–12] Pressures up to 25 pounds per square inch (psi) were more effective than lower pressures, especially the very low pressure produced by a bulb syringe. The efficacy of bacterial removal at 15 psi was significantly greater than that achieved at 10 psi. However, increasing the irrigation pressure to 20 or 25 psi did not significantly improve the result obtained with 15 psi.

Irrigation devices that delivered fluid streams at pressures of 70 psi were developed for dental hygiene in the early sixties. It was not long before surgeons suspected that these devices might provide benefit in cleansing contaminated orificial wounds[13] and traumatic wounds in general.[14–16] The use of the mechanical irrigation device at various pressures from 10 psi to 70 psi were shown to be significantly more effective in removing bacteria and debris from wounds when compared to irrigation with a bulb syringe.[16–18] The use of 70 psi was also found to be more effective in removing wound debris than 25 psi or 50 psi.[16] Using quantitative tissue biopsies, irrigation at 50 psi was shown to more effectively remove bacterial contamination than gravity irrigation from a height of 60 to 65 cm or irrigation by bulb syringe.[19–20]

Some results suggest that the pressure of the irrigating stream is the important component, not whether it is pulsatile or continuous. Experimental studies comparing pulsatile or continuous stream irrigation have not documented the superiority of the pulsatile stream.[10,17,18] In addition, these high pressure, pulsatile, irrigation devices are expensive, cumbersome, and "difficult" to maintain sterile. A more practical and convenient way to produce pressurized irrigation is to deliver the irrigant from a syringe through a needle or catheter. It has been shown that delivery of saline from a 35–mL syringe through a 19–gauge needle delivers a stream of irrigant to the wound surface at 8 psi.[21] Plastic tubing or angiocatheters that do not have a point but have the same bore size as a 19–gauge needle would deliver the same pressure of irrigation fluid but would be safer than the needle due to the potential hazard of accidental needle sticks. When compared to irrigation with a bulb syringe, irrigation with a 35–mL syringe and 19–gauge needle resulted in significantly enhanced removal of bacteria and a significantly reduced incidence of wound infection. This experimental benefit has been confirmed in a human study.[22] Three hundred thirty–five patients who presented to the emergency department with traumatic wounds less than 24 hours old were randomly assigned to wound cleansing by standard bulb syringe (controls, low pressure) or a 12–cc syringe and 22–gauge needle (experimental, 13 psi). Two hundred seventy–seven patients (83 percent) returned for wound evaluation; of these, 117 were in the control group and 151 were in the experimental group. In the control group, 27.8 percent of the wounds were inflamed and 6.9 percent were infected. In the experimental group, 16.8 percent of the wounds were inflamed and 1.3 percent were infected. There was a statistically significant decrease in both wound inflammation and wound infection for wounds cleansed with syringe and needle irrigation (13 psi) compared to wounds cleansed with bulb syringe (0.05 psi).

Other combinations of syringes and catheter sizes can also be utilized. In general, as the size of the syringe increases, the pressure decreases because the force applied to the plunger is distributed over a larger cross–sectional area. For example, with a 19–gauge needle the pressures generated by 6–, 12–, and 35–mL syringes are 30, 20, and 8 psi, respectively. In contrast, increasing the size of the needle increases the pressure because there is greater flow. For example, with a 35–mL syringe the pressures generated with a 25–, 21–, and 19–gauge needle are 4, 6, and 8 psi, respectively.

Recently, irrigation of wounds has been made more convenient by the introduction of battery–powered, irrigation systems (Stryker® Instruments, Kalamazoo, MI; Davol Inc., Cranston, RI). These self–contained, sterile systems insert into an IV bag and pump the sterile saline through a choice of tips at elevated irrigation pressures. The fluid is delivered in a pulsatile stream through the tips. The tips are single orifice or multiple orifice and deliver different spray patterns from streams to showers. The spray tips also contain a suction cone and a vacuum line so that the irrigation fluid can be contained and aspirated into a vacuum canister. The impact pressure generated by these new devices is currently being determined. It is assumed that the manufacturers are aware of the concern about exceeding 15 psi and have engineered their devices to deliver irrigation fluid below that level. Since these devices are relatively new, clinical reports of their performance have not yet been published.

Pressurized irrigation can also be accomplished by applying pressure to the IV bag of a standard irrigation set–up.[23,24] In this situation a standard blood pressure cuff is wrapped around the IV bag and inflated to the desired pressure. The pressure of the exiting irrigation stream can be adjusted by increasing or decreasing the pressure on the cuff. However, applying 15 mm Hg pressure to the blood pressure cuff does not mean that the fluid exiting

Table 2
Irrigation pressures delivered by various devices

Device	Irrigation Impact pressure (psi)
Spray Bottle – Ultra Klenz™* (Carrington Laboratories, Inc., Dallas TX)	1.2
Bulb Syringe* (Davol Inc., Cranston, RI)	2.0
Piston Irrigation Syringe (60 mL) with catheter tip (Premium Plastics, Inc., Chicago, IL)	4.2
Saline Squeeze Bottle (250 mL) with irrigation cap (Baxter Healthcare Corp., Deerfield, IL)	4.5
Water Pik® at lowest setting (#1) (Teledyne Water Pik, Fort Collins, CO)	6.0
Irrijet® DS Syringe with tip (Ackrad Laboratories, Inc., Cranford, NJ)	7.6
35 mL syringe with 19–gauge needle or angiocatheter	8.0
Water Pik® at middle setting (#3)† (Teledyne Water Pik, Fort Collins, CO)	42
Water Pik® at highest setting (#5)† (Teledyne Water Pik, Fort Collins, CO)	> 50
Pressurized Canister–Dey–Wash™† (Dey Laboratories, Inc., Napa, CA)	> 50

* These devices may not deliver enough pressure to adequately cleanse wounds.
† These devices may cause trauma and drive bacteria into wounds. They are not recommended for cleansing of soft tissue wounds.

the tip is at 15 psi. Quantitative testing with standardized (type of cuff, size of IV bag, design of irrigation tip, etc.) would be required to know the direct correlation between cuff pressure and irrigation pressure.

Another concept for conveniently delivering pressurized saline to the wound is from a pressurized canister. It is claimed that the saline is delivered in a 19–gauge stream at 8 psi. Data to support this claim were not available. A clinical study comparing this product to bulb syringe suggested that it was effective in cleansing debris and bacteria from the wound in less time and with less expense than the bulb syringe procedure.[25] It was learned that the pressurized canister needed to be 6 inches from the wound, and the stream must contact the wound at a 45 degree angle to minimize splashing. Similar results were reported in another study comparing the pressurized canister to a 30–mL syringe with a 20–gauge IV catheter.[26]

A common problem with all of these innovative techniques for delivering pressurized irrigation fluid is that the manufacturers do not know what impact pressure their system delivers to the wound surface. In the report by Singer, et al.,[23] the pressure they measured was within the system, not what the impact pressure of the exiting fluid was. The studies by Weller[25] and Chisholm, et al.,[26] claim to be at 8 psi but this value is unsubstantiated. In order to begin to obtain this information my laboratory has established a standardized technique to measure the impact pressure generated by these devices when held perpendicular to the target at a distance of 2.54 cm (1").[27] Preliminary results for a few of the new devices are listed in Table 2.

When using pressurized irrigation the practitioner should always be concerned about splashing the irrigation fluid out of the wound. Because of the significant risk of viral contamination from contact with such fluid it is essential to wear protective clothing, gloves and eyewear during the irrigation procedure. In addition the use of splash shields on the irrigation device or over the wound is also recommended. These splash shields have been shown to significantly reduce environmental splatter.[28] For large cavity wounds it may be practical to seal the wound with a transparent film dressing and irrigate through the film to prevent splashing.[29]

Another complication of high–pressure irrigation is dispersion of fluid into the adjacent tissue or along tissue plains.[13,30,31] The extent of this dispersion is related to the magnitude of the pressure. Fluid dispersion into wound tissue was significantly greater for a 70–psi irrigation stream than for an 8–psi irrigation stream.[30] When a single orifice tip was used to irrigate wounds in dogs, there was extensive penetration of the irrigation fluid into the tissue, especially when the pressure was increased above 30 psi.[31] When a multijet tip (shower head) was utilized, irrigating fluid was not forced into the surrounding tissue. The influence of pressure on tissue penetration was further clarified by a study that compared irrigation at 15 psi to irrigation at 20 psi.[12] Following irrigation of partial thickness wounds on the backs of rats with saline containing one percent aniline blue dye, full thickness wound biopsies were excised and the depth of penetration into the skin was quantitated. When the wound was exposed to 20 psi, the irrigation stream penetrated the entire thickness (100 percent) of skin. In contrast, irrigation with saline at 15 psi only resulted in superficial (10 to 15 percent) penetration of the wound tissue. These results strongly suggest that soft tissue wounds should not be irrigated with fluids delivered at greater than 15 psi.

The efficacy of high pressure irrigation in removing bacteria is decreased with the age of the wound. For acute wounds treated in the emergency room, the majority of bacteria are surface contaminants and are more easily removed than bacteria within the tissue. As the wound ages without appropriate control of wound bacteria, the bacteria invade the tissue and cannot be removed without antibiotics or surgical debridement. Daily irrigation of infected experimental wounds with high–pressure irrigation

was ineffective in significantly reducing the mean level of bacteria within the wound tissue.[32] These results would suggest that irrigation alone will not reduce the level of bacteria within the tissue of chronic wounds. In this situation surgical debridement or topical antibiotics should be considered.

Despite the ability of Saxe, et al.,[32] to obtain significant reduction in bacterial levels in their animal experiment the benefit of irrigation has been shown in one study involving chronic wounds. Diekmann used a dental irrigating device on its lowest setting (6 psi) to irrigate pressure ulcers on eight patients twice a day for two weeks.[33] Eight other patients with similar type pressure ulcers received standard care. Wounds treated with pressurized irrigation had a mean decrease in wound area of 51 percent, while the mean decrease in wound area of the control wounds was only 13 percent. Because of the large standard deviation and small number of wounds in each sample, the difference was not statistically significant. These results are very encouraging and support the contention that clean wounds heal faster than non–clean wounds.

Another form of wound irrigation is the whirlpool bath that contains a pump that generates pressurized streams of water in the bath through jets. The use of whirlpool is recommended for chronic wounds that contain thick exudate, slough, or necrotic tissue. Wound cleansing is enhanced in the whirlpool because of the extended time of contact between the wound and the fluid. This extended soaking time saturates and softens the wound debris and facilitates its removal. The aggressiveness of the irrigation process can be controlled by how close the wound is placed to a jet. The impact pressure generated by the jets has not been determined. The practitioner and the patient should know when maximal acceptable pressure has been achieved.

Using bacteria as a marker for cleansing action, two studies have demonstrated that whirlpool is an effective cleansing technique.[34,35] These studies indicated that a 20 to 30 minute immersion with agitation, followed by 30 seconds of rinsing at maximum force tolerated, was the most effective cleansing technique. Feedar and Kloth recommend whirlpool twice daily in conjunction with interim wound dressings to facilitate debridement of necrotic tissue.[36] However, once the wound has been cleansed of foreign debris the benefits of the whirlpool are outweighed by the trauma to the newly exposed healing tissue. Therefore do not expose clean, granulating wounds to whirlpool therapy.

Wound Disinfection

All chronic wounds are contaminated with bacteria. Unless the patient is severely immunocompromised, these bacteria can be controlled with standard, physiologically–sound management procedures. The single most important parameter in reducing the level of bacterial contamination in the chronic wound is removal of all devitalized material. Bacteria thrive in devitalized tissue and exudate. Aggressive debridement and thorough cleansing are the physiologically–sound procedures for disinfecting wounds. Bacteria do not normally survive in clean, healthy tissue.

identified the species of organisms present in the non–healing wounds and found a strong correlation with the gram–negative organisms such as *Proteus mirabilis*, *Pseudomonas aeruginosa*, *Escherichia coli*, and *Bacteroides* species.[40–42] These studies indicated that *Proteus* species may be more deleterious to wound healing than the other gram–negative organisms.

When high levels of bacteria in the wound are suspected as the cause of non–healing, then a quantitative culture needs to be obtained. Quantitative cultures are different than standard swab cultures since extreme effort is made to thoroughly cleanse the wound surface of contaminants

---

The single most important parameter in reducing the level of bacterial contamination in the chronic wound is removal of all devitalized material.

A chronic wound that has been converted to a clean wound by physiologically–sound procedures should show signs of healing within 2 to 4 weeks.[37–39] If healing is not apparent then the treatment plan needs to be critically reviewed to make sure that pressure relief, adequate nutrition, acceptable blood supply, and proper wound dressings are being provided. If all of these factors have been evaluated and the wound is not healing, then high levels of bacterial contamination in the wound tissue may be inhibiting the healing process.

Although the influence of bacteria on healing is controversial, it seems obvious that viable bacteria in a wound would be competing with the wound healing cells for nutrients and oxygen. Bacteria would also be elaborating metabolic wastes, reactive enzymes, and toxins. All of these agents would be inflammatory, and prolonged inflammation retards would healing.

Several, well–controlled, clinical studies have documented that patients with pressure ulcers and venous ulcers that have high levels of bacteria ($\geq 10^5$) do not heal.[40–45] Other studies involving leg ulcers have reported that healing occurred despite high levels of bacteria.[46–49] However, they did not report the rate of wound healing. Wound healing can occur in the presence of high levels of bacteria, but it is probable that it would have occurred much faster if the level of bacterial contamination had been reduced.

In addition to the level of bacterial contamination, it might be important as to which species of bacteria are present. Several of the bacterial studies

and then obtain a specified volume, weight, or surface area of wound material for analysis. Quantitative cultures can be tissue biopsies, needle aspirates or standardized quantitative swabs.[50] Tissue biopsy, consisting of removal of a piece of tissue with a scalpel or punch biopsy and quantification of the number of organisms per gram of tissue, has been the "gold standard" with which other methods of monitoring tissue bacteria have been compared.[51] Needle aspiration utilizes a 22–gauge needle and 10–cc syringe inserted into the tissue to aspirate fluid that can subsequently be quantified in colony forming units per volume of fluid.[52] Quantitative swab culture was first described by Levine, et al.,[53] and consists of cleansing the wound with nonbacteriostatic saline followed by rotating the end of a cotton tip applicator over a one–square centimeter surface area of the wound with sufficient pressure to express fluid from underlying tissue. Serial dilutions are made on agar plates and results are expressed as organisms per swab or by categorizing from scant to heavy bacterial growth.

Even though tissue biopsy is the "gold standard," there is excellent correlation between the results of tissue biopsies and quantitative swabs, even when semi–quantitative results have been utilized.[53,54] Any microbiology laboratory can perform a semi–quantitative analysis of a swab obtained under controlled conditions. The important component is obtaining the sample according to a specified protocol.[55] It is important to remember that rather than trying to determine the exact

Table 3
Partial list of antiseptic agents that have been used in the false hope of killing bacteria without killing wound cells

Iodine
Peroxide
Hypochlorite
Acetic acid
Chlorhexidene
Boric acid
Alcohols
Hexachlorophene
Formaldehyde
Silver nitrate
Merthiolate
Gentian violet
Permanganate
Aluminum salts

number of organisms, you are determining if there is a high level ($\geq 10^5$) of bacteria in the wound that may be responsible for impaired healing.

If the wound is clean and further debridement and cleansing would not be beneficial, then a short regimen of topical antimicrobial agent should be considered to reduce an unacceptable level of bacteria. The agents of choice are topical antibiotics, not topical antiseptics. Do not use antiseptics in wounds to reduce bacteria in wound tissue. Unlike antibiotics that can selectively kill bacteria without harming tissue, antiseptics do not have a selective antibacterial mechanism, and thus damage all cells upon contact. Therefore, the repeated use of antiseptics in chronic wounds may cause sufficient damage to the cells essential for wound repair that optimal wound healing is delayed.

The scientific literature is replete with documentation of the ability of antiseptics to rapidly kill high levels of bacteria. These favorable results are obtained by exposing bacteria suspended in fluid directly to the antiseptic solution. Thus, there is direct contact between the bacteria and the antiseptic, and the results are optimized. However, a test tube of fluid does not represent a chronic wound. When wound exudate, necrotic tissue, or blood are added to the test tube, the effectiveness of the antiseptics is significantly reduced, if not completely eliminated.

Because of their inability to effectively penetrate tissue, antiseptics are used primarily as prophylactic agents for killing bacteria that are on the surface of tissue. In order to be effective as a therapeutic

agent, an antiseptic has to penetrate into contaminated tissue in an active form of sufficient concentration to provide antimicrobial activity. Because of their chemical reactivity, antiseptics actively bind to many organic substrates present in the wound.[56–58] Thus, antiseptics, when used at clinically appropriate concentrations, might never reach the bacteria in the wound tissue with effective antimicrobial activity. After extensive experimentation, Fleming in 1919 summarized his results as follows: "This would seem to indicate clearly that it is impossible to sterilize a wound with an antiseptic, even if it were possible to keep the antiseptic solution in the wound for a long time without dilution..."[57]

No controlled clinical study has been able to refute Fleming's conclusion that topical antiseptics offer little benefit in reducing the number of bacteria that reside within wound tissue. The benefit that most authors report when evaluating antiseptics as part of a wound management study is most likely due to another aspect of the wound management protocol such as debridement. The majority of wound bacteria resides in necrotic tissue. When more aggressive debridement is instituted as part of a clinical study, the bacterial burden in the wound is reduced, and the wound improves. In uncontrolled studies, the improvement in the wound has been inappropriately ascribed to the utilization of antiseptics.

There are numerous reports in the literature that describe the benefits of different antiseptics (Table 3). However, when all of these reports were reviewed for scientific validity, none of them truly validated the ability of an antiseptic agent alone to decontaminate a pressure ulcer.[59] Even the clinical standard, povidone–iodine, does not have well–controlled studies to validate its efficacy. Several published studies indicate that the use of povidone–iodine decreases bacterial levels and promotes healing.[60–64] None of these studies were controlled by treating a similar group of patients the same way, but substituting saline for the povidone–iodine. When such a study was conducted povidone–iodine was shown to be ineffective.[65]

The antimicrobial efficacy of povidone–iodine solution was evaluated in a prospective, randomized, controlled study compared to saline and the topical antibiotic silver sulfadiazine.[65] Forty–five hospitalized patients with infected pressure ulcers (greater than 10^5 organisms per gram of tissue) were treated topically with silver sulfadiazine every 8 hours, povidone–iodine–soaked gauze every 6 hours, or saline–soaked gauze every 4 hours. Tissue biopsies for quantitative bacteriology were obtained twice weekly. Wound therapy was considered successful when the wound biopsies revealed less than

10^5 organisms per gram of tissue. At the end of the three–week study, 100 percent of the ulcers receiving the topical antibiotic cream had wound bacterial levels of less than 10^5. Treating ulcers with saline–soaked gauze every four hours was also a very effective way of debriding the ulcers and reducing the level of bacteria. The use of saline resulted in 78.6 percent of the ulcers achieving a bacterial level of less than 10^5. The results obtained with povidone–iodine were significantly ($p \leq 0.022$) inferior to those obtained with silver sulfadiazine. For the ulcers treated with gauze soaked with povidone–iodine, only 63.6 percent achieved a bacterial level of less the 10^5. The results of this controlled trial confirm Fleming's original laboratory results that showed that antiseptics cannot kill bacteria within tissue. The results obtained in this study with povidone–iodine were due to the debriding action of wet gauze, not to the antiseptic properties of the povidone–iodine.

Dakin's solution (0.5 percent sodium hypochlorite) is another antiseptic solution that is commonly used to treat chronic wounds. The popularity of Dakin's solution was established by Alexis Carrel in his miraculous treatment of open war wounds in World War I.[66] But under those conditions any agent would have proven beneficial. Despite its long history of clinical use, no controlled studies have documented its antimicrobial efficacy compared to standard practice. The clinical benefit of Dakin's solution is probably due to its ability to dissolve necrotic tissue.[67] Removal of the necrotic tissue would be correlated with a reduction in the level of bacteria in the wound and an improvement in healing. In this situation, Dakin's solution is acting as a chemical debriding agent and as such should be discontinued when the necrotic tissue has been removed. Dakin's solution should never be used to pack a clean wound.

Acetic acid is another agent that has a long history of clinical use. The activity of acetic acid is probably due only to its physiologically unacceptable pH.[68] Because *Pseudomonas* species are extremely sensitive to acidic environments, topical acetic acid (5 percent) has been shown to be of benefit in two uncontrolled trials where *Pseudomonas* infections were present.[69,70]

Hydrogen peroxide is another agent that has an undocumented reputation as an effective antiseptic agent. Hydrogen peroxide has very little antimicrobial activity, but it is very effective in dissolving blood clots. Therefore, under the right condition where blood clots or hematomas are present, hydrogen peroxide acts as an effective chemical debriding agent, not as an antiseptic. The American Medical Association reviewed the literature on

---

Table 4
Topical antibiotics that have been utilized to control bacteria in chronic wounds

Silver Sulfadiazine
Mafenide acetate
Nitrofurazone
Polysporin
Mupirocin
Metronidazole

---

hydrogen peroxide and concluded that it had little bactericidal effect in tissue, but that its effervescence might provide some mechanical benefit in loosening debris and necrotic tissue in the wound.[71]

Conclusion

Even though there is not scientifically valid documentation of the benefits, practitioners continue to use antiseptics in wounds because of tradition. This tradition must stop. Antiseptics are toxic chemicals that, when used in clean wounds, do more harm than good. The volume of literature that documents the extreme toxicity of these agents is overwhelming. It includes *in vitro* tests[72–74] as well as *in vivo* tests in animals[72,75–78] and humans.[79,80]

Accepting the fact that traditional concentrations of antiseptic solutions are too toxic for wound care, some practitioners have assumed that diluting the antiseptic will dilute its toxicity to wound healing cells while maintaining its toxicity to bacteria. Certain reports in the literature support this contention by finding a "magic" dilution of antiseptic that kills bacteria but not wound healing cells.[72,81] These reports are misleading because the antiseptic agents were tested in test tubes with saline that contained no wound materials like exudate or tissue.[82] Even though the basis for diluting antiseptics appears dubious, I fully encourage the process. If everyone that continues to use antiseptics would dilute them 1 : 1000 or 1 : 10,000, they would see a significant improvement in wound healing because they significantly reduced the toxicity of the topical agent they were using.

When an antimicrobial agent is deemed necessary to reduce bacterial levels within the wound, then a topical antibiotic should be utilized. The use of topical antibiotic therapy has been the mainstay of burn care for the past two decades. Some topical antibiotics that have been used for chronic wounds are listed in Table 4. None of these agents are commonly used systemically in clinical practice. Because of the risk for selecting out resistant strains of bacteria, clinically utilized antibiotics should not be used topically on chronic wounds. Even though Bendy, et al. documented the success of topical gentamicin in reducing bacterial levels and promoting healing in pressure ulcers,[40] there are other topical antibiotics that will do a similar job without developing strains of bacteria that are resistant to clinically essential systemic antibiotics.

The use of topical antibiotics in chronic wounds has not been reported very often in the literature. Despite the limited number of studies that have been reported, the results have been very impressive. The use of silver sulfadiazine cream in heavily contaminated pressure ulcers resulted in reduction of bacterial levels to less than 10^5 organisms per gram of tissue in all treated ulcers within three weeks.[65] In another study, ten patients with putrid smelling ulcers and positive cultures for anaerobic organisms were treated twice a day with metronidazole gel.[83] After five days of treatment all odor was eliminated and repeat cultures were negative for anaerobic organisms.

Topical antibiotics can be very effective when used against sensitive organisms. When in doubt about the sensitivity of the organisms in the wound to the antibiotic being used, consult your microbiologist. There are well–defined tests for determining the sensitivity of wound organisms to topical antibiotic preparations.[84,85] In general, topical antibiotics should not be used for more than two weeks and the patients must be monitored for any signs of reaction to the antibiotic.

Following are some helpful hints:
- Effective wound cleansing is essential for effective wound healing.
- The benefits of wound cleansing must always be balanced against the harms inflicted upon the wound.
- Select biocompatible wound cleansers and utilize them in a non–traumatic manner.
- When irrigating wounds keep the irrigation pressure below 15 psi.
- Do not use antiseptic agents in clean wounds.
- For non–healing, clean wounds that contain high levels of bacteria consider a two–week trial of topical antibiotic.

References

1. Rydberg B, Zederfeldt B. Influence of cationic detergents on tensile strength of healing skin wounds in the rat. *Acta Chir Scand* 1968;134(5):317–20.
2. Bettley FR. The toxicity of soaps and detergents. *Br J Dermatol* 1968;80(10):635–42.
3. Custer J, Edlich RF, Prusak M, Madden J, Panek P, Wangensteen OH. Studies in the management of the contaminated wound. V. An assessment of the effectiveness of pHisoHex and Betadine surgical scrub solutions. *Am J Surg* 1971;121:572–5.
4. Edlich RF, Schmolka IR, Prusak MS, Edgerton MT. The molecular basis for toxicity of surfactants in surgical wounds. 1. EO:PO block polymers. *J Surg Res* 1993;14(4):277–84.
5. Bryant CA, Rodeheaver GT, Reem EM, Nichter LS, Kenney JG, Edlich RF. Search for a nontoxic surgical scrub solution for periorbital lacerations. *Ann Emerg Med* 1984;13(5):317–21.
6. Foresman PA, Payne DS, Becker D, Lewis D, Rodeheaver GT. A relative toxicity index for wound cleansers. *WOUNDS* 1993;5(5):226–31.
7. Burkey JL, Weinberg C, Brenden RA. Differential methodologies for the evaluation of skin and wound cleansers. *WOUNDS* 1993;5(6):284–91.
8. Wright RW Jr, Orr R. Fibroblast cytotoxicity and blood cell integrity following exposure to dermal wound cleansers. *Ostomy/Wound Management* 1993;39(7):33–40.
9. Rodeheaver GT, Smith SL, Thacker JG, Edgerton MT, Edlich RF. Mechanical cleansing of contaminated wounds with a surfactant. *Am J Surg* 1975;129(3):241–5.
10. Madden J, Edlich RF, Schauerhamer R, Prusak M, Borner J, Wangensteen OH. Application of principles of fluid dynamics to surgical wound irrigation. *Curr Topics Surg Res* 1971;3:85–93.
11. Rodeheaver GT, Pettry D, Thacker JG, Edgerton MT, Edlich RF. Wound cleansing by high pressure irrigation. *Surg Gynecol Obstet* 1975;141(3):357–62.
12. Foresman PA, Etheridge CA, Thacker JG, Rodeheaver GT. Influence of a pulsatile irrigation system on bacterial removal from and tissue injury to contaminated wounds (unpublished research report). Charlottesville, VA, University of Virginia Health Sciences Center, 1989.
13. Bhaskar SN, Cutright DE, Gross A. Effect of water lavage on infected wounds in the rat. *J Periodontal* 1969;40(11):671–2.
14. Gross A, Bhaskar SN, Cutright DE, Beasley JD 3rd, Perez B. The effect of pulsating water jet lavage on experimental contaminated wounds. *J Oral Surg* 1971;29(3):187–90.
15. Gross A, Cutright DE, Bhaskar SN. Effectiveness of pulsating water jet lavage in treatment of contaminated crushed wounds. *Am J Surg* 1972;124(3):373–7.
16. Grower MF, Bhaskar SN, Horan MJ, Cutright DE. Effect of water lavage on removal of tissue fragments from crush wounds. *Oral Surg Oral Med Oral Pathol* 1972;33(6):1031–6.
17. Green VA, Carlson HC, Briggs RL, Stewart JL. A comparison of the efficacy of pulsed mechanical lavage with that of rubber–bulb syringe irrigation in removal of debris from avulsive wounds. *Oral Surg Oral Med Oral Pathol* 1971;32(1):158–64.
18. Stewart JL, Carlson HC, Briggs RL, Green VA. The bacteria–removal efficiency of mechanical lavage and rubber–bulb syringe irrigation in contaminated avulsive wounds. *Oral Surg Oral Med Oral Pathol* 1971;31(6):842–8.
19. Hamer ML, Robson MD, Krizek TJ, Southwick WO. Quantitative bacterial analysis of comparative wound irrigations. *Ann Surg* 1975;181(6):819–22.
20. Brown LL, Shelton HT, Bornside GH, Cohn I Jr. Evaluation of wound irrigation by pulsatile jet and conventional methods. *Ann Surg* 1978;187(2):170–3.
21. Stevenson TR, Thacker JG, Rodeheaver GT, Bacchetta C, Edgerton MT, Edlich RF. Cleansing the traumatic wound by high pressure syringe irrigation. *JACEP* 1976;5(1):17–21.
22. Longmire AW, Broom LA, Burch J. Wound infection following high–pressure syringe and needle irrigation (letter). *Am J Emerg Med* 1987;5(2):179–181.
23. Singer AJ, Hollander JE, Subramanian S, Malhotra AK, Villez PA. Pressure dynamics of various irrigation techniques commonly used in the emergency department. *Ann Emerg Med* 1994;24(1):36–40.
24. Vadodaria SJ, Parekh DB. An irrigation system for large–wound toileting. *Ann Plast Surg* 1990;25:152–3.

25. Weller K. In search of efficacy and efficiency. An alternative to conventional wound cleansing modalities. *Ostomy/Wound Management* 1991;37:23–8.

26. Chisholm CD, Cordell WH, Rogers K, Woods JR. Comparison of a new pressurized saline canister versus syringe irrigation for laceration cleansing in the emergency department. *Ann Emerg Med* 1992;21(11):1364–7.

27. Beltran KA, Thacker JG, Rodeheaver GT. Impact pressures generated by commercial wound irrigation devices (unpublished research report). Charlottesville, VA, University of Virginia Health Sciences Center, 1994.

28. Pigman EC, Karch DB, Scott JL. Splatter during jet irrigation cleansing of a wound model. A comparison of three inexpensive devices. *Ann Emerg Med* 1993;22(10):1563–7.

29. Chernofsky MA, Murphy RX Jr, Jennings JF. A barrier technique for pulsed irrigation of cavitary wounds. *Plast Reconst Surg* 1993;91:365–366.

30. Wheeler CB, Rodeheaver GT, Thacker JG, Edgerton MT, Edlich RF. Side effects of high pressure irrigation. *Surg Gynecol Obstet* 1976;143(5):775–8.

31. Carlson HC, Briggs RL, Green VA, Stewart JL. Effect of pressure and tip modification on the dispersion of fluid throughout cells and tissues during the irrigation of experimental wounds. *Oral Surg Oral Med Oral Pathol* 1971;32(2):347–55.

32. Saxe A, Goldstein E, Dixon S, Ostrup R. Pulsatile lavage in the management of postoperative wound infections. *Am Surg* 1980;46(7):391–7.

33. Diekmann JM. Use of a dental irrigating device in the treatment of decubitus ulcers. *Nurs Res* 1984;33(5):303–5.

34. Neiderhuber S, Stribley R, Koepke G. Reduction of skin bacterial load with use of therapeutic whirlpool. *Phys Ther* 1975;55(5):482–6.

35. Bohannon RW. Whirlpool versus whirlpool rinse for removal of bacteria from a venous stasis ulcer. *Phys Ther* 1982;62(3):304–8.

36. Feddar JA, Kloth LC. Conservative management of chronic wounds. In: Kloth LC, McCulloch JM, Feddar JA (eds). *Wound Healing: Alternatives in Management*. Philadelphia, PA, FA Davis, 1990.

37. Robson M, Phillips LG, Thomason A, Robson LF, Pierce GF. Recombinant human growth factor–bb for the treatment of chronic pressure ulcers. *Ann Plast Surg* 1992;29:193–210.

38. Robson M, Phillips LG, Thomason A, Robson LF, Pierce GF. Platelet–derived factors BB for treatment of chronic pressure ulcers. *Lancet* 1992;339:23–25.

39. van Rijswijk L. Full–thickness pressure ulcers: patient and wound healing characteristics. *Decubitus* 1993;6(1):16–21.

40. Bendy RH, Nuccio PA, Wolfe E, Collins B, Tamburro C, Glass W, Martin CM. Relationship of quantitative wound bacterial counts to healing of decubiti: effect of topical gentamicin. *Antimicrob Agents Chemother* 1964;4:147–55.

41. Lookingbill DP, Miller SH, Knowles RC. Bacteriology of chronic leg ulcers. *Arch Dermatol* 1978;114(12):1765–8.

42. Daltrey DC, Rhodes B, Chattwood JG. Investigation into the microbial flora of healing and non–healing decubitus ulcers. *J Clin Pathol* 1981;34(7):701–5.

43. Sapico FL, Ginunas VJ, Thornhill–Joynes M, Canawati HN, Capen DA, Klein NE, Khawam S, Montgomerie JZ. Quantitative microbiology of pressure sores in different stages of healing. *Diagn Microbiol Infect Dis* 1986;5(1):31–8.

44. Lyman IR, Tenery JH, Basson RP. Correlation between decrease in bacterial load and rate of wound healing. *Surg Gynecol Obstet* 1970;130(4):616–21.

45. Margraf HW, Covey TH Jr. A trial of silver–zinc–allantoinate in the treatment of leg ulcers. *Arch Surg* 1977;112(6):699–704.

46. Gilchrist B, Reed C. The bacteriology of chronic venous ulcers treated with occlusive hydrocolloid dressings. *Br J Dermatol* 1989;121(3):337–44.

47. Alper JC, Welch EA, Ginsberg M, Bogaars H, Maguir P. Moist wound healing under a vapor permeable membrane. *J Am Acad Dermatol* 1983;8(3):347–53.

48. van Rijswijk L, Brown D, Friedman S, Degreef H, Roed–Petersen J, Borglund E, Ebert HM, Sayag J, Beylot C, Su WPD. Multicenter clinical evaluation of a hydrocolloid dressing for leg ulcers. *Cutis* 1985;35:173–6.

49. Eriksson G, Eklund AE, Kallings LO. The clinical significance of bacterial growth in venous leg ulcers. *Scand J Infect Dis* 1984;16(2):175–80.

50. Stotts NA. Determination of bacterial burden in wounds. *Adv Wound Care* 1995;8(4):2846–2852.

51. Robson MC, Heggers JP. Bacterial quantification of open wounds. *Mil Med* 1969;134(1):19–24.

52. Lee P, Turnidge J, McDonald PJ. Fine–needle aspiration biopsy in diagnosis of soft tissue infections. *J Clin Micro* 1985;22(1):80–3.

53. Levine NS, Lindberg RB, Mason AD, Pruitt BA. The quantitative swab culture and smear: a quick, simple method for determining the number of viable aerobic bacteria on open wounds. *J Trauma* 1976;16(2):89–94.

54. Thomson P, Taddonio T, Tait M, Rice T, Prasad J, Smith D. Correlation between swab and biopsy for the quantification of burn wound microflora. *Proc Int Cong Burn Inj* 1990;8:381.

55. Cuzzell JZ. The right way to culture a wound. *Am J Nurs* 1993;93(1):48–50.

56. Zamora JL, Price MF, Chuang P, Gentry LO. Inhibition of povidone–iodine's bactericidal activity by common organic substances: an experimental study. *Surgery* 1985;98(1):25–9.

57. Fleming A. The action of chemical and physiological antiseptics in a septic wound. *Br J Surg* 1919;7:99–129.

58. Lacey RW. Antibacterial activity of povidone towards non–sporing bacteria. *J Applied Bacteriology* 1979;46:443–9.

59. Morgan JE. Topical therapy of pressure ulcers. Surg Gynec Obstet 1975;141:945–7.

60. Connell JF Jr, Rousselot LM. Povidone–iodine. Extensive surgical evaluation of a new antiseptic agent. *Am J Surg* 1964;108:849–55.

61. Gilgore A. The use of povidone–iodine in the treatment of infected cutaneous ulcers. *Curr Ther Res* 1978;24(7):843–8.

62. Lee BY, Trainor FS, Thoden WR. Topical application of povidone–iodine in the management of decubitus and stasis ulcers. *J Am Geriatr Soc* 1979;27(7):302–6.

63. Sugarman B. Infection and pressure sores. *Arch Phys Med Rehabil* 1985;66(3):177–9.

64. Michael J. Topical use of PVP–I (Betadine) preparations in patients with spinal cord injury. *Drugs Exptl Clin Res* 1985;11(2):107–9.

65. Kucan JO, Robson MC, Heggers JP, Ko F. Comparison of silver sulfadiazine, povidone–iodine and physiologic saline in the treatment of chronic pressure ulcers. *J Am Geriatr Soc* 1981;29(5):232–5.

66. Carrel A, Dehelly G. *The Treatment of Infected Wounds*. New York, NY, 1917.

67. Taylor HD, Austin JH. The solvent action of antiseptics on necrotic tissue. *J Exp Med* 1918;27:155–64.

68. Leveen HH, Falk G, Borek B, Diaz C, Lynfield U, Wyncoop BJ, Mabunda GA, Rubricuis JL, Christoudias GC. Chemical acidification of wounds. An adjunct to healing and the unfavorable action of alkalinity and ammonia. *Ann Surg* 1973;178(6):745–53.

69. Phillips I, Lobo AZ, Fernandes R, Gundara NS. Acetic acid in the treatment of superficial wounds infected by Pseudomonas aeruginosa. *Lancet* 1968;1:11–3.

70. Milner SM. Acetic acid to treat Pseudomonas aeruginosa in superficial wounds and burns. *Lancet* 1992;340:61.

71. *AMA Drug Evaluation, Tenth Edition*. Chicago, IL, American Medical Association, 1994, pp 1620–1.

72. Lineaweaver W, Howard R, Soucy D, McMorris S. Freeman J, Crain C, Robertson J, Rumley T. Topical antimicrobial toxicity. *Arch Surg* 1985;120(3):267–70.

73. Cooper ML, Laxer JA, Hansbrough JF. The cytotoxic effects of commonly used topical antimicrobial agents on human fibroblasts and keratinocytes. *J Trauma* 1991;31(6):775–84.

74. Teepe RG, Koebrugge EJ, Lowik CW, Petit PL, Bosboom RW, Twiss IM, Boxma H, Vermeer BJ, Ponec M. Cytotoxic effects of topical antimicrobial and antiseptic agents on human keratinocytes in vitro. *J Trauma* 1993;35(1):8–19.

75. Branemark PI, Ekholm R. Tissue injury caused by wound disinfectants. *J Bone Joint Surg Am* 1967;49(1):48–62.

76. Brennan SS, Leaper DJ. The effect of antiseptics on the healing wound: a study using the rabbit ear chamber. *Brit J Surg* 1985;72(10):780–2.

77. Cotter JL, Fader RC, Lilley C, Herndon DN. Chemical parameters, antimicrobial activities, and tissue toxicity of 0.1 and 0.5% sodium hypochlorite solutions. *Antimicrob Agents Chemother* 1985;28(1):118–22.

78. Brennan SS, Foster ME, Leaper DJ. Antiseptic toxicity in wounds healing by secondary intention. *J Hosp Infect* 1986;8(3):263–7.

79. Becker GD. Identification and management of the patient at high risk for wound infection. *Head Neck Surg* 1986;8:205–210.

80. Viljanto J. Disinfection of surgical wounds without inhibition of normal wound healing. *Arch Surg* 1980;115:253–6.

81. Heggers JP, Sazy JA, Stenberg BD, Strock LL, McCauley RL, Herndon DN, Robson MC. Bacterial and wound–healing properties of sodium hypochlorite solutions: The 1991 Lindberg award. *J Burn Care Rehab* 1991;12:420–424.

82. Rodeheaver G. Commentary on Heggers, et al. (ref. 81) paper. *Diabetes Spectrum* 1992;5(6):349–350.

83. Witkowski JA, Parish LC. Topical metronidazole gel. The bacteriology of decubitus ulcers. *Int J Derm* 1991;30(9):L660–661.

84. Rodeheaver GT, Gentry S, Saffer L, Edlich RF. Topical antimicrobial cream sensitivity testing. Surg Gynec Obstet 1980;151(Dec):747–752.

85. Nathan P, Law EJ, Murphy DF, MacMillan BG. A laboratory method for selection of topical antimicrobial agents to treat infected burn wounds. *Burns* 1978;4:177–187.

14
Infection and Culturing

Brian Gilchrist, BSc, MSc, RGN

Gilchrist B. Infection and culturing. In: Krasner D, Kane D. *Chronic Wound Care, Second Edition*. Wayne, PA, Health Management Publications, Inc., 1997, pp 109–114.

Introduction

All chronic wounds contain bacteria. This seemingly simple statement encapsulates in a few words all the difficulties faced by the clinician when considering the issue of infection in chronic wounds. If you look, you will find bacteria, but are those bacteria doing any harm?

In fact, most surfaces of the human skin will yield bacteria when suitably sampled, and yet it is clear that infection does not normally occur when the skin is intact. The mechanisms which prevent infection from occurring are well documented: the hard outer layer of the skin provides a physical barrier to invasion by microorganisms; the pH of the skin surface is not conducive to the build up of bacteria in sufficient numbers to cause infection; the skin normally secretes fatty acids and antibacterial polypeptides; and the normal resident flora also plays a role in preventing potentially pathogenic organisms from becoming established.

The presence of a chronic wound, on the other hand, clearly provides a portal of entry for organisms, and the fact that many such wounds are the result of some deficiency in tissue nutrition also suggests that the normal protective mechanisms may not always come into play. In particular, the single most significant predisposing condition associated with the development of potentially harmful wound infection is often the absence of a normal blood supply (e.g. in pressure ulcers or in lower limb ulceration caused by ischemia), and this should always be one of the first factors to be considered.

The Effects of Infection on Healing

Wound healing normally progresses in an orderly sequential fashion, and this sequence can be considerably disrupted by the presence of infection. Although not fully understood, a recent review suggests that the major mechanisms by which an alteration in sequence occurs include disruption and prolongation of the inflammatory phase of healing, depletion of components of the complement cascade, disruption of normal clotting mechanisms, disordered leukocyte function, and less efficient angiogenesis and formation of granulation tissue.[1] Clearly, then, clinical infection will play a major role in the healing of a chronic wound.

The difficulty, however, begins with the decision about whether or not the chronic wound is actually infected. If you take a swab from a chronic wound healing by secondary intention, then most times you will culture at least one (and probably more) species of bacteria,[2] and there is really no way of telling which bacteria are of pathogenic importance and which ones are simply an incidental finding.

The Diagnosis of Infection

If bacterial presence is a normal situation, how can the infected wound be distinguished from the non–infected wound? The first important point to realize is that, for a number of reasons, the taking of a wound swab will not in itself answer the question. First, as has already been stated, the presence of large numbers of bacteria is the "normal" situation; therefore, simply growing bacteria is not in itself a sufficient criterion to say that a wound is "infected"; second, there are problems related to the actual sampling of the bacteria. The bacteria grown may not be representative of the pathogens that are actually present in the wound (especially if the infection is due to anaerobic bacteria), and conversely, the bacteria that are grown

Table 1
Host Reactions[10]

Cellulitis
Abnormal discharge
Delayed healing
Change in pain
Abnormal granulation tissue
Bridging
Abnormal odor

in the laboratory may not themselves be causing any harm. The presence of mixed flora may also restrict growth of certain bacteria in laboratory conditions. Last, in the literature, there appears to be considerable confusion over what exactly constitutes "infection," with the term often being loosely used to simply suggest bacterial presence, while in other reports it implies a very exact measurement of the bacterial burden present.

From a microbiological point of view, it is possible to differentiate between three distinct situations: contamination, colonization and infection.[3]

Contamination is the presence of bacteria without multiplication; colonization includes multiplication, but with no host reaction; and infection is deposition and multiplication of bacteria in tissue with an associated host reaction.

It is the presence of this host reaction which allows us to decide whether or not a wound is clinically infected, as opposed to colonized, which in chronic wounds is the normal situation.

While some authors have suggested that the only way to precisely define infection is by taking quantitative wound biopsies, the key number being $>10^5$ bacteria per gram of tissue or ml of wound fluid,[4] others have shown that numbers greatly in excess of this amount can be found in chronic wounds which do not demonstrate signs of clinical infection (and which go on to heal).[5] Additionally, it has been shown that, " [there is] great variability in bacterial count per gram of tissue across [an] ulcer surface,"[6] and the method has also been questioned as it does not tell you anything about invasion, nor does it take into account the cause and extent of the wound in relationship to the actual patient and the organism involved.[7] As most chronic wound care is undertaken by nurses in the community and there is some concern that the taking of a biopsy may not itself be without risk, it seems likely that at least at present this technique may be restricted to specialist tertiary referral centers.

We are then left with "host reactions." The most obvious ones are the classic signs of cellulitis: heat, redness, swelling and pain. When seen, they are usually very obvious, and it is well accepted that the treatment is systemic antibiotics, with perhaps bedrest and elevation of the limb, as in the case of an infected leg ulcer. However, chronic wounds are often (although not exclusively) seen in the elderly, and in this case the patient may not mount a typical immune response.[8] In addition, patients who are neutropenic or on systemic steroid therapy may have an inadequate inflammatory response.[9]

Other clinical signs of possible infection have also been described (Table 1):[10]

Abnormal discharge. Three types of discharge may indicate possible wound infection: 1) serous exudate with concurrent inflammation, probably due to increased capillary permeability, with the body attempting to deliver white cells to the site of the infection, and coincidentally leaking serum; 2) seropurulent and hemopurulent discharge, as a result of liquifaction of tissues in the presence of microorganisms; 3) and pus, the presence of which is always an indicator of infection, even when no organisms are cultured from the wound. Surprisingly, pus is relatively rare in the case of chronic wounds, probably because they are generally wet and draining, and the pus therefore does not collect in the same way as it might in an enclosed space. Care must also be taken to differentiate between pus and slough, which is simply moist devitalized tissue.

Delayed healing. Infection clearly causes a delay in normal healing, although it must be recognized that it is not the only reason for delay. Nevertheless, if the wound is healing slower than might otherwise be expected, infection should be considered as a possible cause (once it has been re–established that the diagnosis is correct).

Change in pain. Any change in pain, especially the development of a more acute pain, should be taken to indicate that something untoward is occurring in the healing wound, possibly the presence of infection. A note of caution should be sounded, however. Although venous ulceration is commonly associated with chronic pain,[11] the development of an acute pain should not automatically be associated with infection; rather, the presence of significant ischemia should first be eliminated by the repeated measurement of the ankle pressure index.[11] If the measurement has not significantly changed, then the use of systemic antibiotics may be considered. Increased pain in a pressure ulcer might also be associated with an increase in ischemia, and it should first be established that the patient has been placed on an appropriate pressure relieving support surface.

Change in appearance of the granulation tissue. Along with increased wetness, infected granulation tissue may appear a darker color, become more friable, and appear to bleed more easily than normal. Infection by specific organisms may result in a particular discoloration, for example, pseudomonal infections often appear as green or blue discoloration which will flouresce under UV light.

detected when using a specific, specialized technique.[2]

There is considerable evidence that repeated swabbing of chronic wounds will not yield any useful prognostic information as their bacterial flora is quite stable.[13,14] It would therefore appear that the most productive times to take swabs are when the wound is first seen, as a screening device,

---

There is considerable evidence that repeated swabbing of chronic wounds will not yield any useful prognostic information as their bacterial flora is quite stable.[13,14]

Bridging of soft tissue and the epithelium. This is caused by bacteria retarding the growth of new tissue under the epithelium, thus preventing complete healing.

Odor. All chronic wounds have some smell associated with them, but it is generally not too unpleasant. On the other hand, infection by anaerobic bacteria generally results in a highly offensive odor, while wounds containing necrotic material may have a characteristic rotting smell. Care must be taken not to confuse abnormal odors with those often noted on removal of certain dressings, especially the hydrocolloids which often produce a highly malodourous exudate.

What Sample to Take

As has already been discussed, there are those clinicians who advocate quantitative bacteriology as the only accurate method of sampling bacteria in a wound.[4] Nevertheless, it is more likely that a wound swab will be the preferred or more practical method of specimen collection. The precise technique for dealing with specimens will vary according to local policy and practice; a typical system has been described by Lawrence.[12]

Although there is no agreement in the literature as to how the swab should be taken, or from which part of the wound, Lawrence suggests using two serum tipped swabs, and "rubbing across the surface in a zig–zag manner, simultaneously rotating the swab between finger and thumb." One swab is then placed in cooked meat medium, and the other in its container. Provided that they are kept cool (20° C or lower) he states that, "no undue loss of bacteria [will occur] over a 48 hour period." Keeping the swabs cool also allows for the detection of anaerobic bacteria, although studies have shown that a greater numbers of anaerobes can be

to provide baseline information, and if clinical infection is suspected. In particular, it may be prudent to screen initially for *Streptococcus* Group A, as this organism is particularly virulent. Much smaller numbers are needed to induce clinical infection, and there is evidence that the organism may be associated with chronic, large non–healing ulcers.[15] Special media may be advised, and the advice of the microbiology department should be sought. Many centers will no longer process routine swabs without evidence of clinical infection because of the cost, and even in this situation considerable care should be taken in interpreting the results. If an anaerobe is suspected, then a biopsy may be considered; in the case of diabetic foot ulceration it will be prudent to treat for anaerobes even if they are not detected on routine culture.

One other consideration needs to be taken into account: some chronic wounds may actually be caused by infection (as opposed to infection being a complication of an existing wound). Examples are thrombophlebitis, in which case a blood culture will normally allow for the isolation of the causative organism, and osteomyelitis, where it has been suggested that only tissue obtained at operative debridement will yield accurate cultures.[16]

Other new, sophisticated techniques, such as imaging and scanning, are available for the assessment of infection in chronic wounds,[17] but as yet these techniques are not freely available and they remain to be proven in terms of clinical utility, except in very specialized centers.

The Treatment of Patients with Infected Chronic Wounds

Before considering the local treatment of any wound, the clinician must first ensure that any other factors which might lead to an increased risk or susceptibility to infection are either controlled or eradicated. It is thus necessary to ensure that a full and detailed history has been taken and that a clinical examination has been performed. Too often, "treatment" appears to consist solely of sending off a swab and changing the dressing. When the patient's condition fails to improve, the dressing is blamed, and is substituted for a different brand or type. Failure to identify other factors present may be the single most important factor in non–healing of a chronic wound, as it is critical to understand that, "Neither aseptic techniques nor the use of antibiotics has properly recognized that resistance to bacterial invasion depends almost entirely on the efficiency of the host's natural defense mechanisms."[18]

Central to this point is the answer to the question, "What caused this wound?" Chronic wounds are a symptom, not a disease, and before any treatment is contemplated a definitive diagnosis should be attempted. Although this approach may sometimes prove to be rather elusive, in many cases the correct identification of the cause will lead to a rational treatment approach being developed, and subsequent healing will result.

Factors which impair host resistance. There are many factors which have been shown to impair host resistance and to lead to a chronic, non–healing wound.[19] These factors include the presence of a foreign body in the wound (e.g. pieces of dressing, especially gauze and tulle, dirt, suture material, drains); the presence of dead tissue, as it leads to a smaller number of bacteria being needed in the initial innoculum; contused tissue; tissue ischemia; previous or current irradiation; the presence of a hematoma; and the use of vasoconstricting drugs.

In addition there are a number of medical conditions which are well known to predispose to infection: diabetes, cancer, rheumatoid arthritis, excessive alcohol intake, malnourishment, conditions which lead to decreased or absent functioning of the immune system, systemic use of steroids or antibiotics and co–existing distant skin lesions such as exfoliative dermatitis, which themselves easily become the target of superficial infection.[20]

Removal of bacteria. There is little evidence in the literature to show that it is necessary to remove bacteria from the surface of a chronic wound in order for it to heal, and it is now well accepted that sterility of the wound surface is neither a necessary condition for healing, nor is it actually possible.

In experimental wounds, it has been shown that wounds healed despite the presence of large numbers of bacteria in the wound fluid of occluded wounds,[21] while clinical studies on leg ulcers have shown that the presence of bacteria did not hinder wound healing.[2,13,22]

Use of antimicrobial agents. There appear to be a number of reasons why the use of topical antimicrobials is not generally advocated in chronic wound care.[23] They may lead to local cell and tissue damage; systemic toxicity; the development of contact sensitivity and allergic reactions; superinfection and the possibility of the development of antibiotic resistance, caused by disturbances in the normal skin ecology; or interactions with other concurrent drug therapy, especially steroids.

The use of topical antibiotics in chronic wound care has been advocated[24] where it has been shown quantitatively that more than 10^5 bacteria per gram of tissue are present; however, this form of treatment remains controversial as, for example, clinical studies have shown that topical silver sulphadiazine confers no benefit in wound healing over simple occlusion alone[5] even in wounds where counts were shown to be higher than 10^5. A recent authoritative review concluded, "Topical antibiotics are inappropriate for wounds and ulcers although they are widely promoted for this purpose. We know of no controlled trials...showing their superiority."[25]

An exception to this rule may be in the specific case of grossly malodorous wounds, such as fungating malignant lesions, where the use of topically applied metronidazole gel has been shown to be effective in reducing or preventing the odor.[26]

The accepted view would appear to be that at present the use of antibiotics is only advocated where clinical infection is present, and that they should be administered systemically. As stated earlier, it may be prudent to treat for anaerobes, even where none have been demonstrated; however, the specific choice of antibiotic(s) will depend on local prescribing advice and policies. The use of prophylactic antibiotics has been studied in the case of leg ulcers,[27] where it was shown that there was no difference in either the healing rate or the bacterial flora, and it was concluded that changes in the bacterial flora were due to the improvement in the general condition of the wound, rather than the therapy. There is a body of opinion, however, that does advocate the use of antibiotic prophylaxis where *Streptococcus* Group A has been detected because of the possible risk of serious infection, although there is no general agreement. There is similar lack of agreement about whether or not to treat *Pseudomonas aeruginosa* with antibiotics, although there is evidence that it may be possible to eradicate this organism with the use of a hydrocolloid dressing.[2]

The use of antiseptics in chronic wound care continues to be an issue of considerable controversy. In addition to the evidence that chronic wounds do not have to be sterile to heal, there has been an increasing realization that wound fluid contains cells and chemicals, such as antibacterial proteins and live white cells, that are actually beneficial to the wound and that will, in themselves, act as powerful weapons against infection.[28,29] This approach has led to the realization that frequent repeated washing of the wound surface may be undesirable, and that wounds will heal more efficiently if they are left undisturbed for as long as possible. Also, there is a strong feeling that the application of antiseptics may in itself be harmful. "All antiseptics in normal clinical concentrations are toxic to wound cells *in vitro*, and they have been shown to be

exhaustive review by Button failed to show any published research that demonstrated that the use of an " aseptic technique" was associated with a reduction in cross infection.[34]

Dressings and infection. The most significant development in wound care in the past 15 years has been the proliferation of dressings which act by occluding the wound and keeping the surface moist. The principles of moist wound healing are described in detail elsewhere in this volume, as are the dressings; however, it is sometimes suggested that the use of such dressings will promote the development of wound infection, as traditionally

---

...the overwhelming evidence is that occlusion may actually work to reduce the incidence of wound infection.[36]

---

destructive of normal tissue as well. Their ability to kill bacteria is compromised in the presence of blood, wound exudate or tissue so that it is unlikely that antiseptics can effectively kill bacteria that are established in tissue."[30]

Interpretation of the literature is very difficult as many of the studies have been carried out in animal models, which generally have none of the concurrent factors predisposing to infection that are found in the human with a chronic wound. Also, most studies do not include occlusion as part of the protocol, therefore allowing a scab to form and providing protection for the cells underneath.

As there is no evidence that bacteria need to be removed and a strong likelihood that toxic chemicals may cause further harm, it would seem that the best solutions to be used for wound care at present are normal saline or tap water. Evidence from a study on acute traumatic wounds, where the presence of contamination is more likely to lead to increased wound infection, has shown that the rate of infection is not increased where unsterile tap water is routinely used.[31] Our own clinical experience using a large bucket of water for routine wound care in a leg ulcer clinic also suggests that the use of antiseptics is unnecessary.

Further evidence from Tomlinson has shown that the use of different cleaning techniques does not result in a significant reduction in microorganisms present,[32] while others have shown that the optimum pressure required to remove bacteria by irrigation is 25 pounds per square inch,[33] thus suggesting that low pressure irrigation is ineffective at removing bacteria from a wound. Indeed, an

wet gauze dressings or the presence of excess amounts of moisture have been associated with infection. A review of the evidence, however, suggests that this is not the case,[35] and in fact the overwhelming evidence is that occlusion may actually work to reduce the incidence of wound infection.[36] There are a number of mechanisms that contribute to this effect, but the most important one would seem to be support of the body's normal immune function. Occlusive dressings have been shown to promote angiogenesis, thus restoring blood supply, which in turn allows for the delivery of antibacterial systems, and oxygen, which can be utilized by the white cells for bacterial killing. Occlusion prevents the formation of a scab and the subsequent dehydration and incorporation of white cells into that scab; the cells instead remain alive and viable under the dressing. Some dressings have a low pH under them, which may affect bacterial growth, and as they are left in place for longer than conventional dressings, any antibacterial proteins present are retained for longer.

In addition, many occlusive dressings, especially hydrocolloids, suspend free water thus making it unavailable for bacterial proliferation, and are often impermeable to bacteria (and viruses[37]) thus preventing superinfection and perhaps playing a role in infection control. Finally, occlusion has been shown to be a very effective method for promoting wound debridement. Debridement is a crucial factor in controlling and preventing wound infection, as it removes a source of food for bacteria and allows contraction and epithelial migration to take place.

Summary

All chronic wounds contain bacteria, often in very large numbers. There is little evidence to suggest that these bacteria need to be removed in order for the wound to heal, and most methods are very inefficient at doing so. Treatment should therefore be aimed at the following: 1) removal or control of risk factors and underlying etiology, 2) restoration of an adequate blood supply, 3) proper debridement of dead tissue, 4) avoidance of the use of toxic chemicals or topical antimicrobials, and 5) promotion of a moist wound environment.

Above all, attention should be given to the treatment of the patient as a whole, and not just focused on the hole in the skin.

References

1. Robson MC, Stenberg BD, Heggers JP. Wound healing alterations caused by infection. *Clin Plast Surg* 1990;17:485–492.
2. Gilchrist B, Reed C. The bacteriology of chronic venous ulcers treated with occlusive hydrocolloid dressings. *Brit J Derm* 1989;121:337–344.
3. Ayton M. Wounds that won't heal. *Nursing Times* 1985;81(supp):16–19.
4. Robson MC, Heggers JP. Quantitative bacteriology and inflammatory mediators in soft tissue. In: Hunt TK, Heppenstall RB, Pines E, Rovee D (eds). *Soft and Hard Tissue Repair*. New York, NY, Praeger Publications, 1984, pp483–507.
5. Hutchinson JJ. Influence of occlusive dressings on wound microbiology – interim results of a multi–centre clinical trial of an occlusive hydrocolloid dressing. In: Harding KG, Leaper DL, Turner TD (eds). *Proceedings of the 1st European Conference on Advances in Wound Management*. London, England, MacMillan, 1992, pp 152–155.
6. Schneider M, Vildozola CW, Brooks S. Quantitative assessment of bacterial invasion of chronic ulcers. *Am J Surg* 1983;145:260–262.
7. Thomson PD, Smith DJ. What is infection ? In: Kerstein MD (ed). A Symposium: Wound infection and occlusion – separating fact from fiction. *Am J Surg* 1994;167(1A):supp 7–11.
8. Gilchrist B. Wound infection in the elderly. J. Ger. Derm. 1993; 1(3): 130–131.
9. Cutting K. Detecting infection. *Nursing Times* 1994;90(50):60–62.
10. Cutting KF, Harding KG. Criteria for identifying wound infection. *J Wound Care* 1994;3(4):198–201.
11. Cullum N, Rowe B (eds). *Leg Ulcers. Nursing Management*. Harrow, Scutari Press, 1995.
12. Lawrence JC. Wound infection. *J Wound Care* 1993;2(5):277–280.
13. Erikkson G, Eklund A–E, Kallings, LO. The clinical significance of bacterial growth in leg ulcers. *Scand J Infect Dis* 1984;16(2):175–180.
14. Hansson C, Hoborn J, Moller A, Swanbeck G. The microbial flora in venous leg ulcers without clinical signs of infection. *Acta Derm Venereol* (Stockh) 1995;75:24–30.
15. Schraibmann I. The significance of B–haemolytic streptococci in chronic leg ulcers. *Ann R Coll Surg Eng* 1990;72:123–124.
16. Perry CR, Pearson,RL, Miller GA. Accuracy of cultures of material from swabbing of the superficial aspect of the wound and needle biopsy in the preoperative assessment of osteomyelitis. *J Bone Joint Surg* 1991;73(5):745–749.
17. Lazarus GS, Cooper DM, Knighton DR, et al. Definitions and guidelines for assessment of wounds and evaluation of healing. *Arch Derm* 1994;130:489–493.
18. Burke JF. The physiology of wound infection. In: Hunt TK (ed) *Wound Healing and Wound Infection*. New York, NY, Appleton– Century–Crofts, 1980, pp 242–249.
19. Tobin GR. Closure of contaminated wounds. *Surg Clin Nth Am* 1984; 64(4):639–652.
20. Louria DB. Factors predisposing to clinical infections of the skin. In: Maibach HI, Hildick–Smith G (eds). *Skin Bacteria and Their Role in Infection*. New York, NY, McGraw Hill. 1985, pp 75–84.
21. Mertz PM, Eaglstein WH. The effect of a semiocclusive dressing on the microbial population in superficial wounds. *Arch Surg* 1984; 119: 287–289.
22. Blair SD, Backhouse CM, Wright DD, et al. Do dressings influence the healing of chronic venous ulcers? *Phlebology* 1988;3:129–134.
23. Selwyn S. The topical treatment of skin infections. In: Maibach HI, Aly R (ed). *Skin Microbiology. Relevance to Clinical Infection*. New York, NY, Springer–Verlag, 1981, pp 317–328.
24. Robson MC. Plastic Surgery. In: Heggers JP, Robson MC (ed). *Quantitative Bacteriology: Its Role in the Armamentarium of the Surgeon*. FL, CRC Press, 1991, pp 71–84.
25. Local applications to wounds I. Cleansers, antibacterials, debriders. *Drug and Therapeutics Bulletin* 1991;29(24):93–95.
26. Management of smelly tumours (Editorial) *Lancet* 1990;335:141–142.
27. Alinovi A, Bassissi P, Pini M. Systematic administration of antibiotics in the management of venous ulcers. *J Am Acad Derm* 1986;15(2):186–191.
28. Hohn DC, Ponce B, Burton RW, Hunt TK. Antimicrobial systems of the surgical wound. I. A comparison of oxidative metabolism and microbicidal capacity of phagocytes from wounds and from peripheral blood. *Am J Surg* 1977;133:597–600.
29. Hohn DC, Granelli SG, Burton RW, Hunt TK. Antimicrobial systems of the surgical wound. II. Detection of antimicrobial protein in cell–free wound fluid. *Am J Surg* 1977;133:601–606.
30. Rodeheaver GT. Influence of antiseptics on wound healing. In: Alexander JW, Thomson PD, Hutchinson JJ (ed). *International Forum on Wound Microbiology*. Princeton, NJ, Excerpta Medica. 1990:22–26.
31. Angeras MH, Brandberg A, Falk A, Seeman T. Comparison between sterile saline and tap water for the cleaning of acute traumatic soft tissue wounds. *Eur J Surg* 1992;158:347–350.
32. Tomlinson D. To clean or not to clean ? *Nursing Times* 1987;83(9):71–75.
33. Madden J, Edlich RF, Schauerhamer R, et al. Application of principles of fluid dynamics to surgical wound irrigation. *Curr Top Surg Res* 1971;3:85–93.
34. Button D. A Preliminary Investigation Into the Assessment of Nurses' Competence in Performing Aseptic Techniques. Unpublished MSc Thesis, University of Manchester. 1984.
35. Gilchrist B, Hutchinson J. Does occlusion lead to infection? *Nursing Times* 1990;86(15):70–71.
36. Hutchinson JJ, Lawrence JC. Wound infection under occlusive dressings. *J Hosp Infect* 1991;17:83–94.
37. Bowler PG, Delargy H, Prince D, Fondberg L. The viral barrier properties of some occlusive dressings and their role in infection control. *WOUNDS* 1993;5(1):1–8.

15

Wound Care: Putting Theory into Practice in the United Kingdom

Keith G. Harding, MB, ChB, MRCGP and Sue Bale, BA, RGN, NDN, RHV, Dip N

Harding KG, Bale S. Wound care: Putting theory into practice in the United Kingdom. In: Krasner D, Kane D. *Chronic Wound Care, Second Edition.* Wayne, PA, Health Management Publications, Inc., 1997, pp 115–123.

Introduction

Traditionally, lectures and books on wound healing and wound management concentrate on the detailed information that has been gathered by large numbers of people with different professional backgrounds on experimental wounds. While this data is an essential step toward understanding what is happening in a healing wound both biochemically and histologically, it does not necessarily ensure that similar principles can be transferred in the daily care of patients with wounds.

Another problem that exists in wound management is that medical and nursing personnel which make up the clinical staff are not looking carefully and critically at the care plans for the patients. Furthermore, the clinical practitioners do not take the problems encountered in patient care to the basic scientists for suggestions to help solve their problems.

To overcome these problems in wound care, there has to be a greater and closer collaboration between clinicians, laboratory scientists, and manufacturers of wound management materials to ensure that problems in patient care are identified, that the cellular processes are understood, and that materials are available for specific wound problems.

To overcome the traditional inertia in wound care, this chapter details the experience of clinicians in the United Kingdom in the management of a wide variety of granulating wounds. The practical aspects of wound healing that are an essential prerequisite for good clinical practice are addressed by identifying problems and suggesting solutions.

Wound Healing

The cellular and biochemical events that must take place in a coordinated fashion to ensure that prompt and satisfactory wound healing occurs are well described.[1,2] A summary of the major events, as shown in Figure 1, divides wound healing into four interdependent phases. Initially, a normal clotting mechanism is required to trigger succeeding events. The initial stage ensures that hemostasis takes place and, by the release of vasoactive substances, that an inflammatory response develops, which results in polymorphs and macrophages appearing in large numbers in the wound area. This stage is followed by the formation of collagen from the fibroblasts present in the wound area. This collagen matures over a period of time to help restore the tensile strength of the wound.

This very simplified explanation of what happens in the healing wound is not a static process because the collagen already present adjacent to the healing wound is initially broken down in the wound by enzymes known as collagenases. Thus, at approximately 10 to 14 days post–wounding, this wound is at its weakest point. This process is more pronounced in certain tissues and is of most significance in colonic wounds.

While wound healing is designed to return tissues to as near normal as possible, wounds are not normal tissues. As early as the 1950s, studies of

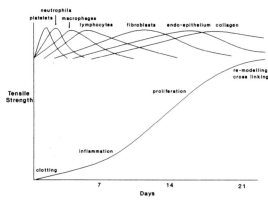

Figure 1. Phases of wound healing.

Table 1
Systemic Factors Affecting Wound Healing

- Age
- Anemia
- Anti–inflammatory Drugs
- Cytotoxic Drugs
- Diabetes Mellitus
- Systemic Infection
- Jaundice
- Malignant Disease
- Malnutrition
- Obesity
- Temperature
- Trauma
- Uremia
- Vitamin Deficiency
- Zinc Deficiency

Table 2
Local Factors Affecting Wound Healing

- Blood Supply
- Denervation
- Hematoma
- Lack of Protection
- Local Infection
- Mechanical Stress
- Radiation
- Surgical Technique
- Suture Material and Technique
- Type of Tissue

---

abdominal wounds in animals showed that at the end of one year, only 70 percent of the pre–wounded tensile strength had been achieved. Wound healing should not be considered "complete" simply when complete epithelialization has occurred. Indeed, work carried out in Cardiff has shown that an incisional hernia can occur up to five years post–operatively.[3]

Unfortunately, understanding experimental wound healing of this type often relies either on the creation of a wound and the post–wounding disruption of it or on using radio–labeled substances to identify rates of production of substances in the wound. The majority of the work performed to date has relied on experiments performed in animals. This work has been justifiably criticized as not reproducing the true clinical situation. In an attempt to overcome this sort of criticism, an experiment was carried out by making abdominal wall wounds in female rats. A condom on the end of a cannula was introduced through the anterior fornix of the vagina at varying times post–wounding. The condom was inflated to reproduce the abdominal distension that takes place post–operatively in patients. Another important experiment used a rabbit ear chamber to observe angiogenesis and to determine the role of oxygen in stimulating healing and the need for a hypoxic drive at the leading edge of the healing wound to stimulate cell division and migration.[4] These experiments demonstrate the lengths researchers have gone to in an attempt to reproduce clinical situations in an experimental model.

Experimental work has produced long lists of systemic and local factors that are known to affect healing (Tables 1 and 2). But the reality is that a patient (no matter how many complicating factors are present) must be cared for. A treatment plan must be designed to ensure that the wound heals as quickly as possible with minimal complications. It is important to recognize that many factors can be controlled in experimental situations that cannot be controlled in patients.

The local factors listed in Table 2 are also of importance, but the requirement for good surgical technique and the appropriate use of surgical materials cannot be ignored by the surgeon performing the operative procedure. Unfortunately, when a wound is slow to heal, the blame is usually placed on the patient, nurse, or the dressing being used to care for the wound. It is vitally important for the surgeon to recognize that good wound healing starts at the time of operation and not when the patient returns to the unit from the operating room. Good surgical technique is one of the most important aspects of wound care that can be controlled;

surgeons must give appropriate attention to this aspect of patient care.

Traditionally, wound healing is classified as healing by either first or second intention to produce a sutured wound or a wound healing by granulation tissue formation. While this classification is adequate to describe the different cellular processes that take place, it does not adequately relate to the problems seen in clinical practice. Alternative classifications include the healing of acute versus chronic wounds; for example, the healing of an appendectomy wound compared to the healing of a venous ulcer is different, if only in terms of time scale. Another possible classification is related to the type of tissue involved, for example, the healing of skin wounds versus the healing of bones. The healing of infected wounds versus the healing of noninfected wounds also merits consideration. Finally, from a practical standpoint, healing wounds in a hospital setting is different than healing in the community, not because the processes are different, but because the amount of support and help that can be provided for patients in the community is different from that which can be provided in the hospital.

Having stated that these alternative classifications should be considered, healing by primary and secondary intention has its merits. In practice, it is usually wounds healing by secondary intention that cause the most difficulty. In addition to the practical difficulties of determining the best way to manage wounds healing by secondary intention and the long time to achieve healing that is often required, it is also important to remember that the development of wound contraction is of potential benefit or harm to the patient and should be considered in planning the care that each patient receives.

Although experiments have been designed and undertaken during recent years to help our understanding of the cellular events that take place, they are no substitute for making direct observations of wounds seen in patients.

Practical Wound Healing in Cardiff, Wales

Organization of wound healing research unit. The University Hospital of Wales, located in Cardiff, Wales, is an 1,000–bed teaching hospital where a granulating wound clinic has been in existence in the department of surgery since 1972.

This wound clinic was set up by Professor L.E. Hughes, the professor of surgery, to help develop new materials for wound management. Over the course of an eleven–year period from 1978 to 1988, 3,349 patients were seen in this granulating wound

Table 3 Staff Structure	
Director of Wound Healing Research Unit	
Nursing Staff	10
Medical Staff	4
Administrative Staff	5
Scientific Staff	6
Educational Facilitator	1

clinic. A range of wound types were seen with pilonidal sinus excision, perianal and abdominal wall wounds being the most commonly encountered. Other wound types included ileostomy closure sites, abscess excisions, melanoma excision sites and wounds resulting from benign breast surgery. Overall, 90 percent of the wounds were healed using wound management materials and interventions other than formal surgical procedures.

Pilonidal sinus wounds were the most common wounds seen in 1988 because, in Cardiff, the favored method of treatment is to excise the area and allow healing to occur by secondary intention. In the wound clinic, only relatively small numbers of leg ulcers and pressure ulcers are seen since there is no guaranteed access to inpatient facilities. It is important to consider the possibility that patients with large or slow–healing wounds may require the increased professional support that is only available on an inpatient basis. The clinic did, however, receive requests for advice on treatment of many patients with these wounds, but they were only seen for a single consultation. There are no data on the outcome of these wounds. The clinic is staffed by a physician, a research bacteriologist, and a research nurse who works with nursing colleagues within the hospital and community environments. In our experience, we have found that the research nurse is the key to ensuring the success of the clinic by linking with other professionals involved in each patient's care.

From 1972 until 1991 this service was provided only on a part–time basis and the salary costs were raised from small research grants given by commercial concerns. This arrangement was unable to provide sufficient support for the demands being made for such a service. To overcome this problem the Wound Healing Research Unit was created in April 1991 to develop the first comprehensive clinical and research unit dedicated to wound healing and wound management.

The unit has four main objectives: 1) to provide a comprehensive clinical service for all patients with wound healing problems; 2) to undertake clinical research to provide information as how best to use modern materials and pharmaceuticals in wound healing; 3) to allow clinicians and scientists to pursue an integrated program in wound care and wound biology to lead to more scientific and innovative approaches to wound management; and 4) to provide a wide range of educational activities for all professionals involved in wound care (Table 3).

Clinical Service

Eleven outpatient clinics are provided during a working week and include a diabetic foot clinic, leg ulcer clinics and acute wound clinics. An inpatient visiting service is available over a wide geographical area and domiciliary visits are made where patients are not well enough to attend as outpatients. During 1994, 1,713 new patients were referred to the Wound Healing Research Unit and 11,666 patient contacts were made.

Clinical Research

An extensive research program is being undertaken in areas ranging from pressure relieving mattresses to dressing materials and other therapeutic devices including pharmacological agents.

Wound Biology

With the continued expansion of the Unit, laboratories are now present on two sites. The initial laboratory is concentrating mainly on molecular biologically–based studies on healing and, using such techniques, has focused particularly on the expression and regulation of dermal collagens during the healing of acute and chronic wounds.

The early studies were concerned with establishing the pattern of expression of the major fibrillar collagens I and II in healing surgical excision cavity wounds and lower limb ulcers. Histological, immunohistochemical, reverse transcription–polymerase chain reaction (RT–PCR), and in situ hybridization techniques were developed in order to analyze the expression of collagens I and III in different wound types, including facial and intra–oral wounds, leg ulcers, excision cavities, and scars. Expression of the pro–inflammatory cytokines IL–1α and 1ß, which regulate collagen gene expression, was also analyzed in these different wounds. These studies demonstrated co–expression of collagens I and III during the healing of surgical excision cavity wounds and spatially differentiated expression of collagens I and III in lower–limb ulcers. Interestingly IL–1ß transcripts were readily identified in most wound types whereas IL–1α expression was only detected in the later phases of healing in the acute wound. More recently we have examined the expression of collagens VII and XII in various wound types. Analysis of the expression of matrix metalloproteinases in human wounds using a combination of immunohistochemical, sinographic, RT–PCR, and in situ hybridization techniques is being undertaken. Preliminary findings indicate differential expression of MMP2 and MMP9 in human wounds.

At new laboratories, we have looked at the differential expression of a number of integrins during healing of wounds of different etiologies using immunohistochemical studies and cell culture experiments. These new laboratories include a Biochemistry laboratory, an Immunohistology and Microbiology laboratory, and Tissue Culture facilities. The major thrust of this component of the Unit is to study cellular interactions within the wound environment and how the wound healing process may be influenced by local factors derived from the inflammatory process and the wound micro–biological flora. In addition, *in vitro* wound models are being established using human cell lines, wound tissue explants, and hydrodynamic models for micro–biological studies. In addition to their use to investigate the basic parameter of the healing process these models are being used to investigate how exogenous therapies may have a beneficial effect on healing.

Educational Activities

For many years the recognition of the department's and more recently the unit's expertise in wound healing has resulted in frequent requests from health professionals throughout the world to visit the clinics to obtain advice and information on a wide range of subjects. The importance of education is recognized by the appointment of an Educational Facilitator within the unit whose major responsibility is to provide a range of educational activities for all healthcare professionals. In addition to short courses it is possible for us to undertake a course that will lead to a university diploma in Wound Healing and Wound Care, which is designed to appeal to a multidisciplinary audience.

In addition to these activities members of the unit advise national and international bodies involved with wound healing activities through membership of advisory boards of journals and through organizing major international conferences.

Members of the unit also produced two text books for a major medical publisher. The unit has been involved in the production of the first educational program on wound healing for medical undergraduates. Over the years we have produced a number of video tapes, some of which have won educational awards. The unit has been commissioned to produce a multi media educational program for Team Care Valleys to help develop wound healing expertise and primary healthcare teams.

Educational Good Practice Guides on wound management have been produced for junior medical staff and senior nurses.

Observations on Wounds

The benefits of seeing a large number of patients with granulating wounds caused by differing etiologies have enabled us to develop a greater understanding of certain fundamental aspects of wound healing.

Wound shape. In order for a wound to heal by granulation, the wound must be of a boat or bowl shape to ensure that granulation tissue fills the base before the epithelial edges of the wound meet. If the shape of the wound does not allow this process to occur, there is considerable risk of premature surface healing, leaving a cavity underneath which will subsequently break down. If wounds created by surgeons are not of satisfactory shape, then the patient is referred back to the surgeon for a further operative procedure.

Wound color. In a number of patients, a yellow, fibrinous membrane develops on the surface of the granulating wound. Wounds that develop this membrane do not become infected. The wound heals at a rate that is considered normal for that wound type. If attempts are made to remove the membrane, it will recur within a few days. Recognition of this variant of normal is important to prevent unnecessary manipulation of the wound.

In contrast, many doctors and nurses feel that the presence of a deep red color to the granulation tissue is a good sign of healing and should be encouraged. However, our experience suggests that certain wound types that develop this livid red surface may be infected and slow to heal.

Wound Examination

Wound examination requires more than just a cursory glance at a wound to ensure that each has a normal shape, size, and color for its specific wound type. Wounds that are tracking away from the surface need to be probed to ensure that free drainage can be maintained. If not, surgery must be performed or a dressing that fills the sinus adequately must be used. Examination of the wound should also include some simple but effective measurement of the wound size. It is extremely easy to measure a wound's length, width, and depth, which should be included in the patient's notes in order to have an objective measurement of progress in wound healing over a period of time. Without consistent recording of these measurements, it is very difficult to determine whether a wound has decreased in size over a period of time. In a number of patients that were referred to the clinic with wounds that were not progressing toward healing, an obvious cause was found when the wound was observed critically as described above.[5]

Expected Healing Times

One of the most difficult questions to answer when dealing with patients who have granulating wounds is "How long will the wound take to heal?" The answer to this question can be extremely variable, and it is apparent to all caregivers involved in clinical care that wounds caused by different etiologies heal at different rates, e.g., the healing rate of a pilonidal sinus wound is different from the healing of a venous ulcer. In wounds of similar etiology, there will be a variation in the healing rates in different patients due to the individual's healing potential. In addition, it is likely that the wound management regime that is followed may also affect the healing rate. Materials, if used inappropriately, are more likely to retard healing rather than improve healing rates.

It is difficult to collect data on all wound types in this respect, but we have evaluated three wound types: pilonidal sinus wounds, vertical abdominal wounds, and axillary wounds. We have been able to show that the healing of these wound types can be predicted with a considerable degree of accuracy.[6] The predictability of healing these wound types enables clinicians to detect when wounds of a similar type are not healing at the normal rate. It also alerts clinicians to the need to look carefully at the wound to identify the reasons why healing is not occurring. In the wound types for which these data are present, infection and underlying systemic diseases such as diabetes and malignancy have been identified as causes for deviation from predicted healing time.

Infection in Granulating Wounds

Infection is a cause of significant delay of healing in pilonidal sinus, abdominal, and axillary wounds.

Table 4
Features of Infection in Granulation Tissue

- Superficial bridging
- Friable tissue
- Bleeding on contact
- Pain in the wound
- Delay in healing

Treatment with antibiotics is necessary to remove organisms and return the healing of the wound to normal.[7] Experience in managing infected granulating wounds of the above types has led us to believe that wound swabbing is only of secondary importance to recognizing the abnormal granulation tissue seen in infected wounds. (The characteristics of unhealthy granulation tissue are listed in Table 4.) In our clinic, before the results of the wound swabs are available, the decision is made to use antibiotics to treat patients with this abnormal granulation tissue. We have found that, in practice, patients with infected granulating wounds require treatment with oral antibiotics for a minimum of two weeks and occasionally for up to four weeks to ensure that the infection has been cleared and that the granulation tissue has returned to its normal healthy appearance.

The antibiotics regime is usually a combination of metronidazole and erythromycin. In pilonidal sinus wounds, the usual organism cultured in infected wounds is of the *Bacteriodes* species[8] and in abdominal and axillary wounds it is *staphylococcus aureus*.

We have also found that granulating wounds appear infected at two stages: either immediately upon presentation at the clinic, approximately 10 days post–operatively, or at the end stage of healing when the wound has progressed satisfactorily but just prior to the point when complete healing becomes indolent with the abnormal granulation tissue described above. In wounds that become infected at this stage, clearing organisms is achieved by using a topical antibiotic or by a 0.5 percent solution of silver nitrate being applied to the wound for a 10 to 14 day period. This regime has been extremely effective in dealing with infection at the end stage of healing.

Use of Antiseptics or Cleansing Solutions

Considerable data have been generated on the harmful effects of chemical agents on the healing of wounds.[9–11] This evidence has been produced mainly in tissue culture and animal experiments. However, it is likely to be of clinical relevance since a great deal of wound cleansing is performed because of a routine that a nurse or doctor has developed over a period of time and not because of any specific requirement for a particular wound. The routine use of antiseptics should, in our opinion, be resisted because it only lowers the bacterial colonization of the wound for a short period and there is no evidence that it produces any significant clinical benefit. The use of these potentially toxic substances by healthcare professionals on a routine basis is not good practice. Healthcare professionals should be encouraged to develop a flexible and thoughtful approach to the procedures they are undertaking for each patient under their care to determine whether each step in a procedure is necessary for the benefit of the patient. All chemical agents have the potential to harm the actively dividing cells that are attempting to heal the wound. Clinicians too often feel that they need to use something "medicated" when sterile water or saline would suffice.

Practicality of Treatment Regime

One of the most important lessons learned in the wound clinic has been that even though the best regime for a patient can be identified on theoretical grounds, if that regime cannot be put into practice, it is of little use to the patient. Factors that influence the execution of a suggested regime are related to the availability and cost of materials, the amount of professional care that can be provided for a patient, and the amount of care that the patient or the patient's relatives are able to provide.

It is obvious that there is a considerable amount of professional input that can be offered in a hospital environment. Twice–daily dressing changes are possible if indicated. However, if the same patient with the same wound was being cared for on an outpatient basis, twice–daily dressing changes may not be practical.

Another situation that may arise is when a patient is offered a regime that involves discomfort. Despite the theoretical benefits of such a regime, the patient may refuse it or be non–compliant and frustrate attempts at healing. While in the majority of wounds the objective is to achieve healing in as short a period of time as possible, in certain situations other objectives must be considered. In a patient with a wound resulting from advanced malignancy, attempts to achieve complete healing are unrealistic. In this situation, the goal should be to relieve pain and odor and to make the patient as comfortable as possible. Patients are very appreciative of attempts to minimize the burden that such wounds place on them.[11]

Another situation seen in a small percentage of patients with chronic wounds (particularly leg ulcers) occurs when all attempts to achieve healing are frustrated by the patient. These patients are often elderly individuals who live alone and whose only contact with society is through their health-care professional. When this situation occurs, a treatment regime should be directed toward offering a simple and inexpensive form of treatment and spending time talking to the patient.

Specific Wound Types

Pilonidal sinus wounds. Patients with pilonidal sinus wounds usually range from 20 to 30 years of age and desire to return to normal activities as quickly as possible. It is important to consider a regime that allows a prompt return to normalcy but reduces the risk of recurrence of this condition by ensuring that the wound does not bridge superficially and that hair or other foreign bodies are not trapped in the wound.

Leg ulcers. In patients with leg ulcers, one of the biggest problems is to accurately establish the etiology of the ulcer. The majority of these wounds result from deficiencies in the venous system of the leg. However, a significant number of these patients have an arterial element of their etiology, which cannot be detected on clinical grounds alone and produces an ulcer of mixed arterial and venous etiology. The use of Doppler measurements to obtain brachial and ankle pressure is necessary and of significant importance in planning treatment, as applying compression to a leg with unrecognized arterial disease is likely to retard the healing process.

In achieving adequate levels of compression on a limb, it is important to consider the ability of the nurse, family, or patient to apply bandages or stockings appropriately. Methods of achieving high levels of compression are of limited benefit if that level is not maintained for a long period of time and, in certain cases, a lower level of compression that can be maintained over a longer period may be more beneficial.

Hidradenitis Suppurativa. This particularly distressing condition affects the apocrine sweat glands found in the axillae and perineal areas of the body and results in recurrent boils and abscesses in these areas. To overcome the problem of recurrence and repeated drainage of abscesses in this condition, radical excision of the area of skin containing these

---

Table 5
Types of Granulating Wounds

- Deep Sinuses
- Cavities
- Exuding Wounds
- Dry Wounds
- Flat Surfaces
- Necrotic Wounds

---

sweat glands has been developed in Cardiff. Although these are large and irregularly shaped wounds, appropriate wound management results in an acceptable cosmetic result with linear scarring and full range of movement.[13] This outcome shows that the phenomenon of wound contraction can be used to the patient's advantage and not produce the problems seen in patients who have wounds such as burns. Although these large wounds may require 8 to 12 weeks to achieve complete healing, with appropriate wound management they can be managed on an outpatient basis for the majority of this healing time.

Evaluation of Dressings for Granulating wounds

Within the last ten years, there has been an explosion in the development of new wound dressings with differing physical properties that have been developed to improve the care of wounds usually dressed with gauze. Since its development as a wound dressing in the 1800s, gauze has become the traditional method of managing granulating wounds. Despite the recognition of problems with its use for many years, it still remains in widespread use today.

In the early 1970s, Terry Turner (see Chapter 16) identified characteristics of an ideal wound dressing. Many manufacturers have attempted to overcome the problems of gauze by developing new dressings that fulfill these criteria. Unfortunately, in many situations, products have been developed based on the performance of materials in a laboratory situation and have not been supported with scientifically organized clinical studies to ensure that they are of clinical benefit. Without sufficient clinical data to identify how, when, and why these dressings should be used, little progress in the management of wounds will be achieved.

In our clinic, we have undertaken various studies to accurately identify the place of some of these materials in the management of wounds.[14,15] These studies involved the use of dressings in a hospital situation and examined the practical aspects of wound management in the community since most wound care in the United Kingdom is offered in the hospital environment.

Both clinicians and manufacturers have been guilty of attempting to produce and prescribe a single product for the management of all wound situations. It is our belief that no single wound dressing will ever be able to deal with all wound situations. The task for all healthcare professionals involved in wound care is to identify the most appropriate dressing for each stage of the healing process.

Although Turner's criteria for an ideal dressing are of great importance, another classification has been used to help identify which dressing to use in specific situations. The simple but practical list of wounds seen in clinical practice (Table 5) enables the clinician to identify dressings of particular types that are of most benefit in various situations, e.g., hydrocolloids are particularly beneficial for dry wounds and sheet foams for flat epithelializing surfaces.

Despite having an increased range of materials with which to dress the wound, there remains a mistaken belief that the dressing alone will heal the wound. Consequently, clinicians often neglect to take into consideration other even more important factors in a particular patient. For instance, in the management of leg ulcers, achieving adequate levels of compression on the limb is more important than the wound contact layer. Inappropriate expectations of dressing performance will not be replaced until healthcare professionals concerned with wound care are educated and clinicians undertake procedures based on logical reasoning.

Educational Issues in Wound Care

While wound care is an essential part of the daily work of many doctors and nurses, there is a considerable lack of knowledge and understanding of what are the most appropriate methods of managing wounds. Doctors do not receive any specific education in wound healing and wound management at the undergraduate level. Once they are practicing, we believe they do not wish to show their ignorance of such a basic aspect of care. Nurses do receive education on wound care, but their teachers often use outdated ideas. Since many nurses do not wish to question their superiors, many old–fashioned and potentially harmful procedures are still being taught and used.

In addition to this lack of information, the responsibilities for wound care are often ill–defined. These responsibilities not only vary from hospital to hospital but also vary between different departments within a hospital. In North America, enterostomal therapy nurses have taken on the responsibilities for wound management. This development has been one of the most significant advances in wound care for many years as it has produced an identified professional group with interest and expertise in this area of patient care. Unfortunately, no such easily defined group exists in the United Kingdom.

While there is a need to educate doctors and nurses, there is also a need to inform other professional groups that may become involved in wound care. The hospital pharmacist often has a role in the purchasing of dressings. In the near future, the potential for incorporating active substances into dressings will increase this role considerably. Hospital managers and those responsible for budgets in other areas of the healthcare systems require an education. They must understand that although some of the newer materials may have higher unit costs, the potential improvement in terms of healing time, health professionals' time and improvement in the patient's quality of life while the wound is healing are all important factors to be considered. Finally, patients should be educated, not only to involve themselves in more of their own wound care, but also to know to complain when the wound care that is being offered is preventing them from quickly returning to a normal lifestyle.[16]

Without the education of all of the groups mentioned, as well as the manufacturers, any attempt to improve wound care for patients is likely to be frustrated. The educational requirement is an area that merits urgent attention.

Conclusion

The aim of this chapter has been to show that a sound knowledge of the stages of wound healing is required by all caregivers involved with wound care. However, having that knowledge alone is not sufficient for clinicians to offer good wound care to patients. The lessons learned and the protocols developed in the Wound Healing Research Unit in Cardiff have helped to enable the staff to offer patients comprehensive and practical wound care. The principles learned from previous experience with surgical wounds are applicable to the more chronic and difficult wounds such as leg ulcers. Also, the potential for using the post–operative surgical wound as a model for wound healing in patients has merit, as the population that suffers from chronic wounds often has a wide variety of other factors that affect wound healing potential in individual patients.

The presence of this type of unit staffed by surgeons, physicians, laboratory staff, and nurses in a university hospital has shown that a team of healthcare professionals is required to offer good wound care. The breaking down of interprofessional barriers is important. Also, the prospect of setting up a wound "intensive care" where patients with particularly difficult wounds have access to all professional groups may become a reality when wound care is recognized as a legitimate area of interest and expertise.

The presence of this type of unit staffed by surgeons, physicians, laboratory staff, and nurses in a university hospital has shown that a team of healthcare professionals is required to offer good wound care.

The potential for using wound management products that have active ingredients that stimulate wound healing and the possibility of introducing growth factors into the wound are interesting developments. In view of the likely expense of such treatments, it is essential that clinical research is performed to ensure that they are used in the most appropriate way for the wounds that will benefit most from them.

The manufacturers of wound dressings should no longer be developing products based solely on what can be achieved in a laboratory. They should consult with clinicians in wound care about the problems they face and then develop products to meet those needs. The industry should also consider producing good quality, unbiased educational programs on wound care to assist the large number of healthcare professionals who could benefit from them.

When educational issues have been addressed and the industry and healthcare professionals involved in wound care can work together to improve standards, only then will patients have access to a high standard of wound care.

References

1. Irwin TT. *Wound Healing – Principles and Practice*. London, UK, Chapman Hall, 1981.
2. Bucknall TE, Ellis H. *Wound Healing For Surgeons*. London, UK, Balliere Tundall, 1984.
3. Harding KG, Mudge M, Leinster SJ, Hughes LE. Late development of incisional hernia: An unrecognized problem. *British Medical Journal* 1983;286:519–520.
4. Hunt TK. *The Wound Healing and Wound Infection – Theory and Surgical Practice*. New York, NY, Appleton Century Press, 1980.
5. Harding KG, Turner TD, Schmidt RJ. *Advances in Wound Management*. London, UK, John Wiley, 1986.
6. Marks J, Hughes LE, Harding KG, Campbell H, Riberio CD. Prediction of healing time as an aid to the management of open granulating wounds. *World Journal of Surgery* 1983;7:641–645.
7. Marks J, Harding KG, Hughes LE. Staphylococcal infection of open granulating wounds. *British Journal of Surgery* 1987;74:95–97.
8. Marks J, Harding KG, Hughes LE, Riberio CD. Pilonidal sinus excision – healing by open granulation. *British Journal of Surgery* 1985;72:637–640.
9. Brennan SS, Leaper DJ. The effect of antiseptics on the healing wound: A study using rabbit ear chambers. *British Journal of Surgery* 1985;72:10.
10. Brennan SS, Foster ME, Leaper DJ. Antiseptic toxicity in wounds healing by secondary intention. *Journal of Hospital Infection* 1986;8(3):263–67.
11. Leaper DJ, Simpson RA. The effect of antiseptics and topical antimicrobials on wound healing. *Journal of Antimicrobial Chemotherapy* 1986;17(2):135–37.
12. Bale S, Harding KG. Fungating breast wounds. *Journal of District Nursing* 1987;5(12):4–5.
13. Morgan WP, Harding KG, Hughes LE. A comparison of skin grafting and healing by granulation following axillary excision for hidradenitis supperativa. *Annals of the Royal College of Surgeons of England* 1983;65:235–36.
14. Harding KG, Richardson G. Silastic foam elastomer for healing open granulating wounds. *Nursing Times* 1979;September 27:1679–1682.
15. Harding KG, Bale S, Mcpake B, Hughes LE. Wound management in the community – comparison of Melolin and Lyofoam. *Care Science and Practice* 1988;6(2):56.
16. Bale S, Harding KG. Education for nurses and patients – leg ulcers. *Nursing Standard* 1989;3:422.

16

The Development of Wound Management Products

Terence D. Turner, OBE, FRPharmS, MPharm, MCPP

Turner TD. The development of wound management products. In: Krasner D, Kane D. *Chronic Wound Care, Second Edition*. Wayne, PA, Health Management Publications, Inc., 1997, pp 124–138.

Introduction

Throughout history many diverse materials of animal, vegetable and mineral origin have been used to treat wounds. They range from the hot oils and waxes reported in the Ebers papyrus[1] through the animal membranes and feces of the Middle Ages to the picked oakum of the nineteenth century. Some of these products have survived; both cotton "wool" and Gamgee tissue were as familiar to the surgeon of 1880 as they are to the physician of today.

Until 1960, advances in the design and efficacy of wound management products had been spasmodic and limited to the adaptation of available materials that were being used for other purposes. The products were primarily of the "plug and conceal" variety and could be considered as *Passive* products that took no part in the healing process. Very little attention was paid to the functional performance of a product and minimal consideration was given to the healing environments required for different wound types.

A new generation of products was potentiated by the advances in knowledge of the humoral and cellular factors associated with the healing process and the realization that a controlled microenvironment was needed if wound healing was to progress at the optimal level. These environmental control dressings are classified as *Interactive* dressings; current developments are directed at bioactive products which will directly or indirectly stimulate some part of the healing cascade (Figure 1).

This chapter will survey the progressive development of wound management products indicating the performance profile of the different product groups with their possible clinical usage. The ever increasing new product appearance in the medical market many of which are "me too" duplicates of other products precludes the use of brand names and allows a broader perspective of the advances in "real term" formulations.

Linteum and oakum. Linteum was the first "woven" fabric to be recognized as a "surgical" material, and in 1816 a sample of "patent lint" was presented by William Cade King, Governor of St. Bartholomew's Hospital, London to the House Committee to consider its adoption within the hospital.[2] It consisted of a cloth which had its nap raised on one side by scraping with a knife to produce a soft pile. With the advent of the Crimean War came power driven machines which stimulated William Bradbury Robinson of Chesterfield to produce a lint machine which gave production equal to six girls on hand machines. The lint was also bleached and purified. It was often formed into Dossils (cylindrical pieces), Pledgets (oval shaped), and Boulsters or tents (conical compresses).

Abraham Rees in 1819 summarized the uses as follows:[3]

1) To stop blood in fresh wounds by filling with dry lint. In large hemorrhages, dip lint into alcohol or oil of turpentine.
2) To agglutinate and heal wounds when spread with ointments.
3) To dry wounds and ulcers, thus forwarding the formulation of a cicatrix.
4) To keep the tops of wounds at proper distance so that they do not hastily unite before the bottom is well digested and healed.
5) To prevent the access of air.

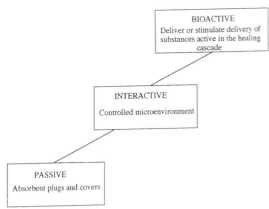

Figure 1. *Classification of wound management product activity.*

He added that it should be noted "that when used to dress deep wounds a thread should be tied to each portion before insertion to assist in its removal." This product was to be used with slight modification for over 100 years.

A similar development on fibrous materials was to be initiated by another war stimulus (Table 1). Dr. Lewis A. Sayre of New York wrote enthusiastically about the use of oakum in the American Civil War.[1] This was a fibrous mass produced by shredding tarred or untarred rope, the former sometimes being referred to as "marine lint" (a name also retained for tow impregnated with fresh Stockholm tar). The *Lancet* of 1870 reported that it "absorbs discharges, destroys bad odors and supersedes the use of lint, ointments and linseed meal or bread poultices." Picking oakum was often considered good occupational therapy for prisoners, with obvious difficulties in producing a good and reproducible quality. In 1871 selected quality rope was being reduced to oakum by "Southall Son and Dymond," manufacturing chemists of Birmingham, England. Joseph Samson Gamgee[4] referred to this material in his clinical lectures at Queen's Hospital, Birmingham in 1876. He told of his extensive use of oakum as an absorbent dressing either by itself or over a thin layer of fine cotton or stitched into gauze bags to make absorbent pads.

Gamgee also noted that in 1870, M. Alphonso Guerin of Paris had reported a method of dressing amputation stumps using "cotton wool." This was raw cotton which although non–absorbent had been washed and carded. Gamgee, wishing to emulate Guerin, obtained the best quality cotton that was available, a material which was prepared as a packing for jeweler's goods and rejected all lesser grades as unsuitable. His interest encouraged the production of better grades in which the fibers had been treated to remove every trace of grease and were thus not only rendered absorbent but had a markedly reduced level of bacterial contamination. In 1880 Gamgee wrote a paper describing experiments in which he had used the cotton pads covered with tiffany, a fine bleached gauze used by nurserymen to stretch under the roofs of their conservatories to protect their plants from the depravation of invading birds. Working in collaboration with Messrs Robinson and son of Chesterfield, England, Gamgee showed that the gauze could be made more absorbent by bleaching and thus formulated the Gamgee tissue which was the forerunner for today's "gauze and cotton tissue." It was the first named pad to be designed using a woven fabric and a fibrous mass with the criterion of function as the basis of the design.

The British Pharmaceutical Codex of 1923,[5] the then only accepted source of quality standards for pharmaceutical products, gave monographs for Gauze and Cotton Tissue, eight different lints, thirteen gauze products and fifteen cotton wools (Table 2). The 1988 British Pharmacopoeia[6] still contained twelve gauze products and three fibrous absorbents but excluded lint and Gamgee tissue (Table 3). Gauze, the survivor of those early fabrics although currently contraindicated as a wound contact dressing, is used widely in surgery. The current European Pharmacopoeia specifies eight different gauze fabrics dependent upon the weight per unit area and number of threads in the warp and weft. These fabrics are available in twelve different sizes and five different plys, giving a possible four–hundred and eighty products of sheet gauze – an exalted position for the humble tiffany greenhouse crop protector (Table 4).

Table 2 Surgical Materials British Pharmaceutical Codex 1923	
Cotton Wools	15
Gauzes	13
Tows	4
Gauze and Cotton Tissue	2
Bandages	9
Protectives (Jaconet etc.)	4
Emplastrums	32
Lints	8

Table 3 Surgical Materials British Pharmacopoeia 1988	
Gauze Products	9
Ribbon Gauze	3
Dressing Pads	5
Fibrous Absorbents	3
Surgical Felts	3
Bandages	20
Surgical Tapes	7
Impregnated Gauze	3
Stockinette	8
Adhesive Dressings	4
Film Dressings	1
Foam Dresings	3

Absorbents[7]

The overall function of clinical absorbents is self explanatory and they have demonstrated minimal development in the past decade. They are required to absorb and retain a wide range of fluids from the blood and serous exudate of damaged tissue to the variable gut content met during surgical intervention.[4,5] They are found in a number of forms: fibrous (staple) absorbents, fabric absorbents, and fiber plus fabric absorbents.

Fibrous absorbents. Fibrous absorbents are made from cotton staple or from the fibers of viscose or cellulose; viscose and cotton and viscose or cotton and acrylic fibers may be admixed.

Absorbent cotton is available in different qualities varying with the length and diameter of the cotton staple. It is available in the form of rolls and balls and is used for cleansing and swabbing wounds, preoperative skin preparation and the application of topical medicaments to the skin.

The absorption, performance, and physical character of absorbent viscose varies markedly with the manufacturing process. It is available in the bright or "dull" form, the latter containing a particulate material such as titanium dioxide within the fiber. The fibers are, in general, a continuous staple with a crenate transsectional profile, but smooth and lumenated forms are available which show different degrees of absorptive capacity and wet tensile strength.

Some fibrous absorbents were developed containing a proportion of acrylamide or other synthetic polymeric fiber. These absorbents frequently enhance the absorptive performance and give "body" to the fleece, thus improving fluid retention and avoiding fluid "squeeze out" which is caused by fleece collapse after wetting.

Cellulose wadding is produced from delignified wood pulp and manufactured in a multiple laminate material form. It is used in large pieces to absorb large volumes of fluid in incontinence but is not used in contact with a wound unless enclosed in an outer fabric sleeve to prevent fiber loss to the wound.

Fabric absorbents. Absorbent lint is a close weave cotton cloth with a raised nap on one side which offers a large surface area for evaporation when placed with the nap upward on an exuding wound. It is generally unacceptable for modern wound management.

Absorbent gauze is the most widely used absorbent and consists of a cotton cloth of plain weave bleached to a good white, clean and reasonably free from weaving defects, cotton leaf and shell. It may be slightly off white if sterilized. It absorbs water readily but its performance may be reduced by prolonged storage or exposure to heat.

Surgical usage of absorbent gauze. Gauze products are primarily absorbents when used preoperatively, perioperatively and postoperativel. Perioperatively, however, they are also required to protect tissue and organs by occluding areas not involved in the procedure, to aid in the application of wet heat which may establish the viability of doubtful tissue, and to assist in blunt dissection where fascias are separated along the lines of cleavage thus avoiding unnecessary cutting.[6]

To contribute to hemostasis the gauze fabric may contain a proportion of viscose incorporated with the cotton either in the warp and the weft or exclusively in the weft. A maximum level of 45 percent of viscose is widely accepted. A range of gauze fabrics exist graded according to the number of threads per 10 cm width of gauze, as shown in Table 4.

Gauze products fall into two broad categories – the "swab" or "sponge" type produced by folding and stitching the cloth and those consisting of the plain cloth. The "swab" type includes swabs, strips, pads and pledgets. The "plain" types include packs and ribbon. They are available with and without a radio opaque (X ray detectable) element, and some are colored for recognition with a suitable fast, non–toxic dye for use by the anaesthetist.

Non woven fabrics include a wide range of products manufactured from synthetic and semisynthetic fibers. Non–woven viscose fabric swabs are available in folded pieces of various dimensions. They are occasionally used in error as a single wound dressing. They have a lower total absorbent capacity than gauze but absorb more quickly because of the random orientation of the viscose fibers. They can replace the more sophisticated cotton swab for general purpose swabbing and cleansing procedures. As fabrics they constitute the outer layer on a number of wound dressing pads sometimes suitably coated with a polymer to reduce adherence at dressing change.

A cellulose sponge is a cavity foam cellulose based sponge available in sheets and thin bands. They are used to absorb at small sites in surgery.

Neuropatties are small squares or strips of non–woven absorbent viscose with thread stitched through the non–woven fabric and left long. They are used as spot absorbents particularly in neurosurgery. They are frequently moistened in saline before application. The threads are left outside the surgical area and on completion of surgery the recovery of each pattie is facilitated by lifting each thread. Products vary in size and shape and there may also be a device for attaching the ends of all the threads, thus producing a mini count rack.

Fiber plus fabric absorbents. Gauze and cellulose wadding consists of a thick layer of cellulose wadding enclosed in a tubular form gauze. The properties of the two separate materials have already been described; combined, the gauze and cellulose wadding tissue is used as an absorbent and protective pad. It should only be used as a wound dressing with a non–adherent layer placed between the pad and the wound. It has a high absorbency, and because of its thickness the additional property of insulation which results in raising the temperature at skin surface has been shown to accelerate the wound healing rate. On a highly exuding surface, there is a tendency for the cellulose wadding element to collapse when wet and become a semi–solid wet mass. This process may cause difficulty in practice. In such fluid loss situations, the gauze and cotton tissue is preferred.

Gamgee tissue is a thick layer of absorbent cotton enclosed in a tubular form gauze. It has the same uses as gauze and cellulose wadding tissue

Table 4
Absorbent Gauze European Pharmacopea

| Type | Threads/10cm | | wt. g/m² |
	Warp	Weft	
13 light	73	5	14
13 heavy	70	60	17
17	100	70	23
18	100	80	24
20	120	80	27
22	120	100	30
24a	120	120	32
24b	140	100	32

but has the advantage of a higher absorbent capacity and less wet collapse. It is also softer in use and thus conforms more readily to the wound surface. It should be used in place of gauze and cellulose wadding tissue on high exudating surfaces such as burns, but as previously stated for gauze and cellulose wadding tissue it should not be used in direct contact with the wound surface but placed upon a non–adherent dressing.

Ideal Wound Dressing

In the 1960s the recognition that gauze was a passive product which plugged and concealed but did little to encourage wound healing resulted in an expression of the minimal criteria for an ideal wound dressing. Such a dressing would allow a wound to heal at the optimum rate concomitant with the physiological state of the patient. Gauze and similar materials did not meet these requirements and their use has diminished relative to the development of new products which meet some but not all of the stated criteria.

The performance parameters of an ideal wound dressing specified in 1979[7] were the result of observations in clinical situations indicating the failure of the then contemporary dressings to optimize wound healing:
• To remove excess exudate and toxic components,
• To maintain a high humidity at wound/dressing interface,
• To allow gaseous exchange,
• To provide thermal insulation,
• To afford protection from secondary infection,
• To be free from particulate or toxic contaminants, and
• To allow removal without trauma at dressing change.

Acceptable handling characteristics were also specified to include a good size range, resistance to tear and disintegration when wet and dry, conformability, sterilizability and disposability.

These parameters have since been extended, but they were the initial stimuli for the development of functionally designed interactive products using both the advances in the technology of materials and our knowledge of the humoral and cellular factors associated with the healing process.

They mark the progression toward the production of an "ideal wound dressing." It should, however, be emphasized that no single dressing will produce the optimum microenvironment for all wounds or for all of the healing stages of one wound. The spectrum of performance requires that the wound is diagnosed and the treatment progressed by prescribing the most suitable dressing.

The first progression toward interactive products was the development of wound dressing pads with a high absorptive capacity, a slow strike through and a low adherence wound contact surface. These were initially available in simple sleeved pads containing cotton, viscose or cellulose fibers with an outer sleeve of gauze or non–woven fabric. They were reformulated as a laminate pad with a multiple layer core, having an outer sleeve of cotton, viscose or non–woven fabric which may have been treated with a polymer (polypropylene) to reduce adherence. The multilayer core is designed to increase absorptive capacity and to prolong usage by delaying strike through to the outer surface. This delay is facilitated by using a fluid retardant layer within the upper and outer sleeve which encourages lateral rather than vertical movement of fluid within the pad. Strike through is undesirable because it provides a band of wet dressing which will allow transmission of airborne organisms to a clean wound or bacteria from an infected wound to the outer dressing surface, thus acting as a possible vector in infection transmission.

Pads with wound contact surfaces designed to be of low adherence were produced for low exudate and drying wounds where high adherence can be expected and high absorptive capacity irrelevant. They vary from aluminum coated fabrics to perforated polymeric films or heat bonded polyethylene films. The wound contact film is attached to an absorbent fibrous mat and an outer woven or non–woven fabric. In some products the polymeric film forms a continuous sleeve on both dressing surfaces. These low adherence, low absorptive capacity dressings are sometimes centered on an adhesive backing to produce an island dressing which is presented as a postoperative adhesive dressing or in the more familiar form of a first aid island or strip dressing for superficial injuries.

Low adherence primary dressing. Manufacturers found difficulties in producing wound dressing pads which would meet all the ideal parameters, in particular that of low adherence. They produced low adherence wound contact products which consisted of a partially open cell structured nylon or viscose fabric which may be finished with a silicone coating. The open cell structure allowed fluid transmission to a secondary superimposed absorbent dressing which could be changed when required without disturbing the primary low adherent contact layer.

The two layer system heralded the concept of a primary and secondary wound management system where the primary dressing would meet the requirements of permeability, non adherence and bacterial impermeability and the secondary the need for absorption, protection and insulation. This concept resulted in a number of products being specified as primary dressings and their associated secondary pads as low or high exudate absorption performers.

Impregnated Dressings

Close weave gauze and open weave tulles are used as carriers of medicated and unmedicated ointments to the wound surface and were developed initially to lower adherence and subsequently as release systems for antibacterials and antibiotics.

Paraffin gauze (Tulle dressing). Paraffin gauze was developed during the 1914 to 1918 European War. It is a bleached cotton or combined cotton and viscose cloth impregnated with yellow or white soft paraffin. It is available as sterile single pieces or multipacks. The paraffin is present to prevent the dressing from adhering to a wound. The gauze which may be leno in nature is coated so that all the threads of the fabric are impregnated but the spaces between the threads are free of paraffin. The material is used primarily in the treatment of wounds such as burns and scalds where the protective function of the stratum corneum is lost and water vapor can escape. Paraffin gauze dressing functions by reducing the fluid loss while the water barrier layer is reforming. The two properties of the paraffin gauze that are most useful are those of non–adherence and semi–occlusiveness.

In addition to burns and scalds the dressing is used as a wound contact layer in lacerations, abrasions and in ulcers where it is used as a packing material to promote granulation. Postoperatively it is used as a vaginal or perineal dressing and for

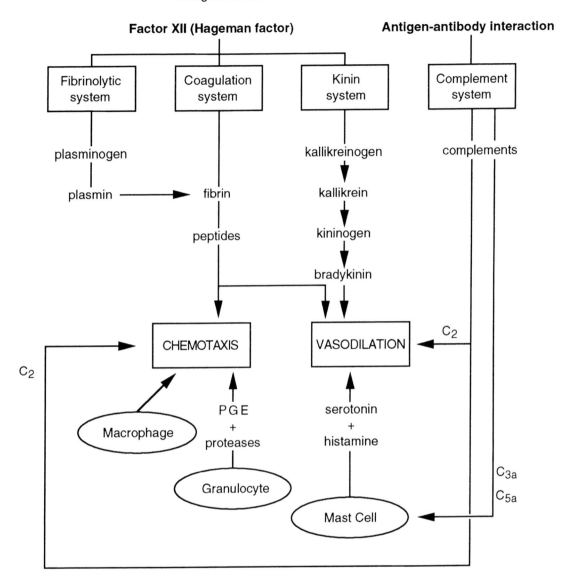

Figure 2. Healing cascade, cellular and humoral factors.

sinus packing. A recent development has been the substitution of cotton gauze with cellulose acetate and a paraffin emulsion impregnation.

Povidone Iodine 10 percent, Chlorhexidine 0.5 percent w/w, Sodium Fusidate 2 percent w/w, 1 percent Framycetin Sulphate, 3 percent Bismuth tri-boron phenate and Cod Liver Oil with Honey are some examples of available impregnations which are recommended for the reduction of infection. Diffusion of the antibacterial agent into or onto an infected and exuding wound has been shown to be minimal. The possibility of development of resistant strains of infective organisms has reduced the usage of these products and has led to the development of antibacterial products containing silver ions. One such material uses a vapor permeable film as a base with a coating of a controlled release polymer that dissolves in either water or water vapor to release silver ions to the wound and the sustained release is said to continue over a period of 5 to 7 days. A similar product in activated carbon dressing is described under deodorizing dressing.

Other impregnations now available include gauze pads saturated with zinc saline, coated with a partially hydrated hydrogel or the "hydrogel" acemannan derived from *Aloe vera, syn. Aloe barbadensis.*

Deodorizing Dressings

These dressings were developed as functionally specific primary dressings. Infected wounds frequently produce obnoxious odors which are embarrassing to the patient and may have a detrimental effect upon the wound management procedure. Fungating carcinomas and venous ulcers are but two of the conditions which would be advantaged by the use of a deodorizing dressing.

These conditions have been formulated from a high gaseous sorptive material, activated carbon, presented as a woven fabric or a fibrous mat backed by a nylon sleeve, a semipermeable film or a polyurethane foam. In each formulation the objective is to reduce odor and the dressings must therefore be large enough to cover the entire malodorous area. One product encourages direct contact of the carbon layer with the wound exudate, and while this contact will limit gaseous absorption it is claimed that the incorporation of bound silver into the charcoal cloth inactivates bacteria which are absorbed onto the fabric surface, thus reducing the infective level which will result in a reduction of odor. It is self evident that once the activated carbon has absorbed serum plus bacteria it will cease to act specifically as a deodorizer.

Polymeric Dressings

In spite of the advances in fiber technology and the better understanding of the physiological parameters associated with wound healing, the fabric dressing development process had failed to provide the optimum microenvironment for wound healing, in particular the controlled absorption of wound exudate to allow a moist environment without tissue sloughing due to excess moisture. The incorporation of new technology fibers such as acrylics and viscose variants and the production of non woven fabrics in swab and pad formulations were the precursors to the use of synthetic and semi–synthetic polymers, having prespecified performance parameters which would produce the required microenvironment for differing wound types at various stages of healing. The first of these Interactive polymeric products appeared in the 1960s and ongoing development has resulted in polymeric films, polymeric foams, particulate and fibrous polymers, hydrogels, xerogels, and hydrocolloids. The polymers used ranged from polyurethane to naturally occurring polysaccharides and collagens.

Polymeric Films[8]

Studies of superficial wounds emphasized the importance of avoiding either dehydration or maceration of a wound surface while maintaining a moist dressing/wound interface and a gaseous exchange system similar to healthy skin.[7,8,9] These requirements potentiated the development of a material which would in part mimic the performance of skin (Figure 2). The resultant products were transparent, synthetic adhesive films generically described as semipermeable adhesive membranes or synonymously as vapor permeable films. They consist of transparent polyurethane or other synthetic film of low reflectance, evenly coated on one side with a synthetic adhesive mass.

The films are adhesive and cohesive, producing intimate adhesion to a dry skin surface and nonadhesion to a wet surface. They have highly elastomeric and extensible properties which contribute to both their conformability and their resistance to shear and tear. The products are sterile and particle free.

The films also possess permeability functions which are essential to their efficacy as wound management material. It should be noted that the removal of the stratum corneum results in a water vapor loss from tissues of between 3,000 and 5,000 G/m^2 over a period of 24 hours. This loss will result in progressive dehydration which could be of great significance, particularly in a full thickness burn situation. The loss through a positioned semipermeable membrane is reduced to 2,500 G/m^2 over 24 hours or less, depending upon the structure of the membrane. This reduction allows excess fluid to be lost by water vapor transmission through the membrane but prevents dehydration and maintains a moist wound interface. Where the volume of exudate produced is significantly greater than the volume removed as vapor, the water impermeability will result in serous effusion accumulating below the film. Obtrusive exudate can be aspirated using aseptic technique and the film puncture repaired by a patch, or the entire dressing can be changed or upgraded to one with greater vapor permeability. Impermeability to water prevents wetting from external sources.

The importance of a moist interface to wound healing is now well recognized. It allows the rapid migration of new epithelium across the wound surface, precludes trauma due to adherence at dressing change and contributes to gaseous diffusion in the damaged tissue. Oxygen and carbon dioxide transfer are accomplished by intramolecular diffusion through the membrane and by solution in the wound surface moisture. The oxygen permeability of the films is variously described as 4,000 to 10,000 $cm^3/m^2/24$ hours at ambient atmospheric pressure. The pO_2 and pH levels of the wound surface are directly related to the gaseous permeability and contribute to cellular activity. The wound is protected against secondary infection by the bacterial impermeability of the film to such organisms as *Pseudomonas aeruginosa*, *Staphylococcus aureus* and *Eschericia coli*.

The physical performance is applicable to the management of superficial tangential wounds such as dermabrasions, split skin, graft donor sites and burns. In a dermabrasion, hemostasis must first be obtained and the margin of the wound dried before the film is applied. Providing the film is correctly positioned, it may be left *in situ* until epithelialization is complete. In its application for the treatment of burns careful disinfection must precede the positioning of the film. It is only recommended for superficial and clinically clean burns and contraindicated for deep burns where it retards the separation of necrotic tissue.

Pressure ulcers can be covered with a vapor permeable film with the added advantage that the film's resistance to shear and low frictional surface properties protect the dermal layers from additional physical abrasion while producing the minimal barrier to normal skin function. This performance allows the film to be used as a prophylactic in areas which are traumatized by pressure but not ulcerated.

The film dressings can also be used for the retention of cannulae and tubes in both operating rooms and patient care units. Specific products have now been produced with a variable water vapor permeability to reduce the build up of moisture beneath the film and the resultant infective hazard.

A recent technological development has resulted in several new "intelligent" vapor permeable films which allow high permeability in high exudate conditions but respond to low exudate by a reduction in the moisture vapor transmission rate, thus maintaining the "moist environment" conducive to the optimization of the microenvironment.

Polymeric Foams

Foam dressings were developed alongside film dressings and, have certain properties in common but differences in their structure and composition, have important implications for their performance in the clinical situation. The dressings are available as sheet dressings and as *in situ* formed foams.

The sheet dressings are mainly polyurethane foams where the absorbency and water vapor permeability are varied either by a physical modification to the foam or by combining the foam with an additional sheet component. They have many of the attributes of an "ideal dressing" with the added advantage that they can be tailored for particular applications, such as that of a tracheostomy dressing, without particle loss to the wound and with the retention of their conformable characteristics.

A partially expanded, modified polyurethane foam was developed by Lock. It comprised a lower layer of open cells and an upper hydrophilic surface with closed impermeable layers which reduced the loss of water vapor and prevented strike through of absorbed fluid. This primary dressing expands when it becomes wet and conforms to the contours of the wound producing an environmental chamber with entrapped solutes and cell debris. It is claimed that this function enhances the inflammatory response of the wound and subsequently stimulates the production of granulation tissue and revascularization. These polyurethane membranes are recommended specifically for the management of stasis ulcers with a superimposed absorbent pad and graduated pressure applied either by stretch bandages or elasticated stockings.

A foam dressing with the prime function of absorbency has been designed for the management of burns. It consists of a highly absorbent hydrophilic polyurethane foam, backed with a moisture permeable polyurethane membrane and bonded to an apertured polyurethane net on the wound contact face. It is capable of absorbing and retaining large volumes of fluid even under pressure. The backing while permeable to water vapor is impermeable to water thus avoiding strike through. As the exudate level decreases, the membrane retains moisture and prevents the drying of the wound. The apertured polyurethane net interface reduces adherence to the wound surface. While recommended for burns these dressings have been used successfully on other exuding lesions.

Low absorptive capacity primary foam dressings have been produced from a carboxylated styrene butadiene rubber latex foam. The foam is bonded to a non woven fabric coated with a polyethylene film which has been vacuum ruptured. The basic foam is naturally hydrophobic and a surface active agent is incorporated to facilitate the uptake of wound exudate. The polyethylene foam layer is particularly effective in preventing adherence, and the dressing is recommended for minor wounds and abrasions where exudate levels are low and adherence a prominent hazard at dressing change.

Foam Cavity Wound Dressings[9]

One of the major problems in wound management is the treatment of large cavity wounds produced either perioperatively (e.g. pilonidal sinus) or by trauma (e.g. pressure ulceration). It is necessary to occlude the cavity by packing to absorb excess exudate and prevent fistula formation and to stimulate the production of granulation tissue, neovascularization and collagen deposition.

The traditional procedure is to pack the cavity with ribbon gauze (see cellulosic absorbents) variously impregnated. The subsequent removal of such a dressing is difficult and the pain and stress associated with the dressing change may require low level anesthesia and the use of a special procedures room or operating room.

An *in situ* formed foam was developed by Dow Corning[8] and found to be clinically superior to the ribbon gauze. Its status in cytotoxic terms was open to question and it has currently been taken off the market, but similar products have now been developed with comparable clinical success.

The Dow Corning material consisted of a two component foam mixed prior to use and poured directly into the wound where the dressing expanded to four times its original volume and set to a soft spongy foam accurately conforming to the contours of the wound cavity. The "stent" was removed twice daily, soaked in a mild antiseptic, rinsed in saline and replaced. A new dressing was formed when required, usually after 7 to 10 days, to rematch the reduction in size of the cavity. It did not adhere to tissue, and the slight pressure produced on the cavity surfaces contributed to the production of granulation tissue. It was indicated for the management of pilonidal sinus, hydradentis suppurata, perianal and perineal wounds and in the management of dehisced abdominal wounds.

Other cavity wound dressing developments have been based upon the "tailoring" of prepacked absorption foam fragments into non woven outers of various dimensions. These foam pillows are positioned directly in the wound and unlike the *in situ* foams have a high absorbency and can be removed and replaced with ease at predetermined intervals.

A recent development is polyurethane–polyacrylic polymer sheet described as a "hydroactive" dressing. It is non–adhesive and, due to its high absorptive capacity when positioned on a wound such as a pressure or venous ulcer, it expands and conforms to the wound cavity. It is maintained in position with a vapor permeable adhesive film.

Along with the vapor permeable films, the foams continue to evolve towards a more precise control of the wound microenvironment with the *in situ* formed foams reappearing as an important cavity wound dressing.

Hydrogels[10]

Hydrogels, or water polymer gels, are three–dimensional networks of hydrophilic polymers prepared from materials such as gelatin, polysaccharides, cross–linked polyacrylamide polymers, polyelectrolyte complexes and polymers or copolymers derived from methacrylate esters. They interact with aqueous solutions by swelling to an equilibrium value and retain a significant proportion of water within their structure. They are insoluble in water. The tissue–like structure of most hydrogels will contribute to their biocompatibility by minimizing mechanical irritation to surrounding cells and tissues. The sheet hydrogels currently used as wound dressings possess most of the properties of an ideal dressing. Their high moisture content maintains a desirable moist interface which facilitates cell migration and prevents dressing adherence. The gels are able to absorb fluid into the polymer matrix and swell in a three dimensional manner, and they maintain a sheet form without intruding into the wound cavity. Water can be transmitted through the saturated gel while the unsaturated gel will have a water vapor permeability comparable with the water vapor permeability of semi–permeable membranes.

The first wound management hydrogel product developed was a cross linked polymer of polyacrylamide and agarose. The mesh size allowed the absorption and desorption of both high molecular weight proteins and low molecular weight solutes. While this performance parameter is essential in its function as an environmental dressing, it could also be utilized to transport compounds to the wound and thus act as the "release component" in a sustained release system. Some success has been evident in using topical antibacterials in this way but it would seem that there may be a greater potential still to be exploited. The ability to sustain release can be seen from the results of the growth curves of L929 and epithelial cells *in vitro* growing beneath a nutrient saturated hydrogel (Geliperm, Geistleib. Pharma, Switzerland). Growth is maintained at a higher level than that observed with the control where the cells are surrounded by media. The cells became a confluent layer adhering to the lower surface of the gel. This property can be utilized to transfer epithelial seed cultures to large partial thickness wound areas and thus supplement the current practice of skin grafting. If the epithelial layer is derived from the patient's own tissue, it would help to avoid problems associated with graft rejection.

Diffusion rates from the hydrogel can also be controlled by the degree of cross linkage. For example, initial cross linking of aqueous solutions of sodium alginate and calcium chloride followed by external cross linking of the produced suspension using poly–l–lysine or poly–ethylene–imine will result in a predetermination of the mesh size and thus control the release rate of sorbed compounds such as polypeptides or growth factors.

Other hydrogel properties could also be utilized as release mechanisms. Gel synepsis at the Theta, 0, critical temperature of temperature sensitive hydrogels results in expansion or collapse of the hydrophilic networks. This process could be used to design a release system for wound management where a drug could be incorporated into the hydrogel structures at one temperature and the active component released abruptly as the critical temperature approaches 32° C when phase separation occurs. pH sensitive hydrogels may be polybasic or polyacidic and will preferentially release compounds in a pH changed environment. This property is used in periodontal medication using glassy hydrophobic hydrogels which become highly hydrated from pH2 to pH6. The pH changes in infected wounds might well be used to initiate the release of topical antibacterials until the pH reverts to normal and the sustained release system ceases to operate. All of these properties have been the subject of investigation with the objective of developing new products.

It has been observed that the positioning of a hydrogel frequently results in a marked reduction in pain response in patients. It is suggested that the high humidity protects the exposed neurones from dehydration and also produces acceptable changes in pH. A secondary effect which may contribute to this response is the property of the gels to immediately cool the wound surface and maintain a lower temperature for up to six hours. In a wound situation this lowering of temperature could result in a reduction of the inflammatory response.

Hydrogel sheets and hydrogel gels of similar composition have been developed to allow continuity of formulation and function in, for example, cavity wounds. The wound volume is filled with the amorphous hydrogel and the hydrogel sheet superimposed.

Hydrogels have recently been developed to produce a moisture "donor" effect for necrotic wounds which require debriding. They are at present available only in the amorphous hydrogel form. Some manufacturers have produced gauze pads "presaturated" and impregnated with a hydrogel. Using a combination of ancient and modern products. Recent developments have been directed at producing hydrogel sheets bonded onto a vapor permeable film to control water vapor transmission and to prevent the possible hazard of "wet" hydrogels becoming "dry" sheets which would be incompatible with a healing surface.

The recommendation for use of these products includes the management of donor sites and superficial operation sites and also the treatment of fresh chronic damaged epithelium. In chronic ulcers they are used to promote autolytic debridement and to encourage granulation and the formation of cellular matrix.

Particulate and Fibrous Polymers[11]

The group of xerogel dressings includes synthetic, semisynthetic and naturally occurring products embracing a range of polysaccharide materials such as alginates and dextranomers. They are in an ongoing state of development with new and "me too" products appearing at frequent intervals.

The xerogel dressings may be regarded as a subgroup of products within the larger group of polysaccharide dressings. The latter contains the well known cellulosic dressing products such as gauze and absorbent cotton (these have been dealt with earlier in this chapter under Absorbents). However, the products which consist of dextranomer beads, dehydrated hydrogels of the agar/acrylamide group, calcium alginate fibers and dehydrated granulated Graft T starch polymers are identified specifically as xerogels,[11] the material remaining after the removal of most or all of the water from a hydrogel (or the disperse phase from any type of simple gel).

Particulate dextranomer. Dextranomer is prepared from dextran, a naturally derived polymer of glucose produced by cultures of a microorganism, *Leuconostoc mesenteroides*. The gel is formed when the dextran molecules comprising the disperse phase of the hydrocolloid are crosslinked by a chemical process utilizing epichlorhydrin and sodium hydroxide.

The dextranomer is supplied in beads of 100 um to 300 um diameter containing poloxamer 187, polyethylene, glycol 300 and some water. A paste formulation is also available which is the dextranomer in polyethylene glycol 600 (PEG 600). The beads are offered as a discrete particle or enclosed in a low adherence pouch for insertion into a cavity wound. One company (Kabi Pharmacia, Uppsala, Sweden) offers a polymeric net which can be placed into a cavity wound before the addition of either granules or paste and facilitates removal and a semipermeable film which is superimposed on the dextranomer dressing to control evaporation and retard the drying of the dextranomer in a low exuding wound. The dextranomer acts as a selective sorbent. The hydrophilic beads will absorb the aqueous component of wound exudate and dissolved materials ranging from inorganic salts to low molecular weight proteins. Dextranomer has a pore size which produces an exclusion limit of 1,000 to 8,000 Daltons which precludes the sorption of viruses and bacteria. Microorganisms are removed from the wound by a capillary action between the beads, a function which is absent from the paste formulation. This function, however, demonstrates a marked increase in absorbing capacity for malodorous elements and pain–producing compounds released during the inflammatory response.

It may be used as a debriding agent on sloughy and exuding wounds where the objective is to produce a clean tissue bed for the production of a granulating tissue. It is not a product which should be used beyond this phase of the wound healing process as its continued application will impair epithelization. Dextranomer is not biodegradable and both granules and paste must be carefully removed with saline to avoid particulate residues and the subsequent development of granulomas.

Fibrous polymers. Alginate fibers are derived from alginic acid which is a polyuronic acid composed of residues of D–mannuronic acid and L–guluronic acid. Alginic acid is obtained chiefly from algae belonging to the *Phaeophyceae*, a species of *Laminaria*.

The isomeric acids are present in varying proportions dependent upon the seaweed source. Calcium alginate is capable of gel formation. The guluronic acid forms an association with calcium providing the stimulus to produce the continuous disperse phase of a hydrogel. Ca^{2+} ion and a phospholipid surface promote the activation of prothrombin in the clotting cascade. Calcium alginate products are used as the source of these ions to arrest bleeding, both in superficial injuries and as an absorbable hemostat in surgery. The rate of biodegradation is related to the sodium/calcium balance in the preparation.

The alginates are produced in fiber form and have been developed as a fleece or layered needled fabric. When applied to a bleeding surface both the availability of the Ca^{2+} ions and the fibrous matrix contribute to coagulation, and serum absorption produces a gel–like mass. The dressings may be removed with a sterile 3 percent sodium citrate solution followed by washing with sterile water.

The "wet" integrity of the dressing which facilitates removal from the wound may be improved by incorporating fibers of greater strength, such as viscose (rayon) staple fiber, or fibers which interact with the alginate fibers when wet, such as chitosan staple fibers.

Alginate gauze and staple products are applied using normal sterile dressing procedures. The frequency of change will be a matter for clinical assessment of the injury and depend on the type of wound and the degree of exudation.

The primary hemostatic usage of calcium alginate is in the packing of sinuses, fistulae and bleeding tooth sockets. the use of calcium alginate as a hemostatic agent dates back to the 1950s. Its subsequent development as a xerogel which is converted to a hydrogel in the presence of wound exudate came in the late 1970s. It was at this stage that the significance of the Ca^{2+} and Na ion ratios became apparent in physical differences between the "gel strength" of products containing high or low Na ion levels. This discovery has led to a range of Ca/Na alginate dressings in the form of fibrous and fabric preparations which have different absorptive capacities and gelling properties. The alginates have also been cross formulated with a Collagen type 1 and chitosan to increase the possible bioactivity.

Recent studies have indicated an auto oxidation property of alginates which stimulates the production of hydrogen peroxide. In addition to containing Ca^{2+} ions, alginates have been identified as contributing to the initial inflammatory response required to "kick start" the healing cascade by causing lysis of mast cells with the subsequent release of histamine and 5HT.

Alginate dressings have been used as a useful non–adherent for lacerations and abrasions and are effective in the management of hypergranulation (proud flesh), interdigital maceration and heloma molle. They are used in hospitals and communities to accelerate healing in intractable skin and pressure ulcers and in the successful management of diabetic ulcers, venous ulcers and burns.

Alginates have also been proven to be useful autolytic debriding agents. When applied to these injury types the alginate must be covered by a secondary dressing of foam or film.

Hydrocolloids[12]

Hydrocolloid dressings have developed from the adhesive flanges used for the long term protection of skin surrounding a stoma. The barrier produced prevented the excretions from eroding or denuding the skin and the flange acted as a base for the adhesive attachment of ostomy collection devices. The development of the hydrocolloid as a wound management product has resulted in new formulations and a range of technologically superior products available in adhesive sheet, granular, and paste forms.

The early hydrocolloid dressings consist of composite products based on naturally occurring hydrophilic polymers. In general they have a pressure sensitive adhesive layer which is composed of a so–called "hydrocolloid," dispersed with the aid of a tackifier in an elastomer, and secondly a film coating, composed of a variable vapor permeable but water impermeable, flexible, elastomeric material. One of the first hydrocolloid dressings described had a pressure sensitive adhesive hydrocolloid layer which consisted of 40 to 50 percent by weight of a mixture of gelatine and sodium carboxymethylcellulose dispersed in polyisobutylene with an antioxidant and a tackifier (mineral oil and terpene resin). This mixture was then laminated with a semi open cell flexible polyurethane foam which had previously been laminated with a closed cell flexible polyurethane film. A currently available hydrocolloid dressing is a flexible mass with an adherent inner face and an outer vapor permeable polyurethane foam. The modified formulation is as follows:

Sodium carboxymethylcellulose	20 percent
Polysiobutylene	40 percent
Gelatine	20 percent
Pectin	20 percent

The product is also available as a paste of similar formulation allowing a continuous "fill" for cavity wounds.

Other hydrocolloid dressings with formulations consisting of sodium carboxymethylcellulose combined with karaya gum or sodium carboxymethylcellulose on its own are also available.

The adhesive formulation of hydrocolloids gives an initial adhesion higher than some surgical adhesive tapes. After application the absorption of transepidermal water vapor modifies the adhesive flow to maintain a high tack performance throughout the period of use. *In situ* the dressings provide a gaseous and moisture proof environmental chamber strongly adhered to the area surrounding the wound and offering protection against contamination from incontinence or other sources. In the wound contact area the exudate is absorbed to form a gel that swells in a linear fashion with a higher moisture retention at the contact surface. This higher moisture retention results in an expansion of the gel into the wound cavity with the continued support and increasing pressure from the remainder of the elastomeric dressing. The larger the volume of exudate, the greater the expansion into the cavity up to the

limitation imposed by the availability of the gel. The advantage of this system is that it applies a firm pressure to the floor of a deep ulcer, a basic surgical maxim for the production of healthy granulating tissue. It is this function that contributes to the recommended usage for venous ulcers.

The formed "colloidal" gel will also produce a sorption gradient for soluble components within the serious exudate and allow the removal of toxic compounds arising from bacterial or cellular destruction. The moist gel is soft and conforms to the wound contours. When the dressing is removed the gel remains in the wound and can be washed away with saline. No damage to the wound results from this procedure. During use the dressing in contact with the wound liquifies to produce a pus–like liquid with a somewhat strong odor. The hydrocolloids are suitable for desloughing and for light to medium exuding wounds, but are contraindicated if an anaerobic infection is present. They have been used successfully in the treatment of chronic leg ulcers, pressure ulcers and as skin barriers in the management of stomas.

As with hydrogels, hydrocolloids can be obtained in both powder and paste form where the powders and pastes have similar formulations to that of the hydrocolloid mass in the sheet dressing. This versatility will allow larger cavity wounds to be treated with a continuous hydrocolloid system.

A recent development for deep exuding pressure ulcer management is a hydrocolloid dressing with a formulation including sodium alginate in the form of a tubular spiral rolled into a round disc which can be positioned in the cavity and covered with a hydrocolloid sheet dressing. A further advance has been the development of "thin" hydrocolloid sheets with improved conformability and a degree of transparency allowing the wound to be observed without removal of the dressing. This latter product is comparable in performance with a vapor permeable film. It should be noted that although the hydrocolloids are considered primarily as Interactive dressings recent work would suggest that some formulations contribute a Bioactive function to the probable advantage of the healing process.

Bioactive Products

When developing Interactive products the environment sought was obtained but some chronic injuries still refused to respond adequately.

Since most wounds when not infected heal spontaneously in endocrinogically and nutritionally normal mammals it had always been considered axiomatic that the rate of healing represents a biologic maximum and therefore could not be accelerated beyond the available capacity of the tissues.

However, the experimental use of processed cartilage and cartilage extracts showed that it was possible to stimulate by topical activation the normal or enhanced activity of the acellular and cellular mechanisms involved in tissue repair.

Such products may be considered to produce a localized systemic intervention and can be defined as "Bioactive" compounds.

Recent work has indicated the importance of polymeric materials such as pectins, alginates and chitosan which act as prooxidants. In other words, in the presence of traces of transition metal catalysts such as iron and copper ions they interact with dissolved molecular oxygen to form superoxide which dismutases spontaneously to form hydrogen peroxide.[13] This reactive oxygen species

---

Since most wounds when not infected heal spontaneously in endocrinogically and nutritionally normal mammals it had always been considered axiomatic that the rate of healing represents a biologic maximum and therefore could not be accelerated beyond the available capacity of the tissues.

A brief re–examination of the healing cascade (Figure 2) is sufficient to identify those parts of the cycle which could be influenced by such materials either by correcting some deficiency in the biochemical pathway or by stimulating the involved cellular elements to increase their activity and accelerate their biofunction.

The initial inflammatory response is predominantly acellular by comparison with the regeneration and repair processes. It is in these two latter processes that the designated "Bioactive" compounds need to perform as the biologic primers for cell proliferation and tissue reconstruction.

Naturally occurring polysaccharides such as hyaluronic acid and chondrotin sulphate are glycosaminoglycans (GAGs) which have been shown to be involved in diverse structural and organization functions in tissues. They and other GAGs such as heparin and dermatan sulphate show a partial specification for cell surface interactions, cell/cell interactions, cell substrate interactions or cell proliferation. They have an important bioactive influence on the microenvironment and therefore on tissue regeneration. Non collagenic proteins such as fibronectin (C1g) laminin and chondronectin are still to be fully characterized but their *in vitro* effects on cell division are well documented. Fibronectin demonstrates chemokinesis on fibroblasts (general stimulation of movement) and, in the presence of a concentration gradient, chemotaxis (directional movement stimulated by a gradient of diffusable substance) and hapotaxis (directional movement stimulated by a gradient of substrate adhesiveness). These Proactive materials are now becoming available having been challenged for their levels of quality, safety and efficacy.

initiates oxidative processes and has been shown at concentrations of 10^{-6} M to 10^{-9} M to stimulate both the proliferation of fibroblasts and the macrophage respiratory burst. The Superoxide Assisted Fenton Reaction is as follows:

$$Fe^{3+} + {}^\bullet O_{2^-} = Fe^{2+} + O_2$$
$$Fe^{2+} + H_2O_2 = De^{3+} + {}^\bullet OH + OH$$

The use of hydrogen peroxide has been discouraged in wound management. Its toxicity in fibroblast cultures and its "tissue destruct" properties *in vivo* have been reported at higher concentrations than those quoted here. At these low concentrations there is a 20 percent increase in murine fibroblast proliferation over a period of 3 to 6 days. Work involving the use of low passage number human fibroblasts have also shown substantially higher increases.

The generation of superoxide also contributes to leucotaxin formation which could reinitiate the inflammatory response in recalcitrant wounds. The resultant influx of monocytes/macrophages would contribute further superoxide and hydrogen peroxide to the wound environment. Following NADPH oxidase activity the higher concentrations of hydrogen peroxide would initially inhibit the proliferation of fibroblasts but as its concentration falls the rate of cell division is enhanced leading to collagen synthesis.

Further investigations both completed and in progress have identified similar antioxidant activity in other hydrogel and hydrocolloid products.[14]

It would appear that the application of antioxidant wound contact materials to soft tissue lesions in patients whose intrinsic antioxidant defenses are compromised by age, dietary deficiency or

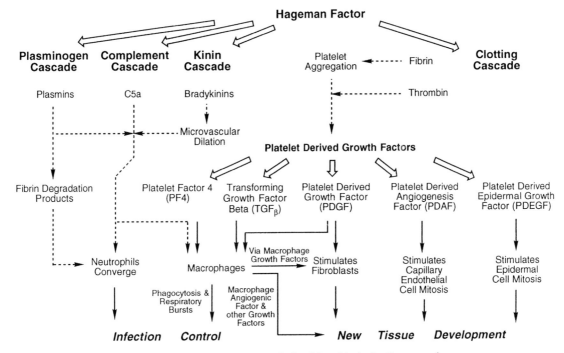

Figure 3. *Platelet derived growth factors and their interrelationship with the healing cascade.*

physiological deficiency, such as diabetes, would contribute to an improved antioxidant status in the wound locality and thus establish and maintain the reducing environment necessary for energy production and hence cell division.[15] This process, plus the maintenance of moist wound healing, could contribute to both the rate of healing and repair of the soft tissue injury by "normalizing" the complete bioenvironment.

Growth factors. 1986 was a landmark in wound healing. This was the year that Cohen and Levi–Montaleini shared a Nobel prize for their work on epidermal and nerve growth factors. This research stimulated many other workers to investigate the potential of other growth factors.

In the last five years over thirty "growth factors" have been identified and reported in the literature. Initially they were characterized as "naturally occurring polypeptides which increased the mitotic index of proliferating cells." Subsequently several growth factors have been identified in wounds but their functions are still a matter of debate.

They have been broadly classified as "paracrine" factors when they act upon a neighboring cell and "autocrine" when they act upon the producing cell.

Three types are recognized based upon the apparent cellular response: proliferative, migratory or producing an alteration in the phenotypic state.

The proliferative response can be stimulated by two factors — one which moves the cell from the resting state inducing DNA replication and thus proving the competence of the cell which is then sensitive to the progressive factor which leads to cell replication. The second type are the chemoattractants which stimulate migration or movement of cells and the third the transforming growth factors which produce a phenotypic alteration. The five principal growth factors are as follows:

EGF: Epidermal growth factor
FGF: Fibroblast growth factor (acidic and basic)
ILG: Insulin–like growth factor
PDGF: Platelet derived growth factor
TGF: Transforming growth factor (alpha and
       beta)

The possible bioactivity of platelet derived angiogenesis factor (PDAF), of platelet derived growth factor (PDGF) and their interrelationship with the healing cascade is summarized in Figure 3.

A recent commentary in the *Lancet* emphasized the clinical potential of the cytokine TGFß which exhibits autocrine, paracrine and endocrine effects. It acts through the heteromultimers of receptors on the cell surface, and the clinical interest has been focused in their role in extracellular matrix deposition and leukocyte infiltration – important factors in wound healing. Their chemotactic effect on fibroblasts stimulates the deposition of collagen and other components of the extracellular matrix. Dermal wounds in rats are reported to heal with reduced scarring and a clinical trial on venous ulcers showed a marked promotion of healing.

The ongoing development of these products and their introduction as pharmacological agents in wound management are dependent upon a number of factors, not least of which is the level at which the increase in cell replication is considered to be therapeutically significant and is further complicated by the difficulty of determining the rate in connective tissue.

The quantitative and qualitative effects must be the subject of new laboratory and clinical assessment procedures. The use of reproducible models, such as skin graft donor sites or implanted wound tissue sampling devices, and bioassy techniques using cell cultures will contribute to our characterization and ultimate usage of these factors.

The clinical expectation of application is wide and the number of organizations involved internationally in research development and production in 1995 was in excess of 200. There would therefore appear to be sufficient interest and available resource to ensure an in depth evaluation of these Bioactive materials which by enhancement or inhibition of inflammation, fibroplasia, epithelization, angiogenesis, connective tissue repair and contraction may act as the "normalizer" in "non–healing" wounds or the "accelerator" in normal wounds.

Future Development. Many of our preconceived ideas on tissue repair will have to be re–examined in the light of the new information these products will reveal. In addition, our clinicians need to re–educate themselves with regard to not only the use of Bioactive products but also the application of the innovative Interactive materials in the management of their patients' wounds. It is a disturbing fact that in spite of the availability of these technologically and clinically advanced products many wounds are still dressed with a gauze fabric — one of the original Passive "out of sight, out of mind" dressings. The famous remark of the French surgeon, Ambroise Pare (1510–1590) "...que je pensay et Dieu la guarist," meaning, "I dressed (the wound) and God healed it" could well be the current fatalistic philosophy of many healthcare providers and produce a delay in the adoption of new products and procedures.

Ongoing developments particularly at the cellular level will hopefully result in the successful and speedy healing of most, if not all, wounds with the resultant alleviation of pain and distress in both man and animals.

References

1. Majno G. *The Healing Hand*. Harvard, MA, University Press, 1975.
2. Bishop WJ. *A History of Surgical Dressings*. London, England, Strangeway Press, 1959.
3. Elliot JR. Surgical materials. *St Bart Hosp J* 1954;58:11–14.
4. Gamgee S. Gauze and cotton tissue. *Lancet* 1876;10:885.
5. British Pharmaceutical Codex. London, England, Pharmaceutical Press, 1923.
6. British Pharmacopoeia. London, England, Pharmaceutical Press, 1988.
7. Turner TD. Hospital usage of absorbent dressings. *Pharm J* 1979;222:421–426.
8. Turner TD. Current and future trends in wound management, 2. *Pharm Int* 1985;6(6):131.
9. Harding KG. Silastic foam. In: Turner TD, Schmidt RJ, Harding KG (eds). *Advances in Wound Management*. New York, NY, John Wiley & Sons, 1986, pp 41–52.
10. Turner TD. Hydrogels and hydrocolloids. In: Turner TD, Schmidt RJ, Harding KG (eds). *Advances in Wound Management*. New York, NY, John Wiley & Sons, 1986, pp 89–95.
11. Schmidt R. Xerogel dressings. In: Turner TD, Schmidt RJ, Harding KG (eds). *Advances in Wound Management*. New York, NY, John Wiley & Sons, 1986.
12. Cherry GW, Ryan TJ. The physical properties of a new hydrocolloid dressing. An environment for healing. In: Ryan TJ (ed). *The Role of Occlusion*. Royal Society of Medicine, 1985, pp 61–68.
13. Schmidt RJ, Turner TD, Chung LY, Andrews AM. Biocompatibility of wound management products, standardization of and determination of cell growth role in Lq2q fibroblast cultures. *J Pharm Pharmacol* 1989;41:775–780.
14. Chung LY, Schmidt RJ, Andrews AM, Turner TD. A study of hydrogen peroxide generation by and antioxidant activity of Granuflex™ (Duoderm™) hydrocolloid granules and some other hydrogel/hydrocolloid wound management materials. *Brit J Dermatol* 1993;129:145–153.
15. Flohe L. Beakman R, Grertz H, et al. Oxygen–centered free radicals as mediators of inflammation In: Sies H (ed). Oxidative Stress. London, UK, Academic Press, 1985, pp 403–428.

Suggested Reading

1. Goldsmith LA (ed). *Biochemistry and Physiology of the Skin, Volumes I and II*. Oxford, UK, Oxford University Press, 1983.
2. Bucknell TE, Ellis H (eds). *Wound Healing for Surgeons*. London, UK, Balliem, Tindall 1984.
3. Peacock EE. *Wound Repair*. London, UK, WB Saunders & Co., 1984.
4. Royal Soc Med Int Cong, Services No. 88. An Environment for Healing. London, UK, Royal Soc. Med., 1984.
5. Westaby S (ed). *Wound Care*. London, UK, William Heinemann Med. Books, 1985.
6. Sedlarik von KM. *Wund–Heilung*. Studtgart, Germany, Gustav Fischer Verlag Jena, 1993.

17

Dressing Decisions for the Twenty–First Century: On the Cusp of a Paradigm Shift

Diane Krasner, MS, RN, CETN

Krasner D. Dressing decsions for the twenty–first century: On the cusp of a paradigm shift. In: Krasner D, Kane D. *Chronic Wound Care, Second Edition*. Wayne, PA, Health Management Publications, Inc., 1997, pp 139–151.

Chance favors the prepared mind.

— *Louis Pasteur*

Introduction

Over the last thirty–five years, we have witnessed a proliferation of wound dressing and covering materials ranging from so–called "sophisticated gauzes" to "intelligent dressings" to synthetic skins. Healthcare professionals are just beginning to understand the clinical implications of using these newer dressing materials. With these advanced product developments, a new mentality for dressing decision–making is emerging. This paradigm shift is certain to change the way wound dressings and coverings are selected and utilized in the twenty–first century. In the midst of these new directions, however, certain product use principles have remained constant. These rules continue to be the cornerstone for dressing decisions in the 1990's. The more clinicians know about dressing categories, their performance parameters and how they affect the wound healing process, the better able they will be to optimize wound care for their patients.

Background

Research of the late 1950's and early 1960's demonstrated that a moist wound environment provides the best microenvironment for wound regeneration and repair and optimizes wound healing.[1–2] This discovery led to the development in the early 1970's of several categories of moisture retentive dressings, most notably transparent films and hydrocolloids. During the '70's and '80's, however, the dressing shelf was still dominated by traditional plug, cover and conceal dressing options, such as gauzes, impregnates and bandages.[3] These are essentially passive dressing options, but attempts were made to enhance their efficacy by using them moist (e.g. wet–to–dry gauze evolved into wet–to–damp or moist gauze dressings) or by combining them with other materials and thereby creating moisture–retentive options (e.g. gauze was combined with transparent films to create island dressings).

New Product Developments

During the 1980's and early 1990's the rapid pace of new product development at least quadrupled the dressing options that are now available for clinical use. The portfolio of available products has expanded to include alginates, foams, and hydrogels, to name a few. The first biologicals and biosynthetics, including collagen and growth factors, are being used clinically, providing a glimpse of what the future may hold.

It seems as if each day new dressings appear on the market and new dressing categories are cropping up faster than ever. As of this writing 36 major generic wound care product categories can be identified (Table 1). It remains true, however,

Table 1
Generic categories of wound care products

Adhesives
Adhesive Removers
Adhesive Skin Closures
Adhesive Tapes
Alginate Dressings
Antibiotics
Antimicrobials
Antiseptics
Bandages
Biosynthetic Dressings
Cleansers
Collagen Dressings
Composite Dressings
Contact Layers
Creams/Skin Protectant Pastes
Dressing Covers
Enzymes/ Debriding Agents
Foam Dressings
Gauze Dressings
Growth Factors
Healthcare Personnel Handrinses
Hydrocolloid Dressings
Hydrogel Dressings
Leg Ulcer Wraps/Compression Bandages/Wraps
Lubricating/Stimulating Sprays
Moisturizers
Moisture Barrier Ointments
Ointments
Perineal Cleansing Foams
Skin Sealants
Sterile Fields
Surgical Scrubs
Surgical Tapes
Transparent Film Dressings
Wound Fillers: Pastes, Powders, Beads, etc.
Wound Pouches

that within a particular category, performance parameters vary widely so that products must be individually evaluated for their actions, safety and efficacy. In other words, a hydrocolloid is not a hydrocolloid is not a hydrocolloid.

While it seems that practicing clinicians have been slow to adopt new dressing materials into everyday practice,[5] the winds of change are upon us. The endorsement of wound healing principles, given by the Agency for Health Care Policy and Research Clinical Practice Guideline, Number 15, entitled *Treatment of Pressure Ulcers*, has done much to spread the message to wound care providers

about moist wound healing and moisture–retentive dressings.[6]

The Paradigm Shift

The paradigm shift for dressing decisions involves the interactive and active use of dressing materials to facilitate the wound healing process.[7,8] In the new paradigm, dressings are akin to drugs, with actions, indications, contraindications and side–effects. The new paradigm holds that by matching dressing performance parameters to a particular phase of the wound healing process, wound healing can be optimized.

A great deal of research is still needed to support this line of thinking. Preliminary research and clinical experience, however, suggest that the new paradigm for dressing decision–making has great clinical utility. If, for example, an informed decision is made to use a dressing that optimizes granulation tissue formation during the granulation phase of wound healing (e.g. an amorphous hydrogel) instead of a dressing that optimizes reepithelialization (e.g. an impregnated gauze), then wound healing outcomes should be improved. Such targeted use of dressing materials will evolve as case studies give way to outcome–focused research on dressing usage. As more refined indications for the use of dressing materials are identified and put into practice, outcome measures such as time–to–healing rates and pain scores should show clinically significant improvements.

Targeted dressing decisions that match interactive and active dressing materials to specific phases of the wound healing process will find their way into algorithms, clinical pathways and care mapping.[9] The challenge will be to base these decisions on the best possible science of the day, but also to be prepared to revise protocols as new information and understanding about dressings emerge from practice and research.

Five Rules of Wound Dressings

While the names, shapes and composition of dressings in the clinician's portfolio are expected to continue to change as the millennium comes to a close, there are several principles or rules of wound dressings that are certain to hold constant well into the twenty–first century. Five of these rules will be addressed and clinical examples given (Table 2).

Rule #1: The Rule of Categorization. *Learn about dressings by generic category and compare new products with those that already make up the category.*

Hundreds of dressings are now available to choose from, so users must develop systematic

Table 2
The five rules of wound dressings

Rule #1: The Rule of Categorization
Learn about dressings by generic category and compare new products with those that already make up the category.

Rule #2: The Rule of Selection
Select the safest and most effective, user–friendly and cost–effective dressing possible.

Rule #3: The Rule of Change
Change dressings based on patient, wound and dressing assessment, not on standardized routines.

Rule #4: The Rule of Evolution
As the wound moves through the phases of the wound healing process, evolve the dressing protocol to optimize wound healing.

Rule #5: The Rule of Practice
Practice with dressing materials is required to learn their performance parameters and related tricks–of–the–trade.

Table 3
The amorphous hydrogel dressing category: A systematic approach

Definition: a non–adhesive, hydrophilic polymer gel product composed primarily of water, may also contain glycerin, co–polymer, and propylene glycol (as a preservative and humectant)

Actions:
• moisture retention
• promotes granulation tissue formation
• hydration
• lightly to moderately absorptive
• insulation
• autolysis of necrotic tissue

Indications:
• used as a primary wound dressing to fill wound cavities or cover exposed surfaces
• may be used for partial– or full–thickness wounds
• may be used for clean, contaminated or infected wounds
• used for autolysis of necrotic tissue (eschar, slough)
• may be used as carrier for topical medications

Contraindications:
• wounds with heavy exudate
• do not use propylene glycol–containing hydrogels for patients with known sensitivity to propylene glycol

Side–effects/Precautions:
• high specific heat, so very soothing, cooling when applied; offers pain relief (+)
• may cause maceration or candidiasis of periwound margins (–)

Additional Information:
• requires secondary dressings
• composition and range of absorbency varies considerably from product to product
• transparency allows for easy wound inspection
• pack a deep wound approximately 2/3 full to allow room for expansion with exudate
• as wound fluid is absorbed, hydrogel viscosity decreases and gel may become liquid
• may be combined with other dressing products (e.g. gauze) or with medications (e.g. metronidazole)

References:
• information from professional peers, patients, clinical experience
• case studies/spec sheets
• clinical studies
• randomized controlled trials

approaches to product selection. Understanding the performance parameters of a dressing category gives the clinician a way to compare, contrast and select products. One method is to approach dressing categories like drugs, outlining their actions, indications, contraindications and side–effects.[10–12] Since interactive and active dressing materials act in many ways like drugs, this analogy is quite appropriate. Table 3 demonstrates this systematic approach to the amorphous hydrogel dressing category.

Sometimes, the optimal dressing is created by combining products from different categories. For example, an amorphous hydrogel may be used to fill a clean cavity wound. To prevent seepage of the hydrogel onto the periwound margin (that could cause a periwound maceration or candidiasis) and for aesthetic reasons (most patients prefer not to be constantly faced with their wound), the hydrogel is covered with a gauze sponge. Finally, to create a semi–occlusive, moisture– retentive environment with an enhanced bacterial barrier, a transparent film is used as a secondary dressing. This film also may allow every other day dressing changes (since the wound in this example is a clean one and the

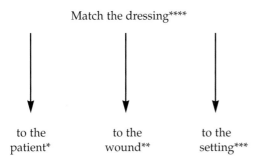

Match the dressing****

to the   to the   to the
patient*   wound**   setting***

*Patient criteria
Systemic factors
Chronic illnesses
Critical illnesses
Immunocompromise/Immunosuppression
Frequency of dressing change
Continence status
Overall treatment plan or goal of therapy
Compliance

** Wound Criteria
Location
Depth (i.e. partial or full thickness)
Dimensions
Configuration (e.g. tunneling)
Clean or necrotic
Amount of exudate
Condition of periwound margins
Presence or absence of infection

*** Setting Criteria
Environmental constraints
Support surface conditions
Independence/Dependence
Caregiver availability and education
Reimbursement

**** Dressing criteria
Absorbency
Adhesive/Non–adhesive
Moisture retentive/ Non–moisture retentive
Occlusive/Semipermeable/Nonocclusive
Frequency of dressing change required
User–friendly vs. User–Intensive
Safety
Efficacy
Cost

Figure 1. Match the dressing to the patient, to the wound and to the setting
© Diane Krasner

patient is not immunocompromised) and facilitates patient hygiene and activities of living, such as bathing and swimming.

Product categories cannot be combined haphazardly; however, the clinician must be certain that products can be safely combined and will not harm the patient. For example, combining certain enzymatic debriding agents with transparent films can cause severe cellulitis and pain. Check the guidelines for use on dressing package inserts for information about safely combining products. If in doubt, contact the manufacturer or your wound specialist for guidance.

As more and more research on dressing categories is conducted, the number of generic dressing categories and our understanding of them will continue to grow. By associating a product with its generic category, a number of questions can be formulated that can guide the clinician in product evaluation and use, for example,

1. How does the action, safety and efficacy profile of product X compare/contrast with other products in that generic category?
2. Does the manufacturer claim product actions that are typical/atypical for that dressing category?
3. If a manufacturer has added another ingredient to the product mix (e.g. adding a hydrocolloid or an alginate to a hydrogel), what is the rationale/new action/new indication?
4. Do the indications for product X match the needs (e.g. the need for exudate absorption, based on a thorough wound assessment performed by a qualified healthcare professional) of patient Y?
5. Are there contraindications or side effects of product X that could be problematic for a specific wound type or a specific patient?

As wound care clinicians better understand dressing performance parameters, their knowledge base is communicated in the professional literature through in–service education and in generic education programs for healthcare professionals. Thus, they will become more capable of matching the most appropriate dressing category to the patient, to the wound and to the setting (Figure 1).

Rule #2: The Rule of Selection. *Select the safest and most effective, user–friendly and cost–effective dressing possible.*

For decades, dressing decision–making has been more of an art than a science. Because no laboratory model for chronic wounds has yet been developed, efforts to test dressing materials on chronic wounds have been hampered. The last decade has seen the evolution of more sophisticated dressing research, including excellent case studies, controlled studies, and randomized prospective trials that strive to demonstrate dressing safety, efficacy, user–friendliness or cost–effectiveness.[13-15] But there has also been too much "pseudo–research" where these outcomes are implied but not conclusively demonstrated.

An excellent example of the practical dressing research that demonstrates enhanced patient and caregiver safety through knowledge–based dressing selection is the 1992 study by Lawrence, Lilly and Kidson. These researchers found in laboratory experiments with a simulated wound model and in selected clinical situations (where measurements were taken) that the airborne dispersal of bacteria was significantly reduced when absorptive hydrocolloid dressings were used instead of gauze.[16] The implications for infection control, cross–contamination and environmental safety are obvious. This study is a model for the sort of dressing research which is urgently needed if science–based dressing decision–making is to become a reality in the twenty–first century.

By using this information about dressings, the clinician can then develop a portfolio of products specific to a facility's needs. The portfolio should reflect the range of wounds encountered (e.g. acute versus chronic; leg ulcers versus pressure ulcers versus diabetic ulcers; exudating versus non–exudating) as well as special requirements of the setting (e.g. Medicare reimbursement constraints for home care and nursing homes). No clinician can have or needs to have every product or even every product category available for use, but by carefully weighing product characteristics and options, a portfolio can be assembled that can facilitate wound care.[17]

As an example of a streamlined dressing portfolio, at the outpatient venous ulcer clinic where I am currently conducting my dissertation research, the vast majority of patients are given a primary dressing and compression from five options (based on an assessment of their wounds and other biopsychosocial factors). These five affordable

---

The need for clinicians to be good consumers and to critically evaluate the product literature on issues related to dressing actions, safety, efficacy, user–friendliness and cost–effectiveness has never been more pressing.

In the meantime, however, the clinician has an enormous responsibility and faces the arduous task of sifting through the literature in an effort to determine dressing actions, safety, efficacy, user–friendliness and cost–effectiveness. Sharing this task with others by forming wound care committees or task forces is one approach to accomplishing the job. Clinicians must insist on obtaining detailed information from manufacturers, suppliers and government agencies [such as the Food and Drug Administration (FDA) for safety and efficacy information and the Health Care Financing Administration (HCFA) for reimbursement information] to obtain the information needed for prudent dressing decision–making. At the very least, one should expect to review several clinical studies in addition to product "spec sheets." If the information obtained is insufficient for decision–making, it is reasonable to request to speak to the manufacturer's national product manager or to see the FDA 510K or PMA application. The need for clinicians to be good consumers and to critically evaluate the product literature on issues related to dressing actions, safety, efficacy, user–friendliness and cost–effectiveness has never been more pressing.

options are readily available to patients in our community. We have seen that the simplicity of the dressing materials chosen minimizes errors and increases compliance in our patient population. The five options are silver sulfadiazene with gauze dressing, hydrocolloid primary dressing, compression stocking, Unna boot, and four layer bandaging system.

Rule #3. The Rule of Change. *Change dressings based on patient, wound and dressing assessment, not on standardized routines.*

Traditional practice called for changing dressings routinely two, three or even four times a day. New thinking indicates that, generally speaking, the natural wound healing process should be disrupted as little as possible. It is common to see dressing changes only once a day or every other day unless the wound is infected or heavily exudating, in which case dressing change schedules will be more frequent. Later in the wound healing process when the inflammatory response has subsided, exudate production is minimal and granulation tissue formation is well underway, it is not unusual to change dressings just twice or once a week.

Table 4
The progression of dressings for an infected sacral Stage 4 pressure ulcer
with yellow necrotic slough and exudate (It is important to address specific wound needs
at various points on the wound healing continuum.)

Wound Healing Phase	Wound Description	Dressing(s)	Rationale
Inflammatory (or reaction) phase	Infected, yellow sloughy wound	Calcium alginate rope	• to absorb wound exudate • to promote autolytic debridement
Granulation (or regeneration) phase	Red, granulating wound	Hydrocolloid paste and dressing	• to fill the wound cavity (dead space) • to provide a moisture–retentive, occlusive micro–environment
Reepithelialization (or remodeling) phase	Pink, resurfacing wound	Hydrocolloid dressing only	• to protect epithelial buds and new epithelium

Yet there are certain circumstances that warrant an immediate investigation and dressing change:
1. patient complaints of pain or discomfort;
2. new or increased edema, erythema, or warmth;
3. strike–through of dressing exudate;
4. channeling, melt–out or lifting–off of occlusive dressings;
5. malodorous or contaminated dressings.

Rule #4. The Rule of Evolution. *As the wound moves through the phases of the wound healing process, evolve the dressing protocol to optimize wound healing.*

Especially for full–thickness and chronic wounds, there is little likelihood these days that the same dressing material will be most appropriate throughout the entire wound healing process. Rather, it is much more likely that dressing choices will evolve as the wound evolves. The emerging standard of care is that dressings are to be carefully matched to the wound, to the patient and to the setting.

An example of the progression of dressings for an infected sacral Stage 4 pressure ulcer with yellow necrotic slough and exudate can be found in Table 4. The example illustrates the need to address specific wound needs at various points on the wound healing continuum. Initially, the focus was on controlling infection and exudate and removing necrotic tissue. When the infection was brought under control, the objective was to fill dead space and provide a moisture retentive dressing. Finally, the goal was to promote wound resurfacing by reepithelialization. These goals of wound care are reflected in the wound healing hierarchy of needs (Figure 2). Additional considerations include systemic factors, nutrition and perfusion.

The Rule of Evolution presupposes that clinicians and their patients have access to a diverse portfolio of dressing products that will meet a variety of performance requirements, such as exudate absorption, thermal insulation, nonadherence or occlusion. "The spectrum of performance requires that the wound is diagnosed and the treatment is progressed by prescribing the most suitable dressing."[18] To date, no single dressing can provide the optimum environment for all wounds at all times in all settings.

We must work hard to assure that patients and their caregivers have access through pharmacies, suppliers and payors to a broad range of affordable wound care products that reflect current standards for wound care.

Rule #5: The Rule of Practice. *Practice with dressing materials is required to learn their performance parameters and related tricks–of–the–trade.*

Dressing wounds, while evolving into a science, is still very much an art. The process requires ongoing experience to hone assessment skills, to keep pace with new product developments and to incorporate the latest findings from clinical and laboratory research. It takes practice to discover and implement the tricks–of– the–trade that can make the difference between dressing success and dressing failure. Timely adjustments of the dressing protocol can determine whether the wound heals or rapidly deteriorates.[19]

Unfortunately, a trend has been seen of delegating or "turfing" dressing change functions to the least prepared member of the healthcare team. The fact is that optimal wound care requires an incredibly sophisticated knowledge base. A team of professionals, including physician and nurse specialists, physical therapists, nutritionists and algologists (specialists in pain) may be required if appropriate wound care is to crystallize for certain patients with complex wounds. We owe it to ourselves and to our patients to practice wound care together in synergy and to share our knowledge and skills across healthcare disciplines. Perhaps then we can ensure that wound care in the twenty–first century is optimized and patient pain and suffering is reduced.

Conclusion

As wound care becomes a more sophisticated science, dressing decision–making becomes more and more complex. Clearly, practicing wound care by tradition alone is no longer an acceptable or reasonably prudent thing to do. The new paradigm suggests that the targeted use of dressing products based on the phase of the wound healing process that the wound is in will help to ensure the best possible patient outcomes. Five rules of wound dressings were presented and discussed. Compliance with these rules and well thought–out dressing decisions will help assure that in the twenty–first century the five dressing rights for patients with wounds are respected and implemented: the right patient, the right dressing, the right time, the right amount, and the right setting.

References

1. Gilje O. On taping, adhesive tape treatment of leg ulcers. *Acta Derm Vener* 1948;28:454–467.
2. Winter GD, Scales JT. The effects of air drying and dressings on the surface of a wound. *Nature* 1963;197:91–92.
3. Alvarez OM, Rozint J, Meehan M. Principles of moist wound healing: Indications for chronic wounds. In: Krasner D (ed). *Chronic Wound Care: A Clinical Source Book for Healthcare Professionals*. King of Prussia, PA, Health Management Publications, Inc., 1990, p. 269.
4. Turner TD. The development of wound management products. In: Krasner D (ed). *Chronic Wound Care: A Clinical Source Book for Healthcare Professionals*. King of Prussia, PA, Health Management Publications, Inc., 1990, pp 31–46.
5. Stotts N, Barbour S, Slaughter R, Wipke–Tevis, D. Wound care practices in the United States. *Ostomy/Wound Management* 1993;39(3):53–70.

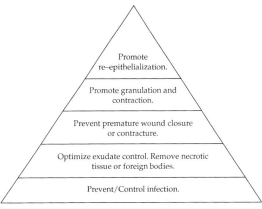

OPTIMIZE SYSTEMIC CONDITIONS

Figure 2. Wound healing hierarchy of needs
© Diane Krasner

6. Bergstrom N, Bennett MA, Carlson CE, et al. *Treatment of Pressure Ulcers*. Clinical Practice Guideline, No. 15, Rockville, MD, U.S. Department of Health and Human Services, Public Health Service, Agency for Health Care Policy and Research, AHCPR Publication No. 95–0652, December 1994.
7. Kuhn T. *Structure of Scientific Theory, Second Edition*. Chicago, IL, University of Chicago Press, 1970.
8. Krasner D. Shifting paradigms for wound care: Dressing decisions; multidisciplinary care; effectiveness. *Durable Medical Equipment Review* 1994;1(2):10–13.
9. Mosher CM. Putting pressure ulcers on the map. *WOCN Journal* 1995;22(4):183–186.
10. Krasner D. Resolving the dressing dilemma: Selecting wound dressings by category. *Ostomy/Wound Management* 1991;35:62–70.
11. Thomas S (ed). *Handbook of Wound Dressings (1994 Edition)*. London, England, Journal of Wound Care, 1994.
12. Hess CT. *Wound Care: Nurse's Clinical Guide*. Springhouse, PA, Springhouse Corporation, 1995.
13. Hutchinson JJ. Prevalence of wound infection under occlusive dressings: A collective survey of reported research. *Wounds* 1989;1(2):123–133.
14. Bolton L, van Rijswijk L: Wound dressings: Meeting clinical and biological needs. *Dermatology Nursing* 1991;3(3):146–161.
15. Xakellis GC, Chrischilles EA. Hydrocolloid versus saline gauze dressings in treating pressure ulcers: A cost–effectiveness analysis. *Archives of Physical Medicine & Rehabilitation* 1992;73:463–469.
16. Lawrence JC, Lilly HA & Kidson A. Wound dressings and airborne dispersal of bacteria. *Lancet* 1992;339(8796):807–808.
17. Krasner D, Kennedy KL, Rolstad BS, Roma AW. The ABCs of wound care dressings. *Ostomy/Wound Management* 1993;39(8):66–86.
18. Turner TD. The development of wound management products. In: Krasner D (ed). *Chronic Wound Care: A Clinical Source Book for Healthcare Professionals*. King of Prussia, PA, Health Management Publications, Inc., 1990, pp 31–46.
19. Cuzzell J, Krasner D. Wound dressings. In: Gogia P (ed): *Clinical Wound Management*. Thorofare, NJ, Slack Incorporated, 1995, pp 131–144.

Appendix 1. A Quick Reference Guide to Wound Care Product Categories*

March 1996
Compiled by Diane Krasner, MS, RN, CETN

This listing of wound care products highlights the importance of generic product categories. Under each generic product category, up to four product examples are given (a mix of old and new products), to help familiarize the reader with each category. No endorsement of any product or manufacturer is intended. Within each category, products must be individually evaluated. All products within a category do not necessarily perform equally. Combination products may be listed in more than one category. Refer to manufacturers' instructions for specifics regarding product usage.

* All product names should be considered copyrighted or trademarked regardless of the absence of an ® or ™.
© Diane Krasner 1996

Alginate Dressings

Product	Manufacturer
CURASORB®/CURASORB® Plus	Kendall
Kaltostat®/Kaltostat® Fortex	Calgon Vestal
Sorbsan™	Dow Hickam Pharmaceuticals

Biosynthetic Dressings

Product	Manufacturer
Biobrane II®	Dow Hickam Pharmaceuticals
Silon®	BioMed Sciences

Cleansers

Product	Manufacturer
a. Saline	Multiple
b. Hydrogen Peroxide	Multiple
c. Skin Cleansers	
Peri-Wash®	Sween
Royl-Derm™	Acme United
Skin Cleanser	Mentor
Triple Care™	Smith & Nephew United
d. Wound Cleansers	
Cara-Klenz™	Carrington
Constant-Clens™	Sherwood Medical
Curasol™	Healthpoint Medical
Dermagran® Spray	Derma Sciences

Collagen Dressings

Product	Manufacturer
ChroniCure™	Derma Sciences
Fibracol® (Collagen/Alginate)	Johnson & Johnson Medical
Medifil™	BioCore
SkinTemp®	BioCore

Composite Dressings

Product	Manufacturer
Alldress®	Scott Health Care
CovaDerm™/CovaDerm™ Plus	DeRoyal
Gentell Covertell®	MKM
Odor-Absorbent Dressing	Hollister

(Continued on next page)

Contact Layers

Product	Manufacturer
Mepitel®	Scott Health Care
Profore®	Smith & Nephew United
Tegapore	3M
Ventex™ Vented Dressing	Kendall

Enzymes/ Debriding Agent

Product	Manufacturer
Elase® (Fibrinolysin/desoxyribonuclease)	Fugisawa
Panifil® Ointment (Papain)	Rystan
Santyl® (Collagenase)	Knoll Pharmaceuticals

Foam Dressings

Product	Manufacturer
Allevyn®	Smith & Nephew United
Flexzan™	Dow Hickam Pharmaceuticals
Lyofoam®/Lyofoam® T	Acme United
PolyMem	Ferris Manufacturing

Gauze Dressings
(see also Composite Dressings)

Product	Manufacturer
a. Woven	Multiple
b. Non-woven	
EXCILON®	Kendall
NATURALON™	Kendall
NU GAUZE General Use Sponges	Johnson & Johnson Medical
SOF-WICK™	Johnson & Johnson Medical
c. Packing/Packing Strips	
(Non-impregnated)	
Kerlix®/Kerlix® Lite	Kendall
NU-BREDE™	Johnson & Johnson Medical
Packing Strips (Plain)	Multiple
TENDERSORB®	Kendall
d. Conforming/Wrapping	
Conform®	Kendall
Elastomull®	Beiersdorf
Kerlix®/Kerlix® Lite	Kendall
KLING™	Johnson & Johnson Medical
e. Debriding	
NU-BREDE™	Johnson & Johnson Medical
TENDERSORB®	Kendall
f. Impregnated Gauze Dressings	
Dermagran™ Wet Dressing	
(Saline)	Derma Sciences
Petrolatum	
Gentell™ Hydrogel Dressing	MKM Healthcare
GRx Saline Wet Dressing	Geritrex Corporation
Vaseline® Petrolatum	Sherwood Medical

(Continued on next page)

Appendix 1. A Quick Reference Guide to Wound Care Product Categories *(Continued)*

g. Non-adherent gauze
      Primapore®   Smith & Nephew United
      Release®   Johnson & Johnson Medical
      Telfa®   Kendall

h. Specialty Absorptive Gauze
      EXU-DRY®   Exu-Dry Wound Care Products
      SURGIPAD® Combine Dressings   Johnson & Johnson Medical
      TENDERSORB® Wet-Pruf Abdominal Pad   Kendall

Hydrocolloid Dressings

Product	Manufacturer
DuoDERM®/CGF/Extra Thin	ConvaTec
RepliCare™	Smith & Nephew United
Restore™/CX/Extra Thin	Hollister
Tegasorb™	3M

Hydrogel Dressings
(see also Impregnated Gauze Dressings)

Product	Manufacturer
SHEET	
ClearSite®	NDM
Elasto-Gel™	Southwest Technologies
Gentell™	MKM
Vigilon®	Bard
AMORPHOUS	
Carrington Gel Wound Dressing™	Carrington Laboratories
DuoDERM® Hydroactive Gel (Hydrogel/Hydrocolloid)	ConvaTec
Hypergel®	Scott Health Care
IntraSite® Gel	Smith & Nephew United

Leg Ulcer Wraps
Compression Bandages/Wraps

Product	Manufacturer
Coban®	3M Health Care
Dome Paste®	Miles
Elastoplast®	Beiersdorf
Setopress®	Acme United

Multi Layered Systems

Product	Manufacturer
Circulon™ System	ConvaTec
Profore®	Smith & Nephew United
Unna-Pak	Glenwood

Skin Sealants

Product	Manufacturer
Preppies™	Kendall
Skin Prep™	Smith & Nephew United
Skin Shield®	Mentor
3M No Sting Skin Protectant	3M

(Continued on next page)

Appendix 1. A Quick Reference Guide to Wound Care Product Categories *(Continued)*

Transparent Film Dressings

Product	Manufacturer
BIOCLUSIVE™	Johnson & Johnson Medical
Flexfilm™	Dow Hickan Pharmaceuticals
OpSite®/Flexifix/Flexigrid	Smith & Nephew United
Tegaderm™/HP	3M

Wound Fillers: Pastes, Powders, Beads, etc.

Product	Manufacturer
Bard® Absorption Dressing	Bard
DuoDERM® Paste	ConvaTec
Iodosorb® Gel	Oclassen
Triad™	Sween

Wound Pouches

Product	Manufacturer
Wound Drainage Collector	Hollister
Wound Manager™	ConvaTec
Adult and Pediatric Sized Ostomy Pouches	Multiple

Not Otherwise Classified (NOC) Product Categories

Adhesives
Adhesive Removers
Adhesive Skin Closures
Adhesive Tapes
Antibiotics
Antimicrobials
Antiseptics
Bandages
Creams
Dressing Covers
Growth Factors
Healthcare Personnel Handrinses
Lubricating/Stimulating Sprays
Moisture Barrier Ointments/Creams/Skin Protectant Pastes
Moisturizers
Ointments
Perineal Cleansing Foams
Sterile Fields
Surgical Scrubs
Surgical Tapes

Appendix 2. A Quick Reference to Wound Care Product Functions and Categories

Developed by Bonnie Sue Rolstad, RN, BA, CETN; Sharon A. Aronovitch, PhD, RN, CETN; and Diane Krasner, MS, RN, CETN

Published by Kendall Healthcare Products Company, Mansfield, MA. Reprinted with permission.

Product Function	Category
Absorb (Products used to absorb exudate)	Absorption beads, pastes, and powders Alginates Composite dressings Foams Gauze (impregnated & non–impregnated) Hydrocolloids Hydrogels (minimal)
Cleanse (Products used to remove purulent drainage, foreign debris, and devitalized tissue that is topically applied)	Wound cleansers
Debride (Autolytic) (Products that cover a wound and allow enzymes in the wound fluid to self–digest eschar and slough)	Absorption beads, pastes and powders Alginates Composite dressings Foams Hydrate gauze Hydrocolloids Hydrogels Transparent films Wound care systems (2–part)
Debride (Chemical) (Products applied topically to breakdown devitalized tissue)	Enzymatic debridement agents
Debride (Mechanical) (Products used to remove devitalized tissue with mechanical force)	Wound cleansers Gauze (wet to dry)
Hydrate (Products used to add moisture to the wound)	Gauze (impregnated or plain, saturated with saline) Hydrogels Wound care systems (2–part)
Maintain a moist wound environment (Products used to manage moisture levels in the wound to maintain a moist environment)	Composites Contact layers Foams Gauze (impregnated or plain saturated with saline) Hydrocolloids Hydrogels Transparent films Wound care systems (2–part)
Manage high output wounds (Products used to manage wounds with excessive amounts of exudate > 100 ml/24 hours or > QID dressing changes	Pouching systems

(Continued on next page)

Pack or fill dead space
(Products used to fill dead space and prevent
premature wound closure or to fill shallow areas
and provide absorption)

Absorption beads, pastes and powders
Alginates
Composites
Foam (pillows)
Gauze (impregnated and non–impregnated)

Protect/cover the wound
(Products used to cover the wound and provide
protection from the external environment)

Composites
Compression bandages/wraps
Foams
Gauze dressings (covers/wraps)
Hydrocolloids
Hydrogels (with covers/borders)
Transparent film dressings
(Contact layers protect the wound from
mechanical trauma during procedures)

Protect periwound skin
(Products used to protect the wound from
moisture and mechanical trauma)

Composites
Foams
Hydrocolloids
Pouching systems
Securement devices
Skin sealants
Transparent film dressings

Provice therapeutic compression
(Products used to provide appropriate levels
of support of the lower extremities in venous
stasis disease)

Compression bandages/wraps

18

Pressure Ulcers: Assessment, Classification and Management

Diane Krasner, MS, RN, CETN

Krasner D. Pressure ulcers: Assessment, classification and management. In: Krasner D, Kane D. *Chronic Wound Care, Second Edition.* Wayne, PA, Health Management Publications, Inc., 1997, pp 152–157.

The mind is like a parachute,
It only works when it is open.

Introduction

The more one knows about pressure ulcers, the more one is awed by their simple complexity. The mechanism of pressure ulcer formation is "simply" pressure, but this is exacerbated by friction, shear, moisture and other individual and environmental factors. Assessment "simply" involves looking at an external wound, but this is complicated by undermining, tunneling, closed pressure ulcers and measurement error. Classification is made "simply" by a four stage system, but this is confounded by wound bed ambiguities, skin pigmentation, reverse staging and by the fact that deeper wounds which extend into bone and joint are not precisely described. Management is accomplished "simply" by a series of basic interventions: pressure relief, topical treatment, pain relief and nutritional support. But this "simple" management scheme challenges healthcare professionals to provide interdisciplinary care; to work synergistically with caregivers, family members and patients; to control costs and resources; and to manage pressure ulcer patients for the long term across the healthcare continuum. In short, pressure ulcers are extremely complex and their assessment, classification and management present enormous challenges for healthcare professionals.

While it has been difficult to determine the actual prevalence and incidence of pressure ulcers, studies conducted during the last ten years have given us a much better handle on these statistics.

Incidence (new cases appearing within a specified period of time) in acute care facilities ranges from 2.7 to 29.5 percent, while prevalence (a cross–sectional count of the number of cases at a specified point in time) ranges from 3.5 to 29.5 percent. In skilled nursing facilities and nursing homes prevalence rates range from 2.4 to 23 percent. And in one study of home healthcare patients, the incidence was 4.3 percent and the prevalence was 12.9 percent.[1] At any given time, over one million Americans are estimated to have pressure ulcers.[2]

Even more distressing are the figures related to specific high–risk populations. In elderly patients admitted to the hospital for femoral fractures, the pressure ulcer incidence was 66 percent, in critical care patients 33 percent, and in quadriplegic patients 60 percent.[1] The number of persons at risk for pressure ulcers has not been accurately determined, but probably runs in the tens of millions in the United States alone.

Pressure ulcers are a significant public health problem, resulting in hospitalizations, institutionalizations, and loss of quality of life. It has been estimated that the national cost of pressure ulcer treatment in the United States exceeds $1.335 billion.[1] Others estimate that the costs to heal a single ulcer range from $5,000 to $65,000 per ulcer. Pressure ulcers are associated with a four–fold increase in mortality risk among geriatric patients and nursing home residents.[3] Pressure ulcers drain personal emotions and finances, strain healthcare system resources and fuel feelings of guilt and blame. Hopefully, a new focus and commitment to prevention, risk assessment and early intervention will help us to overcome this tragedy of modern society.

Table 1

Pressure ulcer risk assessment, assessment and classification systems (listed from earliest to most recent)

Pressure Ulcer Risk Assessment Scales

1. The Norton Scale
   D. Norton et al.
   originally published in 1962
   see Gladstone & Gladstone, *Journal of Advanced Nursing* 1982;1:419–426.
2. The Gosnell Scale
   D.J. Gosnell
   Nursing Research 1973;22:55–59.
3. The Abruzzese Scale
   R.S. Abruzzese
   in Lee BY. *Chronic Ulcers of the Skin.*
   McGraw–Hill, New York, 1985.
4. The Braden Scale for Predicting Pressure Sore Risk
   N. Bergstrom, B. Braden, A. Laguzza, V. Holman.
   Nursing Research 1987;36(4): 205–210.

Pressure Ulcer Assessment/Classification Scales

1. Shea Pressure Sore Classification
   J.D. Shea.
   Clinical Orthop 1975;112:89–100.
2. International Association of Enterostomal Therapy Pressure Ulcer Classification.
   N. Mash. Standards of care of dermal wounds: pressure ulcers.
   IAET, 1987.
3. National Pressure Ulcer Advisory Panel (NPUAP) Pressure Ulcer Classification.
   NPUAP Consensus Development Conference Statement.
   Decubitus 1989;2:24.
4. Yarkony–Kirk Pressure Ulcer Classification
   G.M.Yarkony, P.M.Kirk, C. Carlson, et al.
   Arch Dermatol 1990;126:1218–1219.
5. The Pressure Sore Status Tool
   B.Bates–Jensen
   Decubitus 1992;5(6):20–28.
6. The Sessing Scale
   B.A. Ferrell
   J Am Ger Soc 1995;43(1):37–40.

Mechanisms

A pressure ulcer is "a localized area of tissue necrosis that develops when soft tissue is compressed between a bony prominence and an external surface for a prolonged period of time."[2] Pressure ulcers are also called pressure sores, decubitus and are known colloquially as bedsores. Pressure ulcer is the preferred term because it most accurately reflects the etiology. As the definition suggests, pressure ulcers occur most often as a result of external pressure to an area that compresses the body's soft tissue. This pressure usually – but not always – occurs over a bony prominence. With excessive pressures, capillaries collapse and the flow of blood and nutrients to body tissues is disrupted. This disruption leads to localized ischemia, hypoxia, tissue acidosis, edema, and eventually to the cellular necrosis that is known as a pressure ulcer. Certain conditions caused by immobility, such as paralysis and stroke, place individuals at risk for pressure ulcers. The reader is referred to Chapters 3 and 5 in this source book for more detailed discussions of these problems.

The bony prominences at highest risk for pressure ulcer formation are, from head to toe, the occiput, scapulae, elbows, greater trochanters, ischial tuberosities, sacrum/coccyx, malleoli and heels. Two–thirds of pressure ulcers occur in the pelvic girdle.[4]

Pressure ulcer formation is accelerated in the presence of other mechanisms, most notably friction, shear and moisture. Friction is the mechanical force exerted when skin is dragged across a coarse surface such as bed linens.[1] Epidermal skin layers may be stripped off by friction when patients are pulled across bed linens instead of being lifted. Shear is the mechanical force that acts on a unit area of skin in a direction parallel to the body's surface.[1] When the head of a hospital bed is elevated greater

Assessment

Although pressure ulcers were described as early as ancient Egyptian times,[5] surprisingly it is only since the Second World War that significant interest in pressure ulcers has been found in the healthcare literature. During the last thirty–five years, a number of risk assessment, assessment and classification systems specific to pressure ulcers have been developed (Table 1). For further information on pressure ulcer risk assessment and assessment refer to Chapters 4, 5, 6, 9, and 10 in this source book.

Coordinating such a complex series of assessments and managing the data collected presents enormous challenges for any provider of pressure ulcer related services.

than 30 degrees and the patient slides down in bed, shear often occurs in the sacral area. Moisture, such as that from incontinence of urine or stool or from diaphoresis, weakens the skin's natural barrier through maceration, changes the skin pH and is significantly correlated with the development of pressure ulcers. Not only must pressure, shear, friction and moisture be controlled, but the following factors must also be addressed: immobility, altered activity levels, altered mental status, altered nutritional status and chronic conditions.

The typical pressure ulcer scenario begins with an insult affecting a person's mobility status. Lack of attention to pressure ulcer prevention, inadequate risk assessment and inappropriate pressure reducing interventions often result in an area of redness or nonblanchable erythema (a Stage I pressure ulcer) over a bony prominence, such as the sacrum in a bedbound stroke patient or the ischium in a wheelchair–bound individual. If pressure is not relieved or if friction, shear and/or incontinence are added to the picture, the skin can break down within hours and a significant ulcer can develop within a matter of days. In one extreme case, an elderly woman I cared for had fractured her hip and fell face down on her tiled bathroom floor. She remained face down on the floor for about forty–eight hours, incontinent of urine and stool and becoming severly dehydrated. When she was finally discovered and admitted to the acute care facility, she had stage IV ulcers with eschar on her chin, upper sternum, ribs, iliac crests, and patellae.

In May 1992 and December 1994 two pressure ulcer guidelines were released by the Agency for Healthcare Policy and Research (AHCPR) of the Public Health Service of the U.S. Department of Health and Human Services.[1,6] The first guideline relates to pressure ulcer prediction and prevention and the second to treatment. These guidelines attempt to synthesize the current state of the science of pressure ulcer prevention and care. The reader is referred to Chapters 4, 6 and 10 in this source book for further information on specific guideline recommendations and for information on risk assessment, assessment and documentation.

The current standard for the assessment of pressure ulcer patients involves a series of distinct assessments:

1. Overall history and physical assessment,
2. Ongoing risk assessment,
3. Initial assessment of wounding,
4. Ongoing assessment of healing,
5. Nutritional assessment, and
6. Pain assessment.

Coordinating such a complex series of assessments and managing the data collected presents enormous challenges for any provider of pressure ulcer related services. The development of computerized data management systems for pressure ulcer documentation will certainly assist with this challenge. (See Chapter 6.)

Classification

As mentioned previously, a number of different pressure ulcer classification systems have been developed since 1975 (Table 1). Some of the systems use grades and some use stages. Currently, in the United States, the four stage system, which was accepted at a national consensus development conference sponsored by the National Pressure Ulcer Advisory Panel (NPUAP) in 1989 and adopted for use in the 1992 and 1994 Pressure Ulcer Guidelines by the AHCPR,[1,6] is the most widely accepted classification system for pressure ulcers. The four stages from AHCPR Clinical Practice Guideline Number 15, *Treatment of Pressure Ulcers*, pages 12–13 are defined below and illustrated in Plates 11 to 16.

Stage I. Nonblanchable erythema of intact skin, the heralding lesion of skin ulceration. In individuals with darker skin, discoloration of the skin, warmth, edema, induration, or hardness may be indicators.

Stage II. Partial thickness skin loss involving epidermis, dermis, or both. The ulcer is superficial and presents clinically as an abrasion, blister or shallow crater.

Stage III. Full thickness skin loss involving damage to or necrosis of subcutaneous tissue that may extend down to, but not through, underlying fascia. The ulcer presents clinically as a deep crater with or without undermining of adjacent tissue.

Stage IV. Full thickness skin loss with extensive destruction, tissue necrosis, or damage to muscle, bone, or supporting structures (e.g., tendon, joint capsule). Undermining and sinus tracts also may be associated with Stage IV pressure ulcers.

The following limitations are inherent in these definitions:

1. Because the skin remains intact in Stage I pressure ulcers, these lesions are not ulcers in the usual sense. In addition, Stage I pressure ulcers are not always reliably assessed, especially in patients with darkly pigmented skin. A reliable system to accurately identify Stage I pressure ulcers in individuals with darkly pigmented skin should be developed. Despite these limitations, identification of a Stage I pressure ulcer is critical for indicating the need for more vigilant assessment and preventive care.
2. When eschar is present, a pressure ulcer cannot be accurately staged until the eschar is removed.
3. It may be difficult to assess pressure ulcers in patients with casts, other orthopedic devices, or support stockings. Routine assessment to check for adequate circulation, movement, and sensation may fail to detect pressure ulcers beneath casts. Healthcare providers should (1) assess the skin under the edges of casts, (2) be alert to patient complaints of pressure–induced pain, (3) determine whether casts need to be altered or replaced to relieve pressure, and (4) remove support stockings to assess the skin.

This clinician has found it useful to make a clear distinction between the initial assessment of wounding and the ongoing assessment of healing.

Like many of the other pressure ulcer classification systems, the NPUAP staging system was developed for the initial assessment of wounding by determining the depth of injury. Stage I and II pressure ulcers are partial thickness wounds. Stage III and IV pressure ulcers are full thickness wounds. The depth of ulcers containing necrotic tissue (eschar or slough) cannot be accurately determined and, therefore, the ulcer cannot be accurately staged until the necrotic tissue is removed. Validity and reliability testing for the NPUAP system has not been reported.

Problems have developed due to overuse and misuse of the NPUAP system in the clinical arena. It has been used to classify wounds of varying etiologies although it was developed for use with pressure ulcers only. It has also been used in reverse to describe wound healing, a phenomenon referred to as reverse staging or downstaging. To describe wound healing, clinicians have noted pressure ulcer progression from a Stage IV to Stage III to Stage II to Stage I to healed. Regulatory agencies have also adopted this practice of reverse staging, basing reimbursement and accreditation decisions on the practice. But this is erroneous and does not correspond to the way wounds actually heal, namely by granulation, contraction and reepithelialization. The NPUAP advises, "Reverse staging should never be used to describe the healing of pressure ulcers."[7]

U =	Unstagable; status/ depth cannot be determined
N =	Necrotic tissue present
I =	Infected
D =	Debrided (sharp surgical) during the past 48 hours
G =	Granulating; clean wound
C =	Contracting
R =	Reepithelializing
H =	Healed

***Figure 1.** WHS: Wound Healing Scale®*

Assessment of Wounding Versus Assessment of Healing

This clinician has found it useful to make a clear distinction between the initial assessment of wounding and the ongoing assessment of healing. Initially, when a pressure ulcer develops, a pressure ulcer staging scale should be used to assess the depth of initial wounding. For example, a Stage 4 pressure ulcer is initially a full thickness wound extending into muscle or bone. It is always, at least categorically, a Stage IV pressure ulcer. As the pressure ulcer heals, granulation tissue fills the wound bed, the wound contracts and, finally, the surface is reepithelialized. It is not appropriate to perform an assessment of healing by reverse staging; rather, a wound healing scale should now be used to describe healing. Two wound healing scales have been developed to date, the 1992 Pressure Sore Status Tool (See Chapter 6 in this source book) and the 1995 Sessing Scale.

The Wound Healing Scale®

Recently, this clinician developed the WHS: Wound Healing Scale® in an attempt to find an alternative to reverse staging for the Health Care Financing Administration's (HCFA) Minimum Data Set (MDS), Section M. The MDS has been used extensively since the 1989 passage of the OBRA regulations for data collection in extended care facilities for Medicare patients. Following are the objectives for creating this scale:

- To find a clinically & physiologically acceptable alternative to "backstaging" (reverse staging) for describing wound healing,
- To develop a scale that can be used in multiple settings, by diverse providers,
- To identify a scale that will lend itself to use with large & small data sets, and
- To follow the KISS principle (keep it simple, stupid).

The WHS has eight modifiers that can be used in conjunction with pressure ulcer stages (1 to 4) or with thickness designations (partial [P]/full [F]) for all other wound types, including acute and chronic wounds (Figure 1). For example, 4N = a Stage 4 pressure ulcer with a necrotic base; FG = a full thickness wound with a granulating base. If a wound's status changes from a 3N to a 4D or 4G following debridement, this would be a normal expectation. However, if a wound's status changes from a 3G to a 3N, this should send up a red flag of concern regarding wound deterioration.

Psychometric testing for the reliability and validity of the WHS® will be carried out in 1997. The WHS® offers clinicians a simple, yet comprehensive, tool for describing the status and healing of all types of wounds, not just pressure ulcers.

Pressure Ulcer Management

Given the state of the science about pressure ulcers, most experts advocate the use of consistent interventions for pressure ulcer care in order to achieve optimal patient outcomes. The responsibility for carrying out these interventions may be delegated to any number of healthcare team members. The important point is that someone with expertise and commitment must take responsibility for managing the care of patients with pressure ulcers in a particular facility. The pressure ulcer program may include initial assessment of wounding, ongoing assessment of healing, ongoing risk assessment, ongoing nutritional assessment, ongoing pain assessment, prevention strategies, standards of care and protocols for care, algorithms or critical pathways, and documentation strategies.

Goals of Care

Any pressure ulcer management plan must be consistent with the overall plan of care of the patient. In most cases, the patient will be offered aggressive holistic care, including prevention strategies, pressure reduction or relief, topical treatment, nutritional support and pain relief. In selected patients, such as those with terminal conditions, a team decision may be taken to only provide conservative or palliative care. The reader is referred to *Pressure Ulcers in Adults: Prediction and Prevention*, AHCPR Clinical Practice Guideline, Number 3 (1992) and to Chapter 42 in this source book for further information on this subject.

Prevention

Nowhere is the old adage "an ounce of prevention is worth a pound of cure" more true. With proper risk assessment and prevention strategies most pressure ulcers can be prevented. Readers are referred to Chapter 3 and 5 for detailed information on prevention strategies, including risk assessment and the use of preventive devices.

Management

Aggressive measures to intervene at the first sign of redness over a bony prominence or the slightest skin break can reverse the formation of a serious pressure ulcer. Early intervention is efficient and is probably cost–effective in the long run, although it carries with it a significant price tag for staffing and supplies in the short run. Turning schedules, pressure reducing or relieving devices for support surfaces (beds, chairs, wheelchairs) and topical protective dressings and incontinence supplies are part of the arsenal needed to respond early in the pressure ulcer battle.

Pressure ulcer treatment involves a coordinated, interdisciplinary effort to address the underlying etiology of the pressure ulcer, pressure, nutrition, topical treatment, mobility status, and pain control. Management specifics are detailed in Sections II and III of this source book.

Conclusion

Everyone who is involved in patient care must be attentive to pressure ulcers and committed to their prevention. From the patient to the nursing assistant to the physician, the team must work together to provide the optimal care that is the patient's right – the chain being only as strong as its weakest link. Team members must be familiar with key principles and current research and must have up–to–date knowledge of products, treatments and devices. The pressure ulcer problem challenges us to communicate and to work across professional lines.

Healthcare is changing faster than any of us can comprehend. The next millennium may see critical shortages of nurses and other allied healthcare personnel and reduction in funding for healthcare and research. More efficient systems must evolve to compensate for these trends if we are to continue to reduce the incidence of pressure ulcers. Frequent turning and repositioning, while still the most effective measure for prevention, requires sufficient staffing, which may not be available in the future. Cleaning up quickly after incontinent episodes to prevent maceration and resulting skin breakdown eats up limited manpower hours. Unfortunately, effective pressure ulcer management, as we now know it, is labor–intensive care. Today's "idealized" pressure ulcer care plans must give rise to more realistic protocols for the next millennium.

The physiologic, psychologic, economic, and legal costs related to pressure ulcers are impossible to measure accurately. But one thing is clear: if effective strategies for pressure ulcer prevention and early intervention are implemented, we should seldom have to pay those prices.

References

1. Bergstrom, N, Bennett MA, Carlson CE, et al. 1994. *Treatment of Pressure Ulcers*. Clinical Practice Guideline, Number 15. AHCPR Publication No. 95–0652. Rockville, MD: Agency for Health Care Policy and Research, Public Health Service, U.S. Department of Health and Human Services, December 1994.
2. The National Pressure Ulcer Advisory Panel. Pressure ulcers: prevalence, cost and risk assessment. Consensus Development Conference Statement. *Decubitus* 1989;2:24.
3. Allman RM. Pressure ulcers among the elderly. *New Eng J Med* 1989;320:850–853.
4. Maklebust J, Sieggreen M. *Pressure Ulcers: Guidelines for Prevention and Nursing Management, Second Edition*. Springhouse, PA, Springhouse Corporation, 1996.
5. Rowling JT. Pathological changes in mummies. *Proceedings of the Royal Soc Med* (London) 1961;54:409–415.
6. AHCPR Panel for the Prediction and Prevention of Pressure Ulcers in Adults. 1992. *Pressure Ulcers in Adults: Prediction and Prevention*. Clinical Practice Guideline, Number 3. AHCPR Publication No. 92–0047. Rockville, MD: Agency for Health Care Policy and Research, Public Health Service, U.S. Department of Health and Human Services, May 1992.
7. NPUAP position on reverse staging. *NPUAP Report* 1995;4(2):1.

19

Arterial Ulcers: Assessment, Classification and Management

G. Allen Holloway, Jr., MD

Holloway GA Jr. Arterial Ulcers: Assessment, Classification and Management. In: Krasner D, Kane D. *Chronic Wound Care, Second Edition*. Wayne, PA, Health Management Publications, Inc., 1997, pp 158–164.

Introduction

The underlying message of this chapter is that arterial ulcers occur due to ischemia and that the only effective way to heal these ulcers is to provide an increase in blood supply. In the presence of these ulcers, the patient must be referred to the vascular surgeon or interventionalist for revascularization as other approaches are virtually never effective. Given this overall approach, the chapter then addresses how one evaluates these ulcers, and what adjunctive management techniques may be applicable.

Overview and Etiology

Arterial ulcers are located primarily in the distal lower extremity and rarely in the upper extremity. They occur because of inadequate perfusion of skin and subcutaneous tissue at rest with the consequent death of underperfused cells. Arterial occlusive disease with its accompanying ischemia is a common condition, especially among smokers, diabetics and in the elderly population. It can lead to claudication, rest pain and gangrene as well as localized ulceration. Physicians and other healthcare providers are frequently not well educated in the subject of arterial disease, and as a result are not well acquainted with its natural history and the problems with which it may be associated. Arterial ulcers are one of the complications of arterial insufficiency.[1]

It is important to recognize that arterial insufficiency is rarely a stable condition. It regresses rarely and is almost always a progressive condition which may advance either slowly or rapidly. Hence, ulcers caused by arterial insufficiency are usually progressive, making it important to diagnose and treat as early as possible to avoid further tissue loss.

Assessment – History

The key to the diagnosis of arterial occlusive disease is the history obtained from the patient.[2] In almost all patients, particularly those presenting with pain, the history can indicate the presence of disease and its severity. Patients with early disease may complain of pain when walking. Pain will always occur at a predictable, repeatable distance and may occur in the calves, thighs or buttocks depending upon where in the arterial system the narrowing or blockage occurs. This pain is termed "intermittent claudication" and indicates inadequate blood supply to the area of pain during the stress of exercise. Although this state is frequently stable over long periods of time, it may progress so that shorter and shorter distances walked may bring on the pain, leading eventually to where pain is present even without exercise.[3] This stage is termed "rest pain" and is usually seen in the distal foot and toes. It indicates inadequate blood supply to support the tissues even at rest. Arterial "ischemic" ulcers are most commonly seen at this point. Gangrene of the toes or feet may also occur when perfusion becomes this marginal and may force therapeutic decisions. Ischemic ulcers are usually quite painful but may be masked in the diabetic as discussed below.

The same scenario may also apply in the upper extremity, although less than 10 percent of arterial

Table 1
Characteristics of different ulcer types

	Arterial	Vasculitic	Venous	Diabetic	Pressure
Location:	Usually distal	Below malleolus–foot dorsum	Above malleolus	Pressure areas on foot	Pressure areas
Size:	Small	Small to large	Small to large	Usually small but may be large	Small to large
Shape:	Round	Irregular	Irregular	Round	Round but may be irregular if large
Depth:	Usually relatively shallow	Shallow	Shallow	Shallow to deep, may have tracking and/or undermining	Shallow to deep, may have tracking and/or undermining
Base:	Pale	Necrotic with marked vascularity	Variable, frequently exudative	Variable, frequently necrotic if infected	Variable
Margins:	Smooth	Irregular	Irregular	Usually smooth	Variable
Surrounding skin:	Pale	Hyperemic	Pigmented	Frequently callus	Variable

occlusive disease occurs in this area due primarily to the excellent collateral circulation.[4] Claudication is rarely seen because of this collateral circulation and because the muscle groups are smaller, perform less work and therefore need less oxygen.

Trauma is often a precipitating event for arterial ulcers in either the upper or lower extremity. Stubbing a toe, being run into by a wheelchair or dropping something on a foot are examples of common causes of such trauma. When a traumatic injury occurs, even a small one, an inflammatory response is initiated. In response, local metabolic requirements are increased and a blood supply, which may have been barely adequate to maintain tissue viability, becomes inadequate. Ischemia and infarction of the local tissues occur with tissue loss and/or gangrene. The degree of necrosis is dependent upon the volume of tissue which has inadequate circulation for viability.

The patient should also be questioned about other disease processes which might be confused with arterial occlusive disease and ischemic ulcers. Some of these processes are discussed in more detail in later chapters. Venous insufficiency with venous stasis can lead to ulcers, but these have a different appearance than arterial ulcers. Ulcers associated with a vasculitis, as can be seen with autoimmune disease processes, may emulate ischemic ulcers. They are most often seen in association with patients with severe, deforming rheumatoid arthritis but may be present with other connective tissue diseases. These ulcers frequently arise from small reddened areas which continue to increase in size, coalesce, and are typically extremely painful. Ulcers associated with diabetes mellitus, which should usually be considered pressure ulcers related to the underlying neuropathy, can frequently, although not necessarily, have an ischemic component which must be looked for. These ulcers, despite the ischemic component, are most often painless because of the neuropathy. They usually occur over pressure areas on the plantar or medial and/or lateral aspects of the foot. Physical examination can help to differentiate these ulcers from purely ischemic ulcers. There are other ulcers which can be confused with arterial ischemic ulcers, but they occur less frequently and are beyond the scope of this chapter to discuss in detail. It should also be remembered that ulcers may have more than one etiology, and that each of the above ulcer types may have a component of ischemia superimposed on the primary underlying etiology.

Assessment – Physical Examination

Physical examination of the patient suspected of having arterial ulcers can help to confirm this diagnosis. A general physical exam should be performed to look for obvious problems relating to lungs, heart and nervous system. A focused exam then should be made of the affected extremities and arterial pulses examined. The abdomen above the umbilicus should be palpated for the presence of an aortic aneurysm which could be the source of arterial emboli giving rise to focal ischemia. Femoral, popliteal, dorsalis pedis and posterior tibial pulses should be palpated and described as normal, reduced or absent. Usually an arterial pressure of approximately 80 to 90 mm Hg is necessary to be able to palpate a pulse so that an absent pulse signifies a lower pressure in the artery. Skin in patients with severe ischemia is frequently thin, shiny and pale although dependent rubor may modify this condition. With severe ischemia, elevation of the leg to 30 degrees results in rapid cadaveric pallor of the extremity. When lowered to the dependent position the foot slowly, depending upon the degree of ischemia, refills with blood and becomes reddened or "ruborous" to a degree not seen in the normal foot. This is a simple test that can be performed at the bedside and is an excellent indicator of the presence of severe ischemia. The nails of patients with severe ischemia are also frequently abnormal and may be thickened, yellowed and fragile. Fungal infection of the nails may present a similar picture so that this is not an unequivocal diagnostic sign.

Ischemic ulcers are usually located on the foot although they can occasionally occur above the malleoli. They are usually relatively small and are described as "punched out." They tend to be pale with limited or no surrounding inflammatory response and a base which shows essentially no granulation tissue. This description is in contradistinction to that of the vasculitic ulcer which may occur in the same area and is usually angry looking with intense surrounding erythema and an active base of mixed necrotic and red granulation tissue. Venous stasis ulcers virtually always occur proximal to the malleoli in the gaiter area and are relatively shallow. Usually there are surrounding stasis changes of pigmentation, scarring and edema, and the ulcers tend to be larger with irregular margins.

A summary of the characteristics of some of these different ulcer types is presented in Table 1.

Vascular Laboratory

Confirmation of the diagnosis of an arterial ischemic ulcer can be done by obtaining non–invasive studies of the arterial system in the vascular laboratory. Simplest and most basic are ankle arterial pressures which are similar to blood pressures obtained in the upper arm. Pressures are measured in the ankle by placing a blood pressure cuff on the lower shin just above the ankle. An ultrasonic Doppler, rather than a stethoscope, is used to determine systolic arterial pressure in the dorsalis pedis or posterior tibial arteries when cuff pressure is released, as Korotkoff sounds used to sense arterial pressure in the upper arm cannot be heard at the ankle. The ankle/brachial index (ABI) is determined by dividing the ankle systolic pressure by the brachial systolic pressure obtained at the same time. This normalizes the ankle pressure to the central arterial pressure and compensates for central arterial pressures which may vary markedly in different individuals. A normal ABI should be between 1.0 and 1.2, with anything less than 0.9 being considered abnormal.[5] Intermittent claudication is said to occur at less than 0.8 with severe ischemia being considered to be less than 0.5. It should be recognized that these numbers are not absolute but should be used as clinical guidelines. At the same time, Doppler arterial waveforms (or arterial pulse volume recordings) are recorded to correlate with the ABIs. Frequently in diabetic patients as well as in 10 to 15 percent of non–diabetics, calcification of the medial layer of the peripheral arteries may render them partially or totally incompressible, giving an artificially elevated arterial pressure and index. The Doppler arterial waveforms which are normally triphasic may be biphasic or monophasic indicating more severe disease than is measured by the pressures and indices in incompressible arteries. Measuring pressures and indices at different levels in the legs, called segmental pressures, can determine where the pressure decreases and can therefore help to locate the site or sites of arterial occlusive disease.

In some vascular laboratories, transcutaneous oxygen measurements, T_cPO_2, are used to help determine the degree of microvascular perfusion of an area. This easily performed measurement involves only attaching an electrode to the skin with double sided adhesive tape and allowing approximately 20 minutes for equilibration before reading the results. Empirically, values for T_cPO_2 of less than 20 mm Hg have been associated with either very slow or absent healing and values of greater than 30 mm Hg with adequate healing, with values of 20 to 30 mm Hg being in the "gray zone."[6,7] These measurements may be particularly valuable where ABIs are low, and it is desired to avoid surgical revascularization procedures if possible. A T_cPO_2 of greater than 30 mm Hg in the area of an ulcer suggests that it likely has adequate perfusion to heal, and a trial period of good ulcer management may be a reasonable option. These values can be somewhat variable and are regarded as an adjunct to, and not an absolute in, decision making. T_cPO_2 measurements are not universally available or accepted and thus may not be available to all patients with peripheral ulcers.

If clinically indicated, it may also be reasonable to assess the venous system to determine whether ulcers felt to be arterial might have a venous component and to what degree that might contribute to the problem. Measurement of adequacy of the venous system is not as simple or standardized as in the arterial system. Various plethysmographic tests which involve measuring changes in volume of the involved extremity have been suggested and are in use. These include phleborheography, impedance plethysmography, strain gauge plethysmography, reflectance plethysmography and air plethysmography. All have their advocates and detractors, but none has become a standard at the present time. However, the ultrasonic venous duplex exam has probably become the de facto standard for the evaluation of venous obstruction and particularly deep venous thrombosis (DVT), as well as, to a lesser degree, venous insufficiency. By looking at the ultrasonic B–mode image and the Doppler flow characteristics within a vein, one can determine whether obstruction exists and if there is reflux. However, this reading is at best only semi–quantitative and leaves much to be desired when trying to objectively assess chronic venous insufficiency. This topic is more fully addressed in a Chapter 20.

Clinical Laboratory Studies

Routine clinical laboratory blood studies are usually relatively insignificant in the patient with arterial occlusive disease. However, abnormalities in hematocrit and hemoglobin should be looked for because they are correctable problems which lead to decreased perfusion in a situation of borderline perfusion. Abnormally high or low values can lead to either decreased oxygen transport or localized sludging and/or thrombosis and may worsen a marginal situation with impending or actual ulceration. An elevated WBC can suggest localized or more generalized infection which with its increased metabolic demands may convert a situation of marginal perfusion into one of ischemia with new or worsening tissue loss.

Immunologic studies may also be of occasional value in the patient where the differential diagnosis may include vasculitic ulcers. A markedly elevated erythrocyte sedimentation rate or significantly elevated ANA, Rheumatoid Factor or other more specific immunologic test may tend to support the diagnosis of an underlying vasculitic process rather than arterial occlusive disease.

Classification

Almost all ulcers are, in the end, caused by ischemia which induces tissue necrosis and subsequent ulceration. However, there are different mechanisms which lead to this end result. Arterial insufficiency is the most common form of ischemia and results from arterial obstruction or occlusion of arteries proximal to the ulcer. Atherosclerosis is the most common etiology, but any process which obstructs the arterial inflow can result in ischemia.

Other processes which do not primarily obstruct the arterial system can also cause ischemia. In patients with diabetes and ulceration or infection, arterial insufficiency may be present as it is known that atherosclerosis occurs at an accelerated rate in these patients, but the local effects of infection and inflammation can result in thrombosis in the capillary microcirculation resulting in local ischemia. Ischemia also leads to pressure ulcers. In these patients, pressure applied to a susceptible area results in compression of the capillary microcirculation with decreased or absent blood flow. If this ischemia persists for a long enough period of time, cell death occurs and ulceration will appear shortly thereafter. Skin is the tissue most resistant to ischemia and thus is usually the last to undergo this type of necrosis. Subcutaneous tissue is less resistant and thus when skin necrosis and breakdown do occur, a large area of necrosis may already exist in the subcutaneous tissue.

It also appears that the ulcers associated with venous stasis disease may well have an underlying etiology of ischemia. Increased venous pressure with relatively unchanged arterial pressure results in a decreased pressure differential across the capillary beds with resultant decreased flow. If the venous pressure is sufficiently high, the pressure differential and subsequent flow is markedly reduced and may provide inadequate oxygen to maintain cell viability. The symptoms of pain which are present when a venous stasis ulcer first occurs are very similar to the ischemic pain seen with arterial insufficiency and probably represent a similar process.

Trauma to an area can also result in thrombosis in either the macro– or micro–circulation with accompanying ischemia. Thus it is not uncommon to see skin and tissue breakdown in an area of trauma, especially if circulation to the area has been previously compromised. An example is the elderly patient with preexisting arterial and/or venous insufficiency who is hit lightly by a wheelchair or similar object and develops an ulcer in the area within a few days. Vasculitis can also result in ulcers which are ischemic. With local inflammation and necrosis in surrounding capillary and arteriolar vessels, blood flow to the adjacent skin and subcutaneous tissue is cut off, rendering the area ischemic. As there is continuing inflammation in the microvasculature due to the underlying process, it is not surprising that these ulcers are very painful as this results in continuing ischemia. When the inflammatory process is controlled, pain abates and the ulcers often go on to heal.

period of time to be effective. Clinically it has been noted that if a graft remains patent just long enough for an ulcer to heal, the area may well remain healed even if the graft subsequently occludes. Obstructed arteries from the aorta down to distal vessels in the foot can almost all be replaced either by a vein taken from the patient or by artificial arterial conduits manufactured most commonly from Dacron or PTFE (Teflon®). These procedures include aortic, aorto–femoral, femoro–popliteal and more distal femoro/popliteal–tibial, femoro/popliteal– peroneal, femoro/popliteal–dorsalis pedis and femoro/popliteal–lateral tarsal grafts, the latter commonly referred to as "fem–distal" or "fem–faraway" grafts. In the hands of trained vascular surgeons, these procedures have become quite standard and offer the patient a good chance to heal the ulcer and save the limb. However, it is beyond the scope of this chapter to review in detail different methods and procedures for surgical revascularization and

---

With correction of the ischemic process almost all ulcers will go on to heal quite rapidly. Therefore, the primary goal is to establish adequate circulation to the affected area.

Management – Surgical (Interventional)

Management of ulcers associated with ischemia is, in theory, very simple. With correction of the ischemic process almost all ulcers will go on to heal quite rapidly. Therefore, the primary goal is to establish adequate circulation to the affected area. Surgical revascularization is the mainstay in this area although interventional procedures such as percutaneous balloon angioplasty or stent placement performed by radiologists or other non–surgeons is assuming a larger role.

Any situation of threatened limb loss which includes gangrene, rest pain, or ischemic ulceration is considered to be an absolute indication for surgical intervention providing the patient is in adequate health to be able to withstand the indicated procedure. Improved techniques and methods have resulted in improved results over the past few years, and immediate success rates are in the range of 85 to 90 percent.[8–10] It should be noted that if these procedures are either not done or unsuccessful, further ischemia with subsequent gangrene is the rule and there is a high probability of limb loss within the next several months. On the other hand, a bypass may not have to remain patent for a long

the reader is referred to one of the standard textbooks on vascular surgery if coverage in greater depth is desired.[11]

Interventional procedures have also improved and have become more widely used. These typically include percutaneous balloon angioplasty, percutaneous placement of intra–vascular stents and, less commonly, percutaneous laser angioplasty. These procedures are performed through an intra–arterial catheter and are frequently done at the time of an angiogram indicated to delineate the location and extent of arterial compromise. However, they cannot be used in all circumstances and have generally had less long–term success than surgical revascularization procedures.[12,13] As they are less invasive and have less morbidity than the direct surgical approach, they may be considered as options for selected patients, particularly those with limited lesions or who are considered poor surgical candidates. Success with these procedures is determined generally by location and severity of the lesion or lesions. The more proximal the artery and the shorter the length of obstruction, the better the success. Although some interventionalists report success with totally occluded arteries in certain instances, particularly in those of shorter duration, occlusion is generally felt to be best treated with a bypass graft procedure.

In the past, surgical sympathectomy was considered a procedure which could in some instances increase blood supply to an ischemic region, particularly the foot or distal leg. However, studies have shown that this procedure is generally ineffective and when it is effective the results are frequently short–lived.[14] A more recent technique which has been shown to be effective in some instances with non–reconstructible ischemic disease is Epidural Spinal Electrical Stimulation. In this situation, a multi–polar electrode is placed in the epidural space of the spinal cord either percutaneously through a needle or with a local surgical procedure. Results have shown that in selected patients, not only is there relief of rest pain, but ulcers of 1 cm or less have healed and remained healed.[15] These results have been shown in relatively small studies, but the method may be of use in selected patients where institutional support for the procedure is available.

In the event of failure of the foregoing methods, the presence of gangrene or severe rest pain may necessitate amputation of the involved extremity. An ischemic ulcer may, of course, be managed conservatively providing it is not causing severe pain or that there is no progressive gangrene. Unfortunately, the natural history in most patients indicates that the ischemic disease is progressive and that ulcers will generally increase in size or that the limb will progress to severe rest pain and/or gangrene. Dry gangrene in the absence of severe rest pain may also be managed conservatively and in the patient where attempts are made to avoid surgery, may well represent the best option. If the gangrene remains dry without drainage or evidence of infection, particularly in a digit, the affected part may be covered with a dry dressing and observed. The natural history indicates that in many of these patients, the involved area may mummify and, if a digit, eventually fall off. Although this result may be felt to be socially unacceptable, it represents a very good medical option for the patient.

In the event of ulcer progression, gangrene or severe rest pain, amputation may be the only choice. However, depending upon the patient, this may well be an acceptable, if not good, option. In the patient who does not have significant other disease and who undergoes amputation, particularly at the below–knee level, it is our approach to expect that the patient will be fitted with a prosthesis and that they will be able to resume normal activities in approximately one month. For patients who are elderly, who have significant other illnesses, or who require an above–knee rather than below–knee amputation, this process may be more difficult to accomplish.

Management – Medical

Medical therapy in these patients does not correct the underlying problem, has not generally been proven effective, and is indicated only when surgical therapy cannot be considered an option. Pentoxiphylline (Trental®) has been advocated in patients with claudication, but there is no evidence that it is effective in patients with ischemic ulcers.[16] Additionally, results of studies in patients with claudication have shown that the optimal response occurred in 6 to 8 weeks which is far too long for patients with advanced ischemia. The use of certain prostaglandins has also been advocated, especially prostaglandin I_2 (prostacyclin), which is given intravenously over several days.[17] Although there may be some promise for this therapy, it should still be considered experimental and cannot be recommended for these patients at this time.

Various vasodilators have been used in the past to attempt to bring additional blood flow to areas of ischemia. These vasodilators, as might be expected, have been ineffective and there is evidence that they may even be detrimental to these patients. One of the strongest, if not the strongest, vasodilators known is ischemia. Therefore, ischemic areas already appear to be under the influence of this potent vasodilator, and we should not expect additional dilatation from medications. Additionally, areas which are not ischemic, such as calf muscles, are dilated by these substances and represent low resistance pathways for blood flow. These areas then "steal" the blood from the obstructed, high–resistance pathways supplying the ischemic area and render these areas even more ischemic. Most clinicians working in this area thus consider vasodilators to be contraindicated in cases with fixed ischemia.[18]

Consideration of wound dressings to be used with ischemic ulcers is probably of limited importance. As cells which dry out die, it is clearly beneficial to be certain that wounds are kept moist to prevent additional cell death and necrosis. However, beyond this benefit, nothing that is applied to an ischemic ulcer will cause any improved healing until an adequate blood supply is achieved. The emphasis therefore should be to avoid doing things which will worsen the ulcers such as letting the wound dry out or applying substances which may be toxic to cells. Once there is an adequate blood supply, normal techniques of wound care apply and healing will ensue in most cases if these techniques are followed.

Although infection occurs in some ulcers, it tends to be unusual in arterial ischemic ulcers. This would appear to be at least partially related to the fact that with inadequate arterial perfusion to supply nutrition to the area, there is not enough blood to supply either nutrients for bacteria to multiply in the tissue or elements necessary to mount an inflammatory response. The fact that infection in a gangrenous digit occurs at the border between non–viable and perfused tissue would tend to support this theory. It is also observed clinically that an ulcer which does not appear infected may rapidly become infected when the ischemic extremity is revascularized and adequate perfusion to the area is re–established. If there is clinical evidence of infection, however, customary antibiotic coverage and surgical debridement as indicated should be instituted.

Summary

Arterial ulcers are, by definition, caused by ischemia with subsequent necrosis of tissues in the affected area. The patient with arterial insufficiency almost always presents with pain, and the extent of the vascular problem can usually be learned from a directed medical history. Diagnosis is made from the history and physical examination which, in severe cases, may show changes typical of advanced ischemia. The diagnosis is usually confirmed with studies performed in the vascular laboratory. Although other ulcer types may have a component of ischemia superimposed in the primary etiology, they can be differentiated from arterial ulcers through the patient history, physical assessent and vascular/clinical laboratory tests. Successful treatment is predicated on bringing improved blood supply to the ischemic area. Most commonly this requires surgical revascularization by a vascular surgeon, although other interventional procedures may play a role in selected patients. When an adequate blood supply to the area is achieved, it is expected that virtually all of these ulcers will progress to healing.

References

1. Zink M, Rousseau P, Holloway GA. Lower extremity ulcers. In: Bryant R (ed). *Acute and Chronic Wounds; Nursing Management.* St. Louis, MO, C.V. Mosby, 1992, pp 164–212.
2. Taylor LM, Porter JM. Natural history and nonoperative treatment of chronic lower extremity ischemia. In: Moore WS (ed). *Vascular Surgery; A Comprehensive Review.* Philadelphia, PA, WB Saunders Co., 1993, pp. 223–34.
3. Boyd AM. The natural course of arteriosclerosis of lower extremities. *Angiology* 1960;11:10–14.
4. Edwards JM, Porter JM: Evaluation of upper extremity ischemia, In: Bernstein EF (ed): Vascular Diagnosis, Fourth edition. St. Louis, MO, C.V. Mosby, 1993, pg 630.
5. Carter SA. Role of pressure measurements. In: Bernstein EF (ed). *Vascular Diagnosis, Fourth Edition.* St. Louis, MO, C.V. Mosby, 1993, pp 486–512.
6. McMahon JH, Grigg MJ. Predicting healing of lower limb ulcers. *Aust N Z J Surg* 1995;65(3):173–6.
7. Bunt TJ, Holloway GA. TcPO2 as an accurate predictor of therapy in limb salvage. *Ann Vasc Surg* 1996;10(3):224–227.
8. Whittemore AD, Donaldson MC, Mannick JA. Aortoiliac occlusive disease. In: Moore WS (ed). *Vascular Surgery; A Comprehensive Review.* Philadelphia, PA, WB Saunders Co., 1993, pp 451–64.
9. Veith FJ. Femoral–popliteal–tibial occlusive disease. In: Moore WS (ed). *Vascular Surgery; A Comprehensive Review.* Philadelphia, PA, WB Saunders Co., 1993, pp 465–89.
10. Gibbons GW. Vascular evaluation and long–term results of distal bypass surgery in patients with diabetes. *Clin Podiatr Med Surg* 1995;12(1):129–40.
11. Moore WS. *Vascular Surgery; A Comprehensive Review.* Philadelphia, PA, WB Saunders Co., 1993.
12. Criado FJ, Queral LA, Patten P, Velentin W. The role of endovascular therapy in lower extremity revascularization; Lessons learned and current strategies. *Int Angiol* 1993;12(3):221–30.
13. Wolf GL, Wilson SE, Cross AP, et al. Surgery or balloon angioplasty for jperipheral vascular disease: A randomized clinical trial. *J Vasc Interv Radiol* 1993;4(5):639–48.
14. Rutherford RB. Role of sympathectomy in the management of vascular disease. In: Moore WS (ed). *Vascular Surgery; A Comprehensive Review.* Philadelphia, PA, WB Saunders Co., 1993, pp 300–12.
15. Horsch S, Claeys L. Epidural spinal cord stimulation in the treatment of severe peripheral arterial occlusive disease. *Ann Vasc Surg* 1994;8(5):468–74.
16. Reich T, Cutler BC, Porter JM, et al. Pentoxifylline in the treatment of intermittent claudication of the lower limbs. *Angiology* 1984;35(7):389–95.
17. Hossman V, Auel H, Rucker W, et al. Prolonged infusion of prostacyclin in patients with advanced states of peripheral vascular disease: A placebo–controlled cross–over study. *Klin Wochenschr* 1984;62:1108–14.
18. Coffman JD, Mannick JA. Failure of vasodilator drugs in arteriosclerosis obliterans. *Ann Int Med* 1972;76:35–9.

20

Venous Ulceration: Assessment, Classification and Management

Vincent Falanga, MD, FACP

Falanga V. Venous ulceration. In: Krasner D, Kane D. *Chronic Wound Care, Second Edition*. Wayne, PA, Health Management Publications, Inc., 1997, pp 165–171.

Introduction

Venous ulcers of the lower extremity are often regarded as an easily treatable condition. This view probably comes from comparing the prognosis of venous ulcers to that of other serious ulcerations of the lower extremities, such as arterial and diabetic (neuropathic) ulcers. In contrast to these other chronic wounds, venous ulcers are generally not very painful, do not lead to amputation and, in the opinion of some clinicians, can be healed with relative ease. However, it is clear that the morbidity associated with venous ulcers is substantial, and there is growing appreciation that these chronic wounds do not heal in a predictable and certain time frame, as has generally been thought.[1]

Over the last few years, there has been increasing interest in venous ulceration. In part, this renewed interest is the result of better ways to diagnose venous disease and improvements in the treatment of venous ulcers. Several advances have occurred recently in the care of chronic wounds. The notion of moist wound healing, for example, has revolutionized the way we treat venous ulcers and has helped spun a host of novel biosynthetic dressings. Many of these biosynthetic dressings stimulate autolytic debridement and the formation of granulation tissue.[2] Compression therapy for venous ulcers, too, has undergone a quiet revolution. Rigid compression therapy, such as the Unna boot, is still a cost–effective modality favored by many, but alternatives are gaining ground. Examples are four–layer bandaging, more flexible non–elastic wraps, improved elastic graded stockings, and extremity pumps.[3] Other advances are either gaining acceptance or being evaluated. These include the use of cultured keratinocytes and skin equivalents,[4,5] matrix materials,[6] and growth factors.[7] Moreover, the last decade has seen a number of publications addressing the cause of venous ulceration and the possible pathogenic steps leading from venous hypertension to ulceration.[8–10] In this article, we will discuss these important aspects of venous disease as they relate to present and future treatments.

Epidemiology

Information on the prevalence of venous ulceration and other epidemiological issues comes mostly from countries like Sweden and the United Kingdom, which have a more centralized system of healthcare and data entry. In the most recent study from Skaraborg county (Sweden), the point prevalence of venous ulcers in a population of 270,800 people was 0.16 percent.[11] The male:female ratio was 1:1.6. It was found that 61 percent of the patients had their first ulcer episode before the age of 65, while 22 percent and 13 percent of venous ulcers had developed before the ages of 40 and 30 years, respectively. An ulcer duration of more than 1 year was reported by 54 percent of the patients and the vast majority of patients (72 percent) had recurrent ulcerations. The location of the ulcers was as follows: 44 percent on the left leg, 35 percent on the right leg, and 21 percent on both legs. The medial aspect of the leg, which for many clinicians is the typical location for venous ulceration, was involved in only 61 percent of the cases. At the time of the survey, the median size of the ulcer was

2.6 cm^2 (range: 0.04 to 550 cm^2). Overall, a history of deep vein thrombosis was present in 37 percent of the patients. The same percentage of patients had undergone previous surgery for varicose veins.

Callam, et al. reported the natural history of leg ulceration in a Scottish community.[12] They studied 600 patients with 727 ulcers and found that 76 percent were due to venous ulcers. In 40 percent of their patients the ulceration had developed before the age of 50. Thus, it appears from this study and from the one by Nelzen, et al. that venous ulceration is by no means confined to the elderly. In the report by Callam. et al., 60 percent of the patients had recurrent ulcers, and healing of the ulcers did not occur as easily as commonly thought: half of the ulcers were present for more than 9 months and 20 percent had not healed for more than two years.[12]

It is interesting that the point prevalence (0.16 percent) of venous ulceration, reported by Nelzen, et al. in their survey of a Swedish community, comes very close to predictions made about the prevalence of these chronic wounds in the United States.[11] In the United States, the most extensive survey, done in 1973 in Tecumseh, Michigan, arrived at an extrapolated figure of 400,000 to 600,000 ulcers for the entire American population.[13] A similar conclusion had been reached by Dale and Foster in 1964.[14]

Pathogenesis

A basic appreciation of the physiology of venous return from the lower extremities helps in the understanding of the pathogenesis of venous disease and ulceration.[15–17] The components of the system are the deep veins, the superficial and communicating veins (the latter connect the deep to the superficial veins), and the calf muscles. In the supine position, the pressure in the deep veins is close to 0 mm Hg. In the normal standing situation, the deep vein pressure increases dramatically, generally to about 80 mm Hg. Upon walking, contraction of the calf muscles causes cephalad blood flow from the deep veins, a subsequent decrease in deep vein pressure, and a flow of blood (because of pressure differential) from the superficial veins to the deep veins. Upon muscle relaxation, the vein valves are fully functional and prevent retrograde blood flow. In venous disease, which can develop because of vein damage or faulty muscle pump action, the fall in venous pressure during ambulation or exercise does not occur. This failure of venous pressure to fall is termed venous hypertension, although clearly it does not represent an absolute increase in pressure.

While it is generally agreed that venous hypertension is the fundamental problem in the eventual development of venous ulcers, the pathogenic steps linking venous hypertension to ulceration are largely unknown. Recently, several hypotheses have emerged which emphasize either macromolecular dermal leakage and fibrin formation, or endothelial cell damage and neutrophil activation. In 1982, Browse and Burnand proposed that venous hypertension leads to an increased number of distended dermal capillaries, which causes the leakage of fibrinogen from the vasculature into the dermis. Polymerization of fibrinogen into fibrin would then form pericapillary fibrin cuffs, which would impede the exchange of oxygen and other nutrients between blood and dermis. The resultant anoxia would cause loss of tissue integrity and ulceration.[8] This hypothesis had several merits. Pericapillary fibrin cuffs, though not specific, are almost always present in venous disease.[17] Moreover, the emphasis on fibrin cuffs suggests fibrinolytic agents as a viable therapy. Perhaps more importantly, the hypothesis proposed by Browse and Burnand[8] has stimulated increased interest in venous ulceration and its pathogenesis. In time, however, a number of flaws became apparent in this hypothesis. First, it was found that fibrin cuffs are discontinuous around dermal vessels. Secondly, it became recognized that even highly polymerized fibrin would not have the tight structure needed to be a true barrier for the diffusion of oxygen and nutrients.[10,18] We have recently proposed that the formation of pericapillary fibrin cuffs is merely the result of a more global problem, that is the dermal leakage of macromolecules, such as fibrinogen and α–2 macroglobulin. We have suggested that the leaked macromolecules bind to or trap growth factors and matrix material, thus rendering them unavailable to the repair process.[10] There is some experimental evidence for this hypothesis, including the fact that certain growth factors, such as transforming growth factor–ß 1, may be largely sequestered within fibrin cuffs.[19] A substantially different hypothesis for venous ulceration is one in which adherence of neutrophils to endothelium leads to damage to the dermal vasculature.[9] Regardless of the pathogenic steps involved, clinically one observes a failure of reepithelialization, often in the setting of seemingly adequate granulation tissue. It remains unclear whether the problem resides with the keratinocytes or with the biochemical make up of the wound bed.[1]

In conclusion, a number of hypotheses for how venous hypertension leads to ulceration are presently being tested. This flurry of activity in studying the pathogenesis of venous disease will

Table 1
Clinical Findings and Differential Diagnosis of Venous Ulcers

Clinical and Laboratory Features	VN	AT	NP	CF	PG	VS	AS
History of thrombosis	+	−	−	−	−	−	+
History of recurrence	+	−	±	±	−	±	±
Connective tissue disease	−	−	−	±	±	+	±
Systemic inflammatory conditions	−	−	−	±	+	+	±
Severe pain at rest	−	±	−	+	−	±	±
Numbness, parasthesias	−	±	+	−	−	±	−
Hyperpigmentation	+	−	−	±	−	±	−
Dermatitis	+	−	−	−	−	−	−
Lipodermatosclerosis	+	−	−	−	−	−	−
Atrophie blanche	±	±	−	±	−	+	+
Livedo reticularis	−	−	−	+	−	+	+
Purpura	−	−	−	+	−	+	+
Wound bed eschar	−	+	+	±	±	+	+
Exposed tendons	−	±	±	±	±	−	±

VN = venous ulcer; AT = arterial ulcer; NP = neuropathic ulcer; CF = ulcer due to cryoproteinemia;
PG = pyoderma gangrenosum; VS = vasculitis; AS = anti–phospholipid syndrome.
− = rare; ± = often; + = almost always.

hopefully lead to alternative treatments and novel therapeutic approaches.

Assessment – History

The patient with venous ulceration has a clinical history which is more important for the lack of certain features than for the presence of a specific history or specific symptoms. Table 1 lists some useful points helpful in the differential diagnosis. Not present in venous ulcers is the rest pain or claudication of arterial insufficiency. Contrary to the observation regularly made in patients with arterial ulcers, the pain and discomfort of venous disease is often improved by leg elevation. The neuropathic symptoms of patients with diabetes such as leg and foot numbness, burning, and other parasthesias are also absent. To be sure, there is considerable discomfort associated with venous ulcers, but the severity of these symptoms varies unpredictably with individual patients and with particular ulcers. For example, we have found that the surface area of the ulcer does not correlate well with the presence of pain. On the contrary, our experience suggests that small but deep ulcers, particularly around the malleoli, are the most painful; this increased pain may be the result of periosteal injury. Similarly, it has been our experience that

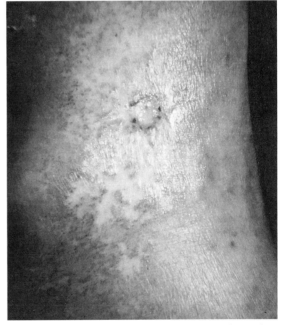

Figure 1. Changes of atrophie blanche around an ulcer located near the medial malleolus. The white atrophic areas contain tiny flat capillaries.

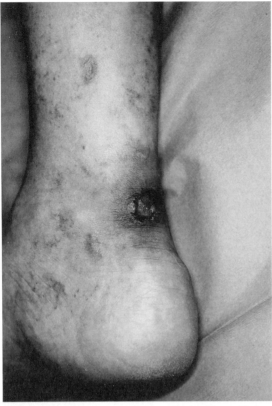

Figure 2. *Necrotic wound bed in a patient with cryofibrinogenemia. Hyperpigmentation and "microlivedo" lesions are present around the ankle.*

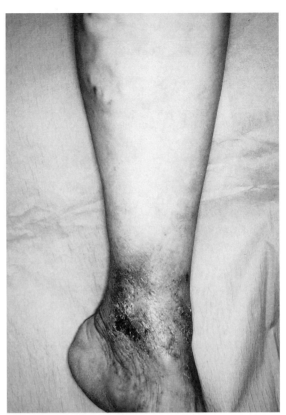

Figure 3. *Several typical features of venous ulceration. The superior portion of the leg has obvious varicosities, while the medial portion of the leg shows changes of lipodermatosclerosis and dermatitis around the ulceration.*

patients with small venous ulcers surrounded by atrophie blanche have a clinical course characterized by more pain and discomfort (Figure 1). Nevertheless, when pain is severe, one should consider the possibility of either cellulitis or a different etiology for the ulceration, such as cryofibrinogenemia (Figure 2). Making the latter diagnosis is particularly important because that condition responds well to treatment with the anabolic steroid stanozolol.[20] In addition to pain, patients with venous ulcers often complain about the odor and copious drainage from the wound and of pruritus in the skin around the ulcer. While by themselves these individual symptoms are rather non–specific, together they are more common in patients with venous ulcers than in those with arterial disease or diabetes. Trauma probably plays an important role in the initiation of venous ulcers, particularly in patients with extensive lipodermatosclerosis (see below). Indeed, ulcers commonly occur within the areas of lipodermatosclerosis (Figure 3). The post–phlebitic syndrome represents a dramatic clinical entity characterized by severe pain and discomfort, swelling, and recurrent ulceration.

Ulcers due to venous insufficiency can occur in patients with only perforator or superficial vein incompetence. However, in the majority of cases, ulcers develop in the setting of deep venous insufficiency. It is estimated that up to 80 percent of patients with a deep vein thrombosis will develop a venous ulcer, although this figure may be high.[21] More importantly, it is useful to find out whether the patient has undergone coronary artery bypass surgery, since the saphenous vein is commonly used for this procedure.

Venous ulcers recur commonly, and a history of recurrence tends to favor a venous etiology for the ulceration. This is especially true if the recurrence is at the same site. A word of caution is needed here. We have found that, in general, patients have a very difficult time and are often inaccurate in their assessment of ulcer duration, healing, and recurrence. This is an important consideration in the design of clinical trials because study protocols often place unrealistic demands on patients' recollections and assessments of their ulcers. Another important part of the history which needs to be examined critically is the use of topical therapy within and around the ulcer. Topical antibiotics, antiseptics, moisturizing lotions and creams and a host of home–made remedies are among the agents used by patients in an effort to improve their ulcers and symptoms. Patients with venous disease have increased sensitivity to topical agents and allergens and tend to develop dermatitis commonly after the use of topical preparations.[17]

Assessment – Physical Examination

The physical examination of patients with leg ulcers is appropriately begun, not at the leg, but rather by a more general assessment. Several pertinent observations should be made before the wound dressing is removed. The clinician must look for joint deformities and other clinical signs of rheumatoid arthritis, which is associated with pyoderma gangrenosum and rheumatoid ulcers. Patients with rheumatoid arthritis or osteoarthritic changes may be taking large doses of aspirin and other nonsteroidal anti–inflammatory drugs, which could further impair healing.

Proceeding with the physical examination, the clinician should check peripheral pulses and look for signs of venous disease: varicosities, hyperpigmentation, lipodermatosclerosis, and dermatitis (Figure 3). The latter, often referred to as stasis dermatitis, is in our opinion the result of topical preparations. There are some notable signs to look for which would make venous disease less likely. For example, the wound bed in venous ulcers rarely, if ever, shows true black necrosis or eschar. Although venous ulcers can be quite deep, the presence of exposed tendons virtually excludes a venous etiology for the ulceration. Livedo reticularis or, more commonly, subtle signs of "microlivedo" are not seen with venous ulcers. Their presence should lead to a consideration of vasculitis, cryoproteinemias, and the antiphospholipid syndrome. The location of venous ulcers is frequently on the medial aspect, but a lateral location or tibial ulcers can be seen.[11,12] In our experience, venous ulcers are rarely found on the foot. Table 1 describes the main clinical features of venous ulceration and its differential diagnosis.

Venous ulcers generally have an irregular outline, while arterial or vasculitic ulcers are often round or punched out. Typically, the skin surrounding venous ulcers is indurated, due to a fibrotic component (lipodermatosclerosis) which precedes the development of ulcers.[22] Other times, lipodermatosclerosis is not present but the ulcer is surrounded by white atrophic skin speckled with tiny blood vessels, referred to as atrophie blanche (Figure 1). In our opinion, atrophie blanche is a non–specific finding and may be seen with other vascular diseases.

The wound edges in venous ulcers either are flat and almost flush with the wound bed or display a rather steep elevation from the ulceration. The latter situation is typical of non–healing ulcers. Not present is the undermining of the edges which is characteristic of pyoderma gangrenosum. Examining the wound edges closely is helpful in other ways as well. Basal cell carcinomas, arising from venous ulcers, appear as seemingly exuberant granulation tissue which tends to roll over onto the wound edges.[23]

The shape of the leg itself is helpful in pointing to a venous etiology. Because of lipodermatosclerosis, which tends to scar down the middle and lower portion of the leg, venous disease gives the leg the appearance of an inverted bottle. On the contrary, lymphatic disease results in legs having a similar diameter from below the knee to the ankle. Commonly, however, venous disease is complicated by poor lymphatic drainage. The telltale sign of this occurrence is the presence of filiform or verrucous epithelial changes on the foot and in the vicinity of the ulceration.

Laboratory Studies

For the most part, the diagnosis of venous ulceration remains a clinical determination. Laboratory studies can confirm the presence of venous insufficiency but, by themselves, cannot be used to decide whether the ulcer is due to venous insufficiency. For example, a patient with a vasculitic or arterial ulcer may have abnormal plethysmographic studies or other findings of venous insufficiency. The ankle/brachial index (ABI) is helpful in excluding severe arterial insufficiency. In this test, the systolic pressures are measured by Doppler with the patient in the supine position. An ABI greater than 0.7 or 0.8 (normal is 1.1) generally indicates no arterial disease. An ABI of 0.5 or less speaks for severe arterial disease. However, the ABI is not fool–proof, especially in patients with diabetes mellitus who may have non–compressible arteries and thus a spuriously elevated ankle pressure. It is said that up to 20 percent of patients with venous disease have some arterial insufficiency as well.[17,21]

Air plethysmography has emerged as an easily performed assessment of venous insufficiency. In this simple and non–invasive test, one can measure the degree of venous reflux and the efficiency of the calf muscle pump. In our experience, this test is abnormal in almost all patients with venous ulcers. With the use of a tourniquet, it can also give information on whether the deep venous system is affected. Additional information regarding venous reflux can be obtained by the use of venous

Doppler ultrasound, which is now available in many centers. Biopsies of the ulcer bed or ulcer's edge can be helpful in excluding basal or squamous cell carcinomas, which can occur in long–standing ulcers.[23] Immunofluorescence studies can detect the presence of pericapillary fibrin or fibrinogen in the vast majority of venous ulcers.[18] The test is highly sensitive, and the absence of fibrin cuffs should cause the clinician to doubt the diagnosis of venous disease. However, the test is not as specific as initially thought.

Treatment

In the opinion of most physicians, compression bandages remain the cornerstone of therapy for patients with venous ulcers. Compression is thought to either correct or improve venous hypertension. However, the best way to provide compression remains a controversial point.[24] Some clinicians prefer the use of rigid compression, as achieved with a traditional zinc oxide impregnated non–elastic bandage (Unna boot). It has been theorized that, during ambulation, the calf muscles press against the rigid bandage, thus insuring more effective action of the calf muscle pump unit. Other clinicians, however, cite the very rigidity of the Unna boot as a flaw. It can be argued that rigid compression does not accomodate the changing volume of the leg during alterations in leg edema. Instead, others prefer flexible elastic bandages, which conform to the leg better and, thus, can continue to provide compression throughout the day, irrespective of the leg volume. There is no simple answer to this controversy. It is important to emphasize that the mechanism of action of the Unna boot, i.e. pressure against the calf muscles during ambulation, is different from that of flexible bandages. Therefore, one should not use measurements of sub–bandage pressures to compare the two.[24] However, as we have mentioned, advantages or disadvantages can be cited for both modes of therapy. Rigid compression offers the definite advantage of insuring the application of pressure by a healthcare worker. In our opinion, it is difficult, if not impossible, for patients to properly apply compression bandages to their own legs. An obvious disadvantage of the rigid Unna boot–like compression is that, because it stays in place several days at a time, it becomes soiled with wound exudate and often produces an uncomfortable odor. On the other hand, flexible compression is easy to use and allows for more frequent dressing changes. More recently, four layer bandaging has been proposed as a more optimal way to achieve compression. This method utilizes four different bandage materials which, in the opinion of the proponents of this type of dressing, provide a more optimal compression environment for the leg.[25] This form of compression looks promising. We have recently advocated the concept of localized supplemental pressure over the ulcer. This procedure can be done inexpensively by the use of additional pads or gauze dressings over the ulceration.[17]

If compression therapy is a universally accepted way to treat legs affected by venous ulcers, there is little agreement on how the ulcer itself should be dressed. Moist wound healing is advocated for these chronic wounds by an increasing number of clinicians. A variety of biosynthetic dressings may be used to keep the venous ulcer bed moist.[2] Our approach has been to use a hydrocolloid when debridement is needed and to rely on foams and films when the ulcer bed is adequate. Hydrocolloids or other dressings are allowed to "adhere" to the skin and should not be removed until they are lifted off by the wound exudate, thus avoiding injury to the epithelium. We prefer foams over films when a non–adherent dressing is more appropriate as, for example, when the skin around the ulcer has dermatitis or appears to be particularly fragile. When dermatitis is a major clinical component we prefer the use of gel dressings, which are often ideal in that situation. In all cases, we try to avoid the use of any topical preparation, including emollients and antibiotics. In our experience, topical agents in patients with venous disease are the cause of the so–called "stasis dermatitis." Thus, we believe that "stasis dermatitis" is not an intrinsic component of venous disease, as is often thought. When topical preparations are discontinued in patients with dermatitis, it generally takes several weeks if not months for the dermatitis to resolve. There are probably some agents that can be used without causing dermatitis in the long run. For example, we have not yet seen dermatitis develop in patients using slow–release topical preparations of iodine, such as cadexomer iodine, which are becoming a common form of therapy.[26] However, for the most part, we tell patients to avoid all topical preparations. Indeed, if a severe contact dermatitis develops around venous ulcers, we generally treat it with systemic rather than topical steroids.

The time needed for venous ulcers to heal with the use of compression bandages alone varies considerably in published reports. In our experience at the University of Miami leg ulcer program, we can expect complete reepithelialization in 35 to 50 percent of patients after four to six months of therapy. However, the rate of closure is probably dependent on such variables as the history of the ulcer, the degree of venous insufficiency, the extent of lipodermatosclerosis, and the presence of cardiovascular disease. Medications such as aspirin and systemic corticosteroids also interfere with healing. We make wide use of in–patient split–thickness skin grafting for those patients who do not respond to compression treatment in the first few weeks or who, for a number of reasons, are very slow in the rate of reepithelialization. We have had a considerable success rate with skin grafting of different types of chronic wounds of the lower extremity, including venous ulcers. At long term follow–up, we have found that 52 percent of ulcers were healed, 26 percent were partially healed, and 22 percent recurred.[27] It is likely that recurrence rates may be tied to risk factors for venous disease.[28,29] Compression bandages are started immediately after grafting and continued throughout treatment. Patients are advised to wear graded stockings (30 to 40 mm Hg at the ankle) for the rest of their lives.

The therapeutic measures we have outlined improve the condition of most patients. New therapeutic modalities, such as rheologic agents (i.e. pentoxifilline), epithelial allografts or skin equivalents, and growth factors, have shown promise. It remains to be seen whether some of these approaches will prove to be cost–effective.

Conclusions

Many advances have been made in the last few years in understanding the pathophysiology of venous ulceration, in the diagnosis and assessment of venous disease, and in dressing materials and compression therapy. New technologies, including bioengineered skin products, growth factors, rheologic and fibrinolytic agents, and probably gene therapy will likely play an important therapeutic role in the next several years. Perhaps most important is the great interest in venous disease and ulceration which we have witnessed recently. This interest promises to bring us more advances in the understanding and treatment of these chronic wounds.

References

1. Falanga V. Chronic wounds: Pathophysiologic and experimental considerations. *J Invest Dermatol* 1993;100:721–725.
2. Helfman T, Ovington L, Falanga V. Occlusive dressings and wound healing. *Clinics of Dermatology* 1994;12(1):121–127.
3. Phillips TJ, Dover JS. Leg ulcers. *J Am Acad Dermatol* 1991;25:965–987.
4. Phillips TJ, Kehinde O, Green H, Gilchrest BA. Treatment of skin ulcers with cultured epidermal allografts. *J Am Acad Dermatol* 1989;21:191–199.
5. De Luca M, Albanese E, Cancedda R, Viacara A, Faggioni A, Zambruno G, Giannetti A. Treatment of leg ulcers with cryopreserved allogeneic cultured epithelium. *Arch Dermatol* 1992;128:633–638.
6. Wethers DL, Ramirez GM, Koshy M, Steinberg MH, Phillips G, Siegel RS, Eckman JR, Prchal JT, and the RGD Study

7. Steed DL and the Diabetic Ulcer Study Group. Clinical evaluation of recombinant human platelet–derived growth factor for the treatment of lower extremity diabetic ulcers. Diabetic Ulcer Study Group. *J Vasc Surg* 1995;21(1):71–8.
8. Browse NL, Burnand KG. The cause of venous ulceration. *Lancet* 1982;2:243–245.
9. Coleridge–Smith PD, Thomas P, Scurr JH, Dormandy JA. Causes of venous ulceration: a new hypothesis? *Br Med J* 1988;296:1726–1727.
10. Falanga V. The trap hypothesis of venous ulceration. *The Lancet* 1993;341:1006–1008.
11. Nelzen O, Bergquist D, Lindhagen A. Venous and non–venous leg ulcers: clinical history and appearance in a population study. *Br J Surg* 1994;81:182–187.
12. Callam MJ, Harper DR, Dale JJ, Ruckley CV. Chronic ulcer of the leg: clinical history. *Br Med J* **year?**;294:1389–1391.
13. Coon WW, Willis PW, Keller JB. Venous thromboembolism and other venous disease in the Tecumseh Community Health Study. *Circulation* 1973;48:839–845, 1973.
14. Dale WA, Foster JH. Leg ulcers: comprehensive plan of diagnosis and management. *Med Sc* 1964;56–58.
15. Goldman MP, Fronek A. Anatomy and pathophysiology of varicose veins. *J Dermatol Surg Oncol* 1989;15:138–145.
16. Stemmer R. Deuxieme loi de Starling et oedemes des membres inferieurs. *Phlebologie* 1966;19:267–276.
17. Falanga V. Venous ulceration. *J Dermatol Surg Oncol* 1993;19:764–771.
18. Falanga V, Kirsner RS, Katz MH, Gould E, Eaglstein WH, McFalls. Pericapillary Fibrin Cuffs in venous ulceration. *J Dermatol Surg Oncol* 1992;18:409–414.
19. Higley HR, Ksander GA, Gerhardt CO, Falanga V. Extravasation of macromolecules and possible trapping of TGF–beta in venous ulceration. *Br J Dermatol* 1995;132:79–85.
20. Falanga V, Kirsner RS, Eaglstein WH, Katz MH, Kerdel FA. Stanozolol in treatment of leg ulcers due to cryofibrinogenemia. *The Lancet* 1991;338:347–348.
21. Katz M, Falanga V, Eaglstein WH. Leg ulcers: a wound healing model. In: Champion RH, Pye RJ. (eds). *Recent Advances in Dermatology*. Churchill Livingstone, New York, NY, 1992, pp 199–218.
22. Helfman T, Falanga V. Stanozolol as a novel therapeutic agent in dermatology. *J Am Acad Dermatol* 1995;32:254–258.
23. Harris B, Eaglstein WH, Falanga V. Basal cell carcinoma arising in venous ulcers and mimicking granulation tissue. *J Dermatol Surg Oncol* 1993;19:150–152.
24. Partsch H. Compression therapy of the legs: A review. *J Dermatol Surg Oncol* 1991;17:799–808.
25. Blair SD, Wright DDI, Blackhouse CM, Riddle E, McCollum CN. Sustained compression and healing of chronic venous ulcers. *Br Med J* 1988;297:1159–1161.
26. Ormiston MC, Seymour MTJ, Venn GE, Cohen RI, Fox JA. Controlled trial of Iodosorb in chronic venous ulcers. *Br Med J* 1985;291:308–310.
27. Kirsner RK, Falanga V. Techniques of split–thickness skin grafting for lower extremity ulcerations. *J Dermatol Surg Oncol* 1993;19:779–783.
28. Scott TE, LaMorte WW, Gorin DR, Menzoian JO. Risk factors for chronic venous insufficiency: A dual case–control study. *J Vasc Surg* 1995;22:622–628.
29. Harada RN, Katz ML, Camerota A. A noninvasive screening test to detect "critical" deep venous reflux. *J Vasc Surg* 1995;22:532–537.

Suggested Reading

1. Bundens WP. Use of air plethysmography in the evaluation and treatment of patients with venous stasis disease. *Dermatol Surg* 1995;21:67–69.

21

Diabetic Wounds: Assessment, Classification and Management

David L. Steed, MD

Steed DL. Diabetic wounds: Assessment, classification and management. In: Krasner D, Kane D. *Chronic Wound Care, Second Edition*. Wayne, PA, Health Management Publications, Inc., 1997, pp 172–177.

Introduction

Diabetic wounds remain a significant problem in the United States, where there are between 11 and 16 million diabetic patients. A diabetic foot ulcer and its complications are a major cause for hospitalization in these patients. Although only six to ten percent of hospitalizations in diabetic patients are for management of foot ulcers, these admissions account for nearly one quarter of the days a diabetic patient is hospitalized.[1] As many as 10 to 15 percent of diabetic patients may be at risk for the development of foot ulcers.[2] Moreover, failure of these ulcers to heal may lead to amputation.[3] There are 50,000 to 60,000 amputations performed on diabetic patients each year in the United States.[4] The cost of care for these patients is difficult to estimate, but is likely to be billions of dollars if one considers the cost of hospitalization, amputation, rehabilitation, prosthetics, lost wages and long term care.

Neuropathy

Diabetic foot ulcers occur most commonly because of peripheral neuropathy and peripheral vascular disease. It has been estimated that 60 to 70 percent of diabetic patients with foot ulcers have peripheral neuropathy as the etiology, 15 to 20 percent have peripheral vascular disease as the cause, and 15 to 20 percent have both.[5,6] The peripheral neuropathy is both a sensory and motor neuropathy. The neuropathy occurs as a complication of prolonged glucose elevation. It may be present in as many as ten percent of patients when diabetes is diagnosed, and nearly half of diabetic patients who have had the disease for more than 20 years. Certainly, the incidence of neuropathy is more common in diabetic patients with foot ulcers. The sensory neuropathy leads to a loss of protective function. Ulcers commonly begin from a minor wound due to a lack of protective sensation. Improperly fitting shoes are a common problem in which the patient develops an area of irritation and may be unaware of it. Other common troubles may derive from foreign bodies entering the foot from walking barefoot, improper trimming of nails, burns from putting the foot in hot bath water or warming their feet on a radiator in cold weather.

The neuropathy in these patients is also a motor neuropathy. The motor nerves which control motion of the foot do not function properly, resulting in failure of the signals which are constantly sent to the small muscles of the foot to keep proper tension and tone in the muscles. In such a case, the tendons do not pull in the proper alignment and deformities develop. These deformities are commonly referred to as Charcot deformities. The diabetic patient develops a "claw" deformity of the foot where the toes are pulled up and thus do not bear weight. This deformity causes the metatarsal heads to become more prominent on the plantar surface and reduces weight bearing from the toes. There may also be thinning of the fat pad on the plantar surface of the foot. The skin beneath the metatarsal heads is a common site of plantar ulceration in diabetic patients, especially so in areas beneath the first and fifth metatarsal heads. The patients also develop midfoot collapse with loss of the plantar arch. The markedly abnormal shape of the foot coupled with the sensory neuropathy makes the diabetic patient at risk for skin breakdown.

Vascular Disease

There are other factors which lead to ulceration in diabetic patients. The patients commonly have peripheral vascular disease. Diabetes is a commonly accepted risk factor for atherosclerosis as are smoking, hyperlipidemia and hypertension. Although there was once debate as to whether diabetic patients had "small vessel disease" with occlusion of very small vessels, that theory has not held. Most clinicians would agree that diabetic patients are at increased risk for typical atherosclerosis. These patients seem to develop a pattern of disease commonly involving the tibial arteries. A classic finding in a diabetic patient is a bounding popliteal pulse with no pulse palpable in the foot. There are other problems in diabetic patients. For example, they do not handle infection as well. These factors all lead to a higher amputation rate in diabetic patients.

Assessment

The assessment of the diabetic patient begins with a thorough history and physical examination. Patients may give a history which suggests generalized atherosclerosis such as a pattern of coronary artery disease or cerebrovascular disease. They may also complain of claudication. As amputation is common in this patient population, they may have had a previous amputation. It is necessary to evaluate the pulses carefully and to look for signs of peripheral neuropathy. A Charcot deformity of the foot is evidence of significant peripheral neuropathy as is muscle wasting in the hands. The degree of neuropathy can be quantified with Semmes–Weinstein monofilaments.[7] A foot which is insensate to the smaller filaments is considered to be at risk for ulceration.

The cause for ulceration in the diabetic foot is often apparent from the location of the ulcer. Ulcers on the tips of the toes or on the foot laterally are commonly caused by improperly fitting shoes. Ulcers between the toes or "kissing ulcers" may be from shoes which are too narrow. Ulcers on the dorsum of the foot and, in particular, on the tops of the toes may be from a claw deformity of the foot causing rubbing on the shoe. Such patients may require an extra depth shoe. Ulcers beneath the metatarsal heads are common and occur because of a claw deformity making the metatarsal heads

more prominent. The areas beneath the first and fifth metatarsal heads are at the greatest risk for ulceration. Ulcers in the middle of the weight–bearing surface beneath the arch suggest a Charcot deformity. Many of these patients have a rocker bottom contour to their foot with maximum weight bearing on the mid portion of the plantar surface. Ulcerations of the heel occur in debilitated patients, especially those with peripheral vascular disease. These ulcers are commonly caused from pressure on the heel. A comatose patient, for example, may develop these ulcers from rubbing on a shoe, a brace, or bed sheets.

Classification

Ulcers may be classified according to their depth and the tissues involved. Mild ulcers involve partial thickness skin and may be simple blisters. Full thickness ulcers involve the skin and subcutaneous tissue. More severe ulcers involve tendon, bone, or joint.

Determining Ulcer Type. Plain films may demonstrate osteomyelitis; however, changes on x–ray become apparent about three weeks after the changes occur clinically. Moreover, it is difficult to separate bony erosions from previous surgery and debridement or neuropathy from the changes of osteomyelitis. Bone scans have been used to diagnose osteomyelitis but indicate inflammation and increased blood flow, not specifically infection. Although many methods are used to determine bony involvement, most are expensive and have many false positives and negatives.[8] Magnetic resonance imaging may be more accurate in determining osteomyelitis, but it too is expensive. Perhaps the most cost effective method to determine osteomyelitis is to probe the wound with a sterile cotton tipped applicator. If the tip can touch bone, osteomyelitis will be present in as many as 85 percent of cases.

Debridement is an important adjunct in the treatment of diabetic ulcers. During debridement the degree of bony involvement can be assessed quite accurately. As these patients commonly have peripheral vascular disease, it is important to assess their pulses. However, local factors may make it difficult to assess the degree of blood flow accurately in these patients. Any patient with a foot ulcer should have non invasive vascular testing unless a pulse is clearly palpable.

In most vascular laboratories, Doppler derived lower extremity arterial pressures are measured and an ankle/brachial index (ABI) is calculated by making a ratio of pressure at the ankle to pressure in the arm. The normal ABI is 0.9 to 1.1.

Claudication occurs as the ABI falls to about 0.7. Ischemic rest pain occurs at about 0.4 and tissue death occurs when the ABI falls to 0.1 to 0.3. However, diabetic patients commonly have falsely elevated ABIs. The atherosclerotic process in these patients leads to severe calcification of the arteries. As the arterial pressure is measured by Doppler using a blood pressure cuff, a portion of the squeeze of the cuff is used to overcome the rigidity of the vessel wall leading to a falsely elevated value. Therefore, some other assessment of flow must be used. Toe pressures reflect blood flow more accurately in diabetic patients, but many labs are not equipped with cuffs small enough to measure toe pressures. Wave forms measured by Doppler or pulse volume recording are also quite helpful. A normal ABI with a markedly dampened wave form suggests calcified vessels and that the ABI is falsely elevated.

Perhaps the most useful tool is a transcutaneous oxygen tension measurement (TcPO$_2$). The TcPO$_2$ is a measurement of perfusion of the skin. It is measured by an electrode placed directly on the skin. For TcPO$_2$ to be normal, the lungs must oxygenate the blood, the heart must pump the blood, an artery must be patent to carry the blood to the skin, and the skin must be intact to allow oxygen to diffuse to the probe. In general, the TcPO$_2$ is about 80 percent of the arterial PO$_2$. The normal TcPO$_2$ is 55 mm Hg or greater. There is evidence that the blood supply for wound healing is adequate with TcPO$_2$ of 30 mm Hg or greater. If the TcPO$_2$ is greater than 30 mm Hg, there is likely to be adequate blood supply for wound healing despite the fact that the patient has peripheral vascular disease and an absent pulse in his/her foot.

Infection. It is important to look for infection in these patients. Signs of inflammation should be present if there is infection. Interestingly, despite the fact that they do not have normal sensation, many diabetic patients complain of pain in their foot when infection develops.

Debridement is also useful in determining infection, as undrained pockets of pus may be found as the wound is unroofed. Quantitative bacteriology may be helpful in determining if the wound is in "bacterial balance." In general, wounds must have less than 10^5 bacteria per gram of tissue to heal. Routine cultures of dry wounds or surface swabs are not helpful in determining the bacteria responsible for cellulitis. These cultures reflect skin organisms and may not identify the organism beneath the skin responsible for the infection. However, cultures of pus or deep wound cultures are helpful in determining the infecting organism.

Mild infections are commonly caused by aerobic gram positive cocci. More serious infections are caused by gram positive cocci, gram negative bacilli, and anaerobes.[9] As many as 25 percent of diabetic patients may have anaerobic bacteria in their wounds. Anaerobic cultures are difficult to perform, thus anaerobic organisms may be present even when cultures have not identified them. Finally, it should be remembered that many diabetic patients have multiple flora in their wounds. Enteric organisms are particularly common in wounds which have been present for more than one month.

Management

Proper treatment can begin after a careful history, a physical examination and a laboratory evaluation, including plain x–rays, noninvasive vascular testing and cultures when appropriate, have been completed.

Preventing weight bearing pressure is critically important in the healing of diabetic ulcers[10] and can be achieved by the use of crutches, a walker, a wheelchair or other such devices. Patients can also be fit with special foot wear, such as a half–shoe, which will allow them to touch the ground for stability yet not bear weight on the ulcer site. It is important to remember that patients are to be non–weight bearing at all times. Occasionally, patients may, for example, get out of bed during the night to use the bathroom and walk on their foot — even several steps may destroy the healing which has been accomplished. Patient compliance is difficult to assess; however, if patients come to the clinic and are using appropriate nonweight bearing devices, it is likely they are complying with their restrictions. Conversely, patients who come to the clinic walking on their foot are likely to be non-compliant.

Antibiotic selection is quite important for these patients. In general, the physician should choose broad spectrum antibiotics. If there are no cultures to direct antibiotic therapy, then antibiotics against enteric organisms and anaerobes are appropriate. Monitoring blood glucose is critical for patients with infection as an elevated blood glucose may be a sign of uncontrolled infection.

Treatment. Wounds must be debrided at the time they are initially evaluated. Many wounds can be debrided in the office setting. Debridement is helpful not only in removing necrotic tissue, but also in assessing the depth of the ulcer and its severity, whether there is bony involvement or undrained pus.[11] Debridement can often be performed under local anesthesia as these patients have sensory neuropathy, yet some patients require no anesthesia. In patients with normal blood supply, bleeding may be significant and the physician performing the debridement must be capable of handling any hemorrhage which occurs. If the patient is found to have bony involvement, the bone must also be debrided.

Osteomyelitis is a disease most effectively treated by surgery. Once the infected bone is removed, the patient requires antibiotics only for control of bacteria in the surrounding tissues and, in most circumstances, does not need six weeks of intravenous therapy. It is difficult at times to know if there is bony involvement at the time of debridement; however, exposed bone is commonly infected bone. Debridement should remove this bone back to solid bleeding bone.

When edema is present, the patient should keep his/her leg elevated; if there is no edema, leg elevation is not necessary. In fact, the patient should keep his/her leg in the position that feels most comfortable. Patients with peripheral vascular disease and arterial insufficiency may feel better with the leg in a dependent position. The patient's desire to keep his/her leg in a dependent position may be a clue that he/she has pain from ischemia.

If the patient does have arterial insufficiency with a reduced ABI and lowered $TcPO_2$ then arteriography may be indicated. Many patients with peripheral vascular disease secondary to diabetes may have renal failure as well. Contrast agents used for arteriography may damage the kidney further if the patient is not well hydrated or if excessive amounts of contrast are used. Revascularization of the lower extremities can be performed with inflow at the level of the groin or knee and outflow in the foot. In situ bypass, using the saphenous vein to the dorsalis pedis or posterior tibial arteries or even their branches, has been successful in salvaging limbs and has patency rates approaching those of more proximal bypasses. One year patency rates of 90 percent have been reported.[12] It must be recalled, however, that these patients have coronary artery disease in many cases, and lower extremity bypass carries some risk of death.

Hyperbaric oxygen therapy may have some benefit in the healing of lower extremity ulcers. However, there are no randomized, prospective, double blind trials with sham treatments suggesting a benefit from this form of therapy in patients with diabetic foot ulcers. There is laboratory evidence that hyperbaric oxygen therapy is of some benefit in moderately ischemic wounds, yet hyperbaric oxygen therapy is only effective if the patient is placed in a whole–body chamber. Topical hyperbaric oxygen therapy has not been shown to have any positive effect on wound healing. If hyperbaric oxygen therapy is to be successful, it should raise the $TcPO_2$ of the wounded extremity when measured as the patient leaves the chamber. If there is no improvement in $TcPO_2$ following a treatment, it is unlikely that any benefit will be achieved from this form of therapy.

Post–Therapy Care. Much controversy exists over the proper care of the diabetic ulcer, and there are no standards of care yet defined. What is the best dressing? How often should the dressing be changed? Should the wound be bathed or soaked? Is whirlpool therapy of benefit? How often should debridement be performed? What is the best cream, salve or ointment? These are some of the questions that remain unanswered.

In general, harsh agents, including undiluted iodine, alcohol and peroxide, which kill healing cells should be avoided. These agents should never be placed undiluted directly into an open wound. There is good evidence that they kill the cells involved in wound healing. Gentle soap such as common bath soap can be used to clean these wounds, remove necrotic tissue and not damage the wound. Topical antibiotic salves will keep the bacterial colony count low while providing a moist wound environment in which healing may occur. It is difficult to separate these topical salves as there have been very few double blind trials comparing these agents. Saline moistened gauze will also provide a moist wound environment. If the gauze is allowed to dry, necrotic material will adhere to the gauze and will be removed from the wound with the gauze. If this effect is required, the gauze should not be soaked off the wound. Newer agents, such as hydrocolloid dressings, have been developed and may play a role in the treatment of these ulcers.

Debridement of the diabetic foot ulcer is an important adjunct in getting these wounds to heal[13]. Debridement establishes the depth of the wound and whether tissues such as tendon and bone are involved. Proper debridement removes necrotic devitalized tissue which contains bacteria and is of benefit by helping to control infection and bring the tissues into bacterial balance.[14] If debridement is taken to the level of healthy viable bleeding tissue, some degree of bleeding occurs. Platelets are activated to control hemorrhage. These same platelets also contain growth factors which begin the healing process. Debridement is also of benefit in that it removes necrotic material and allows the proliferative phase of wound healing to begin.

Sharp surgical debridement is quite effective in removing necrotic debris. There is an element of risk in that it is a surgical procedure and may be associated with pain, bleeding, and transient bacteremia. Saline soaked gauze, when placed on a wound and allowed to dry, will remove some necrotic tissue. This technique is quite effective yet simple to perform. Enzymatic debriding agents can remove necrotic tissue from a wound. It is difficult to remove large amounts of necrotic tissue using this technique. Material digested by these agents may serve as a medium for growth of bacteria and irritate surrounding tissues. These debriding agents are probably no more effect than a surgeon's knife. Occlusive dressings placed on a wound will allow some degree of autolysis from lytic enzymes present in wound fluid.

Recently, there has been much interest in agents which manipulate the cellular environment of the wound. Growth factors are potent agents involved in wound healing. They are found in nearly every tissue of the body, are easily harvested from the platelet, and enter most wounds at the time of injury as platelets are called into the wound to control hemorrhage. Growth factors can be harvested as a "platelet releasate" by extracting the platelet pellet from a peripheral blood sample. The growth factors are found in the alpha granules of the platelet and can be released using thrombin. The growth factors found in the platelet then are likely to be the ones involved in wound healing. The growth factors found in a platelet releasate are also likely to be present in the proper ratio. However, not all growth factors promote wound healing, and some factors may signal wound healing to stop. The question arises of how concentrated to make the platelet releasate so as to maximize the concentration of the healing factors without concentrating the factors that stop wound healing. Also, if one harvests platelets from one individual and gives his releasate to another individual, can infectious agents such as cytomegalovirus, hepatitis virus, or the AIDS virus be transmitted?

As an alternative, one can make an individual growth factor by recombinant DNA technology. Although this technology may be expensive, if a growth factor were proven to be effective and made in large quantities the cost would likely be less. The question arises then as to which growth factor is best. Using one growth factor to heal a wound is not nature's plan. Any growth factor developed must be proven efficacious, thus requiring randomized prospective double blind trials which may not be easy to perform as so many factors in wound healing remain undefined.

There have been several reports of improved diabetic ulcer healing using Platelet Derived Wound Healing Formula (PDWHF). PDWHF is a platelet releasate. When platelets are taken from the patient him/herself, an autologous preparation can be made. There has been some suggestion that PDWHF improves wound healing; however, there has also been a report that wounds worsened using this therapy.[15,16]

An isolated growth factor may be effective in healing diabetic ulcers. The question that arises is which growth factor should be studied? A growth factor which influences many different cells such as Platelet Derived Growth Factor (PDGF) or Transforming Growth Factor–beta (TGF–ß) may be helpful in healing these ulcers. A randomized prospective double blind trial of recombinant human PDGF has been reported to be successful in improving the healing of refractory diabetic neurotrophic foot ulcers when used in the context of good care.[17] As yet, no trials of TGF–ß have been reported. It is possible that other growth factors will prove to be beneficial.

Summary

In summary, the diabetic ulcer is a significant healthcare problem affecting more than one million patients at some point in their lives. Inadequate or improper therapy may lead to such trauma as limb loss. Aggressive treatment including proper footwear, nonweight bearing, appropriate antibiotics, debridement, aggressive revascularization and careful monitoring may lower the amputation rate in these patients. For the refractory ulcer, new therapies are being developed which might have a significant benefit in lowering the amputation rate.

References

1. Bild DE, Selby SV, Sinnock P, Browner WS, Braveman P, Showstack JA. Lower extremity amputation in people with diabetes; epidemiology and prevention. *Diabetes Care* 1989;12:24–31.
2. Levin ME. Diabetic foot ulcers: pathogenesis and management. *JET Nurs* 1993;20:191–198.
3. Most RS, Sinnock P. The epidemiology of lower extremity amputation in diabetic individuals. *Diabetes Care* 1983;6:87–91.
4. Miller OF. Essentials of pressure ulcer treatment, the diabetic experience. *J Dermatol Surg Oncol* 1993;19:759–63.
5. Pecoraro RE, Reiber GE, Burgess EM. Pathways to diabetic limb amputation: basis for   prevention. *Diabetes Care* 1990;13:513–21.
6. Boulton AJ. The diabetic foot: neuropathic in aetiology. *Diabetic Med* 1990;7:852–8.
7.   Sosenko JM, Kato M, Soto R, Bild DE. Comparison of quantitative sensory threshold measures for their association with foot ulceration in diabetic patients. *Diabetes Care* 1990;13:1057–61.

8. Keenan AM, Tindel NL, Alavi A. Diagnosis of pedal osteomyelitis in diabetic patients using current scintigraphic techniques. *Arch Intern Med* 1989;149:2262–6.

9. Wheat LJ, Allen SD, Henry M. Diabetic foot infections: bacteriologic analysis. *Arch Intern Med* 1986;146:1935–40.

10. Boulton AJ, Hardisty CA, Betts RP. Dynamic foot pressure and other studies as diagnostic and management aids in diabetic neuropathy. *Diabetes Care* 1983;6:26–33.

11. Taylor LM, Porter JM. The clinical course of diabetics who require emergency foot surgery because of infection or ischemia. *J Vasc Surg* 1987;6:454–9.

12. Lo Gerfo FW, Gibbons GW, Ponposelli FB. Trends in the care of the diabetic foot: expanded role of arterial reconstruction. *Arch Surg* 1992;127:617–21.

13. Witkowski JA, Parish LE. Debridement of cutaneous ulcers: medical and surgical aspects. *Clin Dermatol* 1992;9:585–591.

14. Robson MC, Stenberg BD, Heggers JP. Wound healing alternations caused by infection.*Clin Plat Surg* 1990;19:485–92.

15. Steed DL, Goslen JB, Holloway GA, Malone JM, Bunt TJ, Webster MW. Randomized prospective double blind trial in healing chronic diabetic foot ulcers. *Diabetes Care* 1992;15:1598–1604.

16. Krupski WC, Reilly LM, Perez S. A prospective randomized trial of autologous platelet– derived wound healing factors for treatment of chronic nonhealing wounds: a preliminary report. *J Vasc Surg* 1991;14:526–36.

17. Steed DL, Diabetic Ulcer Study Group. Clinical evaluation of recombinant human platelet–derived growth factor for the treatment of lower extremity diabetic ulcers. *J Vasc Surg* 1995;21:71–81.

22

Fundamental Strategies for Skin Care

Cathy Thomas Hess, BSN, RN, CETN

Hess CT. Fundamental strategies for skin care. In: Krasner D, Kane D. *Chronic Wound Care, Second Edition.* Wayne, PA, Health Management Publications, Inc., 1997, pp 178–183.

Introduction

Today, healthcare providers are strategically building state–of–the–art wound and skin care systems that best support clinical practices across all care settings and patient populations. The nursing diagnosis, Skin Integrity, Impaired,[1] is associated with patients who have skin disruptions and supports the need for comprehensive wound care systems. Common occurrences such as pressure ulcers, skin maceration secondary to incontinence or drainage, and dry skin are just a few examples often associated with this diagnosis.

The Agency for Health Care Policy and Research (AHCPR) identified the need to develop clinical practice guidelines for the prevention and treatment of pressure ulcers, a segment of wound and skin diagnoses.[2,3] This need was driven by the magnitude of the pressure ulcer problem, evident in human suffering, and the economic burden stressing the healthcare system of today and the future. The AHCPR guidelines document the prevalence of pressure ulcers in skilled care and nursing home facilities at approximately 23 percent, with the prevalence in acute care facilities at 9.2 percent. Pressure ulcers alone, excluding all other wounds, are estimated to be an $8 billion dollar a year industry.

Statistics on dry skin, another factor affecting skin integrity, indicate that skin dryness affects 59 to 80 percent of the elderly population.[4] These documented statistics further support the need for providers to closely examine current skin care practices. Additionally, the clinical diagnosis of urinary incontinence, affecting 15 to 30 percent of non–institutionalized persons over age 60 (and at least half of the 1.5 million nursing home residents), also leaves this aging population at risk for impaired skin integrity and maceration secondary to moisture.[5]

The fundamental building blocks addressing prevention of skin breakdown are generally overshadowed by the deluge of intervention strategies touted for patients with chronic wounds. It is paramount that providers take these proactive steps in clinical practice to develop sound skin care prevention strategies preceding intervention strategies. Education is the basis for the development of these clinical strategies. The clinician must understand the anatomy and physiology of the skin; current clinical practice guidelines; and indications and contraindications of skin care products utilized in clinical practice. When used effectively, the proactive building blocks of early prevention and intervention strategies make the potential for cutting the cost of pressure ulcers in half extremely viable.

Skin

The skin is the first line of defense in protecting the body from constant changes in the environment. Far too often, the attention needed for the skin is only realized after the integrity has been disrupted. It is important that the clinician be aware of factors affecting the characteristics of the skin in order to apply the proper proactive strategies. These factors include aging, bathing, cleansers, dryness, friction, lotions, moisturizers, nutrition, soaps and shearing forces. The clinician's knowledge of the skin, coupled with the knowledge of how these factors affect the skin, is essential in preventing damage to the skin's integrity.

The Layers of the Skin

In order to provide a proper skin care assessment and to effectively develop a plan of care for the patient's skin, a thorough understanding of the skin is essential. This knowledge base will assist the clinician in appropriate prevention and treatment strategies for the patient's skin.

The skin is the largest organ of the body, constituting approximately 10 percent of the body's weight.[6] The skin's functions include protection, sensation, thermoregulation, excretion, metabolism and communication (body image). Comprised of two layers, the skin is defined by an outer epidermis and an inner dermis which is anchored to muscle and bone by the connective tissue.

The epidermis is thin, avascular and normally regenerates every 4 to 6 weeks. Its primary function is to maintain the body's skin integrity, acting as a physical barrier to toxic agents, dirt bacteria, mircoorganisms and physical insults. The pH (potential hydrogen) of the skin is slightly acidic, normally preventing microorganisms from becoming pathogenic.

The epidermis is layered with cells called keratinocytes or epidermal cells and is comprised of five sublayers. The first layer is called the stratum corneum. This layer is composed of dead keratinized cells. These cells, called keratinocytes, are completely filled with the durable protein keratin and function as a protective barrier. Following the stratum corneum is the stratum lucidum, stratum granulosum, stratum spinosum, and lastly, the stratum germinativum or the basal cell layer. The fifth sublayer is anchored to the second thicker layer of skin, the dermis. The dermis provides strength, support, blood and oxygen to the skin. Deep in the dermis arise the sweat glands, sebaceous glands, hair follicles, and small fat cells. Sebum, secreted by the sebaceous glands, maintains hydration of the skin by providing a protective lipid layer which minimizes fluid loss through the epidermis.[6] Hypodermis, also known as the superficial fascia, attaches the dermis to the underlying structures. Its function is to promote an ongoing blood supply to the dermis for regeneration.

Factors Affecting the Skin's Condition

There are many factors playing a role in structural changes of the skin. It is important that the clinician be cognizant of these physical changes when assessing the skin and implement an appropriate protocol for prevention of skin breakdown.

Age. The evolutionary process of aging has the potential to alter the immune system, cardiovascular system, urinary system, respiratory system and inevitably the integumentary system. Therefore, it is logical that as people age, the skin ages too.

Aging causes the dermis to decrease in thickness. Epidermal regeneration increases with age, leaving the skin at great risk for irritation. Sensation and metabolism decrease in the aging population as do subcutaneous tissue, sweat glands and vascularity, which cumulatively affect the thermoregulatory system. The junction between the epidermis and dermis also changes in the aging process, affecting skin integrity.[7] This weaker link leaves the skin more vulnerable to mechanical trauma. Additionally, the hypodermis thins, leaving the aging population at risk for wounds such as pressure ulcers. Lastly, the visible wrinkling of the skin, occurs as a result of the loss and thinning of underlying tissues.

Skin cleansing strategies. There is no conclusive evidence documenting appropriate skin cleansing interventions, such as showering, tub baths, or sponge baths for patients. Many variables discussed in this chapter play an important role in bathing strategies. The use of certain soaps and cleansers for bathing may promote dry skin. The clinician should recognize that reducing the frequency of the bathing schedule may assist in controlling the skin's dryness.

It is also important for the clinician to recognize the importance of bathing techniques, the use of topical products, frequency of application, the psychosocial approaches for bathing and the function of the bath. These factors should be individualized for the patient's needs in the plan of care.[8]

The AHCPR guideline recommends the following interventions for skin cleansing:

* *Skin cleansing should occur at the time of soiling and at routine intervals. The frequency of skin cleansing should be individualized according to need and/or patient preference. Avoid hot water and use a mild cleansing agent that minimizes irritation and dryness of the skin. During the cleaning process, care should be utilized to minimize the force and friction applied to the skin.*

Rationale: Daily activities result in metabolic wastes and environmental contaminants accumulating on the skin. For maximum skin vitality, these potentially irritating substances should be removed frequently. If unexpected contamination occurs, such as fecal or urinary incontinence, the skin should be cleansed as soon as possible to limit chemical irritation. As a person ages, the frequency of routine skin cleansing may decrease because there is less sebum and perspiration. The reduced frequency of cleansing lessens the magnitude of trauma experienced by the more sensitive skin.

Skin injury due to excess thermal energy or the accelerated metabolic activity induced by elevated temperature should be minimized by only using wash water that is comfortable (slightly warm) to the skin.

During the cleansing process, some of the skin's "natural barrier" is removed. The more the barrier is removed, the drier the skin becomes and the more susceptible it is to external irritants. Under most conditions, the individual's skin is minimally soiled and can be properly cleansed with a very mild cleansing agent that does not disrupt this "natural barrier."[2]

Dry skin. Dry skin has been reported to affect between 59 and 80 percent of the aging population. Factors contributing to the presence of dry skin including humidity, loss of sebum, age, excessive perspiration, exposure to the sun, smoking, stress, and systemic dehydration. Dry skin is the loss of moisture from the stratum corneum.[4] Losing this moisture from the stratum corneum leaves this layer less pliable and more prone to skin alterations, such as cracking. Dry skin may appear cracked, rough, scaly (raised or uplifted skin edges), flaked (desquamation), chapped and itchy (pruritus).[4]

The AHCPR clinical practice guideline addresses the need for providers to minimize environmental factors leading to the dryness of skin. Two examples mentioned in the guideline, low humidity (less than 40 percent) and exposure to cold, promote dry skin. The guideline further suggests treating dry skin with topical moisturizers. Clinicians must also be aware that the use of soaps and cleansers as well as frequent bathing may be associated with drying of the skin. These products and techniques are discussed further in this chapter.

The AHCPR guideline recommends the following interventions for dry skin:

Minimize environmental factors leading to skin drying, such as low humidity (less than 40 percent) and exposure to cold. Dry skin should be treated with moisturizers.

Rationale:Preliminary research evidence suggests that a weak association may exist between dry, flaky, or scaling skin and an increased incidence of pressure ulcer development. It also appears that adequate hydration of the stratum corneum helps protect against mechanical insult. The level of stratum corneum hydration decreases with ambient air temperature, particularly when the relative humidity of the ambient air is low. Further, the development of clinically dry skin may result from a decreased level of relative humidity in the ambient air.

Decreased skin hydration results in reduced pliability, and severely dry skin is associated with fissuring and cracking of the stratum corneum. Also, a number of studies have shown that both the clinical picture of dry skin and measures of stratum corneum hydration generally improve with the application of various topical moisturizing agents. Although efficacy of any specific moisturizing agent has not been established, it would appear prudent to treat clinical signs and symptoms of dry skin with a topical moisturizer. Further, although there is no direct evidence to support efficacy in preventing pressure ulcers, maintenance of ambient environmental conditions (relative humidity and temperature) appear to be prudent in facilitating stratum corneum hydration and minimizing the occurrence of dry skin.[2]

Frictional and shearing forces. The force of friction pulls back the skin of the body while the weight of the body slides it forward. This activity may be seen in patients who wear braces, orthotics, splints, traction, and inappropriately fitting shoes. The wound caused by friction presents as an abrasion. Friction is a contributing factor to the epidermal stripping of the skin thereby decreasing the fibrinolytic abilities of the dermis. This sequence of events leaves the skin at risk for pressure necrosis. Interventions to prevent mechanical stripping include lubricants, transparent film dressings, skin sealants, hydrocolloids and protective dressings.

Shearing forces occur when the patient's skeletal frame slides down toward the foot of the mattress. At the same time, the sacral coccygeal area remains in a fixed position on the bed linens. The result of this force presents as an ulcer with possible tunneling or undermining. Interventions to reduce the activity of shearing include limiting the head of the bed to no more than a thirty degree angle and raising the knee gatch when the patient is positioned at a thirty degree angle.

The AHCPR guideline has the following recommendations for skin injury due to frictional and shearing forces.

Skin injury due to friction and shear forces should be minimized through proper positioning, transferring, and turning techniques. In addition, friction injuries may be reduced by the use of lubricants (such as corn starch and creams), protective films (such as transparent film dressings and skin sealants), protective dressings (such as hydrocolloids), and protective padding.

Rationale: Shear injury occurs when the skin remains stationary and the underlying tissue shifts. This shift diminishes blood supply to the skin and soon results in ischemia and tissue damage. Most shear injuries can be eliminated by proper positioning.

Friction injuries to the skin occur when it moves across a coarse surface such as bed linens. Most friction injuries can be avoided by using appropriate techniques for moving individuals which prevents dragging across linens.

Voluntary and nonvoluntary movements by the individuals themselves can lead to friction injuries, especially on elbows and heels. Any agent that eliminates this contact or decreases the friction between the skin and the linens will reduce the potential for injury .[2]

Skin Exposure to Moisture. The appropriate use of topical skin care products is essential to

Table 1
Common Ingredient Reference Guide for Skin Care Products*

Classification	Purpose	Type
Antimicrobial	Destroys or inhibits bacterial growth	Benzalkonium chloride Benzethonium chloride Hexylresorcinol Methylbenzethonium chloride
Detergent	Surfactant which cleans by emulsifying oils and suspending particulate soil	Ammonium lauryl sulfate DA–lauryl sulfate Disodium oleamido MEA sulfosuccinate Sodium laureth sulfate Sodium lauryl sulfate
Emollient	Softens and soothes skin	Almond oil Aloe vera Apricot kernel oil Clycomethicone Dimethicone copolyol Glyceryl stearate Jojoba oil Lanolin Mineral oil Phenyl trimethicone Silica
Humectant	Absorbs, holds and retains moisture	DL Panthenol Propylene glycol Sodium PCA
Moisturizer	Adds moisture to the skin	Water
Preservative	Protects products from spoilage by microorganisms	Disodium EDTA Imidazolidinyl urea Quanternium–15 Methylparaben Propylparaben Potassium sorbate
Skin Protectant	Protects injured or exposed skin from harmful stimuli	Allantoin Aluminum hydroxide gel Calamine Cocoa butter Cornstarch Dimethicone Glycerine Kaolin Petrolatum Shark liver oil Sodium bicarbonate
Surfactant	Lowers surface tension between two or more incompatible phases	Poloxamer 188 Potassium palmitate Polysorbate 20

Adapted with permission from Common Ingredient Reference Guide. © 1993 Renaissance Pharmaceutical/Acme United Corporation, Fairfield, CT.

maintain the skin's suppleness and to prevent skin dehydration and maceration. Far too often, clinicians are presented with the challenge of maintaining intact skin in the presence of moisture due to incontinence, perspiration or wound drainage.

The AHCPR guideline has the following recommendations for minimizing skin exposure to moisture:

Minimize skin exposure to moisture due to incontinence, perspiration, or wound drainage. When these sources of moisture cannot be controlled, underpads or briefs can be used that are made of materials that absorb moisture and present a quick–drying surface to the skin. For information about assessing and managing urinary incontinence, refer to Urinary Incontinence Adults: Clinical Practice Guidelines.5 Topical agents that act as barriers to moisture can also be used.

Moisturizers

Moisturizers are most often applied to hydrate dry skin and are available in forms such as creams, lotions and bath oils, ointments and pastes.

Creams. Creams are preparations of oil in water. The main component of a cream is water, causing it to be of a thinner consistency. Because creams are less viscous, they are less occlusive than ointments and, therefore, must be applied much more frequently to maintain their effectiveness.

Lotions. Lotions are comprised of powder crystals dissolved in water. They are held in suspension by surface active agents. The high water content in lotions produces a coolant effect on the skin. Lotions do not have occlusive properties and, therefore, must be applied frequently to hydrate the skin.

Clinicians must be cognizant of the ingredients within skin care products when applying these products to patient's skin.

Rationale: An individual's skin may be exposed to a variety of substances that are moist: urine, stool, perspiration, or wound drainage. Although these substances may contain factors other than moisture that irritate the skin, moisture alone can make skin more susceptible to injury. Underpads and briefs are often used to protect the skin of individuals who are incontinent of urine or stool. Because these products are designed to reduce injury attributed to the moisture associated with urinary and fecal incontinence, it is not unreasonable to assume they would serve a similar function in those instances where the source of moisture is perspiration or wound drainage.[2]

Topical skin agents. Maintaining the integrity of the patient's skin is critical throughout the continuum of care. Clinicians utilize topical skin care products to prevent skin breakdown and "treat" impaired skin integrity from diagnoses such as incontinence and wound drainage. Skin care products are a critical piece in the plan of care to preserve skin integrity. Products such as moisturizers, barrier creams and cleansing agents should be selected based on the patient's skin type, desired outcome, application and removal of product, and cost.

Clinicians must be cognizant of the ingredients within skin care products when applying these products to patient's skin (Table 1). Topical skin care products have indications based on their ingredients and contraindications/warnings indicating when products should not be used/applied.

Bath oils. Bath–oil and tap–water bathing have been studied to determine the hydration status of the skin and skin surface lipids.[9] In one study by Stender, Blichmann and Serup, the authors concluded that there was no major difference in the hydration of the epidermis after a 30 minute emersion in an oil–bath compared to that of the tap–water bath.[9] The skin surface lipids following the oil–bath lasted at least three hours which was comparable to an application of a moisturizer. The authors determined that the use of moisturizing lotions may be more advantageous than the use of oils.

Ointments. Ointments are comprised of water in an oil base. Typical oil components are either lanolin or petrolatum. Ointments are generally characterized by their occlusive properties.

Pastes. Pastes are created when powders are added to ointments. Pastes are more vicious and enduring than ointments. One common complaint of clinicians using paste is the difficulty of removing the paste from the patient's body. Clinicians may find it helpful to utilize mineral oil when attempting to remove the paste from the skin's surface.

Conclusion

It is critical that clinicians utilize the most current clinical practice guidelines within their practices and institutions in order to achieve positive patient outcomes. Far too often, topical skin care products are applied to a patient's skin, as a proactive and reactive strategy without the provider clearly understanding the purpose of the product. A comprehensive understanding of skin and topical products is often the best defense in maintaining the patient's skin integrity, controlling costs and accelerating the healing process.

References

1. Alfaro R. *Applying Nursing Diagnosis and Nursing Process: A Step–by–Step Guide.* Grand Rapids, MI, J.B. Lippincott Company, 1994.
2. Panel for the Prediction and Prevention of Pressure Ulcers in Adults. *Pressure Ulcers in Adults: Prediction and Prevention. Clinical Practice Guideline, No. 3.* AHCPR Publication No. 92–0047. Rockville, MD: Agency for Health Care Policy and Research, Public Health Service, US Department of Health and Human Services; May, 1992.
3. Bergstrom N, Bennett MA, Carlson CE, et al. *Treatment of Pressure Ulcers. Clinical Practice Guideline, No. 14.* AHCPR Publication No. 95–0642. Rockville, MD: Agency for Health Care Policy and Research, Public Health Service, US Department of Health and Human Services, December 1994.
4. Frantz R, Gardner S. Clinical concerns: Management of dry skin. *Journal of Gerontological Nursing* 1994;20(9):15–18.
5. Urinary Incontinence Guideline Panel. *Urinary Incontinence In Adults: Clinical Practice Guideline.* AHCPR Pub. No. 92–0038. Rockville, MD: Agency for Health Care Policy and Research, Public Health Service, US Department of Health and Human Services, March 1992.
6. Hess CT. *Nurse's Clinical Guide to Wound Care.* Springhouse, PA, Springhouse Publications, 1995.
7. Wysocki A. Skin integrity. In: Bryant RA (ed). *Acute and Chronic Wounds: Nursing Management.* St. Louis, MO, Mosby, 1992, pp 2–10.
8. Rader J. To bathe or not to bathe: That is the question. *Journal of Gerontological Nursing* 1994;20(9):53–54.
9. Stender JM, Blichmann C, Serup J. Effects of oil and water baths on the hydration state of the epidermis. *Clinical and Experimental Dermatology* 1990;15:206–209.

23

Skin Care for the Oncology Patient

Anne E. Belcher, PhD, RN, FAAN

Belcher AE. Skin care for the oncology patient. In: Krasner D, Kane D. *Chronic Wound Care, Second Edition*. Wayne, PA, Health Management Publications, Inc., 1997, pp 184–190.

Introduction

Patients with cancer may experience disruptions in skin integrity related to the disease or its treatment. Shaffer in 1994 summarized the causes of impaired skin integrity in persons with cancer including "immobility, malignant skin lesions, infectious skin lesions, nonspecific rashes, irritation from urinary and/or fecal incontinence, abrasions resulting from scratching and shearing forces, invasive therapeutic procedures, radiation skin reactions, 'recall' skin reactions, chemotherapy extravasation, lymphatic and/or vascular obstruction, decubiti, and/or malnutrition."[1]

Disease–related causes of skin problems include primary skin cancers, such as malignant melanoma, basal cell or squamous cell carcinoma, Kaposi's sarcoma and mycoses fungoides. Skin integrity may also be disrupted by metastatic tumors, such as chest wall recurrence in breast cancer or leukemic and lymphomatous infiltrates. Petechiae, purpura and ecchymoses may cause increased skin fragility.

Treatment related skin problems may result from chemotherapy, biologic response modifiers, radiation therapy, surgery and other invasive procedures. For example, chemotherapy may cause drug extravasation, alopecia, hyperpigmentation, hyperkeratosis, photosensitivity, ulceration and radiation "recall" reactions. Biologic response modifiers (such as colony–stimulating factors, interferons and interleukins) may cause toxic erythema (generalized or localized), hypersensitivity, phototoxicity, and pruritus. Radiation therapy may cause dry or moist desquamation. Surgical incisions and invasive procedures such as biopsies and vascular access devices may also impair skin integrity. See Table 1 for general principles of skin management in persons with cancer.

Management of Pruritus

Pruritus or itching may result from the cancer itself or from treatment, that is, reactions to chemotherapy or radiation therapy. Disorders linked with pruritus include leukemias, lymphomas, renal failure or hepatic dysfunctions. This frequently discomforting symptom can be managed in the following ways: 1) by encouraging the patient to increase fluid intake in order to maintain sufficient hydration; 2) by applying water–soluble lotions and emollients to damp skin; 3) by providing a humidified environment; 4) by teaching the patient to keep fingernails short and smooth; it may be necessary to provide cotton gloves or socks for the patient's hands as a reminder not to scratch irritated skin; 5) by instructing the patient to wash hands frequently to lessen the likelihood of contaminating open areas when scratching; 6) by using methods of skin stimulation such as pressure, massage, vibration, and cold compresses to lessen the sensation of itching; 7) by having the patient avoid tight, irritating, nonabsorbant clothing; 8) by preventing or managing vasodilatation with cool baths and showers; 9) by advising the patient to avoid alcohol and caffeine–containing beverages and food; and 10) by using distraction techniques, such as guided imagery, relaxation exercises, or yoga.

Medications which may be prescribed to manage pruritus include antihistamines, corticosteroids, tranquilizers, and topical agents. Symptomatic supportive care also includes the use of colloidal oatmeal powder baths twice a day, topical water–trapping agents such as petrolatum and menthol lotions. Early and consistent management of pruritus can effectively prevent disruptions in skin integrity.

Table 1
General Principles of Skin Management in Persons with Cancer

- Assess skin areas at risk for damage; focus on color, moisture, texture and temperature.
- Use preventive measures to maintain skin integrity, including meticulous skin hygiene.
- Maintain or attain adequate nutrition.
- Avoid or provide immediate intervention for incontinence.
- Prevent the hazards of immobility.
- Manage pruritus.
- Provide patient and family education regarding skin hygiene and assessment.

Table 2
Skin Care During Radiation Therapy

- Clean the skin with lukewarm water as needed and pat rather than rub the skin dry with a soft towel.
- Use only nondeodorant, unperfumed soaps.
- Do not apply powders, perfumes and deodorants to the irradiated area.
- Avoid the use of cornstarch in the axilla, groin, and gluteal folds.
- Avoid shaving the treatment area with a razor blade.
- Protect the treated skin from cold, heat and sun.
- Wear only loose–fitting cotton clothing close to the skin.
- Avoid placing adhesive tape on the irradiated skin.[2]

Management of Treatment Effects

Radiation Therapy. Before the patient receives radiation therapy, his/her usual skin and hair care should be assessed as the use of contraindicated products can enhance skin reactions. In addition, both the patient and family should be instructed in appropriate skin care during treatment (Table 2).

Skin effects associated with radiation therapy are localized and depend on the area treated, the volume of tissue irradiated, fractionation, total dose, type of radiation and individual skin differences. The time between radiation exposure and the observed effects can vary from days to weeks to months; early reactions occur during or within weeks after treatment, with some symptoms not subsiding until two or more weeks after treatment has ended. Delayed reactions can occur months or years after treatment. Strohl in 1988 noted that erythema may appear after the patient has received 3000 to 4000 rads (generally during the second or third week of treatment), with dry and/or moist desquamation developing after 4500 to 6000 rads.[3]

Skin reactions tend to be more extensive in areas receiving large doses of radiation. Electron beams produce more intense reactions due to superficial concentration of the radiation. Skin reactions are less severe with megavoltage therapy treatments, which have skin sparing features. Treatments may involve the use of a bolus material placed on the skin to increase the skin dose. Treatments delivered from a tangential angle as opposed to perpendicular to the treatment site can increase the skin reaction.[4]

Sitton in 1992 indicated that areas of the skin such as those covering bony prominences, the skin on the face, or surgical wounds tend to be more sensitive.[4] Because of increased warmth and moisture and lack of aeration, areas with skin folds, such as the axilla, perineum, groin and gluteal fold and under the breasts, are also likely to develop skin reactions. Skin reactions can occur where the radiation exits the body, that is, on the side of the body opposite from where treatment is delivered. Chemotherapy being administered concurrently with radiation increases the patient's risk of a skin reaction. The severity of radiation effects on the skin correlates with the volume of tissue irradiated. As the treatment area increases, skin tolerance decreases. A fractionation schedule (total dose of radiation divided into fractions given daily) allows for some recovery of normal skin between doses.

Individual differences among patients also impact the skin effects of radiation therapy. For example, a malnourished patient in negative nitrogen balance will heal more slowly, with delayed tissue repair. Elderly or debilitated patients with dry skin may not tolerate therapy as well and may require a reduced daily dose to keep skin and other side effects at a tolerable level.

Patients receiving pelvic irradiation after low anterior or anterior–posterior resection for rectal cancer need special attention. Not only is the surgical wound site at increased risk because it is in the treatment field, but the presence of a stoma with appliance and skin barrier can also act as a bolus material. The radiation therapist may tape the patient's buttocks apart during treatment to lessen the skin reaction. Removal of the appliance and skin barrier may also be necessary.

Transient early erythema may develop within a few hours of exposure to radiation, increase in intensity with cumulative doses, and subside in 24 to 48 hours. This early reaction is inflammatory and results from activation of proteolytic enzymes and increased capillary permeability. There may also be increased pigmentation related to activation of the melanocytes. Main erythematous skin reactions may occur three to six weeks into treatment and are related to loss of epidermal basal cells. The erythema ranges from mild, light pink to deep and dusky. Slight edema and increased skin sensitivity may also be noted. This skin reaction may progress with continued treatment, and dry desquamation (dry, itchy and flaky skin) may develop. Mild to severe moist desquamation may be observed where the epidermal layers of the skin slough, leaving a raw, painful area that may drain serous exudate. These areas usually heal in a matter of weeks.

Dry desquamation often causes tenderness and itching. In addition to prior suggestions regarding the management of pruritus, Iwamoto in 1994 recommended the use of a nonperfumed hydrophilic moisturizing lotion that does not contain heavy metals.[5] Lotion which has not been absorbed should be removed with a soft washcloth prior to treatment to prevent an enhanced treatment reaction.

Normal saline irrigations or cool compresses three to four times a day soothe the skin of the patient with moist desquamation. Bucholtz in 1992 suggested cleansing with one half–strength to one third–strength hydrogen peroxide and saline followed by a saline rinse.[6] A thin layer of A&D Ointment® (Schering Corporation, Kenilworth, NJ), lanolin or Aquaphor® (Beiersdorf, Inc., Norwalk, CT) may be applied. In some cases of moist desquamation, treatment should stop and zinc oxide or silver sulfadiazine cream should be applied either directly to the skin or via a nonadherent dressing such as a Telfa® pad (Kendall Healthcare Products Company, Mansfield, MA). Hydrocolloid dressings have also been found to be effective; they can be left on the irritated skin for up to five days without increasing the risk of infection.[7] Wet dressings with such astringents as BluBoro® (Herbert Laboratories, Irvine, CA) or Domeboro® (Miles, Inc. West Haven, CT) cleanse, dry and seal exudative surfaces. Aluminum acetate solutions also help to prevent bacterial and candida overgrowth. Soaks may be administered for one half hour, three to four times daily, with dressings remoistened and reapplied every 10 to 15 minutes.

In one study, hydrogel dressings (i.e. ClearSite®, New Dimensions in Medicine, Dayton, OH) were used by nurse specialists[8] to treat more than twenty patients with desquamation. A sheet hydrogel dressing was chosen because of its moist wound healing properties, ease of application and atraumatic removal. Therapeutic results were obtained in all of the patients. Less than one–third of the subjects had therapy suspended because of the severity of the desquamation. Providing a moist environment with minimal trauma during dressing changes led to impressive healing. Change procedures were performed by both patients and caregivers. According to the authors, "Re–epithelialization and pain relief occurred even when radiation treatment was continued."[8]

When moist desquamation develops in the perineum, sitz baths, perineal compresses and protective emollients can all be used. The perineum may be dried with a hand–held blow dryer set on the cool setting. Treatment may be stopped for a period of time to allow for tissue healing.

Once the patient has completed treatment, skin healing usually occurs within a few weeks; however, the patient may retain tanned skin within the treatment field which will eventually subside. The irradiated area may remain more sensitive to heat or cold and may develop a sunburn more quickly than untreated areas. The patient should continue to avoid direct sun exposure by wearing scarves, hats and other protective covering. A sunblock with a high sun protection factor (SPF) should be applied before sun exposure. Dry skin may be an ongoing problem after treatment. Mild soap and bath oils can be used during bathing for relief. Lubricants such as petrolatum, mineral and baby oils, and Eucerin® (Beiersdorf, Inc., Norwalk, CT) are helpful. Patients may prefer such dry skin lotions as AlphaKeri® (Bristol Myers, Princeton, NJ), Lubrex® (T/I Pharmaceuticals, Inc., Irvine, CA), Lubriderm® (Warner–Wellcome Company, Morris Plains, NJ); creams such as Nivea® (Beiersdorf, Inc., Norwalk, CT) or AlphaKeri® (Bristol Myers, Princeton, NJ), or thicker preparations such as Eucerin® (Beiersdorf, Inc., Norwalk, CT) or Aquaphor® (Beiersdorf, Inc., Norwalk, CT).

Delayed radiation effects include fibrosis and atrophy of the skin, altered pigmentation, ulceration, necrosis, telangiectasia, and lymphedema due to fibrosis of the lymph glands. Heavily irradiated skin may heal with thinner, smoother epithelium and little or no hair, sweat glands or sebaceous glands. Loss of elasticity, dryness, increased vulnerability to injury and limited ability to repair damage characterize the previously irradiated area. The "recall" phenomenon may occur months to years after radiation therapy; skin, mucous membrane, or pulmonary reactions may develop within the treated area if certain chemotherapeutic agents such as dactinomycin and doxorubicin are administered systemically after the completion of radiation therapy. While more severe than the initial reactions, "recall" reactions usually subside within two weeks. Tepid wet compresses and topical corticosteroid preparations are used for the relief of pain, erythema, and edema; topical antibiotics such as silver sulfadiazine or bacitracin may be prescribed for ulceration, should that occur.

treatment will prevent spillage of cancer cells during surgery, thus lessening the likelihood of local recurrence of the disease. In some instances, ablative surgery may be performed in a previously irradiated field. The risk of wound breakdown and infection is high, thus tension free closure of all skin and mucosal suture lines is essential.[9] The use of vascularized flaps from beyond the irradiated area may be required. Early debridement should be performed when wound breakdown does occur, followed by transfer of healthy, well vascularized tissue into the wound. As Wornom in 1995 notes,

---

The major categories of chemotherapy–induced cutaneous toxicity include alopecia, hyperpigmentation, nail disorders, photosensitivity, extravasation injury and hypersensitivity reactions.

Late ulcerations occur in areas of previous radiation therapy as a consequence of ischemia, skin breakdown and secondary bacterial invasion. These areas occur most often in the head and neck, chest wall, and perineum. Patients describe wounds as extremely painful. Wornom in 1995 identified the following principles to guide wound management: adequate debridement, local wound care with topical antibacterial agents, and wound coverage with healthy, well–vascularized tissue, such as muscle or omentum.[9] Dead bone or cartilage which is exposed within the wound should be removed until viable tissue is reached. When osteoradionecrosis of the mandible or chest wall occurs, surgical removal of large segments of these structures may be necessary. Hyperbaric oxygen therapy may be useful; increasing the vascularity of the remaining wound bed improves a flap's ability to adhere to the wound and may shrink the area of debridement required. Prosthetic material should be avoided in the reconstruction of these defects. If mandibular reconstruction is implemented, it is best done with free vascularized bone flaps such as the fibula.

The time between debridement and wound closure should be minimized, as these wounds are likely to become infected. Both procedures are frequently carried out in one operation. After closure, wound pain is often dramatically reduced, resulting in a rapid decrease in the patient's need for narcotic analgesics.

Preoperative radiation is most often used to treat cancers of the head and neck but may also be used to treat other cancers and sarcomas. The rationale for this approach is the belief that this preoperative

"This is particularly important if major blood vessels such as the carotid artery are exposed in the wound because spontaneous rupture of these vessels can occur leading to exsanguinating hemorrhage."[9]

Chemotherapy. The major categories of chemotherapy–induced cutaneous toxicity include alopecia, hyperpigmentation, nail disorders, photosensitivity, extravasation injury and hypersensitivity reactions. While alopecia is one of the most psychologically devastating side effects of chemotherapy, it will not be discussed in this chapter. There are many excellent resources, including reports of research–based interventions, to guide the healthcare provider in the support of the patient experiencing hair loss.

Hyperpigmentation is commonly caused by the alkylating agents and antitumor antibiotics. Changes occur in both localized and diffused patterns and may involve the skin, teeth, nails, hair and mucous membranes. The problem usually subsides over time and may resolve completely.

Nail changes include the appearance of transverse white bands or nail depression (Beau's lines), onycholysis (partial separation of the nail plate from the bed), or brittle and dystrophic nails.

Photosensitivity creates signs and symptoms which include exaggerated sunburn–type reactions, often causing the patient to complain of stinging and urticaria. Certain chemotherapeutic agents, as well as photodynamic therapy (an intravenous photosensitizing agent followed by laser treatment), may cause severe erythematous phototoxic reactions.

Hypersensitivity reactions are infrequent but may be Type I (immediate–hypersensitivity reaction with urticaria and angioedema which may be associated with anaphylaxis) or Type III (serum–sickness reactions). A variety of chemotherapeutic agents cause macular papular eruptions.

The accidental infiltration of irritant or vesicant chemotherapeutic drugs from the vein into the surrounding tissues at the intravenous site is termed extravasation. An irritant is a drug capable of producing venous pain at the IV site and along the vein with or without an inflammatory reaction. A vesicant is a drug that can produce a blister and/or tissue destruction. Extravasation can cause sloughing of tissue, infection, pain, and loss of mobility in an extremity. Factors which determine the degree of tissue damage include drug vesicant potential, drug concentration, the quantity of drug extravasated, duration of tissue exposure, vein–puncture site/device, needle insertion technique and individual tissue responses.[10] High–risk extravasation sites include joint spaces, underlying tendons and neurovascular bundles, especially because these areas lack thick subcutaneous fat layers. Once the chemotherapeutic agent has leaked out of the vein, it binds to DNA in the tissues, causing cell death. Continued release of the drug leads to progressive ulceration.

Tissue destruction can be subtle and progressive with initial signs and symptoms including pain or burning at the IV site, progressing to edema, erythema, and superficial skin loss. Tissue, tendon and muscle necrosis may develop as late as one to four weeks after the extravasation.

Treatment strategies include the use of specific antidotes and guidelines for immediate action to minimize tissue damage. The key aspects of successful management are prevention of the extravasation and prompt intervention. Aspects of prevention, as identified by Otto in 1992, include 24 hour vesicant infusion via central venous access only, testing vein patency before administering chemotherapeutic agents, providing adequate drug dilution, careful observation of the access site and extremity during the infusion, verification of blood return from the IV site before, during and after drug infusion, and reminding the patient of symptoms of drug infiltration to be reported.[10]

Should extravasation occur at a peripheral site, the drug infusion should be stopped with the needle left in place. Residual drug and blood in the tubing, needle or catheter should be aspirated; the IV antidote should be instilled using the prescribed technique and frequency. Application of topical ointment, dressings and compresses, and elevation of the extremity should proceed according to protocol. The area should be assessed at regular intervals for erythema, induration and necrosis, and the patient should be asked to describe the presence and characteristics of pain. Surgical consultation should be requested within 72 hours if pain persists and extensive debridement may be needed.

Biotherapy. Interferon has been linked with a pruritic eruption extending over the trunk and extremities; it responds to antihistamines. Other cutaneous reactions include mild alopecia or cyanosis of the nail bed and oral mucosa. Granulocyte–macrophage colony stimulating factor may cause a rash. Interleukin–2 (IL–2) may cause erythematous reactions.

Palliative Care. Grocott in 1991 identified the following priorities for wound management in palliative care: control of pain, prevention of complications such as infection or bleeding, control of exudate, control of odor, minimal disturbance to the patient because of frequent dressing changes, removal of dressings without trauma, restoration of body symmetry, and cosmetic acceptability.[11] She describes the challenge of caring for terminally ill patients whose wounds are extensive and filled with necrotic material, producing exudate which is difficult to control, visible and exuding (such as a facial lesion), or difficult to dress because of their location (such as breast/head and neck lesions). The author recommends that dressing regimens for such patients consist of materials such as hydrocolloids and alginates held in place by molded, highly absorbent, light, secondary materials such as foam latex. She challenges specialists to create such dressings to better control the wounds of patients receiving palliative care. For further information on this topic, the reader is referred to Chapter 42 in this source book.

Collinson in 1992 focused on the problems identified by patients and their caregivers in the management of a malignant fungating wound and the development of an appropriate protocol for alleviating these problems.[12] Excess exudate, odor and bleeding were found to be the most common and distressing problems for both patients and their caregivers. Two protocols were developed over a period of four years of experience with the management of approximately 350 patients. One protocol included cleansing via irrigation with warm normal saline, debriding with an amorphous hydrogel dressing (Intrasite® Gel, Smith & Nephew United, Inc., Largo, FL), and dressing with semi–permeable film daily at first and then less frequently as debridement occurs. Necrotic tissue starts to liquefy within 24 hours after this protocol is implemented. It is very effective on eschar and may be used during radiation therapy. Intrasite® Gel acts by rehydrating and liquefying necrotic tissue; it has fluid handling properties which ease application, especially on large wounds. The other protocol included cleansing via irrigation with warm normal saline, primary dressing with an alginate dressing (Sorbsan™, Dow Hickam Pharmaceuticals Inc., Sugar Land, TX), and secondary dressing with a foam dressing (Lyofoam®, Acme United Corporation, Fairfield, CT) or semi–permeable film, with frequency of dressing change dependent on the amount of exudate. This procedure debrides areas of soft sloughy necrotic tissue, controls capillary bleeding, and may be used during radiation therapy.

Summary

The cancer patient may require special skin care for a variety of reasons which are related to disease and/or treatment. Maintenance of skin integrity and early management of skin reactions in persons receiving radiation therapy are of particular concern. Chemotherapy extravasation presents unique problems and requires interventions specific to the drug and agency protocol. Patients undergoing surgery often have radical procedures that result in large incisions with complex drainage systems. The terminally ill patient may have wounds presenting special challenges to the healthcare provider and caregiver. Wound care in these patients is often complicated by their impaired immune status, thus particular care is required to prevent infection while controlling common symptoms like itching and pain, as well as problems like odor and drainage.

References

1. Shaffer S. Protective mechanisms. In: Otto S. (ed). *Oncology Nursing* . St. Louis, MO, Mosby, 1994, pp 698–719.
2. Dow K., Hilderl, L. *Nursing Care in Radiation Oncology.* Philadelphia, PA, W.B. Saunders, 1992.
3. Strohl RA. The nursing role in radiation oncology: symptom management of acute and chronic reactions. *Oncology Nursing Forum* 1988;15(4):429–434.
4. Sitton E. Early and late radiation–induced skin alteration. Part I: Mechanisms of skin changes.*Oncology Nursing Forum* 1992a;19(5):801–807.
5. Iwamoto R. Radiation therapy. In: Otto S. (ed). *Oncology Nursing.* St. Louis, MO, C.V. Mosby, 1994, pp 467–492.
6. Bucholtz J. Radiation therapy. In: Ziegfeld CR (ed). *Core Curriculum for Oncology Nursing.* Philadelphia, PA, W.B. Saunders, 1992.
7. Margolin S, Breneman J, Denman. Management of radiation–induced moist skin desquamation using hydrocolloid dressing. *Cancer Nursing* 1992;13:71–80.
8. Fisher E. Malone, MJ, Hebert T. Treatment of Desquamation in Radiated Skin. Twenty–fifth Annual Wound, Ostomy and Continence Conference, San Antonio, Texas, July 10–15, 1993.
9. Wornom IL. The Management of the Irradiated Wound. The 4th Annual Wound Care Symposium, Richmond, Virginia, April 2–5, 1995.
10. Otto S. Chemotherapy. In: Otto S (ed). *Oncology Nursing.* St. Louis, MO, Mosby, 1994.
11. Grocott P. Application of the principles of modern wound management for complex wounds in palliative care. In: Harding KG, Leaper DL, Turner TD (eds). *Proceedings of the 1st European Conference on Advances in Wound Management.* Cardiff, September 4–6, 1991, pp 88–91.
12. Collinson G. Improving quality of life in patients with malignant fungating wounds. In: Harding KG, Cherry G, Deale, C, Turner TD (eds). *Proceeding of the 2nd European Conference on Advanced in Wound Management.* Harrogate, October 20–23, 1992, pp 59–63.

Appendix 1. Chemotherapeutic Vesicant Drugs with Recommended Antidotes

<u>Drug</u>

<u>Antidone</u>

Alkylating Agent
Mechlorethamine (nitrogen mustard)

Isotonic
Sodium thiosulfate
- Dilute 1.6 ml sodium thiosulfate 25% with 8.4 ml of sterile water; inject 1 to 4 ml through existing IV access; inject subq if IV access is removed; apply ice pack and or cold compresses.

Antibiotics
Actinomycin D
Dacarbazine
Daunorubicin
Doxorubicin
Epirubicin
Esorubicin
Idarubincin
Mithramycin
Mitomycin C
Piroxanthrone

Hydrocortisone 100 mg/ml
- Inject 0.5 ml IV through existing IV line and 0.5 ml subcutaneously into extravasated site; apply cold compresses.

Dexamethasone 4 mg/ml
- Inject 0.5 ml IV through existing IV line and 0.5 ml subcutaneously into extravasated site; apply cold compresses/ice packs immediately; do not apply pressure.

Alternative protocol

Topical DMSO 1 to 2 ml of 1 mmol DMSO 50 % to 100%
- Apply topically one time at the site; apply cold compresses.

Bisantrene

Sodium bicarbonate 1 mEq/ml
- Mix equal parts of sodium bicarbonate with sterile normal saline (1:1 solution); resulting solution is 0.5 Eq/ml; inject 2 to 6 ml (1 to 3.0 mEq) IV through existing IV line and subcutaneously into the extravasated site; apply cold compresses.

Vinca Alkaloids
Vinblastine
Vincristine

Hyaluronidase (Wygase) 150 U/ml
- Add 1 ml sterile sodium chloride; inject 1 to 6 ml (150 to 900 U) subcutaneously into the extravasated site with the multiple injections; apply warm compresses.

Local Antidote
(may be used for daunorubicin, doxorubicin, and mitomycin

- Topical cooling may be achieved using ice packs, cooling pad with ice water circulating, Cryogel packs changed frequently; cooling of site to patient tolerance for 24 hours.
- Elevate and rest extremity 24 to 48 hours.

Reprinted with permission from Otto S. Oncology Nursing. Mosby–Year Book, Inc., 1994.

24

Cutaneous Complications of Wound Healing

Jeffrey Hurley, MD

Hurley J. Cutaneous complications of wound healing. In: Krasner D, Kane D. *Chronic Wound Care, Second Edition*. Wayne, PA, Health Management Publications, Inc., 1997, pp 191–195.

Introduction

Wound healing represents one of the most intriguing and intricate processes in all of mammalian biology. The factors that govern it are similar, if not identical, in all organs, irrespective of the type of wound or its genesis. Indeed in healthy individuals, wounds, once produced, will begin to heal promptly and proceed unimpededly to complete resolution assuming other influences do not interfere with the healing process. The "filler" material, or scar tissue, while morphologically and functionally not the equal of the original parenchyma and stroma it has replaced, will nonetheless adapt over time to accommodate fairly well to the needs of the organ.

Fundamentally a wound is simply a break in the surface continuity of the organ. Wounds vary widely in depth, size and shape. From the tiny circular wound of a needle puncture or a linear erosive fissure of a xerotic dermatitis to a burn wound covering 80 percent of the body surface or a deep, irregularly-shaped osteomyelitic ulcer, wounds run the gamut of morphologic defects.

From the anatomic, physiologic and biological perspectives, the dynamics of wound healing have been elegantly reviewed elsewhere.[1–4] The purpose of this chapter is to consider the cutaneous complications of wound healing, the unexpected and unwanted developments that delay or adversely alter healing so that it cannot be completed or results in an imperfect or problematic scar.

In discussing the complications of wounds, it is impossible to overemphasize the importance of the healing capabilities of the host. Whether genetic or acquired, defects in the host's ability to resist or control the forces or agents that alter the healing process predispose the patient to one or more of these complications. It is well to recognize that such complications may compromise wound healing at any stage of the process, early or late, and may thus produce somewhat different effects on the given wound.

The cutaneous complications of wound healing may be categorized as follows: Infectious, Inflammatory, Degenerative, Traumatic, Neoplastic, and Proliferative.

Infectious Complications

Wounds, more than most tissues, are vulnerable to invasion and colonization by pathogenic microorganisms. Because of their moist, serosanguinous bases, wounds provide an ideal milieu for a great variety of microorganisms. The list of transient organisms that survive temporarily on the skin include virtually all the organisms, pathogenic and non–pathogenic, with which man can possible come into contact. Most cannot mount enough of an attack to survive. Coagulase–positive *Staphylococci* and *Streptococci* are among the most likely transients to infect wounds, and certain gram–negative organisms, especially *E. Coli*, *Proteus* species, and *Pseudomonas* can pose special problems, especially in wounds of long–standing. Fungal and yeast forms, such as *Candida*, *Cryptococcus*, *Aspergillus*, and *Penicilium* are regarded as opportunistic, for they require a locally or systemically weakened host. Intrinsic defense mechanisms of the host, including humoral and

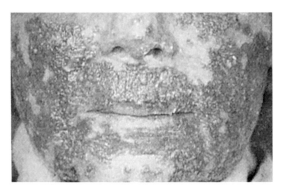

Figure 1. Outbreak of cutaneous herpes simplex in a patient after undergoing a chemical peel.

Reprinted with permission from Plastic and Reconstructive Surgery. Perkins SW, Sklarew EC. Prevention of facial herpetic infections after chemical peel and dermabrasion: New treatment strategies in the prophylaxis of patients undergoing procedures of the perioral area. September 1996. © 1996, Waverly.

cellular mediators, inflammatory cell products and immunologically activated agents, normally resist such invasion.

The noscomial origin of pathogens is always a major concern in the management of wounds. Outside the hospital, sources such as unwashed hands, the axillary, oral, nasal, perianal and periorificial skin, other patients and animals with cutaneous infections, contaminated fomites and water all represent important reservoirs of organisms that can infect wounds. It is worth emphasizing that the use of topical or systemic antibacterial agents that selectively suppress some organisms, may permit or induce the colonization and growth of other organisms resistant to such agents. This is especially true for gram–negative bacteria.

Clinically, bacterial infection of wounds, regardless of the offending organism or type of wound, usually presents with the same characteristic picture. Commonly, there is a spreading erythema of varying degree surrounding the wound. Streaks of erythema may extend from the area proximally, corresponding to efferent lymphatic channels. The patient usually feels pain, and tenderness is easily elicited by the examiner. Coincident warmth and swelling complete the inflammatory picture. A tender regional adenitis may also be present and fever is not uncommon.

Details of the basic pathophysiologic events of wound infection and the laboratory findings can be found elsewhere. See Chapters 9 and 12. The treatment of an infected wound involves both local and systemic approaches. If the wound can be treated adequately on a local basis, therapy may include appropriate local compresses, topical antibiotics

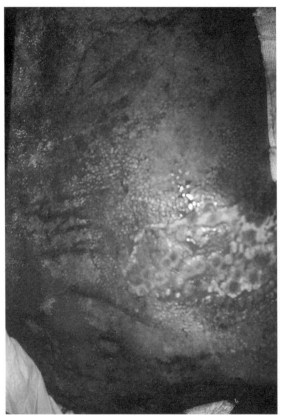

Figure 2. Opportunistic colonization of Penicillum sp. in healing erosive wounds of patients with toxic epidermal necrolysis.

Reprinted with permission from Journal of Geriatric Dermatology. Shelley WB, Shelley D, Kosarek C. Photovignette: Opportunistic mold colonization of toxic epidermal necrolysis. September 1995. © 1995, Health Management Publications, Inc.

and surgical intervention, e.g. debridement, incision and drainage. One must recall that in the pre–Fleming era, this type of therapy was all that practitioners had to offer (excluding topical agents). If there are signs of worsening infection, such as cellulitis, lymphangitis, fever and chills, appropriate oral or parenteral antibiotic therapy is indicated.

Other forms of pathogens may opportunistically invade the healing wound during susceptible periods as well. Viruses, especially Herpes simplex virus (HSV), can occasionally colonize the wound and can add a great deal of morbidity for the patient. For example, patients that undergo dermabrasion for facial scarring are highly susceptible to HSV wound infections either from autoinoculation or person to person contact. As a result, these patients are routinely treated prophylactically with oral acyclovir because the risk for HSV contamination is so high.

When infection does occur, the wounds are clustered with herpetic vesicles that tend to be very painful and render the wound even more susceptible to secondary bacterial infection of the types already discussed. Such wounds may heal with disfiguring and/or hypertrophic scars and can be chronically painful. These same complications are currently being encountered with the increasingly popular facial rejuvenation procedures using chemical peeling agents (Figure 1) or skin resurfacing carbon dioxide lasers.[5]

As mentioned above, fungal infection can compromise a wound at times. The predisposing influence is usually a weakened cell–mediated immunity and if left untreated, will result in less than optimal wound healing. More commonly, however, more aggressive and faster growing pathogens, such as bacteria, outcompete fungal organisms in the wound healing bed. Yeasts or molds must also be mentioned as possible opportunistic or secondary pathogens and can include *Candida*, *Aspergillus*, and *Penicillium* species (Figure 2).[6]

Because of the inherent risks of infection in any healing wound, whether from the myriad of bacterial invaders or the less frequent but still threatening viral and fungal pathogens, antiseptic precautions and ever–vigilant surveillance of clinical changes must be undertaken to assure uneventful and optimal healing.

Inflammatory Complications

Wounds cannot proceed to complete healing without the necessary cascade of inflammatory factors that contribute to the entire healing process. These components of inflammation and the steps by which they enter into healing are thoroughly detailed in other chapters in the text. In unusual circumstances, however, inflammation can, either by excess or a reactive process, effect the final healing result negatively. For example, the disfiguring facial scarring seen in acne conglobata, an intense and deep inflammatory form of acne, reflects the severity of the inflammation. Autoimmune diseases, including some of the blistering disorders of the skin, such as pemphigus vulgaris or bullous pemphigoid, may arise in sites of trauma or healing wounds and may thus interfere with normal healing.[7] Pemphigoid, especially, has been known to arise at enterostomal sites, complicating the routine care of these areas (Figure 3).

Degenerative Complications

Wound complications may also develop as a result of degenerative changes brought on by

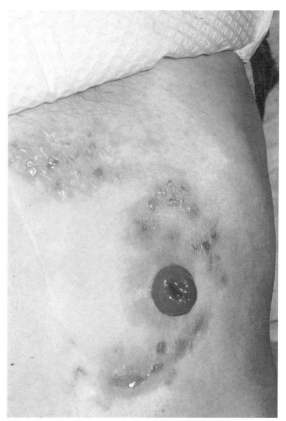

Figure 3. Erythematous bullous eruption surrounding colostomy site. Biopsy consistent with bullous pemphigoid.

intrinsic metabolic problems within the host. Diabetes mellitus and nutritional deficiencies are examples of such conditions. In addition, external influences, such as drugs or radiation, may similarly alter the healing of wounds.

Patients with diabetes, especially cases that are poorly controlled, more commonly experience delayed wound healing.[8] This likely stems from the associated poor nutrition and deficient wound oxygenation secondary to diabetic microangiopathic and connective tissue changes in the dermis. A more susceptible area for local wound infection is created. When these wounds finally do heal the resulting scars tend to be more atrophic and less acceptable cosmetically.

Nutritional deficiency states have long been known to hinder wound healing.[9] The influences of scurvy in vitamin C–deprived British sailors in the 17th century in the production of non–healing wounds and bleeding gums are well–known. Protein deficiency and other deficiencies of vitamins such as A, B, and K have also been amply documented in the literature as factors predisposing patients to poor wound healing.

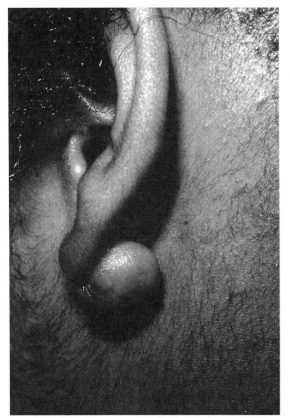

Figure 4a. Keloidal scarring posterior ear lobe resulting from pierced earrings.

Courtesy of Ernest Benedetto, MD, Drexel Hill, PA.

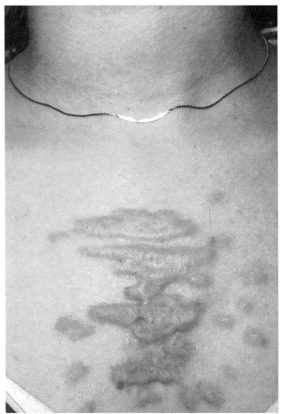

Figure 4b. Keloidal scarring overlying sternum.

Courtesy of Ernest Benedetto, MD, Drexel Hill, PA.

Certain medications can also impede wound healing.[10] Glucocorticoids are the most noteworthy among the drugs known to have such effects. The pathophysiologic changes in wounds caused by steroids are numerous and include decreased fibroblast proliferation, decreased collagen synthesis, altered neutrophil and macrophage chemotaxis, and retarded epidermal regeneration. The effects of other medications known to delay wound healing, such as anti–neoplastic drugs, anticoagulants, anti–inflammatory agents such as Cyclosporine A, Colchicine, and antiprostaglandins have been thoroughly reviewed elsewhere. Their actions on the healing process may be different, but the less than optimal end result is the same.

Patients who have been treated with radiation may also experience characteristic degenerative changes in and/or around their wounds, including atrophy, loss of hair, hypo– or hyperpigmentation and telangiectasia. Ulcers may develop in the treated area along with varying degrees of fibrosis.

Traumatic Complications

It is obvious that any trauma to a wound will delay healing. An accidental re–injury or the removal of a gauze dressing are common examples of such problems. A factitial injury caused by self–inflicted mutilation of a wound will also interfere with the skin's ability to repair itself. The resultant complications include a more disfiguring scar and the increase in morbidity imposed by longer healing time. Precautions must be taken to reduce the risk of trauma to a wound, but the inevitability of accidental injuries is recognized and physicians must be on guard for these unfortunate complications.

Neoplastic Complications

Rarer still are the unusual instances when a malignancy complicates a healing wound. Squamous cell carcinoma has been known to develop in ulcer beds (Marjolin's ulcer) as well as in burn scars, radiation treated skin and vaccination scars. Other tumors such as basal cell carcinomas and dermatofibrosarcoma protoberans have been known to arise in scars as well.

Proliferative Complications

The growth of granulation tissue is a normal phase of open wound healing and it presages reepithelialization. In certain circumstances, however, either because of trauma or hormonal influences, e.g. pregnancy, there is an overgrowth of granulation tissue. The lesion arising in these situations has been improperly termed "pyogenic granuloma." This term is incorrect because the lesion does not produce pus nor is it composed of granulomatous inflammation. It is however a local proliferation of highly vascularized connective tissue with a dense mixed inflammatory infiltrate consistent with granulation tissue. If this process is not corrected, reepithelialization cannot occur and wound healing cannot proceed normally.

Keloids and hypertrophic scars are other examples of wound tissue overgrowth.[12,13] (Figures 4a and 4b). Keloids can occur at any site of trauma or surgery but are most common on the shoulders, chest and back. The earlobe and scalp are other common sites of keloid formation that develop secondary to earlobe piercing or scalp folliculitis. The latter is seen more often in blacks. These lesions are inflamed, firm, disfiguring overgrowths of scar tissue and may extend well beyond the boundaries of the original injury. They are often pruritic and can be painful. Hypertrophic scars differ from keloids in that they generally stay within the confines of the original wound, are usually linear and are less bothersome symptomatically. Hypertrophic scars tend to soften or regress after six to nine months. The treatment of keloids is difficult and results are often disappointing. Intralesional corticosteroids, pressure garments and even radiation therapy have been used with varying success. The local application of a silicone sheet for several months has also been recommended for keloids and may even be used prophylactically if a keloidal tendency is known. Surgical removal of such lesions usually results in another, often larger, keloid and should be avoided.

Summary

Although uneventful healing is the usual course with most wounds, complications that delay or prevent healing occur occasionally and can present a significant challenge to the healthcare team. In this chapter, the possible cutaneous complications of healing wounds and their prevention and treatment are considered. Anticipation of impending untoward developments during healing should permit appropriate steps in management that will minimize or prevent such complications. Once present, these complications can be treated effectively if the fundamental principles governing the pathologic physiology are understood and corrective measures based on this understanding are instituted. With new knowledge and therapeutic approaches that derive therefrom, the treatment of abnormal healing wounds should improve still further in the years to come.

References

1. Clark RAF. Mechanisms of cutaneous repair. In: Fitzpatrick TB, et al. (ed). *Dermatology in General Medicine*. New York, NY, McGraw–Hill, Inc., 1993, pp 473–486.
2. Clark RAF. Cutaneous tissue repair: Basic biologic considerations, I. *J Am Acad Dermatol* 1985;13(5):701–725.
3. Reed BR, Clark RAF. Cutaneous tissue repair: Basic biologic considerations, II. *J Am Acad Dermatol* 1985;13(6):919–941.
4. Cohen IK, Diegelmann RF, Lindblad WJ (eds). *Wound Healing: Biochemical and Clinical Aspects*. Philadelphia, PA, W. B. Saunders, 1992.
5. Rapaport MJ, Kamer F. Exacerbation of facial herpes simplex after phenolic face peels. *J Dermatol Surg Oncol* 1984;10:57–58.
6. Shelley WB, Shelley D, Kosarek CA. Photovignette: Opportunistic mold infection of toxic epidermal necrolysis. *J Geriatric Derm* 1995;3(6):A15.
7. Salomon RH, Briggaman RA, Wernikoff SY, et al. Localized bullous pemphigoid. *Arch Dermatol* 1987;123:389–392.
8. Dchnider SL, Kohn RR. Effects of age and diabetes mellitus on the solubility of and non–enzymatic glcosylation of human skin collagen. *J Clin Invest* 1981;67:1630.
9. Pollack SV. Wound healing. A review III: Nutritional factors affecting wound healing. *J Dermatol Surg Oncol* 1979;5:615–619.
10. Pollack SV. Wound healing. A review IV: Systemic medications affecting wound healing. *J Dermatol Surg Oncol* 1982;8:667–672.
11. Burkhardt BR, et al. Dermatofibrosarcoma protuberans: A study of 56 cases. *Amer J Surg* 1966;111:638–44.
12. Murray JC, Pollack SV, Pinnell SR. Keloids: A review. *J Am Acad Dermatol* 1981;4:461.
13. Ketchum LD, Cohen ID, Masters IW. Hypertrophic scars and keloids. A collective review. *Plast Reconstr Surg* 1974;53:140.

25

Moisture Control and Incontinence Management

Diane Kaschak Newman, RNC, MSN, FAAN; Donald W. Wallace, MD and
Joyce Wallace, RNC, MSN, CRNP

Newman DK, Wallace DW, Wallace J. Moisture control and incontinence management. In: Krasner D, Kane D. *Chronic Wound Care, Second Edition*. Wayne, PA, Health Management Publications, Inc., 1997, pp 196–201.

Introduction

Healthcare providers have long suspected that a relationship exists between excessively moist skin, the development of pressure ulcers, and the presence of urinary and/or fecal incontinence. It is thought that moisture reduces the resistance of the skin to ulceration and infection and thus increases the risk of pressure ulcer formation. The evidence that such a cause and effect relationship is real is mounting, but is not yet clearly established. This chapter will discuss the known relationships between these conditions and provide information that leads to a more rational therapeutic approach to their treatment.

An Overview of Incontinence

Incontinence can be defined as the primary dysfunctional symptom of a disorder of the genitourinary or lower intestinal system that leads to the development of the involuntary loss or leakage of urine or fecal material, respectively. Urinary and fecal incontinence are very common among the elderly. Urinary incontinence can effect 10 to 35 percent of adults in the general population and about half of the patients in a nursing home or those receiving skilled nursing visits in their homes.[1] This disorder is more prevalent among women than among men and there is an increasing incidence of urinary incontinence with age. Urinary incontinence and fecal incontinence in the nursing home or home care setting often occur together and

are more severe than in patients who are in an ambulatory healthcare setting.[1] Incontinence is associated with increased morbidity and it has a major adverse social, psychological and economic impact on society.

The pathogenesis of urinary incontinence involves several factors. Most patients with urinary incontinence will suffer from either a gynecological, neuro–functional, or psycho–behavioral disorder as the underlying basis for their incontinence.[2] Fecal incontinence may be caused by bowel disease, obstruction, neurologic disorder or some other gastrointestinal malady.[1,3]

Urinary incontinence is difficult to treat in some patients, with the usual modes of treatment through either a behavioral, pharmacological, or surgical approach being of no benefit. Typically, such persons reside in long–term care facilities or are homebound and have cognitive or physical impairments that cannot allow them to learn or perform learned strategies which prevent urine leakage.[4] In long–term care facilities, this population is largely cared for by a nonprofessional nursing staff who may or may not be directly supervised by a registered nurse. Others are cared for at home, most often by family members. Currently, continence care for such persons usually involves management of the incontinence through the use of collection devices or containment by using disposable or reusable products, which may increase the risk of skin breakdown.

Fecal incontinence is the inability to control the expulsion of stool which results in the loss of feces at an inappropriate time and place. Fecal inconti- nence occurs in about one percent of elderly per- sons, but in nursing homes it has been reported in 23 to 66 percent of the residents. Although pressure ulcer formation is commonly seen in patients with incontinence, maintaining intact skin is a nursing care problem.

Incontinence and Pressure Ulcers

The role that incontinence plays in the develop- ment of pressure ulcers in patients is not yet ade- quately defined in terms of a clearly recognized and statistically significant clinically documented association with each other. But uncontrolled or poorly managed incontinence can lead to the pre- disposition of patients to skin irritation and subse- quently lead to the formation and inhibition of the healing of pressure ulcers.[5] Skin moisture and wet- ness from incontinence is a mediator for skin breakdown. Potential sources of excessive moisture on the skin include urinary incontinence, fecal incontinence, frequent washings, non–absorbent and/or poorly ventilated padding on the skin, and skin occlusion.

Because of the substantial increase in morbidity in patients with pressure ulcers [6–9] and a potential association of the development of pressure ulcers with incontinence, the need to adequately treat incontinence is very important. Unfortunately underemphasis is all too often placed on the signif- icance of aggressive treatment of incontinence in hospitalized, homebound or nursing home patients. Patients with incontinence and concurrent medical problems such as cerebrovascular acci- dents or myocardial infarctions are justifiably given more attention throughout the duration of the patient's healthcare provision. Of course, these con- current illnesses are serious and should receive the most urgent attention. However, predisposition of the skin to form pressure ulcers under excessively moist or wet conditions may cause further compli- cations in these patients if advanced stage pressure ulcers develop and require treatment.

Relationship Between Incontinence and Skin Breakdown

As mentioned earlier, the exact relationship between incontinence and the development of pressure ulcers has not been firmly established in a direct manner. The most compelling scientific and clinical support of a link between incontinence and pressure ulcers comes from the known relation between excessively moist or wet skin and the breakdown of the normal, healthy integrity of the

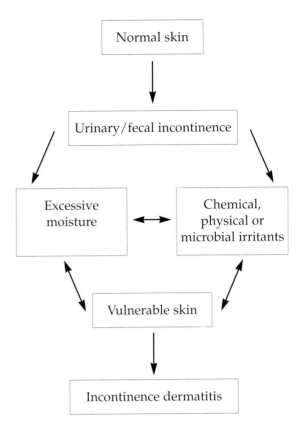

Figure 1. Proposed mechanism of incontinence dermatitis.

skin. The pathophysiology of the dermal injury caused by excessive moisture is itself not entirely understood but is believed to involve a very com- plex cascade of events that can act upon one anoth- er in a self perpetuating cycle (Figure 1).

Experimental data appears to demonstrate that fecal incontinence and its contact with the skin pro- vides evidence of a more direct connection between incontinence and skin irritation.[13,14] Both urinary and fecal incontinence occurring together may increase the risk for the development of pressure ulcers.

While the exact role that excessive moisture plays in the development of dermal injury is not entirely understood, it is believed to involve a com- plicated series of pathophysiologic events that con- tribute and/or cause the skin to breakdown and lead to loss of skin function and integrity. Normal skin has many protective homeostatic mechanisms that maintain its function as a barrier to external sources of attack, such as excessive moisture, microscopic organisms, mechanical disruptions, chemical irritants, or other forces. Excessive mois- ture contact with skin is believed to directly effect the skin's coefficient of skin friction.[12] A serious alteration of the skin's coefficient of friction can lead to increased skin chaffing, maceration, and thus, skin irritation and breakdown.[13]

The skin is usually slightly acidic. In normal healthy individuals, skin pH ranges from 4 to 6.8, with a mean of 5.5 pH.[13,14] The acidic pH is a major factor that helps to prevent colonization of the skin by microorganisms, particularly yeast and fungus. This factor is often referred to as the "protective acid mantle" of the skin. Furthermore, the presence of excessive skin surface moisture can contribute to microbial overgrowth. When combined with alteration in skin pH (into the alkaline range), the effect can be particularly devastating.[13]

absorbent products and the correct use of skin cleaners, protection creams, and powders, tools are available for supporting the management of urinary incontinence in chronically ill persons.[4] The judicious use of products to contain urine loss and maintain skin integrity is a first–line defense in these cases.

The Clinical Practice Guidelines for *Pressure Ulcers in Adults: Prediction and Prevention* defines a pressure ulcer as any lesion, loss of integrity to the skin or damage to underlying tissue that is caused by the presence of unrelieved pressure to the area of concern.[5] The guideline recommends that proper skin care should minimize the skin exposure to

---

There is no doubt that excessive moisture may make the skin more susceptible to skin irritation and inflammation, both of which have the potential to lead to pressure ulcers of the skin.

An alkaline pH of the skin is known to also adversely effect the normal keratinization of the skin, further enhancing the loss of normal skin integrity in the patient whose skin is already compromised by factors already considered.[14] When the patient's skin is subject to moisture from urine in combination with fecal incontinence, further alkalinization is produced by conversion of urea (from the urine) to ammonia by fecal bacteria. All of these factors, including skin maceration, skin alkalinization and increases in skin friction, are believed to work in concert to weaken the skin. Weakened skin, in turn, is more susceptible to irritation, breakdown and microbial infection, further weakening the skin. This is a self–perpetuating cycle of events (Figure 1) which can predispose the skin to pressure ulcer formation.

Treatment Considerations

Although the precise mechanism and connection between incontinence and pressure ulcers is still under investigation, it remains very important to control the moisture and wetness on the skin of chronically ill, frail, immobilized patients. There is no doubt that excessive moisture may make the skin more susceptible to skin irritation and inflammation, both of which have the potential to lead to pressure ulcers of the skin. According to the 1996 AHCPR Clinical Practice Guideline Update, *Urinary Incontinence in Adults: Acute & Chronic Management*, with the continued improvement of

moisture due to incontinence. Every effort must be made to maintain a normal amount of moisture and humidity at the surface of the skin. For patients with pressure ulcers that are believed to be associated with incontinence, the ideal strategy for treating them may involve a combination of aggressive incontinence and skin care management. Depending on the etiology of the incontinence and the stage of the pressure ulcer, management of the incontinence may involve a combination of strategies, for example, behavioral therapy with pharmacological therapy and diet management or a surgical procedure. In addition, an increase in the frequency of absorbent product changes may be required to help keep a patient's skin away from excessive moisture contact.

In terms of skin care management, the approach to dealing with the prevention and treatment of pressure ulcers and patients with incontinence should focus on the proper use of appropriate skin products, topical antimicrobials (when indicated), gentle pH balanced cleansers, correct barrier products and effective use of incontinence pads. It is also important to select skin care products which are non–irritating, non–sensitizing and pH balanced. It should be noted that FDA does not require manufacturers of skin care products to document that their products are indeed non–irritating, non–sensitizing and pH balanced. Such testing is completely voluntary and not always conducted. When in doubt, ask the manufacturers to provide written documentation of such testing.

NEWMAN, ET AL.

4. Fantl JA, Newman DK, Colling J, et al. *Urinary Incontinence in Adults: Acute and Chronic Management.* Clinical Practice Guideline, No. 2, 1996 Update, Rockville, MD: US Department of Health and Human Services. Public Health Service, Agency for Health Care Policy and Research, AHCPR Publication No. 96–0682. March 1996.

5. Bergstrom N, Bennett MA, Carlson CE, et al. *Treatment of Pressure Ulcers.* Clinical Practice Guideline, No. 15. AHCPR Publication No. 95–0652. Rockville (MD): US Department of Health and Human Services. Public Health Service, Agency for Health Care Policy and Research;   December 1994.

6. Bergstrom N, Braden B. A prospective study of pressure sore risk among institutionalized patients. *J American Geriatric Society* 1992;40:747–758.

7. Brandeis GH, Morris JN, Nash DJ, Lipsitz LA. The epidemiology and natural history of pressure ulcers in elderly nursing home residents. *JAMA* 1990;264(22):2905–2909.

8. Allman RM, Laprade CA, Noel LB, et al. Pressure sores among hospitalized patients. *Annals of Internal Medicine* 1986;105: 337–342.

9. Berlowitz DR, Van B, Wilking S. Risk factors for pressure sores – A comparison of cross sectional and cohort derived data. *J American   Geriatrics Society* 1989;37:1043–1050.

10. Berg RW. Etiologic factors in diaper dermatitis: A model for development of improved diapers. *Pediatrician* 1987;14 suppl(1):27–33.

11. Berg RW, Buckingham KW, Stewart RL. Etiologic factors in diaper dermatitis: The role of urine. *Pediatric Dermatology* 1986;3(2):102–106.

12. Zimmerer RE, Lawson KD, Calvert CJ. The effects of wearing diapers on skin. *Pediatric Dermatology* 1986;3(2):95–101.

13. Berg RW. Etiology and pathophysiology of diaper dermatitis. *Advances in Dermatology* 1988;3:75–98.

14. Bryant R, Wysocki A. *Acute and Chronic Wounds: Nursing Management.* St. Louis, MO, Mosby Year Book, Inc. 1992.

15. Jeter K, Lutz J. Skin care in the incontinence patient. *Journal for Prevention and Healing Advances in Wound Healing* 1996;9(1):29–34.

16. Grove G, Lutz JB, Burtin SA, Tucker JA. Assessment of diaper clogging potential of petrolatum–based skin barriers. Poster presentation at the Multi–Specialty Nursing Conference on Urinary Continence. Phoenix, AZ, 1994.

26

When a Wound Isn't a Wound: Tubes, Drains, Fistulae, and Draining Wounds

Nancy A. Faller, RN, MSN, CETN

Faller NA. When a wound isn't a wound: Tubes, drains, fistulae and draining wounds. In: Krasner D, Kane D. *Chronic Wound Care, Second Edition*. Wayne, PA, Health Management Publications, Inc., 1997, pp 202–208.

Introduction

Tubes, drains, fistulae, and draining wounds, at first glance, seem to have nothing in common. However, on closer scrutiny, it becomes apparent that there is in fact a link: skin and tissue integrity. With each of these conditions — tubes, drains, fistulae, and draining wounds — an underlying nursing priority is prevention of altered skin and tissue integrity at the stoma, os, or opening.

This chapter investigates both the demographics and the associated risk factors of these conditions collectively as well as the management options for these conditions individually. The demographics section explores the issues related to the location of the tube, drain, fistulae, or draining wound, as well as the risks to skin and tissue integrity. The management section explores the modalities available for skin protection as well as other condition specific considerations. In addition, these nursing interventions address the nursing goals of monitoring intake/output by containing drainage for measurement, maintaining patient comfort by containing odor, and minimizing healthcare expenditures by containing cost.

Demographics

Tubes. Tubes may be placed in the gastrointestinal (GI) tract, in the genitourinary (GU) tract, or in an abscess cavity or space. Tubes may be placed for one of two reasons: input or output. Input tubes are placed for the input of feedings (GI), irrigations, or medications. Output tubes are placed for drainage. Tubes are identified by the organ or cavity they enter. Some examples of GI tubes are esophagostomy tubes, gastrostomy tubes, jejunostomy tubes, cecostomy tubes, and biliary tubes. Some examples of GU tubes are nephrostomy tubes, ureterostomy tubes, and vesicostomy tubes. Some examples of abscess tubes are pancreatic tubes, peritoneal tubes, and pleural tubes.

Drains. Drains may be placed following any surgical procedure. They promote drainage of serous or purulent exudate. Drains are frequently placed during incision and drainage (I&D) procedures.

Fistulae. Fistulae are abnormal openings between one hollow organ and the skin or between two hollow organs. Both of these types of fistulae present risks for altered skin and tissue integrity. Fistulae which communicate between one hollow organ and the skin are called external or cutaneous fistulae. Fistulae which communicate between two hollow organs are called internal fistulae.

Like tubes, fistulae are identified by the organs involved. Some examples of external fistulae are colo–cutaneous fistulae and vesico–cutaneous fistulae. Some examples of internal fistulae are colo–vesical fistulae, colo–vaginal fistulae, vesico–colic fistulae, and vesico–vaginal fistulae. Although the latter group are "internal" fistulae, they frequently drain through the anatomic perineal orifices. This drainage often presents a situation of fecal or urinary incontinence.

Draining wounds. Draining wounds include any wound with excessive drainage which can not be contained with conventional dressings or which

Table 1
Methods of Skin Protection and Tube Stabilization

Reference	Equipment	Manufacturer	Change Interval	Cost per Week*
Conwill J[a]	Sure–fit wafer $1^{3}/_{4}$ x 4 x 4 Sure–fit convex insert $1^{1}/_{2}$ x $1^{1}/_{8}$ Tape, adhesive 1 x 10 Tape, paper 1 x 8	ConvaTec (reuse)	5 to 7 days	$5.52
Davis B[b]	Stomahesive 2 x 2 (Comfeel 2 x 2)	ConvaTec (Coloplast)	7 days	$.84 ($1.37)
Fitzgerald J[c]	Stomahesive 3 x 3 SkinPrep wipe Alcohol pad Tape, paper 1 x 6	ConvaTec Smith+Nephew United	7 days	$2.35
	SkinPrep wipe (Skin gel wipe) Tape, Microfoam 3 x 8 Gauze, split 4 x 4	Smith+Nephew United (Hollister) 3M	3 x week	+$2.49 =$4.84
Gillen P[d]	Sure–fit wafer $1^{1}/_{2}$ x 4 x 4 Sure–fit convex insert $1^{1}/_{2}$ x $^{7}/_{8}$ SkinPrep wipe Baby bottle nipple Tape, adhesive 1 x 3 Tape, paper 1 x 20	ConvaTec (reuse) Smith+Nephew United (reuse) Water soluble lubricant, packet	1 to 2 x week	$6.58
Guidos B[e]	DuoDerm 4 x 4 x 2 Skin gel Gause 4 x 4 Povidone–iodine swab Tape, paper 1 x 56	ConvaTec Hollister	not specified	$12.04 each
Hogan K, Van Rensselser L[f]	Stomahesive 4 x 4 Tube anchor Dermastik SkinPrep wipe	ConvaTec Kells (reuse) Smith+Nephew United	5 to 7 days	$4.22
McKee C, Sherr S[g]	ReliaSeal 2 x 2 Gauze 4 x 4 Skin sealant Tape, paper 2 x 8	Bard	1 x week	$5.36 each
Powers M, et al.[h]	Drain/tube attachment device	Hollister	6.3 days (wear time)	$8.23
			p.r.n.	$7.39 each

Table 1
Methods of Skin Protection and Tube Stabilization *(continued)*

Reference	Equipment	Manufacturer	Change Interval	Cost per Week*
Sage S[i]	Transparent adhesive dressing 6 x 8 Gauze 4 x 4 x 2 Suction catheter tubing			
VanDriel J[j]	Stomahesive 4 x 4 SkinPrep wipe Peri–Wash Gauze 4 x 4 x 4 Bacitracin ointment packet Povidone–iodine wipe Tape, paper 1 x 56	ConvaTec Smith+Nephew United Sween	4 to 5 days	$7.47
Faller N, Lawrence K[k–m]	Lyofoam 2 x 2 (from 6 x 8) Molnar disc Hypafix tape 4 x 4	Acme United Smith+Nephew United VPI/Cook (reuse)	7 days	$1.47

Bibliography

a. Conwill J: Management of long–term percutaneous catheters. *J Enterostom Ther* 1986;13(4):163–164.
b. Davis B: Effective and inexpensive management of a PEG tube. *Ostomy/Wound Management* 1989;24:62–65.
c. Fitzgerald J: Hospital and home care of sutureless percutaneous catheters. *Ostomy/Wound Management* 1989;25:42–45.
d. Gillen P: Stabilizing a gastrostomy tube. *J Enterostom Ther* 1983;10(3):108–110.
e. Guidos B: Preparing the patient for home care of the percutaneous nephrostomy tube. *J Enterostom Ther* 1988;15(5):187–190.
f. Hogan K, Van Rensselser L: An improved method of anchoring a gastrostomy tube. *Nutritional Support Services* 1983;8(3):12–14.
g. McKee C, Sherr S: Maintaining percutaneous nephrostomy catheters and the management of intractable leakage at the insertion site. *J Enterostom Ther* 1987;14(3):125–128.
h. Powers M, Brant R, Anderson M, Kissil M: A clinical report on the comparison of a drain/tube attachment device with conventional suture methods in securing percutaneous tubes and drains. *J Enterostom Ther* 1988;15(5):206–209.
i. Sage S: Nephrostomy dressing change procedure. *Ostomy/Wound Management* 1991;32:32–36.
j. VanDriel J: Care of the percutaneous nephrostomy tube. *J Enterostom Ther* 1986;13(6):246–248.
k. Faller N, Lawrence K: *Clinical Case Updates: Selected case studies of wounds treated with Lyofoam.* Acme United Corporation 1991;2(3):1–4.
l. Faller N, Lawrence K: How to stabilize a percutaneous tube. *Nursing* 1992;22(7):52–54.
m. Faller N, Lawrence K: Stabilizing a percutaneous nephrostomy catheter or suprapubic tube. *Urol Nursing* 1992;12(3):115–116.

can be contained with conventional dressings but require frequent changes and use an excessive amount of nursing time. Some examples of draining wounds are abcess cavities or spaces, exophitic tumors, and necrotic ulcers.

Risk factors associated with demographics.

Gastrointestinal tract. The risk of altered skin integrity in the GI tract is contingent on the location of the tube or fistulae. Active enzymes, such as salivary enzymes, gastric enzymes, small bowel enzymes, pancreatic enzymes, or biliary enzymes, will traumatize intact skin.

Genitourinary tract. The risk of altered skin integrity in the GU tract is maceration. As opposed to the GI tract, the intensity of this risk does not depend on the location in the GU tract.

Abscess cavities or spaces. The risk of altered skin integrity in abscess cavities or spaces is contingent on the type of drainage. Lymphatic, dissolving hematoma, or abscess drainage is usually macerating.

Table 2
Policy and Procedure for Applying Stabilizing Disc
(VPI Silicone Disc Placement: Biliary, Gastrostomy, Nephrostomy, or Supra–Pubic Tubes)

Policy:
Biliary, gastrostomy, nephrostomy, or supra–pubic tubes will be stabilized with a VPI silicone disc, on physician's order, by an ET nurse or GI nurse.
Stabilizing discs will not be removed from biliary or nephrostomy tubes.
Stabilizing discs may be removed from gastrostomy or supra–pubic tubes 8 wks post insertion, on physician's order.

Purpose:
To prevent displacement of the percutaneous biliary or nephrostomy tube.
To prevent displacement of the percutaneous gastrostomy or supra–pubic vesicostomy tube until the tract has matured.

Equipment:
wash cloth
tap water
VPI silicone disc, the same or one size smaller than the tube
VPI tie
2 x 2 foam dressing (LyoFoam®, Acme United Corporation, Fairfield, CT)
scissors
4 x 4 stretch cloth tape (Hypafix*, Smith & Nephew United, Inc.)

Procedure:
1.   Wash hands
2.   Place patient in supine position
3.   Slit foam dressing to middle; slit stretch cloth tape to middle & cut out $1/4$" circle.
4.   Position patient semi–sitting.
5.   Wash & dry para tube skin.
6.   Remove sutures if present, tube should not move more than $1/4$", in or out. Do not let go of tube/disc until tape in place.
7.   Apply foam dressing around tube, against skin, smooth, shiny side down.
8.   Apply disc around tube, on top of foam dressing.
9.   Apply tie around disc in groove of collar and ratchet tight.
10.   Hold disc down and gently check that there is no movement of tube, by gently pushing in.
11.   Remove backing from stretch cloth tape & apply over disc.

However, abscess drainage from the pancreas can be extremely caustic if it contains pancreatic enzymes.

Tubes, drains, fistulae, or draining wounds which communicate with the pleural cavity may present an additional problem. If the skin opening communicates with a functioning lung, there may be an air leak which must be factored for in planning management.

Tubes

Besides the goal of skin protection, tubes must be stabilized to prevent their displacement. Skin protection and tube stabilization may be accomplished in a number of ways (Table 1). In one study, the method described by Faller and Lawrence[1–3] was shown to be the most cost effective.[4] This method utilizes a foam dressing (Lyofoam®, Acme United Corporation, Fairfield, CT), a silicone disc (MolnarDisc, Cook Urological / VPI, Spencer, IN), and stretch tape (Hypafix*, Smith+Nephew United, Inc., Largo, FL) (Plate 23, Tables 2 and 3). The skin is protected by the foam dressing, which absorbs caustic or macerating drainage. The tube is stabilized by the disc and the stretch tape. The use of a nonadherent foam allows the dressing to be easily changed by the patient, family member, or caregiver. Commercial devices are available. Unfortunately, none of them provide a mechanism for absorbing drainage, thus limiting their application.

Table 3
Policy and Procedure for Changing Foam Dressing
(Dressing Change: Biliary, Gastrostomy, Nephrostomy, or Supra–Pubic Tubes)

Policy:
Biliary, gastrostomy, nephrostomy, or supra–pubic tube dressings will be changed 48 hours after insertion, to inspect insertion site, by ET nurse or GI nurse .
Gastrostomy & supra–pubic vesicostomy tube dressings will be changed once a week x 8 wks post insertion.
Biliary tube or nephrostomy dressings will be changed once a week.
Biliary, gastrostomy, nephrostomy, or supra–pubic tube dressings will be changed if leaking.

Purpose:
To prevent displacement of the percutaneous biliary or nephrostomy tube.
To prevent displacement of the percutaneous gastrostomy or supra–pubic vesicostomy tube until the tract has matured.
To protect the skin.

Equipment:
wash cloth
tap water
2 x 2 foam dressing (LyoFoam®, Acme United Corporation, Fairfield, CT)
scissors
4x4 stretch cloth tape (Hypafix*, Smith & Nephew United, Inc.)

Procedure:
1.   Wash hands
2.   Place patient in supine position
3.   Slit foam dressing to middle; slit stretch cloth tape to middle.
4.   Remove old tape & foam dressing carefully; stabilizing disc/bolster should not move more than $1/4$", in or out. Do not let go of disc/bolster until tape in place.
5.   Wash & dry under the disc/bolster, lifting only one side at a time; again, stabilizing disc/bolster should not move more than $1/4$", in or out.
6.   Slide new foam dressing under disc/bolster, smooth, shiny side down.
7.   Remove backing from stretch cloth tape & apply over disc/bolster.

As well as stabilizing the tube at skin level, it is necessary to stabilize the tube at the opposite or free end. This additional stabilization provides a second safeguard against accidental tube displacement. Tape may suffice for the purpose of stabilization; however, commercial devices are available. There are two types: those which allow access to the opposite or free end of the tube and those which do not. Choice will be dictated by the need to access the opposite or free end of the tube for feedings, irrigations, or drainage. As with other wound products, it is necessary to read the directions carefully. Therefore, specific intricacies of a device should be known before use is attempted in a clinical situation (Table 4).

Tubes and Drains

When the drainage around a tube or a drain cannot be contained with the previously described foam dressing method or with any other other conventional dressing system, the tube or the drain must be pouched. Management is divided into two situations: simple pouching, where the tube or drain does not need to be accessed, and complex pouching, where the tube or drain must be accessed for feedings, irrigations, drainage, or movement in or out.

Pouching simple. Simple pouching is used when the drainage around a tube or a drain can not be contained with a dressing and the tube or the drain does not need to be accessed. The tube or

Table 4
Commercial Devices for Stabilizing the Opposite or Free End of a Tube

Cath–secure®, MC Johnson, Naples, FL
Feeding tube attachment device®, Hollister Inc., Libertyville, IL
Flexi–trak®, ConvaTec, Princeton, NJ
Horizontal tube attachment device®, Hollister Inc., Libertyville, IL
NG Strip®, Genetic Laboratories, St. Paul, MN
Suction tube attachment device®, Hollister Inc., Libertyville, IL

the drain is pouched with a urostomy pouch (versus a drainable pouch). The spigot opening on a urostomy pouch facilitates emptying liquid drainage (versus the wide clip opening on a drainable pouch, which is suitable for more viscous material).

In cases where the opposite or free end of the tube is large or where the drain has pins, it is best to leave the paper backing in place when applying the pouch. The paper backing is slit and the pouch is applied over the tubes or drains. After the pouch is in position the paper backing is removed prior to sealing the system to the skin (Plates 24 and 25).

Pouching complex. Complex pouching is used when the drainage around a tube or a drain can not be contained with a dressing and the tube or the drain does need to be accessed. Pouching modalities are different for tubes and drains.

Pouching tubes. If a tube must be accessed for feedings or irrigations, it is necessary to exit the tube through the side of the pouch. This can be accomplished in a number of ways. The first and least expensive option is to use a hydrocolloid wafer. Two 1" x 1" "buttons" are placed on the inside and on the outside of the pouch, at the desired exit site, directly over each other. A hemostat is used to pierce the hydrocolloid–pouch–hydrocolloid sandwich from outside to inside. The hemostat is then used to grasp the free end of the tube, pulling it back through the pouch. The opening in the pouch can be caulked with a hydrocolloid paste, before sealing it with waterproof tape. (Plate 26).

A second option for exiting a tube through a pouch is the use of a baby bottle nipple. The nipple is attached to the pouch with an upside down "convex flange" insert (Plate 27) or with tape. The tube is then passed through the nipple using the technique previously described for hydrocolloids.

The third option for exiting a tube through a pouch is the use of a commercial exit port. The previous caveat on reading instructions applies also to these devices. If tube access is only needed on an

intermittent basis, the modality for pouching drains (discussed in the next section) may be considered.

Pouching drains. If a drain must be accessed for movement in/out or for irrigations, a two piece or window pouching system is indicated. There are a number of commercial choices for both two piece and window pouching systems, both with and without attached solid, hydrocolloid skin barriers.

Fistulae

Fistulae are managed based on typology. External or cutaneous fistulae are pouched or suctioned. Internal fistulae are drained.

External or cutaneous fistulae. Besides the goal of skin protection around external, cutaneous fistulae, clinicians may wish to collect GI effluent for refeeding. Techniques for replacing nutrients have been described in the literature.[5,6]

Pouching external fistulae. The management of external cutaneous fistulae is the same as the simple pouching system previously described for tubes and drains. However, the wide clip opening on a drainable pouch will be needed for fistulae in the lower GI tract, if thick drainage does not flow freely through the spigot opening on a urostomy pouch.

On many occasions, fistulae open into an abdominal wound or onto an abnormal location where pouching is hindered by a less than level (i.e. concave or scarred) surface. In these two situations, molds may be considered to flatten the skin surface, thus facilitating pouch application.[7]

Suctioning external fistulae. In addition to pouching external, cutaneous fistulae, suctioning has been described.[8–11] This system drains the effluent immediately drawing the enzymes away from the granulating wound and reportedly speeding the rate of wound contraction. This system creates a vacuum seal with a transparent adhesive dressing. The system must be checked after application to assure that adequate suction has actually been achieved or the seal will quickly undermine.

Internal or perineal fistulae. The goal of managing internal, perineal fistulae is to collect the stool or urine preventing contact with the skin. A number of options have been described in the literature.

Draining internal fistulae. The first option is the use of a catheter in the bladder, vagina, or rectum.[12] The use of a catheter in the rectum has been discouraged in all but terminal cases as the risk of traumatizing the continence mechanism becomes apparent.

The second option is for use with vaginal fistulae. A diaphragm or pessary attached to a catheter is inserted in the vagina.[13,14] The fistulae must be proximal to the level of the cervix and the diaphragm must be fitted by a gynecologic practitioner.

The third option is also for use with vaginal fistulae. A Bardic® Uro–Sheath® (Bard Patient Care Division, Murray Hill, NJ) is inverted, attached to straight drainage, then inserted in the vagina[15] (Plate 28). Again, as previously noted, the fistulae must be proximal to the level of the cervix.

The fourth and final option is also for use with vaginal fistulae. A flexible, ostomy pouch can be applied to the perineum.[16] Conversely the Female Incontinence Pouch (Hollister, Libertyville, IL) could be considered. It must be fitted carefully over the vaginal and urethral opening and attached to straight drainage to prevent leakage. The previous caveat on reading instructions is again appropriate.

Draining Wounds

Draining wounds are managed with a pouching system. The principles suggested in the Tubes and Drains section again apply. The use of a urostomy pouch with a spigot for drainage facilitates emptying.

Summary

The primary nursing goal in the management of tubes, drains, fistulae, and draining wounds is the preservation of skin and tissue integrity at the stoma, os, or opening. The secondary nursing goals are to monitor intake/output by containing drainage for measurement, to maintain patient comfort by containing odor, and to minimize healthcare expenditures by containing cost. The nursing interventions described in this chapter allow the nurse to meet both the primary and the secondary nursing goals.

References

1. Faller NA, Lawrence KG. How to stabilize a percutaneous tube. *Nursing* 1992;22(7):52–54.
2. Faller NA, Lawrence KG. Stabilizing a percutaneous nephrostomy catheter or suprapubic tube. *Urologic Nursing* 1992;12(3):115–116.
3. Faller NA, Lawrence KG. Selected case studies of wounds treated with Lyofoam. *Clinical Case Updates* (Acme United) 1991;2(3):1–4.
4. Faller NA, Lawrence KG. Hold that tube ... cost effectively. *Ostomy Wound Management* 1992;38(9):37–40.
5. Blaylock B, Murray M. A jejunal fistula in a granulating wound and jenunal refeeding. *Ostomy Wound Management* 1992;38(6):8–14.
6. Baranoski S, Polyak E. Management of patients with a tracheoesophageal fistula. *Ostomy Wound Management* 1987;16(fall):34–37.
7. Smith DB. Abdominal fistulas. *Journal of ET Nursing* 1984;11(3):116–121.
8. Harris A, Komray RR. Cost–effective management of pharyngocutaneous fistulas following laryngectomy. *Ostomy Wound Management* 1993;39(8):36–44.
9. Faller NA, Zanella A. Management of an enterocutaneous fistula in Uruguay. *WCET Journal* 1991;11(2):36–37.
10. Jeter KF, Tintle TE, Chariker M. Managing draining wounds and fistulae: New and established methods. In: Krasner D (ed). *Chronic Wound Care: A Clinical Source Book for Healthcare Professionals.* King of Prussia, PA, Health Management Publications, Inc, 1990, pp 240–246.
11. Wooding–Scott M, Montgomery BA, Coleman D. No wound is to big for resourceful nurses. *RN* 1988;51(12):22–25.
12. Smith DB. Abdominal fistulas. *Journal of ET Nursing* 1984;11(3):116–121.
13. Grogan JL, Wells PR. A nursing intervention for intractable incontinence. *Journal of ET Nursing* 1993;20(5):228.
14. Fitzgerald J. Vaginal fistulas: one method of management. *Journal of ET Nursing* 1982;9(5):25.
15. Guidos B, Folkedahl B. Options in practice: Perineal skin protection with an enterovaginal fistula. *Journal of ET Nursing* 1993;20(5):220–221.
16. North A. Nursing management of an enterovaginal fistula. *Ostomy Wound Management* 1985;8(Summer):12–13.

Suggested Reading

1. Clemence BJ. Innovative nursing for a "worst case" wound. *RN* 1981;44(7):20–24.
2. Felice MM. Draining wound management: Techniques for skin preservation. In: Krasner D (ed). *Chronic Wound Care: A Clinical Source Book for Healthcare Professionals.* King of Prussia, PA, Health Management Publications, Inc, 1990, pp 247–252.
3. Irrgang S, Bryant R. Management of the enterocutaneous fistula. *Journal of ET Nursing* 1984;11(6):211–225.
4. Jackson BS, Powers ML, Rush–Martin C, Hedrick J, Laughton N, Kissil MT. A case control clinical trial of two wound drainage collection systems. *Journal of ET Nursing* 1988;15(5):191–195.
5. Krasner D. Managing draining wounds: fistulae, leaking tubes, and drains. *Ostomy Wound Management* 1988;19:79–85.
6. McClees N. A method of pouching a paracentesis or incision and drainage site prior to the procedure. *Journal of ET Nursing* 1984;11(3):198.
7. Tonn J. Management of fistula care with a wound drainage collector. *Journal of ET Nursing* 1988;15(2):87–90.
8. Schaffner A, Hocevar BJ, Erwin–Toth P. Options in practice: Small bowel fistulas complicating midline surgical wounds. *Journal of ET Nursing* 1994;21(4):161–165.
9. Wessel L. Management of a wound with multiple drains. *Journal of ET Nursing* 1989;16(1):26–28.

27

Management of Deterioration in Cutaneous Wounds

Bonnie Sue Rolstad, RN, BA, CETN and Ann Harris, MSN, RN, CS

Rolstad BS, Harris A. Management of deterioration in cutaneous wounds. In: Krasner D, Kane D. *Chronic Wound Care, Second Edition*. Wayne, PA, Health Management Publications, Inc., 1997, pp 209–218.

Introduction

Whether acute or chronic, wounds require close scrutiny to monitor for signs of impaired healing or problems in clinical care. Wound deterioration indicates the need for timely re–evaluation and treatment. Not all wounds will heal since some factors that impede wound healing are not correctable. In these situations, nonhealing wounds or wound decline are the expected outcomes. This chapter discusses the importance of ongoing patient and wound evaluation, identifies factors that negatively affect the wound and explores clinical management approaches for wounds that are under treatment and in declining status.

Recognizing Deterioration

Deterioration is a negative course. While all wounds are at risk for deterioration, the extent and duration of decline varies. In pressure ulcers, deterioration is a failure to heal, as shown by wound enlargement that is not brought about by debridement.[1] Clinically, a decline in wound condition may also be demonstrated by dehiscence, increased odor, increased exudate, onset of tunneling or undermining, wound base or edge tissue necrosis, periwound skin maceration or inflammation, to identify a few. A deteriorating wound is distinguished from the static wound in that deterioration results in further tissue destruction, while the static wound remains unchanged.

Re–Evaluation of Wounds

Wound care is designed based upon knowledge of the patient, an understanding of the physiology of wound healing, and the clinician's expertise in the management of wounds. Wounds require systemic and local conditions that promote healing or avoid further tissue deterioration. The patient requires comprehensive evaluation, individualization and education as the approach to care is developed.

When a wound is deteriorating, several issues need to be examined. If the host is severely compromised or in a hospice program, deterioration may be the expected outcome. Conversely, in a healthy patient, a deteriorating wound is not the expected outcome. However, both types of patients need to be re–evaluated. The following discussion explains the use of an interventional model that provides an orderly construct during re–evaluation of the wound in deterioration (Figure 1).

Patient assessment may be comprehensive or brief depending upon the degree of wound decline. A medical history and exam may be indicated and should include a history of the wound chronicity and recurrence. A nutritional evaluation, hematologic workup, vascular studies or radiological studies may also be indicated. Wound assessment includes measurement of height, width, depth, tunneling or undermining as well as attention to other key criteria. Wound base characteristics are addressed noting in percentages the amount of granular tissue, slough and eschar present. The type of exudate (serous, serosanguinous, or purulent) and estimated amount are noted. Of particular

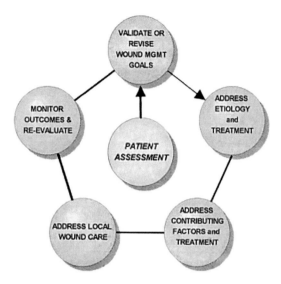

Figure 1. Interventional model for management of deterioration in wounds

Table 1
Contributing Factors in Wound Deterioration

<u>Extrinsic factors</u>

- Concomitant illness (e.g. diabetes, COPD, distant malignancy, lupus erythematosus, rheumatoid arthritis)
- Pharmacologics (e.g. glucocorticoid steroids, chemotherapeutic agents)
- Malnutrition
- Advanced age
- Obesity

<u>Intrinsic factors</u>

- Ischemia
- Wound infection
- Venous stasis
- Non–viable tissue/foreign bodies
- Mechanical trauma
- Radiation
- Malignancy
- Non–physiologial wound care

importance is the onset of increased exudation (in the absence of autolytic debridement) or malodorous exudate. The periwound skin is evaluated for induration, warmth, erythema, maceration and candidiasis.

An interview with the patient and caregiver is essential. The discussion focuses upon how wound care procedures are being performed and any problems encountered. In many situations, the patient is the caregiver. However, if there is another person providing the care, that individual should be included. The patient and caregiver are sometimes considered "silent partners" in wound care. However, lack of inclusion of these partners may tip the scale from success to failure.

Goals in wound management are established based on patient assessment including assessment of general health, values, lifestyle and the caregiver. As conditions change, the goal of management may change. There are three general goals or outcomes in wound management: healing, maintenance and symptom control. While healing is the preferred biologic outcome, wound maintenance or symptom control may be realistic goals when the patient is severely compromised.

Understanding the condition of the host and the potential for healing provides the benchmark to establish anticipated outcomes for the wound. In the healthy host, the goal is usually healing. These patients are generally evaluated and treated more aggressively because of the potential for wound closure. Moist wound healing and debridement generally provide the foundation for management with adjunctive therapy that may include aggressive

nutritional support, vascular surgery, electrical stimulation, hyperbaric oxygen, biologic dressings or growth factors.

However, the compromised host may have limited healing potential because of a multiplicity of risk factors, some of which may not be correctable (Table 1). In these cases, the expected outcome for the wound may be delayed healing, maintenance or symptom control. An example of wound maintenance as the expected outcome of wound care is demonstrated in the inoperative patient with arterial disease who has a distal toe ulcer. These types of wounds may exist for years. The plan of care includes infection control, pain management, and simple, cost–effective topical wound management.

When symptom control is the management goal, wound care objectives are directed toward infection control, odor management, pain control and unintrusive care. The terminal host with a wound may be in a hospice program and severely compromised. Living life fully and as comfortably as possible is the philosophy. Hence, the treatment plan is usually conservative. Remarkably, wounds do heal in the final phases of life. However, the more frequently expected outcome is a nonhealed or deteriorating wound (Figure 2).

Reconsideration of current management, etiology, and contributing factors of the wound is also undertaken. Review of the patient's general health

ROLSTAD AND HARRIS

status may have revealed a general decline or a previously undetected diagnosis, such as a malignancy, anemia or diabetes that requires medical treatment. In some cases, concomitant health problems exist as in the case of the insulin–dependent diabetic who also requires steroids for rheumatoid arthritis. These factors inhibit wound healing and may result in nonhealing or contribute to wound deterioration. The care plan for a patient with a sacral pressure ulcer may have omitted interventions to decrease shear forces, which are a contributing factor in pressure ulcer development. The revised care plan would incorporate proper seating and transferring techniques. Elimination of the etiology and contributing factors is not always possible. However, with a limited correction of these factors, healing or a halt to deterioration may result.

As conditions within the wound change, modification or validation of local wound care treatments is indicated. The underlying cause of decline may be straightforward, as demonstrated by tissue necrosis secondary to desiccation of the local wound environment. A hydrating wound dressing may be the only change required to debride necrotic tissue and restore a granular wound base.

However, the diabetic patient with peripheral vascular disease and a deteriorating foot ulcer may require an interdisciplinary team including a surgeon, orthotist, and diabetic educator in addition to the primary medical physician and wound care specialist. Strategies for problem–solving vary depending upon the problem, its complexity and goal for management. A deteriorating wound may exhibit tunneling or tracts. This new characteristic usually indicates the need for a wound packing dressing (e.g. impregnated or plain strip gauze, calcium alginate). Wounds in declining status are frequently more odorous with increased exudate. They may become clinically infected.

Dressings alone do not heal wounds. The host must provide the resources necessary for wound healing or to ward off infection. However, dressings and wound care techniques can optimize healing. Careful selection and use of dressings can reduce healing time and the incidence of infection.[2]

Monitoring outcomes and re–evaluation of the patient occurs intermittently. Van Rijswijk states that all pressure ulcers should be evaluated weekly.[3] In the early stages of autolysis, frequent assessment is warranted. Some clinicians would assess every one to two days until significant debridement has occurred. This technique allows for modification of the protocol to address changes in the wound. If wound healing is the goal, a pressure ulcer should show signs of improvement within two weeks. These signs may include reduction

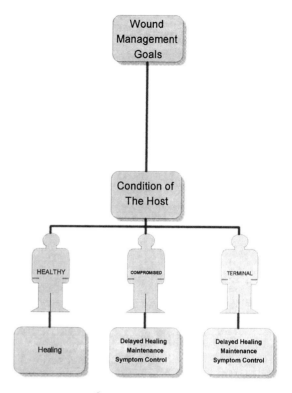

Figure 2. Wound management goals based upon the condition of the host

in erythema surrounding the wound; granulation tissue ingrowth and reduction of slough, necrotic tissue and debris; decreasing size of the wound; decrease in odor in a previously malodorous wound; wound margin attachment beginning where undermining once prevailed or reduction in pain.[4] In the deteriorating wound, signs of improvement may not lead to healing. However, indicators of improvement may include decreased odor, exudate control, decreased necrotic tissue or pain control. The following is a discussion of problems commonly seen in deteriorating wounds and recommendations for treatment.

Clinical Implications

Problem: Wound infection. All cutaneous wounds are contaminated with bacteria, yet healing does occur because of neutrophil and macrophage responses of the host. However, in the deteriorating wound, infection is always suspected since it represents the primary reason a wound does not heal.[5] In practice, wound infection occurs when more than 100,000 bacteria per gram of tissue are present, depending upon the organism. This results in a prolonged inflammatory response and delayed collagen synthesis. Epithelialization is prevented and healthy tissue is injured.[6] At particular risk are the compromised host, highly contaminated areas (e.g. contaminated surgical cases), large wounds with necrotic tissue and diabetics with foot ulcers. Studies indicate that approximately 25 percent of nonhealing pressure ulcers are infected. Newman and associates found underlying osteomyelitis in 68 percent of diabetic foot ulcers when diagnosed by bone biopsy and bone culture.[7]

The use of moist wound healing and occlusive dressings has given rise to concerns about an increased incidence of wound infection in these environments. However, in a retrospective review, Hutchinson reported that the rate of wound infection with occlusion was 2.6 percent and with conventional dressing was 7.1 percent.[8] In most patients, moist wound healing approaches are utilized effectively for contaminated and infected wounds. However, in the infected wound, occlusion is not always appropriate. A non–occlusive dressing may be indicated or an occlusive dressing changed daily. Caution is recommended in the inoperative patient with an ischemic wound. The potential for gangrene may exist and may be exacerbated when moisture–retentive dressings are used. Many clinicians recommend dry dressing protocols for these patients.

Management approaches. Early assessment of patients at high risk for wound infection is essential. Risk factors include immunosuppression, diabetes, large necrotic wounds or large areas of contamination. Signs and symptoms of systemic wound infection include fever, pain, leukocytosis and bacteremia whereas local wound infection may exhibit local warmth, erythema, edema, increase in exudate, purulent exudate and uncharacteristic odor.

Prevention of wound infection is a universal goal in wound care. Universal precautions are used to prevent cross–contamination between patients and caregivers. Single use equipment (e.g. scissors) is preferable with dressing materials and wound measuring guides properly disposed of after each use.

Clean technique or no–touch technique is followed in most types of wound care. Clean gloves are used and changed after removal of soiled dressings. In some highly contaminated wounds, it may be necessary to changes gloves 3 to 4 times during a wound irrigation and dressing change. Good hand washing technique is observed.

Wound debridement is the removal of nonviable tissue, which usually results in a larger wound. The technique selected is dependent upon the urgency, risk of infection and condition of the patient. Debridement of lower extremity ulcers is approached only with knowledge of the vascular status of the limb. In the deteriorating wound, debridement takes on particular importance since the presence of nonviable tissue predisposes to infection, may cause odor and hinders assessment. Tissue may be removed with sharp debridement where a scalpel and scissors are utilized. This is a rapid, effective approach, but requires a skilled professional and may require anesthesia and hemostatic techniques. Mechanical debridement involves whirlpool, high pressure irrigation and wet to dry dressings. While they are easy to perform, pain and nonselective debridement may also result. Chemical debridement using enzymes is useful in select long term situations where maintenance or healing is the goal. Enzymes are easy to use, yet represent a slower form of debridement that requires a prescription and may irritate surrounding skin.[9] Autolytic debridement is achieved through use of moisture–retentive dressings. Wound fluid is held at the site and enzymes in the fluid are able to self–digest devitalized tissue. This is an effective form of debridement alone or in combination with mechanical or sharp debridement. It does not require a prescription and can be done in all health-care settings. Autolytic debridement requires close monitoring, is slower than sharp debridement and is not indicated when the risk of infection is high.

Wound cleansing removes bacteria and surface contaminants. In the deteriorating wound, cleansing is imperative since necrotic tissue and increased exudate are commonly present. Chemical and mechanical trauma to the wound bed should be minimized by selection of the appropriate cleansing solution and mechanical means of delivering solution to the wound. Wounds with adherent materials may benefit from the use of commercial wound cleansers. However, saline is the most physiological and frequently used irrigation solution. (In the home setting saline may be prepared by mixing 2 teaspoons table salt with 1 quart of water. Remaining solution should be discarded.) The amount of pressure delivered using irrigation varies according to the equipment used. When a bulb syringe is used, the irrigation pressure is about 2 psi (i.e. pounds per square inch). This procedure is appropriate for a clean, granular wound. The Agency for Health Care Policy and Research (AHCPR) guideline for treatment of pressure ulcers suggests 4 to 15 psi for safe and effective irrigation. This recommendation may change depending on the type of wound and degree of necrotic tissue. A 35 ml syringe and 19–gauge needle or angiocatheter provide approximately 8 psi which is an effective high pressure irrigation technique that is most frequently used. Water–resistant gowns, protective eyewear and, occasionally, a face shield are indicated with

ROLSTAD AND HARRIS

high pressure irrigation. Whirlpool should be considered for cleansing wounds with thick exudate, slough or necrotic tissue that encompass large areas. For further information refer to Chapter 13 in this book.

The benefits of using antiseptic solutions (i.e. povidone iodine, hydrogen peroxide, acetic acid) in highly contaminated wounds should be weighed against the potential harm to healthy tissue. With the compromised patient in hospice, use of an antiseptic solution to decrease bacteria and odor may be necessary. However, in most situations, these substances are not recommended for wound care.

Dressing materials selected for the uninfected wound will protect the site from further contamination while providing a thermal barrier. Occlusive dressings selected may include transparent films, hydrocolloids, polyurethane foams and composite dressings. Dressings are selected based upon characteristics of the wound. For example, a wound with depth will usually require a filling agent (alginate, hydrocolloid powder/paste, plain or impregnated gauze).

Occlusive dressing changes are usually indicated every 3 to 4 days, depending upon exudate levels in the wound. Fewer dressing changes allow less airborne dispersal of bacteria, protect peri-wound skin, and are less disruptive for the patient and more cost-effective.

Management of the infected wound includes the above general interventions as well as the following recommendations:

A culture is done if signs and symptoms of wound infection are present. A needle aspiration, biopsy or swab culture may be taken prior to initiation of antibiotic treatment.

Systemic wound infections are best treated with systemic antibiotics. When oral antibiotics are used, monitor for gastrointestinal reactions such as diarrhea and nausea.

Topical antibiotics may be indicated. Examples for gram negative and positive organisms include bacitracin zinc, polymyxin B and bacitracin zinc, polymyxin B, bacitracin zinc and neomycin (also effective against pseudomonas), and silver sulfadiazine 1 percent cream (also effective against yeast). Metronidazole gel 0.75 percent is effective against anaerobes and mupirocin 2 percent is effective against MRSA and gram positive organisms, such as staphylococcus aureus and streptococcus.[10] There are other effective antimicrobials that may be purchased over-the-counter.

Topical antiseptics (e.g., Dakin's solution, povidone iodine, acetic acid) are not recommended for routine use, but may be effective for odor control in the hospice patient or in other select cases.

Non-occlusive, moist wound conditions are usually preferred with daily dressing changes. Depending on conditions within the wound, dressings used may include impregnated gauzes, alginates, hydrocolloid powders and pastes, gauze packing strips and foams. The secondary cover dressing may include gauze or island dressings.

Case study (Plate 18). A 78 year old male with congestive heart failure and an extremely irregular heart rhythm who is two years status post femoral popliteal bypass of the right leg, presents with ischemia of the right foot and a wound on the great toe. He is confined to bed and lives with his wife who is also his caregiver. A home care nurse visits twice per week to monitor the patient's condition. The vascular surgeon recommended a below the knee amputation, but the family refused. Based upon collaboration with the surgeon and family physician, conservative wound care procedures were instituted.

The primary goal for the wound was wound maintenance, since there was little hope of healing. The treatment objectives were to prevent infection and provide a simple dressing procedure for the caregiver. Daily dressing changes of wet to moist gauze were used with a conforming gauze wrap for protection. A petrolatum impregnated gauze would also have been a good choice. The wound was cleansed with normal saline. On several occasions, green, thick exudate was present. At those times, topical silver sulfadiazine was used. There were two episodes of increased erythema and pain reported. Treatment then included a two-week course of oral antibiotics and topical silver sulfadiazine, rather than the wet-moist dressing. Dressings were changed daily. The patient was maintained on this protocol for two years before his death which was secondary to heart failure.

Problem: Pain control. Albert Schweitzer once said, "Pain is a more terrible lord of mankind than even death itself." Chronic, uncontrolled pain destroys quality of life and may erode the will to live. Intermittent pain may result in limited functioning, sleeplessness and lost work days. As such, pain is a primary assessment in patients with wounds. Pain in the deteriorating wound originates primarily from malignancy, ischemia, infection, reinjury, desiccation, and topical wound procedures and products. While most patients with wounds do not suffer from chronic pain, those with ischemic wounds, leg ulcers of mixed etiology, and malignant wounds may report debilitating levels of intermittent or chronic pain. Leg ulcer patients have reported significant pain when their wounds are debrided. On a scale of 0 to 10 the median is 8.4. Yet, with proper planning and medication, this pain can be relieved or significantly reduced.[11] For cancer patients with or without wounds, pain and the fear of pain is one of the greatest concerns. Fifty percent of patients in the early stages of disease report pain related to their disease and its treatment. When cancer is in its final stages, approximately 70 percent of patients report persistent and intense pain. When preventive pain management is used, 80 to 90 percent of patients report the pain is bearable or alleviated.[12]

Varying levels of discomfort or pain may also occur during dressing changes. Dry dressings forcefully removed from wounds for debridement purposes generally result in pain. Simple manipulation of tissue during dressing changes may also elicit a pain response. Occasionally, products applied to the wound, such as some cleansers or antimicrobials, will result in stinging or burning.

Management approaches. When wound deterioration occurs, ongoing assessment and monitoring of pain is essential. Assessment of the patient and underlying cause, location, type and intensity of the pain provides baseline information. Use of a pain intensity scale provides a more objective assessment.

Approaches based on pharmacologics, nursing care, or a combination of the two can effectively relieve unnecessary patient suffering. For pain resulting from ischemia with peripheral vascular disease, surgery is the primary intervention. However, if the patient is not a surgical candidate or until surgery is scheduled, effective analgesics are indicated. Severe pain from ischemia is managed with combination opioid/NSAID preparations. In the ischemic foot ulcer, when medication can no longer control the pain, amputation may be indicated.

Chronic pain that may occur in malignancy is best managed by an individualized approach. The AHCPR guideline for pain management offers a three–step analgesic ladder that is useful.[13]

Premedication approximately one–half hour before painful or uncomfortable procedures is recommended. Relaxation, distraction and imagery may also be used to reduce anxiety and help control pain. Opioids, non–steroidal anti–inflammatory drugs (i.e. NSAIDs) or topical 2 percent xylocaine gel may be indicated, based on anticipated level of pain.

Pain related to positioning and support surfaces requires intervention while the patient is in bed or sitting in a chair. For the patient with a pressure ulcer, a pressure reduction or relief device may provide comfort while managing pressure. In cancer patients, an appropriate support surface can eliminate the risk of microtrauma to the bone, which generates metastatic pain. Thin patients with protuberant bony areas in the elbows, spinal areas and trochanters can experience increased comfort with support surfaces that decrease pressure and frequent repositioning. In the immobilized patient, positioning off wound sites and frequent repositioning with pillows or foam wedges increases patient comfort.

Significant decrease in pain perception is reported when moisture–retentive dressings, rather than traditional gauze, are used in wound care. Not only is there less discomfort at dressing removal, but there is less pain while the dressing is in use. This is thought to occur because of a reduction of inflammation and protection of nerve endings. Further, moisture retentive dressings provide more comfort because they are flexible while providing protection for the wound.[14]

Wound care procedures and dressings that provide clinical efficacy and simplicity are particularly important. Short dressing change protocols (approximately 5 to 10 minutes) done once or twice a week are ideal, when possible. The patient receives appropriate wound care with the least amount of tissue manipulation, discomfort and disruption to daily activities. With the hospice patient, pain may be the most important goal in wound care. Lengthy wound care procedures done several times during the day are exhaustive for patient and caregiver and may result in noncompliance. Dressings changed twice a week (e.g. hydrocolloid, and foams) may be useful. For larger granular wounds requiring packing, wound contact layers may be indicated. The contact layer is positioned over the wound base and absorptive layers (e.g. gauze) are then placed over the contact layer. At dressing change, the contact layer is left in place and the gauze is changed as needed. The contact layer is usually changed weekly. This technique decreases tissue manipulation at the wound base.

Avoid further injury to fragile periwound tissue by prepping skin prior to the use of tape, or by using a nonadherent dressing. With leg ulcers, a wrapping gauze may be used with tape applied to the gauze to secure the wrap. Tube elastic bandage or tubenetting may also be used. Select a dressing that will provide the best features needed. For example, when high levels of exudate are present, an alginate or foam dressing may provide better absorption than a hydrocolloid. This protocol will also increase the wearing time of the dressing and decrease the number of dressing changes.

Teach the patient self–care and the rationale for wound care procedures. Increasing patient control when possible may result in decreased anxiety, pain or discomfort. When the patient is unable to do

ROLSTAD AND HARRIS

self–care, a trusted caregiver may be instrumental in decreasing anxiety and thereby increasing patient comfort.

Case study (Plate 19). A 72 year old female had a right lateral lower extremity wound secondary to trauma from a wheel chair. The management goal was healing. Initially, a wet to dry saline dressing protocol with BID changes was used. The peri-wound skin became erythematous from gauze rubbing against the skin. The patient complained of pain at dressing changes because of skin sensitivity and the dressing embedded in the wound. Even when the dressing was moistened with saline, the patient reported pain at dressing removal. Therefore, premedication was ordered. However, in the nursing home, she did not always receive the medication prior to procedures. The procedure was revised to an amorphous hydrogel (Intrasite* Gel, Smith & Nephew United, Inc., Largo, FL) and a non–adherent dressing (Telfa®, Kendall Healthcare Products Co., Mansfield, MA). A conforming gauze was used to wrap the wound. The dressing was changed every day without pain and a healed wound resulted.

Problem: Exudate management. Wounds in declining status may exhibit an onset of increased exudation, recognized by dressing leakage, soiled clothes and odor. The management of wound exudate can often be a challenge in terms of number of times per day a dressing requires changing and maintenance of periwound skin.

Management approaches. Exudate management occurs via moisture vapor transmission (e.g. transparent film and polyurethane foam dressings), absorption (e.g. polyurethane foam, hydrocolloid, alginate, gauze dressings) and a combination of the two. These dressing categories represent varying levels of fluid handling capabilities. For example, a film dressing is indicated for use on dry wounds or those with minimal exudate, while an alginate is indicated for wounds with moderate to heavy drainage.

Some dressings may be layered upon themselves (i.e. alginates, gauze) and covered with a secondary absorbent dressing (e.g. Exu–Dry® Wound Dressing, Exu–Dry Wound Care Products, Bronx, NY). The secondary dressing is used to increase absorption and protect the wound. Always refer to the manufacturer's package insert for proper usage.

Highly exudative wounds require close monitoring of the periwound skin to avoid overgrowth of candida and tissue maceration. A liquid polymer skin prepping agent, solid form skin barrier or ointment, may be indicated to protect the skin in these situations.

Draining wounds and fistulas of the abdomen, chest and neck may exudate heavily. When exudate is equal to more the 100ccs in 24 hours or when patient comfort is an issue, pouching the site with an ostomy or draining wound pouch offers a useful solution. This intervention also offers good odor control, protection of periwound skin, increased patient comfort and the ability to measure output.[15]

Case study (Plate 20). This 43 year old male with cancer of the pharynx underwent a radical neck dissection that resulted in a pharyngocutaneous fistula. The management goal was healing. However, the wound was deteriorating based on increased wound size and increased exudate. During hospitalization, the high amount of saliva drainage was managed by a red rubber catheter that was placed into the site and connected to continuous suction. The distal portion of the wound was dry and required a hydrating dressing, i.e. amorphous hydrogel. The proximal portion was approximately 10 cm in length with heavy drainage. An alginate was used at this site. A cover gauze and a transparent film were used to secure the dressing and provide a closed system to facilitate the suction. The dressings were changed BID with complete granulation in three weeks.[16]

Problem: Odor control. When odor control is a problem, physiological and social issues are involved. Odor occurs because of high bacteria levels in the wound. Social isolation or depression may result because of the unpleasant aspects of having family, visitors and caregivers in close proximity. Odor is generally not a problem in granular wounds. However, patients with deteriorating wounds have odor because the wound is highly colonized, infected or exhibiting tissue necrosis. Deliberate and effective intervention is recommended early on in order to reduce or eliminate the problem.

Management approaches. Odor management is achieved based upon the cause of the problem. The wound may require increased dressing changes, more aggressive cleansing, debridement, an odor absorbent dressing or a pouching system.

Devitalized tissue is an odor source. Therefore, debridement is usually recommended. The type of debridement selected may include sharp, autolytic, or enzymatic debridement. Mechanical debridement, as with wet–to–dry dressings or mechanical scrubbing, is generally not recommended since it is a nonselective removal of tissue. Healthy granulation tissue or epithelial cells may also be removed. Mechanical debridement may also result in patient discomfort or pain.

Wound cleansing is an effective method for decreasing bacterial levels in the wound. In the deteriorating wound, wound cleansing is a particularly important consideration. Once again, toxicity of irrigation solutions must be considered.[17] Techniques for wound cleansing were covered earlier in this chapter and in Chapter 13. One wound cleanser, Puri–clens® (Sween Corporation, N. Mankato, MN), may be sprayed onto gauze and applied to the wound to decrease odor.

More frequent dressing changes also promote removal of bacteria from wounds. If a hydrocolloid is in use with dressing changes twice a week, depending upon exudate levels, a change in dressing to once a day and use of a hydrogel or alginate changes may be effective.

Casual attention to wound care may result in dressing leakage or dressings overdue for change that remain intact. Upon removal, the caregiver may note a stronger odor than usual. This problem can be managed by reassurance that the wound is not infected, with encouragement that dressings must be changed on a specific schedule. In these situations, odor may be a difficult problem in that the patient may have poor olfactory senses.

Products used in wound care may be the source of odor. Hydrocolloid dressings may have a noticeable chemical odor upon removal. Antibacterial dressings may decrease odor from the wound, but may emit a chemical odor. If the odor is bothersome to the patient or caregiver, other options are available.

Synthetic dressings with a charcoal layer also decrease odor. They are available as absorptive wafers and nonabsorptive pads.

Air fresheners or odor eliminators may also be beneficial.

Case study (Plate 21). This 58 year old female has a fungating breast wound. The ulcerations and proliferation arose from malignant tumor cells that infiltrated and eroded the skin. Tissue necrosis resulted secondary to hypoxia with anaerobic and aerobic bacteria proliferation. Odor and exudate levels were problematic. Fragile capillary structures predisposed to bleeding. The management goal was symptom control. Treatment approached focuses on control of hemorrhage, pain control, and odor and exudate management. Control of tumor growth and hemorrhage may require treatment with surgery, radiotherapy, laser therapy, and chemotherapy. Systemic medication is usually recommended to control infection and pain. Odor and exudate management initially included the use of a topical metronidazole alone or in combination with a hydrogel.[18] The formula included 15 cc of 4 percent xylocaine topical, 15 cc metronidazole and 15 cc viscous hydrogel. The gel was thickened to the desired consistency using a hydrocolloid powder and applied to the wound BID. A cover was then applied using a gauze dressing and secured with a tube netting or tank top. No tape was used. As odor and exudate levels decreased, the gel was discontinued and an odor–absorbent dressing (e.g. polyurethane foam and carbon layer) was instituted with daily dressing changes.

Problem: Prevent further injury. Wound care treatments are intended to improve or stabilize the condition of the wound while protecting the periwound skin. However, sometimes the care we provide may actually be injurious and cause delayed healing or further injury. Knowledge regarding common pitfalls in wound care is useful and a few are discussed below. Within this discussion, it is assumed that primary interventions for the wound have been addressed by correcting or controlling the extrinsic and intrinsic factors that may contribute to wound deterioration (Table 1).

Management approaches. Maintenance of periwound skin tissue integrity by frequent assessment and early intervention is key. The area may be dry and require moisturizing to avoid cracking that could result in ulceration. Conversely, moisture in the periwound area may promote proliferation of *staphylococci* and *candida albicans*. If the risk of periwound skin maceration is a concern, a dressing with increased fluid handling characteristics (e.g. polyurethane foam, alginate) or a skin protectant on the surrounding skin (e.g. liquid copolymer, skin barrier) is indicated. It may be necessary to increase dressing change intervals in these situations.

Mechanical injury to the wound may occur because of shear, pressure and friction.[19] Interventions that may be effective in treating these problems include proper positioning and transferring techniques to avoid or minimize shear; pressure reduction/relief support surfaces to reduce or eliminate pressure; and proper removal of adhesives with skin prepping in areas where frequent adhesive removals are anticipated. Mechanical injury may be iatrogenic and occur during dressing removal or with wound cleansing, disinfection and packing. Dressing removal is indicated at regular intervals depending on the dressing in use or if leakage (strike through) occurs. To avoid stripping injuries, adhesive is removed in the direction of hair growth. The edge of the dressing is lifted and gently pulled parallel to the skin while gentle pressure is applied to adjacent skin for support during removal. This dressing may be rolled off the skin. If the dressing is imbedded in the wound surface, a gentle irrigation with normal saline to avoid traumatic removal and an alternative dressing are recommended.

High pressure wound irrigation may damage granular tissue in the wound. Review of this topic is found in the Wound Infection section earlier in this chapter and in Chapter 13.

The use of antiseptics in wound care is discouraged because of cytotoxicity. Review of this topic is found in the Wound Infection section earlier in this chapter and in Chapter 13.

Wounds with depth, undermining or tunneling will generally require packing. Packing is used to obliterate dead space and avoid premature wound closure. Overpacking so that dressing materials are piled above the wound can cause pressure when the body position is shifted and can cause maceration of periwound skin. Tight packing techniques may also result in ischemia. Therefore, packing materials are loosely placed into the wound touching all surfaces in the defect while extending only to the skin level. Packing materials include gauze (e.g. plain, impregnated, strips) alginates, foam pillows, hydrogels (e.g. gel, impregnated gauze, strip) and hydrocolloid powders. A secondary dressing is then used to cover the wound.

Case study (Plate 22). This 72 year old female was diagnosed with bone cancer and subsequently developed a sacral pressure ulcer. She also had fecal incontinence that required a skin protectant. The management goal was symptom control. In order to prevent further injury to the wound and periwound skin as well as to decrease pain, a pressure relief specialty bed was ordered. Caregivers were instructed to maintain no more than a 30 degree laterally inclined position. The wound was referred for instrumental debridement; however, the family refused further intervention. In order to manage odor and exudate and provide unobtrusive care in this terminal patient, the wound was filled with an alginate, and a hydrocolloid dressing was used as a cover dressing. The patient died three days later with only one dressing change having been performed.

Educational Considerations

Management of deteriorating wounds involves knowledgeable team members. Communication among team, patient and family is crucial to timely intervention. Educational is directed toward patient, family, caregiver, healthcare professionals and insurance companies. In particular, education is provided for patients and families, since much of the wound care in the deteriorating wound is provided at home. Discussion of rationale for treatments and written, detailed instruction are a must. When noncompliance is encountered, it is frequently the result of incomplete education, lack of support and motivation or inability to perform recommended procedures. Patients, like wounds, are dynamic and, as such, require frequent, ongoing monitoring, education and support.

Members of the healthcare team also require education about how to assess, document and treat wounds. Interventions discussed in this chapter are predicated upon early referral and treatment. Therefore, the healthcare professional needs to understand patient risk factors that may precipitate deterioration in wounds.

Cost Containment

In this cost containment era, the clinician is obligated to consider the total cost of wound care. Costs may be accrued from dressings, specialty equipment (i.e. beds, pumps), medications, professional visits and facilities. Cost savings regarding prediction and prevention in pressure ulcers has been well documented. Acute care and long term care alike have benefited from this information.

In general, the least expensive approach to wound care, when possible, is guided self–care. It requires a capable, willing patient or caregiver in addition to understandable and easy to use dressings. Close monitoring from an experienced healthcare professional is a key provision of safe and effective wound care.

Consideration is given to the overall cost of wound care, rather than per unit cost. Specialty dressings are frequently more expensive per unit than gauze. However, they are usually changed less frequently which provides a cost savings in comparison to gauze.

When all factors are equal, selection of the least expensive approach is indicated. This requires knowledge of wound care and treatment costs. An example of a cost consideration case is a patient receiving care with moist wound healing and a goal of maintenance. There are numerous methods available to provide a moist wound environment. One method is use of a wet to moist saline dressings; however, use of a petrolatum impregnated dressing may be less expensive by requiring fewer dressing changes.

Many patients with chronic healthcare problems are choosing to stay at home which has created great demand in the home healthcare sector. While home care is less expensive than stays in a nursing home or skilled nursing unit, costs of care at home should consider all equipment as well as the home healthcare nursing charge, which may be $80 to $150 per visit.

Educating the patient on reimbursement issues can be cost–effective. In some situations, expenses are the limiting factor on how a wound is managed. Currently, when a person is on Medicare, 80 percent of qualifying wound care dressings are reimbursed if the wound has been debrided. However, if the patient is not knowledgeable in product reimbursement and thinks the recommended products will be out–of–pocket expenses, dressings may not be purchased because of lack of funds. Additionally, there are wound care products which are excluded from reimbursement and identified by Medicare as non–covered items. Current examples of non–reimbursed items under Medicare guidelines include compression stockings, wound cleansers, skin sealants, moisturizers and other miscellaneous, yet quite necessary, items. These are out–of–pocket expenses. Therefore, if the patient or family is not willing or able to make these purchases, products will not be purchased not protocols followed. This creates a dilemma for patient and clinician alike. Reimbursement for product is changing; therefore, the patient and clinician are encouraged to communicate directly with local equipment distributors.

Conclusion

Deteriorating wounds require close scrutiny to monitor for signs of impaired healing or problems in clinical care. Within the framework of an interventional model, the patient is reassessed and a general goal for the wound of healing, maintenance or symptom control is determined based upon the condition of the patient. The treatment plan is then developed by addressing the etiology of the wound, contributing factors and local wound care approaches. Dressings and topical treatments alone do not make wounds heal. The cause of deterioration and contributing factors must be addressed. However, providing the appropriate topical treatment can provide a clinically acceptable result and a more comfortable patient.

References

1. Bergstrom N, Bennett MA, Carlson CE, et al. *Treatment of Pressure Ulcers*. Clinical Practice Guideline, No. 15. Rockville, MD: U.S. Department of Health and Human Services. Public Health Service, Agency for Health Care Policy and Research. AHCPR Publication No. 95–0052. December 1994.
2. Kerstein MD. Moist wound healing: The clinical perspective. *Ostomy/Wound Management* 1995;41(7A Suppl): 37S–45S.
3. van Rijswijk L, Polansky J. Predictors of time to healing deep pressure ulcers. *WOUNDS* 1994;6(5)159–165.
4. Brown–Etris M. Measuring healing in wounds. NPUAP Proceedings. *Advances in Wound Care* 1995;8(4)53–58.
5. Lawrence WT. Clinical management of nonhealing wounds. In: Cohen IK, Diegelmann RF, Lindbland WJ (eds) *Wound Healing, Biochemical & Clinical Aspects*. Philadelphia, PA, W.B. Saunders Company, 1992, pp. 541–561.
6. Madden JE, Edlich RF, Custer JR, et al. Studies in the management of the contaminated wound, IV. Resistance to infection of surgical wounds made by knife, electrosurgery and laser. *Amer J Surg* 1970;119:222–4.
7. Newman LG, Waller J, Palestro CJ, et al. Unsuspected osteomyelitis in diabetic foot ulcers, diagnosis and monitoring by leukocyte scanning with indium in 111 oxyquinoline. *JAMA* 1991;266(9):1246–51.
8. Hutchinson JJ, Lawrence JC. Wound infection under occlusive dressings. *J Hosp Infect* 1991;17:83–94.
9. Fowler E, van Rijswijk L. Using wound debridement to help achieve the goals of care. *Ostomy/Wound Management* 1995;41(7A Suppl):23S–36S.
10. Bolton LL, Johnson CL, Fattu AJ. Topical medications and pharmacological agents in wound healing. In: Gogia PP (ed). *Clinical Wound Management*. Thorofare, NJ, Slack, Inc., 1995, pp. 55–71.
11. Holm J, Andrén B, Grafford K. Pain control in the surgical debridement of leg ulcers by the use of a topical lidocaine–prilocaine cream, EMLA™. *Acta Derm Venerol* (Stockholm) 1990;70:132–136.
12. Melzack R. The tragedy of needless pain. *Scientific American* 1990;Feb:27–23.
13. Jacox AK, Carr DB, Payne R, et al. *Management of Cancer Pain*. Clinical Practice Guideline. Rockville, MD, U.S. Department of Health and Human Services. Public Health Service, Agency for Health Care Policy and Research. AHCPR Publication No. 94–0592, March, 1994.
14. Field CK, Kerstein MD. Overview of wound healing in a moist environment. *Am J of Surg* 1994;167(1A Suppl):2–6.
15. Rolstad BS, Wong WD. Nursing considerations with intestinal fistulas. In: MacKeigan JM, Cataldo PA (eds). *Intestinal Stomas, Principles, Techniques and Management*. St. Louis, MO, Quality Medical Publishing, Inc., 1993, pp. 307–328.
16. Harris AH, Komray R. Cost–effective management of pharyngocutaneous fistulas following laryngectomy. *Ostomy/Wound Management* 1993;39(8):36–44.
17. Foresman PA, et al. A relative toxicity index for wound cleansers. *WOUNDS* 1993;5(5):226–231.
18. Grocott P. The palliative management of fungating malignant wounds. *J of Wound Care* 1995;4(5):240–242.
19. Harris AH. Putting pressure ulcer prevention in motion. *Advance for Directors in Rehabilitation* 1995;4(10):69–74.

28

Alternative Topical Therapies for Wound Care

Cecilia R. Rund, RN, CETN

Rund CR. Alternative topical therapies for wound care. In: Krasner D, Kane D. *Chronic Wound Care, Second Edition*. Wayne, PA, Health Management Publications, Inc., 1997, pp 219–226.

Introduction

Practically every substance known to man has been used for wound care. In the past, wound care practices have been based on mystery, magic and religion, not on common sense, observation and logical deduction. Even today, one finds ancient beliefs difficult to change. This article reviews various non–conventional therapies that have been used for wound care and explores the rationale for use of each. However, before deciding which form of treatment, if any, may be appropriate, both the patient and the wound must be thoroughly evaluated. Reviewing lab values, Doppler studies, culture reports and even the patient's eating patterns may offer suggestions as to why a wound is not healing as expected. One must also keep in mind the basic principles of wound care when attending to chronic wounds. Simply stated, the wound should be kept clean, moist and protected from both chemical and mechanical trauma. Therefore, the type of topical treatment may not be as important as addressing the general principles of wound healing. If these principles are carefully considered, the choice of topical treatment may readily identify itself. Also, any product used for wound care should be FDA approved and used within the stated indications.

Aloe Vera

The use of the aloe plant was mentioned in the Bible, recorded in the writings of Alexander the Great and Hippocrates, and found in an Egyptian papyrus dating to about 150 B.C. Its use has also been recorded in early ancient Polynesian and Indian literature.[1] The Greeks used aloe as a purgative.[2]

Aloe is derived from the aloe vera plant, a green, succulent, cactus–like plant belonging to the lily family. The substance, aloe vera, is derived from thin–walled mucilaginous cells of the inner central zone of the leaf. It is this gel that is thought to have emollient and moisturizing effects and therapeutic properties.

Robson and colleagues examined pure aloe vera extract and found that it contained glucose, uric acid, salicylic acid, creatinine, alkaline phosphate, cholesterol, triglycerides, lactate, calcium, magnesium, zinc, sodium, potassium, and chloride.[3] Roboz and Hangen–Smith analyzed the gel of a Hawaiian aloe vera plant and found fat, protein, crude fiber, sugars (mannose and glucose), mucilage, crude aloin oil, and resin.[3]

Both positive and negative results have been reported using aloe vera in wounds. Aloe vera gel was used in the 1930s on severe radiation dermatitis.[1] Treatment included applying the whole leaf of aloe to the affected area which reportedly reduced burning and itching and led to wound healing without scarring. In 1953, Lushbaugh and Hale found that aloe seemed to hasten both the degenerative and the reparative phases of the tested irradiated sites in albino rabbits.[3] In 1988, Kaufman and colleagues used aloe vera gel in second degree burn sites on guinea pigs and compared its use to that of one percent silver sulfadiazine cream.[4] They discovered that the aloe–treated wounds epithelialized at a slower rate and that contraction was significantly higher. Several years later in 1991,

Schmidt and Greenspoon used a standard wound protocol to treat 21 post–operative female patients whose wounds were healing by secondary intention.[5] The protocols were identical except that one included aloe vera gel and the other did not. They found that the aloe vera–treated group showed a significant delay in wound healing. Finally, in 1994, Davis and co–workers extracted mannose–6–phosphate from aloe vera gel and applied it to wounds in mice.[6] Their experience revealed an anti–inflammatory effect and overall improved wound healing in the mannose–6–phosphate treated wounds compared to wounds treated with saline gauze.

Because of the varying reports regarding the use of aloe in wound healing, continued research is needed to investigate aloe vera gel and its components in order to discover the possible healing mechanisms of this natural plant material.

Animal Fats/Vegetable Oils

From time to time, persons caring for their loved ones have turned to home remedies such as animal fats and vegetable oils that are available and economical to use for the care of wounds. The use of grease, honey and lint salve for wound care is discussed in the writings of the Smith papyrus from the Egyptians. The grease kept the wound moist and prevented the bandages from sticking to the wound, thus preventing further trauma to the wound.[7] The same theory holds true today. Animal fats seal out harmful, external contaminants and provide a moist environment.

Whether anyone will undertake randomized, controlled clinicals to study the safety and efficacy of animal fats and vegetable oils is doubtful. And when better options exist, they should be employed. However, in cases where resources are extremely limited, animal fats and vegetable oils certainly provide a better environment for wound healing than dry gauze or even paper towels.

Antacids

A common method for treating gastric and/or peptic ulcers is by digesting antacids via the gastro–intestinal system. However, somewhere in the history of wound care, someone discovered that placing antacids onto skin caused a drying effect. It was also observed that if one placed these antacids into superficial, open wounds, the antacid seemed to absorb some of the serous drainage, creating a somewhat dry surface.[8] This practice has taken hold mostly in ostomy care where dry surfaces are needed to attach ostomy appliances. Antacids increase pH and decrease acid production.

However, there is no pharmacologic indication for the use of these products on the skin or in open wounds.[9]

The use of antacids for chronic wound care has no scientific basis at this time since there is no available research regarding the use of antacids and their effect upon tissues in open wounds. Since antacids have a drying effect and moist wound healing is an accepted practice for chronic wound care today, antacids are of questionable utility.

Benzoyl Peroxide

Benzoyl peroxide is an oxidizing agent that has antimicrobial, antifungal and antipruritic activity along with keratolytic properties.[10] It is available in both a lotion and a gel and has been most widely used in the treatment of acne vulgaris. Studies from 1929 show that this agent was studied in the treatment of burned patients as a possible promoter of wound healing.[10] Since that time, benzoyl peroxide in a lotion base has been studied in both full– and partial–thickness wounds to enhance wound healing in pigs. One such study resulted in a more rapid re–epithelialization over a seven day period in keratome wounds on this animal model.[11] However, concentrations of over 20 percent benzoyl peroxide, whether in a gel or lotion base, have retarded re–epithelialization. Other negative results from using benzoyl peroxide in wounds include inhibited wound contraction and contact dermatitis.[11]

Betadine and Sugar Preparations

One choice of wound treatment that resurfaces throughout the years is the sugar and povidone–iodine mixture. This preparation has been both praised and defamed by the healthcare profession.

The ability of sugar to accelerate wound healing has been documented in ancient and modern day medical papers. Sugar is hypertonic, which allows it both to inhibit and destroy the growth of bacteria. Sugar lowers the water activity level of a wound, which inhibits growth of microorganisms. Sugar also alters wound pH, which further discourages invading microorganisms.[12] Because of its wide range of germicidal activity and effective antifungal properties, povidone–iodine was added to the sugar therapy for wound treatment.[13]

Few studies of the use of this mixture exist. Perhaps the most well known is the work done by Dr. Knutson and colleagues. A sugar/povidone–iodine solution and a sugar/povidone–iodine compound (sugar, povidone–iodine solution and povidone–iodine ointment) were used to treat patients with wounds, burns and ulcers. This topical treatment was used in combination with whirlpool, antibiotic therapy, surgical wound debridement and other supportive therapies. This study concluded that wounds improved dramatically when treated with the sugar/povidone– iodine solution or compound. Evaluation of the wound after initiating treatment yielded clean wound beds without odor, absence of surrounding erythema, and rapid growth of granulation tissue.[13]

One must consider whether the improvement in these wounds was actually due to the sugar and/ or the adjunctive therapies. Healthcare providers who are wary of such a mixture utilizing povidone–iodine reflect upon the studies of George Rodeheaver and others who have studied the toxic effects of povidone–iodine. One must consider whether the benefits outweight the cytotoxic effects. The reader is referred to Chapter 13 for further discussion of this subject.

Dilantin (Phenytoin)

After phenytoin was introduced in 1937 as an antiseizure medication, it was noted that approximately 20 percent of persons taking phenytoin developed gingival hyperplasia. Because of this overgrowth of tissue, it was postulated that phenytoin could promote tissue growth when applied topically to wounds. Tissue cultures reported that phenytoin could increase collagen deposition by decreasing collagen degradation.[14]

In a recent study, Pendse and colleagues worked with 75 patients who had chronic skin ulcers in a controlled trial.[15] The treated ulcers included burns, post cellulitis wounds, traumatic wounds, amputation stumps, post–operative wounds and other non–specific wounds. Forty of these patients were treated with topical phenytoin and 35 were treated with saline dressings. This research reported a greater reduction in wound area and the appearance of healthy granulation tissue earlier in the phenytoin group than in the saline–treated group. Wound swab cultures were performed at day zero and then every seven days thereafter. By the end of the first week of treatment, 50 percent of the phenytoin group had negative cultures, while only seven percent of the control group had negative cultures. Complete ulcer healing (defined as 100 percent covered with new epithelium) occurred in 73 percent of the phenytoin treated group and in 28.5 percent of the control group. No signs of phenytoin toxicity were observed. Some patients complained of a burning pain with the application of phenytoin that persisted for 30 minutes. Hypertrophic granulation tissue growth was observed in 10 percent of the phenytoin group.[15]

Further controlled studies are needed prior to recommending topical phenytoin as a wound healing agent.

Gentian Violet

The dye, gentian violet, stains tissues and is now most commonly used on intact skin as a skin marker. In the past, it had been used in the treatment of wounds. Gentian violet has an astringent affect due to its preparation in a 10 percent alcohol base.[16] Gentian violet also shows some antimicrobial activity against gram positive organisms and candida. Recent studies have demonstrated gentian violet to be carcinogenic when used in open wound tissue and on mucous membranes.[16,17]

Heat Lamps

Wounds must have an adequate blood supply to heal. Perhaps this is why (through the years, using various modalities) caregivers have diligently tried to increase the blood supply to wounded areas through the use of alternative therapies. One such method has been through the use of heat lamps. Heat, when applied to healthy skin, causes vasodilatation. With vasodilatation, there is increased perfusion and increased delivery of oxygen to tissues. However, using this method on ischemic tissue may actually depress oxygen tension because of the increased demand for oxygen subsequent to increased metabolism. Also, heat applied to periwound skin may actually exacerbate the inflammatory response, leading to tissue necrosis from thermal overload.[18] Applying such a method directly into open wounds desiccates wound tissues, leading to tissue destruction.

Heat lamps should be used on intact skin, with a specific rationale in a controlled environment by a skilled healthcare provider. The lamp must be a 60 to 100 watt bulb and be no closer than 2 to 3 feet from the treated area. Treatment time should not exceed 20 minutes in duration. Contraindications for heat lamp therapy include combative and/or disoriented patients and patients suffering with sensory deprivation. Heat lamps are also contraindicated on postoperative sites, as heat increases metabolic demands and can prolong wound healing and cause further discomfort to the patient.[19]

Honey

The use of honey to promote wound healing has been documented since the Egyptians who referred to honey in their wound care remedies hundreds of times. Components of honey include glucose (40 percent), fructose (40 percent), water (20 percent), and amino acids. Honey also contains inhibine, an enzyme secreted by the pharyngeal glands of the bee. Inhibine breaks down into hydrogen peroxide and gluconolactone. Hydrogen peroxide is a mild disinfectant, and gluconolactone equilibrates with gluconic acid, a mild antibiotic. It is interesting to note that inhibine can be destroyed by light or heat; however, if honey is attacked by excessive light and/or heat, another ingredient, propolis, gives honey its antimicrobial effect. Propolis is a sticky material which is used to repair or patch cracks in a hive. This substance is gathered by the bees from buds of plants. The active ingredient in propolis is galangine, which is a food preservative.[7] Thus, honey is a natural antimicrobial agent.[20] In 1992, Efem and colleagues published a report on honey's antimicrobial activity. Efem's group isolated pure cultures of *Streptococcus pyogenes, Enterococcus faecalis, Staphylococcus aureus, Escherichia coli, Klebsiella pneumoniae, Proteus mirabilis, Proteus species, Pseudomonas aeruginosa, Bacteroides fragilis, Clostridium tetani, Clostridium welchii* and *Clostridium oedematiens* and plated them on dishes containing appropriate media. Wells were made in the media prior to placement of the bacteria. Two drops of unprocessed honey were then placed into the wells and the specimens were incubated for 24 to 72 hours. The *Bacteroides* and *Clostridial* specimens were incubated within an anaerobic environment. The unprocessed honey inhibited the growth of all bacteria except *Pseudomonas aeruginosa* and *Clostridium oedematiens*. Similar cultures were done using fungi. Unprocessed, undiluted honey inhibited the growth of *Aspergillus fumigatus, Penicillin citrinum, Trichophyton rubrum, Trichophyton tonsurans,* and *Candida albicans.*[21]

Those who advocate using honey in wounds claim that it sterilizes the wound and seems to promote wound healing. Honey–treated wounds revealed debridement of necrotic tissue, reduction of edema, reduced periwound maceration and promotion of both granulation tissue and epithelialization. Added benefits included a reduction in wound odor and wound pain and reduced scarring and wound contraction.[20]

Application procedures for the use of honey are simple. Honey can be poured directly into a wound, or gauze material can be saturated with honey and then packed or placed in the wound. Wounds should be irrigated thoroughly with saline between dressing changes. Contraindications for the use of honey would be allergies to bees and/or honey.

Honey may seem like the ideal dressing; however, there are certain issues of concern. Unprocessed,

raw honey is not considered to be a sterile product. Bees may carry pesticides and other chemicals which may contaminate the honey. Controlled research on honey as a wound dressing is needed. Honey has survived from the days of the great healers of Egypt until the present. Certainly, this natural wonder deserves a closer look.

Impregnated Gauzes

Impregnated gauzes are gauze materials that have been impregnated with a substance or a solution and are available in individually wrapped sterile packages (usually a foil wrap). The substances which impregnate gauzes vary and can be anything from petrolatum to antiseptics. The solutions used to impregnate gauzes can also vary and may include saline or antiseptic solutions. Impregnated gauzes have been used to create a moist wound environment, to prevent dressings from adhering to a wound, to mechanically debride wounds and to establish bacterial balance within a wound. Three specific impregnated gauzes are discussed:

Scarlet red. Scarlet red impregnated gauze contains a blend of scarlet red, white petrolatum, lanolin and olive oil. Scarlet red is a lipid–soluble aniline dye that has been touted as a healing agent since the early 1900's.[14] Fisher, a German investigator, reported observing increased mitosis of epithelial cells after injecting scarlet red into a rabbit's ear.[22] In 1910, scarlet red was reported to stimulate healing of burn wounds without causing wound contraction.[22] Since 1943, scarlet red gauze has been used to treat donor sites.[10,23] In 1962, Russian investigators, Vasiliev and Cheung, studied scarlet red injected rabbit ears in an attempt to discover its mechanism of action. The data suggested that the rapid proliferation of epithelial cells may be a result of the stimulatory action of inflammation.[24]

In 1985, Watcher and Wheland found that scarlet red, among other topical agents, significantly stimulated epithelial proliferation in their porcine model. The mechanism for its mitogenic effect is still unknown and warrants further investigation.[10]

Xeroform. Xeroform impregnated gauze contains bismuth tribromophenate in a petrolatum blend. Indications for use include superficial wounds, second and third degree burns, donor sites and abrasions.[23] Studies regarding the use of impregnated gauzes have included both scarlet red and xeroform gauze. Salomon and colleagues studied xeroform and scarlet red on donor sites of rats and concluded that epithelialization proceeded more quickly under xeroform and scarlet red than under plain gauze dressings.[24] However, Gemberling and associates found no difference in epithelialization rates in humans with the use of xeroform, scarlet red, plain gauze or petrolatum gauze.[13]

Petrolatum. Gauzes impregnated with petrolatum have been used on a variety of wounds. Indications for use include minor burns, skin donor sites, suture lines, abrasions, lacerations, skin tears and other post–operative procedures. Reasons for using this dressing include creating a moist wound environment and preventing other dressings from adhering to healthy tissues. Petrolatum gauze dressings need to be changed regularly enough to prevent the petrolatum from drying and adhering to the wound. Since petrolatum impregnated gauzes can interfere with wound drainage absorption, wounds that are heavily exudating may need a different type of dressing material altogether.

It seems that the final word on impregnated gauzes is not yet available. Clinicians should use these products judiciously and watch for further research that supports or refutes their safety and efficacy.

Insulin

Insulin has been used both topically and subcutaneously in an attempt to treat wounds. Insulin is purported to play a role in the transport of amino acids into cells, thereby aiding in the healing process. Studies using animal models have produced mixed results. Some studies reported no difference in healing times and others reported both a delay and a reduction in healing time. Both Udopa and Chansouri reported an increase in the bursting strength in rat wounds after injecting subcutaneous protamine zinc insulin.[26] Rationale for this study was based on the assumption that insulin probably improved collagen strength. Rosenthal and Enquist concluded that neither topical nor subcutaneous insulin expedited the wound healing process.[1]

Van Ort and Gerber published research in which insulin was used in the treatment of pressure ulcers.[27] Their pilot study performed in 1976 concluded:

"We believe that topical insulin therapy is, at present, a questionable therapeutic intervention and should not be used to treat pressure sores because the efficacy of the treatment is unknown, the drug–related therapy is of questionable safety, and there is insufficient scientific rationale and lack of sound research to support its use."[27]

Insulin has been approved by the FDA for intravenous and subcutaneous use. It should not be used topically without FDA approval. The prudent practitioner should await further investigative studies prior to considering insulin as an alternative treatment for chronic wounds.

Mercurochrome

Mercurochrome is a mercury compound. Mercury compounds have their origins with Arabian physicians during the Middle Ages. These mercury compounds were used to prevent sepsis in open wounds. Mercuric chlorides became commonly accepted following Robert Koch's experiments in 1881.[28] In these experiments, Dr. Koch trialed 70 chemicals and found that mercuric chloride in high concentrations destroyed spores quickly, making it an effective fungicide.

Mercury has also been found to have bacteriostatic activities. Because of reports of mercury toxicity, anaphylaxis, and aplastic anemia, many clinicians have found this product to be unacceptable for use as a fungicide and/or bacteriostatic agent.[16]

Oxygen Therapy

Oxygen is a required element for wound healing. Increased oxygen tension in a wound stimulates phagocytosis and enhances degradation of dead tissue structures and the synthesis of new tissue structures. Epithelial cells depend upon oxygen to replicate. Fibroblasts require oxygen to synthesize collagen, and collagen maturation seems to be dependent upon aerobic activities.[29] Because of these findings, various methods of delivering oxygen to a wounded site have been investigated throughout the years. If oxygen is known to be necessary for wound healing, then perhaps, delivering increased concentrations of oxygen and/or increased concentrations of oxygen under pressure to a wound may, indeed, expedite the healing process. Oxygen therapy is an adjunctive therapy which can be delivered directly to the wound bed (topical) or systematically by breathing oxygen (hyperbaric).

It is most important to differentiate between hyperbaric and topical oxygen therapy, as both the delivery and the mechanism of action are quite different. Hyperbaric oxygen (HBO) treatment, as described by the Undersea Medical Society, occurs when a patient breathes 100 percent oxygen intermittently while the pressure of the treatment chamber is increased to a point higher than sea level pressure.[30] Such treatments place a patient into a monoplace (single body) chamber or more than one patient into a multiplace chamber. The monoplace chamber is pressurized with 100 percent oxygen which the patient directly inhales. A multiplace chamber requires that the entire cabin be pressurized while the patient breathes 100 percent oxygen via a mask, a head tent, an endotracheal tube, or a tracheostomy. Therefore, a patient must inhale 100 percent oxygen within a pressurized chamber to receive true HBO therapy. HBO therapy improves wound healing by increasing the amount of oxygen dissolved in the plasma and tissues. The use of HBO to treat difficult and/or chronic wounds has been well documented.[31] See Chapter 33 for further information.

Topical oxygen therapy is delivered by exposing a body part to a pressurized oxygen flow. The patient is not breathing oxygen, rather the oxygen is delivered directly to the wounded area under a set pressure. This is accomplished by using a portable device such as a soft, plastic sleeve or a hard, plastic chamber that can be secured to a body surface or around an extremity which creates an airtight seal. Topical oxygen therapy is relatively simple to use, can be carried to the patient, and does not cause toxic pulmonary effects.

There is controversy as to the effectiveness of topical oxygen therapy. It is the opinion of some healthcare professionals that topical oxygen, even under pressure, can only increase oxygen tension to the superficial dermis.[32] Is this enough to affect wound healing? Topical oxygen is more effective when wounds are clean, free of necrotic matter and have a good vascular supply. Accounts of increased microcirculation, decreased bacterial count and a reduction in tissue edema have been reported. Conversely, there are those who report that topical oxygen does not penetrate well through the skin and that blood flow can be compromised due to the external pressure.[29]

Steroids

Steroids have long been used to treat dermatologic inflammatory conditions. Since steroids retard dermal collagen synthesis, there are clinicians who have recommended the use of topical steroids to decrease the amount of granulation tissue growth within a wound.[18] Studies in human skin fibroblast culture reveal that corticosteroids inhibit collagen synthesis and protein synthesis. Steroids may also promote collagen degradation since the deposition of serum proteins that inhibit collagenase may be reduced by steroid therapy.[33]

Steroids have a negative effect upon tissue growth within a wound. One important cellular component of connective tissue, the fibroblast, is the target for topical corticosteroid action in the wound healing process. Fibroblast proliferation is decreased.[34] Bolton and Fattu reported that topical steroids seemed to inhibit epithelialization in animal studies although they found no studies to support this observation.[35]

Hydrocortisone is an endogenous glucocorticoid, but topical application results in higher than normal circulating levels *in vivo*. This results in side effects such as dermal atrophy, thymic involution and suppression of adrenal, hypothalamic and pituitary function. More potent, synthetic hydrocortisone analog will pronounce these side effects.[36]

Bodnor and colleagues examined the effects of soft steroids in mouse fibroblast cultures and the effects of soft steroids in wound healing in mice. Soft drugs were defined as "therapeutically useful, biologically active chemical compounds, characterized by predictable and controllable *in vitro* metabolism to nontoxic moieties after performing their therapeutic role."[34] The soft steroids were designed to have a high *in vivo* anti–inflammatory activity, yet not produce systemic and local toxic activity. The soft steroid control group revealed more fibroblasts with normal cell morphology. Mice wounds treated with soft steroids healed slightly faster than the untreated lesions and much faster than in the standard steroid group.[34]

If such anti–inflammatory drugs are to be used in a wound, they must be used with careful consideration. The new soft steroids may offer some benefit, but standard steroids will definitely lead to a delay in the wound healing process.

Sugar

Sugar is derived from the juices of various plants such as the sugarcane, sugar beet, the date palm, and the maple tree. Sugar juice is extracted from these plants, heated, and concentrated via an evaporation process which then produces molasses and crystals of sugar. Sugar can be made into a granular, tablet, or powdered form, and into varying degrees of brown sugar. Because of these various forms of sugar, it is difficult to interpret how raw sugar was used in wound healing throughout history.

Sugar is thought to enhance wound healing by debriding the wound and destroying bacteria. Debridement and bactericidal effects are achieved through the osmotic action of sugar. High concentrations of sugar alter the wound pH, which produces a toxic environment to invading microorganisms. The hypertonicity of sugar relieves the edema surrounding the wound, thereby allowing serum and nutrients to enter the wound tissues. There is speculation that sugar undergoes a fermentation process within a wound, which results in certain alcohols that may act as antiseptics. The presence of sugar in wounds also lowers the water activity level to one in which microorganisms cannot proliferate.[36]

Clinical studies advocating the use of sugar and sugar pastes have appeared throughout the years.

These are small, independent studies that lack controls. One article, which appeared in a 1985 issue of *Lancet* discussed the development of a complicated sugar paste which was used to pack large abscess cavities.[37] This paste seemed to aid in desloughing necrotic wounds and promoting the growth of granulation tissue. Another *Lancet* report in 1987 reported using such a sugar paste in a deep infected wound, only to have the patient develop renal failure with severe hyponatremia.[38] Szerafin and co–workers used granulated sugar in the wounds of nine patients suffering from post–operative mediastinitis after open heart surgery. These wounds were infected, and, after being treated with sugar, they became clean, filled with granulation tissue and healed.[39]

It should be noted that granulated sugar is not sterile and may contain additives such as cornstarch or one percent tricalcium which prevents caking of the packaged sugar. How these additives impact the wound healing process is not known. Further research is needed to investigate the effects of using sugar in wounds.

Vinegar

Vinegar (acetic acid) has been used as a flavoring agent in foods, as a wart remedy, an astringent mouthwash and as an antiseptic agent for open wounds.[25] It is still used in a variety of settings as an antiseptic for wound care, especially where *Pseudonomas* is suspected. A common concentration for use in wound care is 0.25 percent. The effectiveness of acetic acid solutions has probably been overrated since research studies have proven that 78 percent of *Staphylococcus aureus* survived after a 24 hour exposure to such solutions.[40] McKenna's work involved using a 0.0025 percent acetic acid solution, a concentration nontoxic to fibroblasts, with *Staphylococcus aureus, Pseudonomas aeruginosa, Escherichia coli,* group D *Enterococcus* and *Bacteroides fragilis* bacteria.[40] The 0.0025 percent concentration of acetic acid solution resulted in the slight inhibition of *Staphylococcal* growth, moderate inhibition of *Pseudonomas,* but no effect against the other organisms. There was no bactericidal effect against any of these organisms.

Acetic acid is toxic to healthy human cells, unless diluted to a strength where it no longer affects bacteria. Cooper and associates studied the toxic effects of acetic acid on cultured human fibroblast and keratinocytes and found the 0.25 percent concentration to be toxic, the 0.125 percent concentration to be less toxic, and the 0.025 percent concentration to be even

less toxic to these cells.[39] It is not until one dilutes acetic acid to a 0.0025 percent concentration that it becomes non–cytotoxic. However, it also becomes useless as an antiseptic.

Conclusion

Although there are many topical therapies used in the care of wounds, one must remember that prior to deciding which therapy should be used the caregiver must thoroughly assess the patient and the wound. After a thorough assessment, one should be able to make a decision regarding a therapy based on solid, scientific data and shared clinical experience. Healthcare providers must cease the indiscriminate use of topicals. Gone are the days of using a product for wound care because one simply heard from another that it was "good." Another pitfall is adhering to the phrase "It really works…we had good results." Without qualifying these statements, one may carelessly choose to use a therapy that may, in fact, be harmful. Informing oneself regarding the current wound care therapies will empower caregivers to make prudent decisions regarding alternative treatments. Hopefully, this information has provided the reader with new perspectives regarding some alternative therapies for wound care.

References

1. Rund C: Alternative treatments – alternative settings, in Krasner D (ed.): *Chronic Wound Care: A Clinical Source Book for Healthcare Professionals.* King of Prussia, PA, Health Management Publications, 1990, pp 309–316.
2. Haggard HW: *Mystery, Magic and Medicine: The Rise of Medicine from Superstition to Science.* Garden City, NY, Doubleday, Doran & Co., Inc., 1930, p186.
3. Klein AD, Penneys NS: Aloe vera. *J Am Acad Dermatol* 1988;18:714–720.
4. Kaufman T, Kalderon N, Ullman Y, et al.: Aloe vera gel hindered wound healing of experimental second–degree burns: A quantitative controlled study. *J Burn Care Rehabil* 1988;9(2):156–159.
5. Schmidt JM, Greenspoon JS: Aloe vera dermal wound gel is associated with a delay in wound healing. *Obstet Gynecol* 1991;78(1):115–117.
6. Davis RH, Donato JJ, et al.: Anti–inflammatory and wound healing activity of a growth substance in aloe vera. *J Amer Podiatric Med Assoc* 1994;84(2):77–81.
7. Majno G. *The Healing Hand: Man and Wound in Ancient World.* Cambridge, MA, Harvard University Press, 1982.
8. Broadwell DC, Jackson BS: *Principes of Ostomy Care.* St. Louis, MO, The CV Mosby Co., 1982, pp 698–699.
9. Ofner A: *Nursing '95 Drug Handbook,* Springhouse, PA, Springhouse Corp., 1995, pp 624–631.
10. Watcher MA, Wheeland RG: The role of topical agents in the healing of full–thickness wounds. *J Dermatol Surg Oncol* 1989;15(11): 1188–1195.
11. Reed BR, Clark RA: Cutaneous tissue repair: Practical implications of current knowledge, II [Review], *J Am Acad Dermatol* 1985;13(6): 919–941.

12. Anania WC, Rosen, RC, Wallace JA, et al. Treatment of diabetic skin ulcerations with povidone–iodine and sugar. *J Am Pod Med Assn* 1985;75:472–474.

13. Knutson RA, Merbitz LA, et al. Use of sugar and povidone–iodine to enhance wound healing: A five year experience. *South Med J* 1981;74:1329–1335.

14. Cohen K, Diegelman RF, Linblad WJ: *Wound Healing: Biochemical and Clinical Aspects*. Philadelphia, PA, WB Saunders Co., 1992, pp 134– 138, 159, 189, 306–307, 348, 349, 503, 552, 553, 570.

15. Pendse AK, et al.: Topical phenytoin in wound healing. *Inter J Derm* 1993;32(3):214–217.

16. Dealy C: *The Care of Wounds*. Oxford, Blackwell Scientific Publications, 1994, pp 11–17.

17. Ryan TJ: Wound healing and current dermatologic dressings. *Clin Derm* 1990;8(3–4):21–29.

18. Kloth L, McCulloch JM. Physical modalities used in wound management. The Eighth Annual Symposium on Advanced Wound Care, April 30, 1995, Health Management Publications, Inc.

19. Name HK, Park YS. A study on comparisons of ice and heat lamp for the relief of perineal discomfort (Korea). *Kanho Hakhoe Chi (J Nurs Academ) Soc* 1991;21(1):27–40.

20. Harris S. Honey for the treatment of superficial wounds: A case report and review. *Primary Intention* 1994;Nov:18–23.

21. Efem SE, Udoh KT, Iwara CI. The antimicrobial spectrum of honey and its clinical significance. *Infection* 1992;20(4):227–29.

22. Davis JS: A further note on the clinical use of scarlet red and its component, amidoazotoluol, in stimulating the epithelialization of granulating surfaces. Presented as a paper before the Johns Hopkins Medical Society, April 3, 1911.

23. Britton S: *Use and action of scarlet red*. R&D Dept., Sherwood Medical, Feb. 28, 1992.

24. Salomon JC, Diegelmann RF, Cohen IK. Effect of dressings on donor site epithelialization. *Surgical Forum* 1974;25:516–7.

25. Wenniger JA, McEwen GN: *CTFA Cosmetic Ingredient Handbook, Second Edition*. The Cosmetic, Toiletry and Fragrance Assn., Washington, DC, 1992.

26. Torrence C: *Pressure Sores: Aetiology, Treatment and Prevention*. Croom Helm, London, 1983, pp 95–99.

27. Gerber RM, Van Ort SR: Topical application of insulin to pressure sores: A questionable therapy. *Am J Nurs* 1981;1159.

28. Gilson G: *Topical Agents for Open Wounds*. Support Systems International, Inc., 1991, pp 1–4, 16–1.

29. Gogia PP (ed.): *Clinical Wound Management*. Thorofare, NJ, SLACK Inc., 1995 pp 185–193.

30. *Hyperbaric Oxygen Therapy: A Committee Report*. Undersea and Hyperbaric Medical Society, revised 1992.

31. Kindwall EP: Uses of hyperbaric oxygen therapy in the 1990's. *Cleveland Clinic J of Med* 1992;59(5): 517–526.

32. Gruber RP, et al.: Skin permeability to oxygen and hyperbaric oxygen. *Arch Surg* 1970;101:69.

33. Cohen K, Diegelman RF, Linblad WJ. *Wound Healing: Biochemical and Clinical Aspects*. Philadelphia, PA, WB Saunders Co., 1992.

34. Bodnor NS, Kiss–Buris ST, et al. Novel soft steroids; effects on cell growth in vitro and on wound healing in the mouse. *Steroids* 1991;58(8):434–9.

35. Bolton L, Fattu AJ. Topical agents and wound healing (Review). *Clin Dermatol* 1994;12(1):95–120.

36. Podrasky DL, Flynn KT: Topical sugar for healing: Kitchen magic or science? *Ostomy/Wound Management* 1988;(Spring):24–28.

37. Gordon H, Middleton K, et al.: Sugar and wound healing [Letter]. *Lancet* 1985;2(8456):663–665.

38. Debure A, Gachot B, et al.: Acute renal failure after use of granulated sugar in deep infected wound [Letter]. *Lancet* 1987;1(8540):1034– 1035.

39. Szerafin T, Vaszily M, Peterffy A: Topical treatment using granulated sugar in advanced mediastinitis following open heart surgery [Review, Hungarian]. *Orvosi Hetilap* 1990;131 (13): 691–695.

40. Doughty D: A rational approach to the use of topical antiseptics. *J WOCN* 1994;21(6):224–231.

29
Debridement

Karen Lou Kennedy, FNP, RN, CS and Daniel L. Tritch, MD

Kennedy KL, Tritch DL. Debridement. In: Krasner D, Kane D. *Chronic Wound Care, Second Edition*. Wayne, PA, Health Management Publications, Inc., 1997, pp 227–234.

Introduction

Debridement is defined in *Taber's Cyclopedic Medical Dictionary* as "the removal of foreign material and dead or damaged tissue, especially in a wound." Debridement of devitalized tissue is considered the most important single factor in the management of contaminated wounds. Any necrotic tissue observed during the initial (or subsequent) assessment of the wound should be debrided from the wound if this intervention is consistent with overall patient goals. Because several methods of debridement are available, the clinician should select the method most appropriate to the patient's condition and goals. Regardless of the method selected, the need to assess and control pain should always be considered.[1]

Wound healing cannot take place until necrotic tissue is removed. Devitalized tissue is a medium for infection. Most devitalized tissue supports the growth of pathological organisms which can cause infection or retard wound healing. To promote healing, it is essential for the ulcer to be clean and free from necrotic tissue. Devitalized tissue refers to slough or eschar. Slough is necrotic (dead) proteinetious material such as collagen, fibrin and elastin and is usually yellow in color. Eschar is thick, leathery, necrotic, devitalized tissue and is often black, brown or gray. It is well understood, but often forgotten, that a critical phase of wound healing is the debridement process in which debris and dead tissue are removed from the wound by autolysis and phagocytosis.[2] However, in patients with chronic illnesses, surgical wound dehiscence, dehydration or infection, the body's ability to debride itself may be compromised. In some cases necrotic tissue may accumulate faster than the body can debride it.

When To Debride

Debride a wound when there is deep eschar, purulence, infection or a large area of necrotic tissue. Any necrotic tissue in a wound should be debrided from the ulcer unless it is contraindicated given overall patient goals.[1]

Ulcers cannot heal with necrotic tissue present. Protein is lost through ulcer exudate and the necrotic tissue becomes a breeding ground for microorganisms. There is also an increased risk of septicemia, osteomyelitis, limb amputation and death, which are carefully weighed against patient goals and vascular status.

The following co–factors may reduce the individual's capacity to heal: peripheral vascular disease, diabetes mellitus, immune deficiencies, collagen vascular diseases, malignancies, psychosis, and depression.

When Not To Debride

Clean non–infected wounds free of necrotic tissue, foreign matter or fibrin and collagen slough do not need debridement. A stable wound may not need debriding. A stable wound is a clean, free of necrotic tissue, dry, non–tender, non–fluctuant, non–erythematous, non–suppurative wound. If the wound has healthy granulation tissue and has no necrotic tissue, it should not be debrided. If a wound does have necrotic tissue and the overall goal for the patient is not to heal the ulcer, but rather to maintain comfort (which may be an appropriate goal for a terminally ill patient), it may not be appropriate to debride the ulcer.

Do not debride in the presence of dry gangrene or a stable, dry, ischemic wound until the patient's vascular status can be improved. Heel ulcers with dry eschar need not be debrided if they do not have edema, erythema, fluctuance, or drainage.[1] This eschar provides a natural protective cover. If signs of complications occur, debridement may be necessary. A pulseless limb usually should not be debrided. Wounds with these qualities need to be assessed daily. However, if signs of infection, such as edema, erythema, fluctuance or purulent drainage are present, debridement may be necessary.

The major debridement categories, mechanical, autolytic and enzymatic debridement, will be discussed in this chapter as well as biologic debridement, one of the first types of debridement.

Selective Versus Non–Selective Methods

Selective methods of debridement remove only necrotic tissue. Non–selective debridement removes both healthy and non–healthy tissue. Selective methods include sharp/surgical, enzymatic and autolytic debridement. Non–selective debridement methods include wet–to–dry dressings, wet–to–wet dressings, inappropriate wound irrigations and whirlpool.

Selective and non–selective debridement methods can be ranked from aggressive to passive. The most aggressive method is surgical debridement, done with instrumentation by a surgeon or physician, usually in an operating or special procedures room. Sharp debridement, which is slightly less aggressive, is also done with instrumentation (scissors and scalpel). It may be performed by a physician or other licensed, trained healthcare professional, such as a nurse or physical therapist.

Mechanical Debridement

Mechanical debridement is the removal of foreign material and devitalized or contaminated tissue from a wound by physical forces rather than by chemical (enzymatic) or natural (autolytic) forces. Types of mechanical debridement include sharp/surgical debridement, wet–to–dry dressings, dextranomers, irrigation, and whirlpool. (See Chapter 13 on Wound Cleansing, Wound Irrigation and Wound Disinfection in this source book.)

Sharp/Surgical debridement. Sharp debridement is the fastest of the debridement categories. It is selective, causing little or no damage to healthy tissue (unless a minimal amount of healthy tissue is excised as a precautionary measure sometimes known as a wide excision). It can be used alone or combined with other techniques. The purpose of sharp debridement is to remove thick, adherent eschar and devitalized tissue in extensive ulcers.

Small wounds can be debrided at the bedside, in the home, or in the clinician's office. Larger wounds that require significant hemostatis or anesthesia might well require an operating room or special procedures room.

The surgical debridement of wounds is one of the oldest methods of wound treatment. The Chinese were the first to document surgical debridement some 5,000 years ago. Since the wars of antiquity, physicians, surgeons, and their assistants have utilized debridement with sharp instruments to aid in wound healing.

Sharp debridement with scalpel–like instruments is mentioned in Caesar's Gaelic wars, which was written about 44 BC. The word debridement was coined by Napoleon's Chief Surgeon during the Napoleonic Wars. During the American Civil War sharp debridement of wounds was the primary method available to promote wound healing. Multiple references to battlefield wound debridement at Gettysburg, Shiloh, and Bull Run demonstrate the confidence of 19th century surgeons and nurses in the sharp debridement technique. Unfortunately, the skilled personnel necessary to implement debridement were not usually available for the large masses of casualties who would have benefited. These wounds were often complicated by lead and steel fragments, topsoil, and bits and pieces of debris which, of course, also needed rapid debridement.

When surgical or sharp debridement to remove necrotic or mucoid tissue is the debridement of choice, it may not always be feasible; thus, another method such as autolytic or chemical (enzymatic) debridement is often substituted. Sharp debridement may be painful to the patient, so pain control measures should be initiated prior to debridement for patient comfort. Sharp debridement is usually performed on Stage III and IV ulcers with large amounts of necrotic tissue. Removal of foreign material or devitalized tissue is accomplished with a sharp instrument, such as a scalpel. Laser debridement is also considered a type of sharp debridement.[3] Surgical excision is the most efficient method of eliminating devitalized tissue.[3]

Sharp debridement is indicated in advancing cellulitis with sepsis, in the diabetic patient, when infection threatens the patient's life, or when there are large amounts of necrotic tissue or large pieces of slough in the wound. It is often considered for immunocompromised patients, such as those with diabetes mellitus or cancer.

Sharp debridement is contraindicated when the patient is on anticoagulant therapy or has a coagulapathy (i.e., Hemophilia), when the patient cannot remain stationary during the procedure, when a consent form is unobtainable, or when appropriate anesthesia, if indicated, cannot be provided.

One complication which can occur during sharp debridement is hemorrhage due to arterial bleeding. This can be controlled by ligation or cautery. Venous hemorrhage can be controlled with direct pressure to the bleeding area.

The main advantages of sharp debridement are that it is the most rapid method of debridement and it may be done at the bedside either in the home or nursing home. Surgical debridement more than any other method allows for the quick removal of large amounts of devitalized tissue. Large, thick eschar can be removed most appropriately by surgical debridement. If the patient becomes acutely ill from advancing cellulitis or sepsis, then sharp debridement becomes the imperative method of choice. Sharp debridement is quite selective in that little or no damage is done to healthy tissue if the debrider is skilled and cautious. Surgical debridement occasionally involves removal of small amounts of healthy tissue as a precautionary measure to insure that all the necrotic tissue is removed. This is called "wide debridement or excision."

Disadvantages of sharp debridement are that it requires skill, it may require the use of an operating room or special procedures room, sterile instruments are needed, and it may be painful. The law in some states restricts the practice to specific types of healthcare providers.

In *Ostomy/Wound Management*, a survey performed by Fowler, et. al. of practices in thirty states indicated that sharp debridement was considered to be within the confines of nursing practice. Of the thirty states surveyed, three states placed the procedure under an advisory/informed consent rubric and offered strict criteria. One state interpreted the procedure as a category two activity, placing it under simple implementation of special procedures. Seven states indicated the need for advanced or specialty preparation, and four states interpreted instrument debridement of nonviable tissue as an overlapping medical procedure. Four states said it was not within the scope of nursing practice. Most states referred to their nurse practitioner acts to make the determination. In truth, irrespective of state laws, healthcare professionals must obtain hands–on skills by working with the person skilled in instrument debridement. No written test or laws can determine when such a trainee is ready to debride on his or her own. The mentor must make this decision. Most other forms of debridement can largely be learned by textbook.

Sharp debridement can be performed by a clinician in a state that allows it or by an attending physician, surgeon or plastic surgeon. Sharp debridement is a skill learned and perfected through collaboration between healthcare professionals that can benefit both patients and caregivers.[5] Sharp debridement performed by non–physician providers requires review of state practice acts and institutional clearance.

Sharp debridement should be stopped when there is tendon exposure, penetration of fascia plane or excessive bleeding. In such cases, if the debridement is being done by a non–physician, the patient's physician should be notified. A good rule of thumb is to stop when a gut feeling tells you to or when you have any doubt about proceeding. Debridement should also be stopped when holes in necrotic tissue that obstruct vision are encountered or when extensive undermining which would cause loss of visual contact is present. If there is gross purulence or cellulitis, appropriate cultures should be taken. Other factors which will limit debridement are abscess formation or unexpected bleeding. Sharp debridement should be discontinued when the pain tolerance of the patient has been reached or if fatigue of the person doing the debridement occurs. Several short debridement sessions are frequently more appropriate than one longer session and may improve patient comfort. Sharp debridement should be considered when progressive demarcation of the wound is noted.

Basic techniques. Basic sharp debridement techniques include debriding one layer at a time, applying traction to the dead tissue, cutting parallel to the plane of the wound and being careful of tendons and other special tissues or structures. Sharp debridement will almost always make the wound larger. Technical aspects to consider are pain medication, proper lighting, gauze, hemostatic support and additional help. The tools needed for sharp debridement include a scalpel, scissors (serrated edges are most helpful) or other sharp instrument to remove devitalized tissue. Use clean, dry dressings for 8 to 24 hours after sharp debridement associated with bleeding, then reinstitute moist dressings.[1]

Once the debridement location is established, instruments are assembled before beginning debridement. Whether sharp debridement is to be a sterile or clean procedure is currently a matter of considerable debate. At this juncture it is best to use clinical judgment based on an evaluation of the patient's overall health status and immune function, the severity of the wound and environmental factors.

Three basic types of scissors are useful for debridement: tissue scissors, dissection scissors and bandage scissors. Four inch iris or tissue scissors, both curved and straight, are useful in wound debridement and revision. These scissors are sharp and appropriate for use in situations requiring control. Bandage scissors are useful for cutting dressing materials for appropriate size. Surgical scissors, preferably those with serrated edges, are always necessary. Note that all scissors can be serrated at minimal additional cost by indicating this preference to the manufacturer. Drapes (sterile or non–sterile) may be used to isolate the wound or ulcer.

Several different types of forceps are also necessary for rapid debridement. The use of forceps without teeth is discouraged because their flat surfaces tend to crush tissue quite easily. Forceps are more useful if they have teeth which allow less force to be applied to the tissue during debridement. To minimize damage to healthy tissue, use forceps to grasp only necrotic tissue. Different sizes are helpful if removal of necrotic tissue from different levels of the ulcer is to be accomplished. A standard scalpel with a #15 blade is small and works better for precise debridement, a #10 is useful in the removal of thick heavy tissue and for larger incisions, and a #11 blade is commonly used for incision and drainage.

Pain management. Once the appropriate instruments are arranged, then the patient is positioned for his or her comfort as well as for the comfort of the individual performing the debridement. The patient needs to be prepared with appropriate analgesia before the procedure begins. Occasionally simple verbal reassurance is all that is necessary before beginning debridement. Hypnosis is also being used to assist in wound debridement at a number of medical centers in the United States. Analgesia can be provided safely outside of the operating room using local infiltration of anesthetic with regional anesthesia or by employing behavioral (non–drug) methods. Systemic pain relief is often required to provide optimal pain control during and after the procedure.

Only when the realistic fear of cardiorespiratory collapse is present should analgesia be withheld for a painful debridement procedure. The presence of a condition that could result in cardiovascular or hemodynamic collapse is not an absolute contraindication to systemic analgesia, but obviously careful monitoring must be provided.

No anesthetic or analgesic agent should be used unless the clinician understands the proper technique of administration, dosage, side effects, and treatment of overdose. The intravenous route is often the preferred method for delivering the agent because of its rapid onset and more reliable dosing. Intravenous administration avoids the unpredictable absorption, onset, and duration of action associated with intramuscular administration. An intravenous cannula may be quite easily placed following an intradermal injection of lidocaine. Morphine titrated carefully with 5 to 10 minutes observation generally provides a safe and adequate analgesia. Intravenous morphine doses of one to ten milligrams, depending on the age, weight, and pain intensity, provide safe anesthesia in the absence of respiratory problems.

Morphine administered intravenously has certain contraindications including chronic obstructive pulmonary disease or other types of significant lung disease, pregnancy, or any disease which impairs the monitoring of side effects. Since respiratory depression is strongly related to the degree of sedation, stimulation of the patient as well as the administration of small amounts of Naloxone may be adequate to reverse hypoventilation. One needs to be able to utilize the bag and mask if hypoventilation does become severe. Ultimately, endotracheal intubation may be necessary for severe respiratory depression. Nausea, hypotension, and low heart rate may also be noted and the methods of treatment for each of these need to be reviewed in advance. Hydromorphone is another medication that can help control the pain.

Meperidine may also be useful for brief anesthesia, but it is not a satisfactory drug for prolonged use. Fentanyl may be used in small doses and has the additional side effect of inducing chest wall rigidity. Please note that all opioids may cause an acute Parkinson–like syndrome, particularly in older patients.

Nonsterodial anti–inflammatory drugs have minimal analgesic effect and are not useful during debridement.

Benzodiazepines are useful adjuncts to opioids. Although they have no analgesic function, they reduce anxiety and induce amnesia which is especially useful if multiple procedures need to be employed over several days. The combination of benzodiazepines and opioids requires intense monitoring as the incidence of respiratory problems is increased over using either drug separately. The reader is referred to Chapter 43 on Chronic Wound Pain in this source book for further information on this subject.

Wet–to–dry dressings. Wet–to–dry debridement involves moistening one layer of wide–mesh 100 percent cotton gauze with normal saline, wringing it out until it is just damp, applying it to the wound surface, and allowing it to dry before removing. Wet–to–dry dressings are used on full thickness and

Stage II, III and IV pressure ulcers with necrotic tissue and moderate amounts of exudate. Wet–to–wet debridement is the same as wet–to–dry debridement except the dressing is not allowed to dry out before removal. Wet–to–wet debridement is less painful and less traumatic, but it will not lift as much debris from the wound bed.

Wet–to–dry debridement is nonselective and may actually interrupt the wound healing process as emerging granulation tissue is dehydrated and new vessels are disrupted by the removal of an adherent dry gauze. Wet–to–dry debridement is fast and aggressive, but it is non–selective and can be painful and cause bleeding of the wound when the dried gauze is removed. Wet–to–dry and wet–to–wet debridement must be performed with 100 percent cotton gauze sponges.

One advantage of wet–to–dry debridement is that it can be used as the initial form of debridement while the patient is being prepared for surgical debridement. The major disadvantage is that it is non–selective. Wet–to–dry debridement removes viable tissue as well as nonviable tissue. It can be potentially traumatic to granulation tissue and especially to new epithelial tissue. This method may cause bleeding (which essentially begins the wounding process all over again). It should be discontinued when the wound is clean and granulating. At this time if gauze dressings are continued, the gauze should be moistened to promote healing by secondary intention. Removal of the dry dressing may be painful and requires adequate analgesia.

Dextranomers. Dextranomer beads (e.g. Debrisan® Johnson & Johnson Medical, Inc. Arlington, TX) may be inserted directly into the wound either as granules or as a paste. They absorb wound exudate which turns the beads into a gel that continues to clean the wound through its absorptive capabilities. One gram of hydrophylic beads can absorb up to 4 grams of water. The granules do not digest bacteria or necrotic tissue, but they draw bacteria away from the wound bed. The absorption of the exudate, dead cells and bacteria helps to clean and debride the wound. It is essential that the gel be irrigated with normal saline to prevent the formation of granulomas. To help maintain the gel hydration, a semipermeable film may be superimposed on the gel or paste. Dextranomers can be effective in promoting autolysis of necrotic tissue, although the biochemical interaction between these materials and the wound surface is unclear. Dressings are usually changed daily. The wound should be cleansed with normal saline between dressing changes, and care should be given to assure they are thoroughly evacuated from the wound at each dressing change. [7] Dextranomer beads and paste should be discontinued when the wound is clean. One disadvantage of their use is that they may be difficult to apply if the patient cannot be positioned so that they can be poured into the wound.

Autolytic Debridement

Autolytic debridement is a process of debridement that utilizes the body's own digestive enzymes to break down necrotic tissue. Autolysis is accomplished by keeping the wound moist with occlusive or semiocclusive moisture retentive dressings, such as transparent films, hydrocolloids, and hydrogels, that allow the body's own enzymes, (i.e. collagenases, gelatinases and stromelysins) to liquefy necrotic tissue. Eschar and necrotic debris are softened, liquefied and separated when the process works optimally. The ability of the body's own enzymes to facilitate debridement is to an extent dependent upon the available moisture present at the wound site. This is another reason why adequate hydration is important, provided there is normal kidney function. If, for some reason, the wound is not kept moist by the dressing covering, autolytic debridement will not take place.

This method is highly selective, usually painless, but slower than sharp debridement. It can be used with full thickness wounds and Stage III and IV pressure ulcers with small to moderate amounts of exudate and necrotic tissue. Transparent films and hydrocolloids retain wound fluid on the wound site and promote autolysis. Hydrogels will generally hasten the autolytic process by quickly rehydrating and softening necrotic tissue.

Autolytic debridement aids the body's natural wound fluid to soften and separate the dead tissue. Although slower than other methods, autolytic debridement may be appropriate for patients who cannot tolerate other methods and are not likely to develop infections. Autolytic debridement can be used to enhance debridement in patients whose medical and nutritional status is fairly stable. Dressings are usually changed on a daily or prn basis. The wound is cleansed with normal saline or a nonionic surfactant wound cleanser. Autolytic debridement is an appropriate choice for patients who cannot tolerate other forms of debridement. Autolytic debridement is noninvasive and selective. There is minimal discomfort and it takes minimal expertise to perform. Autolytic debridement would be appropriate for patients who are on anticoagulant therapy and for whom sharp debridement is contraindicated.

The disadvantages are that autolytic debridement takes longer than other methods of debridement. The wound must be watched closely for signs of infection. Autolytic debridement is contraindicated if the wound is infected.[1] Occlusive dressings are contraindicated in infected wounds with the potential for anaerobic infection. Occlusive dressings are usually contraindicated in immunosuppressed patients since they might not work as well and must be used with care on patients with wound infection. The wound should be monitored closely for complications of infections, such as abscess, sinus tract, meningitis, and endocarditis.

Enzymatic Debridement

Chemical or enzymatic debridement is the use of proteolytic substances (enzymatic agents) that stimulate the breakdown of necrotic tissue. This form of debridement should be considered when the individual cannot tolerate surgery, in long–term care facilities, or when the patient is receiving care at home, and when the wound does not appear infected. If infection spreads beyond the wound (e.g., advancing cellulitis, sepsis), there is urgent need for sharp debridement.[1] Chemical debridement is less aggressive and slower than sharp debridement. It is usually performed on full thickness wounds, such as Stage III and IV pressure ulcers, with large amounts of necrotic tissue. It can be used to penetrate though hard eschar after scoring or crosshatching. Scoring or crosshatching refers to using a sharp instrument or scalpel to cut through the depth of the eschar in a crosshatch fashion allowing the enzymatic agent to penetrate through to the wound more quickly.

Enzymatic debriding agents liquefy necrotic wound debris. There are several types of enzymatic debriding agents. Collagenase (Santyl®, Knoll Pharmaceutical Company, Mount Olive, NJ), Fibrinolysin (Elase® Parke–Davis, Morris Plains, NJ) and Fibrinolysin and deoxyribonuclease (Elase® with Chloromycetin, Parke–Davis).

Collagenase, an FDA licensed biologic causes debridement of necrotic tissue. Research findings indicate that collagenase promotes debridement and growth of granulation tissue within 3 to 30 days. Santyl is a sterile enzymatic debriding ointment which contains 250 collagenase units per gram of white petrolatum USP. The enzyme is derived from fermentation by *Clostridium histolyticum*. Collagenase possesses the unique ability to digest native and denatured collagen in necrotic tissue. It is recommended that thick eschar be crosshatched with a #10 blade prior to initiating treatment. The

optimal pH range is 6 to 8 lower and higher pH conditions will decrease enzyme activity. The action of the enzyme may be stopped, if so desired, by the application of Burrow's solution USP (pH 3.6 to 4.4) to the wound bed. Collagenase should be applied once a day until debridement is complete and granulation tissue is well established.

Elase contains two lytic enzymes, fibrinolysin and deoxyribonuclease; in addition, Elase with Chloromycetin contains fibrinolysin and deoxyribonuclease combined with chloramphenicol in an ointment base. These chemical debriding agents (also known as enzymatic debriding agents or pharmacological agents) help loosen and remove slough or eschar from the wound. Choloamphenicol is a broad–spectrum antibiotic originally isolated from Streptomyces venezuelae. It is therapeutically active against a wide variety of susceptible organisms, both gram–positive and gram–negative. Desoxyribonuclease attacks DNA and fibrinolysin principally attacks the fibrin of blood clots and fibrinous exudates. Enzymatic action produces clean surfaces which prepare the wound for healing. Fibrinolysin and deoxyribonuclease combined with chloramphenicol adds a broad spectrum antibiotic that is primarily bacteriostatic and acts by inhibition of protein synthesis by interfering with the transfer of activated amino acids from soluble RNA to ribosomes.

Fibrinolysin and desoxyribonuclease combined with chloramphenicol is indicated for use in the treatment of infected lesions such as burns, ulcers and wounds where the actions of both a debriding agent and a topical antibiotic are desired. Chloromycetin can cause bone marrow hypoplasia. Recommended application is at least once a day, preferably two to three times daily. Dense, dry eschar, if present, should be removed surgically before enzymatic debridement is attempted.

Panafil® (Rystan Co., Inc., Little Falls, NJ) contains standardized papain 10 percent, urea U.S.P. 10 percent and chlorophyllin copper complex 0.5 percent in a hydrophilic base. Papain, the proteolytic, active enzyme, is a potent digestant of nonviable protein matter, but is harmless to viable tissue. The urea denatures the protein to allow the papain to work. Panafil has the unique advantage of being active over a wide pH range of 3 to 12. It may be inactivated by the salts of heavy metals (lead, silver, mercury, etc.) Contact with medications containing these metals should be avoided. A small percentage of patients may experience a transient "burning" sensation on application of the ointment. Recommended dosage is once or twice a day.

Accuzyme™ (Healthpoint® Medical, Fort Worth, TX) is a papain–urea debriding ointment. It contains papain (1.1 x 10^5 USP units of activity) and 100 mg urea in a hydrophilic ointment base composed of purified water, emulsifying wax, glycerin, isopropyl palmitate, potassium phosphate monobasic, fragrance, methylparaben and propylparaben. It is active over a pH range of 3 to 12. Accuzyme is indicated for debridement of necrotic tissue and liquefication of slough in acute and chronic lesions such as pressure ulcer, varicose and diabetic ulcers, burns, postoperative wounds, pilonidal cyst wounds, carbuncles and miscellaneous traumatic or infected wounds. There can be a transient "burning" sensation experienced by a small percentage of patients upon applying the product. The wound should be cleansed with Curasol™ Wound Cleanser (Healthpoint Medical, Fort Worth, TX) or saline and reapplied one or two times per day.

Granulex® (Dow Hickam Pharmaceuticals, Inc., Sugar Land, TX) is sometimes mentioned as a debriding agent or listed under the enzymatic debriders. However, it is a topical wound dressing which contains castor oil, balsam peru and the enzyme trypsin. Though the therapeutic use of trypsin is as a debriding agent that does not harm healthy tissue, the amount present in Granulex is only sufficient to maintain balance in a clean wound. The recommended usage is once or twice a day. Some product classifications list Granulex as a debriding agent; however, Granulex should not be classified as a debriding agent or wound cleanser.

Enzymatic debridement is more specific than surgical and mechanical debridement. It is less expensive than the surgical method and is easier to perform in long term care and home care settings. Enzymatic debriding agents may be used on most wounds that need debridement. It can be used for bedridden patients and all dermal ulcers, including diabetic ulcers, atherosclerotic ulcers and venous stasis ulcers. Enzymes can be used alone to break down the eschar, after sharp debridement, or in conjunction with mechanical debridement.[1]

If topical antimicrobials are to be used with enzymatic debriding agents, care should be given in selecting a compatible drug. Caregivers should refer to the package insert of enzymes to determine compatibility with antimicrobials. The following antimicrobials are compatible with most enzymatic debriding agents: Silver sulfadiazine, neomycin, bacitracin, gentamicin, mafenide acetate. Enzyme–incompatible denaturing agents include povidone–iodine, hydrogen peroxide, hexachlorophene, silver nitrate solution, nitrofurazone, benzalkonium chloride, thiomiersol and mercury.

Gauze should be used as the secondary dressing with an enzymatic debriding agent. There are no studies that indicate whether hydrocolloid dressings and/or semipermeable membrane dressings can be utilized with debriding enzymes.

Chemical debriding agents should be discontinued when sufficient debridement has taken place.

Biological Debridement (Maggot Therapy)

The use of fly larvae to debride wounds and promote healing was a common surgical practice in the 1930s.[8] Over the past 60 years Maggot Debridement Therapy (MDT) has been used as an alternative to sharp debridement. Maggots are used for wounds which have irregular edges or are deep and narrow, where surgical debridement would cause major losses of healthy surrounding tissues. Maggots aid wound healing and debride in diverse ways; however, the exact mechanisms of how fly larvae selectively digest only necrotic tissues without breaking down viable tissue are not known.

It is thought that maggots stimulate wound healing by promoting the production of a serous exudate by the host. This fluid reduces the concentration of bacteria. The movement of organisms is also thought to promote granulation tissue formation. In addition, the larvae secrete proteolytic enzymes that tend to break down and digest necrotic tissue. The liquefied tissue is then ingested by the larvae as a source of nutrition. Also, maggots secrete calcium salts and other antimicrobial agents. It appears that the maggots secrete an enzyme cocktail containing collagenases which readily hydrolyzes denatured proteins but is ineffective against native proteins. A secondary benefit of maggot debridement therapy is the presence of antimicrobial factors, produced and secreted by maggots, (related to royalisn, the honey bee antibacterial protein).

The first physician to regularly use and promote maggot therapy was William Baer. During the 1920s Baer demonstrated that maggots could be sterilized first by placing their eggs in a solution of alcohol, hydrochloric acid, and mercury bichloride, and then raising the larvae on a sterile food source. In 1934, Steward noted that shallow lesions with a large amount of necrotic tissue responded best to maggot therapy. Other observers noted that an average of 30 larvae could consume about 1 gram of necrotic tissue per day.

Summary

From acute care to long term care and home care, there is a mechanism and product that would meet the needs and goals of every patient with pressure ulcers that needs debridement. In an era

of advanced technology and multiplicity of biochemical products, debridement of pressure ulcers
remains a necessity to promote healing.

References

1. Clinical Practice Guideline, Number 15, *Treatment of Pressure Ulcers*. U.S. Department of Health and Human Services, Public Health Service. Agency for Health Care Policy and Research, 1994.
2. Cooper, D. The physiology of wound healing: An overview. In: Krasner D (ed). *Chronic Wound Care: A Clinical Source Book For Healthcare Professionals*. King of Prussia, PA, Health Management Publications, Inc., 1990, pp.1–11.
3. Ginsburg SB, Ginsburg LJ. Seeing a difficult problem in a new light:The role of the Laser in pressure ulcer manage-ment. In: Krasner D (ed).*Chronic Wound Care: A Clinical Source Book For Healthcare Professionals*. King of Prussia, PA, Health Management Publications, Inc., 1990, pp. 410–414.
4. Bryant R. *Acute and Chronic Wounds, Nursing Management*. St. Louis, MO, Mosby Year Book.
5. Troyer–Caudle J. Debridement: Removal of non–viable tissue, *Ostomy/Wound Management* 1993;39(6):24–32.
6. Macklebust J, Sieggreen M, *Pressure Ulcers Guidelines for Prevention and Nursing Management*. West Dundee, IL, S–N Publications, 1991.
8. Jeffrey JJ. Collagen degradation. Wound Healing. *Biochemical & Clinical Aspects*. Philadelphia, PA, W.B. Saunders Company,
9. Clark RAF. *The Molecular and Cellular Biology of Wound Repair, Second Edition*.
10. Parks W. The Production, role, and regulation of matrix met-alloproteinases in the healing epidermis. *WOUNDS*;1995;7A:23A–35A.

30
Surgical Repair

Dean P. Kane, MD, FACS

Kane DP. Surgical repair. In: Krasner D, Kane D. *Chronic Wound Care, Second Edition*. Wayne, PA, Health Management Publications, Inc., 1997, pp 235–244.

Introduction

The history of wound healing is first documented in 1700 BC in the Smith Papyrus. The ancient physicians of Greece, Egypt, India and Europe provided debridement and cleansing, removal of foreign bodies, covering and protection, and wound closure to hasten healing and protect their patients from limb loss and loss of life. Wound healing evolved through centuries of caustic and gentle treatments often carried out on the battle field by history's famous field surgeons, but mostly depended on the body's natural ability to heal itself. Boiling oil, hot cautery and scalding water were aggressive 14th century reactions to the use of gun powder and bullet injuries. Salves and gentle care were espoused by Ambroise Paré in the 1500s. Not much has changed in 3700 years, yet with a better understanding of the wound healing process, occlusive, moist environments and surgical reconstruction hasten the wound healing process to achieve the body's first priority, a sealed differential barrier from the outside environment.

Improved patient outcomes, cost containment, comfort and quality of life are all buzz words for wound healthcare in the 1990s. It is expected that the U.S. population age 65 and older will double from 35 million to 65 million by the year 2010.[1] Reviewing the best estimates, 20 to 25 percent of those individuals within an acute care hospital, intermediate nursing facility or assisted living environment will develop a chronic wound. The rest of society is walking and working with painful non–healing ulcers which affect their personal and economic livelihoods.

Priorities

A comprehensive evaluation of the entire patient is necessary at the time of local wound assessment. Co–factors including concurrent illnesses, such as pneumonia, congestive heart failure, urinary tract infection, diabetes, malnutrition, neurologic incompetence, dementia, immobility, incontinence, and prognosis for activities of daily living (ADLs) and ambulation, will affect each patient's individual management plan and wound healing goals.

The current goals of would care include 1) reversing wound progression in order to save life and limb, 2) achieving a stable closed skin barrier which will protect the patient from infection, reduce the number of dressing changes and diminish hospital or nursing intensity, 3) reaching a functional outcome to return the patient to his or her maximal activities in the shortest possible time, 4) providing the most cosmetic match of skin tissues and reducing scars to a minimum, 5) providing comfort and reducing pain, 6) performing these goals in a cost effective manner.

Reconstructive options should be considered for those selected patients whose length of healing would be extraordinarily long in months or years and whose health status is appropriate for more rapid healing options.

Today, many patients with chronic, debilitating neurologic maladies, malnutrition and immobility may never heal a chronic wound. While ongoing assessment and wound maintenance is necessary, these patients may never become suitable candidates for reconstruction. For these patients, compassionate local management and holistic, comfort care are reasonable goals.

Making the Diagnosis

Accurate diagnosis of the wound is necessary in order to provide the correct healing course. While all wounds need closure of the skin's surface, many wounds require other management dependent upon their pathophysiology.

Pressure Ulcers

Over 1.3 billion dollars in healthcare costs were consumed treating an estimated 2.1 million pressure ulcers in 1990.[1] These bed sores, pressure ulcers or decubitus ulcers occur when unrelieved pressure causes soft tissue necrosis between the underlying bed surface and the overlying bony prominence. Patients with central neurologic maladies, such as stroke or Parkinson's disease as well as peripheral nerve injuries including such polyneuropathys as diabetes or spinal cord lesions (paraplegics and quadraplegics), have a high risk of immobility, and therefore pressure ulcer formation is common. Mean capillary pressure is considered to be 32 mm Hg. Any pressure above this amount will cause ischemia and subsequent necrosis of surrounding tissues.

Debilitated patients are usually more dehydrated and have less tissue turgor with diminished oncotic pressures allowing for ischemic injury to occur at less than mean capillary pressures. In addition to local pressure ulcer care and considerations for reconstruction, the total management scheme includes nutrition, hydration, pain control, pressure relieving or pressure reducing surfaces and a turning schedule which adequately maintains patient mobility and tissue perfusion.

The outward signs of pressure ulcer formation are typically described as the "tip of the iceberg." The redness, blistering or small necrotic eschar first visualized on the outer skin overlying sacral, ischial, trochanter, scapular, posterior heel, elbow and occipital bed sores are always smaller than the underlying cone–shaped zone of necrosis which includes epidermis, dermis, subcutaneous fat, fascia and muscle and, if severe enough, participates with the underlying periosteum, bone, and joint.

Prevention of these wounds remains the mainstay of care. Neurologically incompetent, cardiac, orthopedic and spinal cord injured individuals with high risk for pressure ulcer formation should begin with mobility, turning schedules and pressure relieving mattresses or therapeutic beds. Should an eschar develop, autolysis with an occlusive dressing such as a hydrocolloid wafer or transparent film is recommended.

Rapid coagulation necrosis with infection of soft tissue planes may occur. Should this be a source of infection and sepsis, then surgical debridement and drainage of infected tissues is required. Topical and systemic antibiotics may be recommended. Local care is indicated and may include staged debridement of necrotic tissue until such time that the wound has progressed through the inflammatory stages of wound healing hastening the wound healing goals, achieving a clean granulation base free of infection.

Surgical versus non–surgical options are now considered to achieve a closure of the wound. Occasionally, given the appropriate environment, wounds go on to complete healing by secondary intent. Surgical alternatives are considered when reconstruction will hasten the healing process, provide greater pain reduction or reduce costs. The risk/benefit ratio must be clearly discussed with the patient and family.

Flap reconstruction provides well vascularized composite tissue reconstructions lending greater durability to sites with bony prominences. But many patients are not appropriate candidates for such surgical options. For these individuals, the secondary goal of wound care, which is to promote a stable, chronic, aseptic wound including comfort measures and reduced pain, is essential. These patients may have multi–organ failure causing malnutrition, immobility and multiple pressure ulcers and may be non–rehabilitatable. Functional patients may require an interim period of rehabilitation including activities of daily living in order to regain nutrition, strength, range of motion and mobility. During this time the wounds are stabilizing after debridement and drainage of infection. Once optimized, these patients with better prognostic outcomes would undergo excision of the ulcer including the underlying bone, creating an acute non–infected "round" wound. They would then immediately undergo myo–fascio–cutaneous flap reconstruction, filling the defect and closing the donor site in linear fashion. Six weeks following flap reconstruction, these patients may continue their rehabilitation to optimize function.

Patients who have the highest pressure ulcer acuity include diabetics with incontinence and sacral pressure ulcers. These patients frequently become septic necessitating broad spectrum antibiotic coverage for the multi–bacterial flora at the time of debridement. Should incontinence of stool continue, a diverting colostomy must be considered in order to reduce chronic, septic recurrences whether or not flap reconstruction is offered.

Many well vascularized and durable flaps are available based upon the axial circulation of the region.[2–4] Gluteal myocutaneous and gluteal fascio-cutaneous flaps are used in the sacral region. Tensor fascia lata fasciocutaneous flaps reconstruct hip ulcers. Biceps femoris myocutaneous flaps fill ischial sores. Latissimus dorsi myocutaneous and lumbar fasciocutaneous flaps cover scapula wounds.

Posterior heel wounds are the most difficult pressure ulcers to heal due to the end arterial blood supply based on the peroneal vessels laterally and the posterior tibial vessels medially of the foot. Once the dermal blood supply has been interrupted by full thickness necrosis, no collateral circulation is available and healing by secondary intent frequently fails. Debridement many times leads to wet gangrene due to distal peripheral vascular disease. In these cases, it is recommended by this clinician that "multipodis" splints or pillows under the calves lift the heels off all hard surfaces while desiccating the wound with an antiseptic, such as povidone–iodine. Many patients with posterior heel dry gangrene will subsequently lose their limbs to wet gangrene if not monitored often. A stable chronic dry wound may be the best option for many of these patients.

Lower Extremity Ulcers

Lower extremity wounds include a great breadth of arterial, venous, diabetic and vasculitic or skin cancer chronic wounds. Many of these wounds occur together and necessitate a combined management course. Diagnosis is the initial step of management.

Arterial Ulcers. Arterial ulcers develop from inadequate arterial perfusion to the lower extremity. These ulcers may compound pressure ulcers and diabetic neuropathic ulcers, but, if isolated, arterial ulcers typically present themselves with gangrene or necrosis of the most distal aspects of the leg and foot. The wounds themselves appear to be round and punched out from lack of end arterial perfusion. Many patients experience claudication or ischemic pain during their presentation. Increased rubor or erythema of the extremity is noted as collateral circulation occurs at the subdermal level.

If a lack of circulation is palpated or dopplered, non–invasive testing, such as arterial pulse volume recordings, is indicated to identify the level of arterial occlusion. This testing may lead to arteriogram and subsequent angioplasty or revascularization. A treatment plan must be coordinated between the vascular surgeon and the reconstructive surgeon. If infection is present, debridement to reduce the septic burden is necessary while improved perfusion is

rendered. Once increased blood supply is provided and the wound is free of infection with healthy and clean granulation tissue, reconstructive options can by offered. Split thickness skin grafts, full thickness skin grafts and flap reconstructions may be considered.

While revascularization is often short lived, limb loss may have been averted by healing the wound during the interval of good perfusion.

Ischemic pain presents as acute to chronic, unrelenting and knife–like in quality. Immobility, contractures, and total patient withdrawal from full function is likely when ischemic pain occurs. If unable to be revascularized, these patients would be best off undergoing amputation prior to unrelieved ischemic pain to reduce the syndrome of phantom limb pain which will affect their every day's existence.

Venous Ulcers. Venous insufficiency is seen in a large proportion of the ambulatory working population. Venous drainage of the lower extremity returns to the heart through deep and superficial veins which are connected by veins perforating the deep fascial layer. These perforating veins have valves which drain the superficial to the deep venous system, but not vice versa unless they become incompetent from phlebitic obstructions in the deep venous system. Pelvic masses and obesity may worsen deep venous obstruction, causing chronic swelling and lymphedema. Many theories of how venous insufficiency causes skin ulceration are discussed in Chapter 20 of this source book.

Management of venous insufficiency ulcers necessitates control of infection, wound closure and redirection of blood flow from the superficial to the deep venous system.

Associated phlebitis may require anti–coagulation. Associated cellulitis may need acute hospitalization and antibiotics. On occasion, debridement is necessary to control wound infection. Leg elevation and toe to knee compression for edema control is always necessary. Sequential compression garments, typically used to reduce thrombophlebitis during prolonged operative procedures are often useful at the bedside to reduce venous swelling and properly compress the superficial veins for return of blood flow to the heart via the deep venous system. Ultimately, graded leg compression will be necessary with the use of stockings or ace wraps for the patient's entire life.

Diagnosis using duplex venous doppler, contrast venograms or other diagnostic testing may be warranted to identify obstruction. Vascular consultation may be necessary to ligate, sclerose or remove incompetent perforator veins and/or superficial varicosities.

Unna boots have been the mainstay of venous insufficiency wounds for many years. These dressings may be messy and time consuming for many patients. New techniques including multi–layered compression dressings have in fact reduced the pain and swelling of venous insufficiency and ulcerations, allowing for the patients to return to their ambulatory status with quicker healing outcomes.

I have found the majority of venous insufficiency ulcers to maintain epithelial islands within their irregular distal leg wounds which when properly managed will re–epithelialize with no surgical intervention. On occasion, split thickness skin grafts are necessary. They may be performed as outpatient procedures as long as the patient has adequate home support to maintain leg elevation and minimized ambulation during the 3 to 6 weeks of skin graft healing.

Split thickness skin grafts are typically harvested from the lateral thigh although other donor sites are available. Current techniques allow for expansion of these grafts prior to placing them on the non–infected well granulated wound bed. Five to seven days of compression are necessary and most patients are maintained on prophylactic antibiotics while the dressings are in place. Seven days of healing provide minimal, if any, collagen anchoring of the skin grafts to their bed, and immediate ambulation after initial "take" of the skin grafts will lead to skin graft loss. These patients require compression and elevation for 3 to 6 weeks depending upon their level of activity following venous stasis ulcer skin grafting.

Diabetic Ulcers. Diabetic wounds are multifactorial in origin. Patients with diabetic wounds develop polyneuropathy creating motor, sensory and proprioceptive abnormalities. Skin surfaces become insensate and foot clawing creates abnormal joint positions, placing greater pressure over bones and joints previously unaccustomed to such stresses. Combined with vascular disease and immunosuppression, diabetics have a higher incidence of pressure ulcers, traumatic injury and infected progressive wounds over that of the normal population.

Because of their multifactorial ulcer formation, a diabetic workup consists of arterial evaluation for circulation, bone evaluation for osteomyelitis, and a suspicion of deeper and more progressive undermining soft tissue wounds than other arterial and venous insufficiency sores.

Limb salvage is dependent upon pressure relief, maintaining therapy for ADLs and maximizing function, staged debridements and multiple assessments of any continually demarcating wound infections. Intravenous and topical antibiotics or antiseptics are prescribed according to the multibacterial flora cultured from such wounds.

Diabetic infections take longer to heal due to the delayed introduction of macrophages as well as diminished leukocyte migration which causes prolongation of the inflammatory phase. This process allows for progressive bacterial invasion and results in longer lengths of hospital stays. Once infection and osteomyelitis or pyarthrosis are controlled, reconstruction is dependent upon wound location. For weight bearing surfaces, durable tissue in the form of flaps are recommended. Non–weight bearing surfaces may be allowed to heal by secondary intent or, depending upon their size, grafted with split of full thickness skin.

With the majority of diabetic wounds beginning within the toe web spaces or plantar metatarsal phalangeal joint prominences, amputations should be limited and used only for extensive soft tissue injury in the face of systemic sepsis. Patience is a virtue here. Saving one's limb will protect the patient as well as prevent stress on the remaining leg, plantar surfaces, posterior heels and pressure areas during ambulation, sitting and lying. While amputation may be a quicker opportunity for wound healing, it also accelerates the deterioration of functional outcomes for these patients. Transmetatarsal, Ray, Syme, below knee or above knee amputations should be the last resort.

Skin Cancers. Non–healing bleeding wounds, whether heaped with granulation tissue, pigmented or punched out and exudating, must be suspected as possible skin cancers, particularly those noted on sun exposed body surfaces. These lesions must be biopsied for definitive diagnosis and, depending on the pathologic result, widely excised and reconstructed.

Basal cell cancers are less aggressive and not metastatic. Large basal cell cancers can become quite deforming. Wide excision with skin grafting or random flaps are options. Full thickness skin grafts and adjacent tissue random flap reconstruction provide the best color and texture match when considering the exposed areas of the face, neck and hands. Other options include Moh's surgery with similar reconstruction or radiation therapy.

Squamous cell cancers tend to be more ulcerating and may be highly metastatic. Chronic pressure ulcers and burn scars of prolonged duration have been known to degenerate into squamous cell carcinomas. They necessitate wide excision with wound closure. Again, if on the face, reconstructing the anatomic defect with skin matched for color, texture and quality will provide the greatest aesthetic appearance. If these wounds appear on a pressure bearing area, then a durable myofasciocutaneous flap is indicated. Regional lymph node dissection may be necessary to assess for metastatic disease.

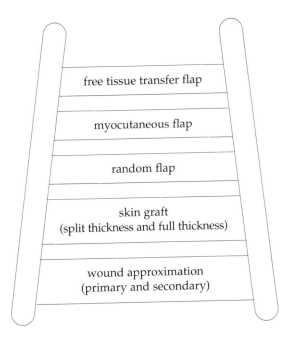

Figure 1. *The reconstructive ladder 5 of surgical wound healing options. Based upon the technical complexity of wound resurfacing, surgeons consider the fastest, most cost effective, durable, least painful, most functional and best aesthetic reconstructive option appropriate for the patient's need.*

By far, melanomas are the most fatal of the skin cancers. If extensive, they may appear as pigmented or nonpigmented ulcerated necrotic lesions on any body surface. Incisional or excisional full thickness biopsies are necessary for diagnosis. Depending upon tissue depth, a prognosis is offered and treatment management options discussed. When located on the distal extremities, if cure is possible, Ray amputation or partial limb amputation may be offered. Surgical and medical oncology recommendations are requested for this uniquely individual problem.

Surgical Wounds

Postoperative surgical wounds will usually heal when placed in traditional midline or well vascularized sites. Many wounds are complicated by vasculitis, tobacco use, diabetes and other circulatory limiting problems. Initially, epidermolysis and erythema may be noted. As wound healing deteriorates, full thickness necrosis, serous discharge, infected exudate and ultimately wound dehiscence occurs.

Consideration should be given to improved perfusion, nutrition and free radical destruction using hydration, vitamins, protein and caloric repletion as well as non–steroidal anti–inflammatory drugs.

WOUND MODELS

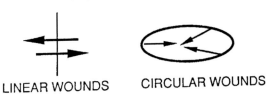

Figure 2. *Round versus linear wound healing model. Round wounds are those wounds which heal spontaneously through the wound healing curve necessitating large amounts of substrate and immunocompetence. Linear wound healing reflects the surgeon's ability to approximate wound edges which will accelerate wound healing by reducing many of the steps needed for spontaneous closure.*

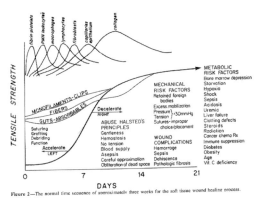

Figure 3. *The wound healing curve[9] noting acceleration (left shift) of the wound healing process and deceleration (right shift).*

Early intervention such as revision of the wound closure back to "bleeding edges" may salvage wound dehiscence before it occurs. Debridement and local care which allow for healing of the wound by secondary intent or by other approaches ascending the reconstructive ladder should be entertained (Figure 1).

Wound Care or Repair?

The wound specialist should seek the consultation of a plastic surgeon when he or she feels that a wound will not spontaneously heal given an optimized wound environment. Surgical closure is called for when a more efficacious outcome is expected by a more intensive surgical approach.

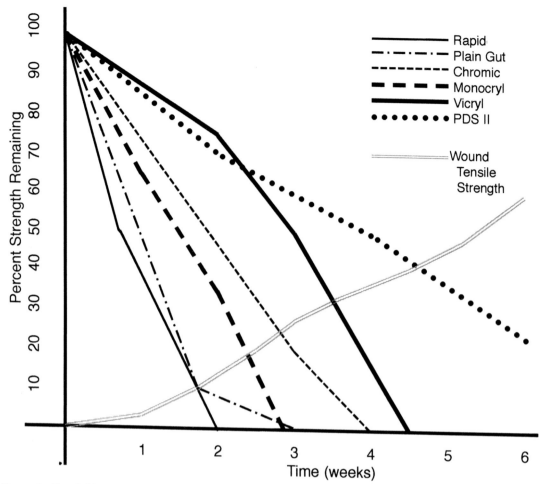

Figure 4. Absorbable suture strength compared to wound tensile strength. Matching the suture to the wound will provide the strength necessary to keep the wound supported during collagen synthesis, remodeling and improving tensile strength. (Adapted from the clinical insert materials, Ethicon, Inc., Somerville, NJ)

Debridement

Debridement is initially performed if infection, exudate, eschar, necrosis, drainage, undermining wounds and sinus tracks are present in order to achieve a more acute wound environment which is devoid of infection, foreign body or debris.

Healing by Secondary Intent:
Kane's Wound Healing Analogy

Spontaneous closure or healing by secondary intent has been well described. Much like building a home (Plate 1), the foundation of the wound is developed through granulation tissue during the inflammatory phase of wound healing where polymorphonuclear leukocytes (the initial ground cleaning crew) clean residual debris and bacteria. Angiogenesis develops a capillary bed of circulation

(the plumbing) for transport of wound healing cells. The frame of the house is developed when fibroblasts (framers of the house) deposit collagen and create a scaffold during the proliferative phase. Wound contracture occurs by the myofibrocytes. Finally, epithelialization is much like placement of the roof's shingles or siding on the outside of the house. This process creates a water tight barrier which seals the external environment from the internal.

Often round wounds larger than the diameter of a quarter dollar (approximately 2.5 cm) will not heal. Epithelial migration over 1 cm is usually thin and unstable.

A reconstructive ladder of surgical wound healing options is considered by all wound professionals once the wound has been optimized (Figure 1).[5]

If a round wound will not heal or remains unstable within 6 weeks, then linear wound repair is indicated (Figure 2).

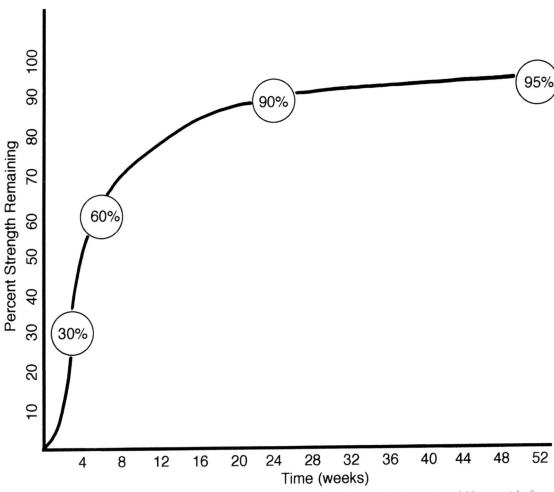

Figure 5. Tensile strength versus time. 30 percent strength in 3 weeks, 60 percent in 6 weeks and 90 percent in 6 months in the well–nourished immunocompetent patient. The reconstructive surgeon must consider tensile strength when selecting the sutures and when mobilizing the patient.

Excision of the wound creates an acute sterile environment and primary closure will approximate skin and soft tissues. By aligning the skin edges properly, collagen synthesis binds the edges together, accelerating the healing curve (Figure 3). The production of collagen does not peak for three weeks. In fact, a wound is weakest at 2 weeks as it is held together by the sutures which keep it from separating (Figure 4). Tensile strength is 30 percent in 3 weeks, 60 percent in 6 weeks, and 90 percent in 6 months in the well nourished immunocompetent host (Figure 5). If it is anticipated that activities or mobility of the patient may stress the wound closure, then it is recommended to wait 6 weeks or longer prior to subjecting tension to the wound.

Split Thickness Skin Grafts

When large superficial injuries occur, much like the shingles blowing off the house, a split thickness skin graft is indicated to resurface the wound (Plate 29). Healing is rapid and stable, providing the defect with the epithelial and partial dermal components. As with all reconstructive options, a donor site is left as is the defect site. Split thickness skin graft donor sites heal by migration of the epithelial cells left behind in the dermal adnexal appendages such as sweat glands and hair follicles. If the donor site is void of such adnexal appendages as seen in elderly patients without hair bearing thigh skin, then a secondary chronic wound at the donor site can be expected (Plate 30). In such a case, consideration should be made for

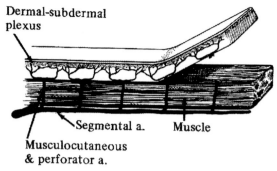

Dermal-subdermal plexus

Segmental a.   Muscle

Musculocutaneous & perforator a.

Figure 6. Random pattern skin flap.[11] Tissue reconstruction based on the underlying subdermal vascular network generally allows closure of "small" defects based on limited vessel circulation. Such flaps are useful when tissue redundancy in one direction allows for linear closure of the donor site and advancement or rotation of tissues to fill the defect needs. (Reprinted with permission from Grabb WC, Smith JW. Plastic Surgery, Third Edition. Little, Brown and Company, 1979, p 39.)

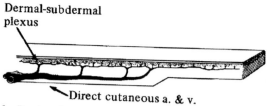

Dermal-subdermal plexus

Direct cutaneous a. & v.

1. Peninsular Axial Pattern Flap

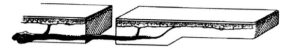

2. Island Axial Pattern Flap

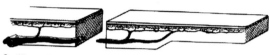

3. Free Flap

Figure 7. Axial pattern skin flaps.[11] A "tongue." of tissue leashed on its own blood supply including skin, subcutaneous tissue, fascia, muscle, bone, nerves or combinations is known as an axial flap. Axial flaps are useful when large or specialized tissue defects necessitate well vascularized composite tissue. (Reprinted with permission from Grabb WC, Smith JW. Plastic Surgery, Third Edition. Little, Brown and Company, 1979, p 39.)

full thickness skin grafting or expanded meshed split thickness skin grafting to both the defect and the donor site.

Skin graft "take" is a process in which the harvested paper thin layer of skin which is now without circulation becomes attached and viable to the defect site. Plasmatic imbibition, a transfer of cell fluids, nutrients and toxins, occurs during the first three days. Inosculation, a process where the cut capillary edges of the skin graft match up with those of the recipient site, and begins the process of re–vascularization. Initially, arterioles attach causing congestion of the split thickness skin graft. Greater tissue weight is noted as well as cyanosis and swelling. When the venules have approximated and tissue decongestion occurs, the skin graft turns pink and pale.

As previously mentioned, it takes 3 weeks of collagen formation to develop 30 percent tensile strength, 6 weeks for 60 percent tensile strength and 6 month for 90 percent tensile strength. Clinically those skin grafts which have initially taken but subsequently failed may have been caused by the misconception that a taken skin graft is fully healed. Should the patient be remobilized, remember that the graft is not fully healed until scar or collagen anchoring of the skin graft has occurred (3 to 6 weeks).

Full Thickness Skin Grafts

A full thickness skin graft includes the epidermis and full thickness dermis. On occasion, composite grafts also include underlying fat or fascia. These grafts replace a total skin deficit as might occur on the nose from a skin cancer excision. Full thickness skin grafts will contract less and blend better due to equal texture and color if "donated" from surrounding redundant tissues (Plates 31 and 32). Due to their extra thickness and perfusion needs, full thickness skin grafts need longer immobilization in order to take. On occasion, epidermolysis may occur due to delayed perfusion of the epidermal layer. Because of the adnexal appendages left in the full thickness skin graft, re–epithelization will occur.

Random Flaps

The next level in wound reconstruction complexity is that of adjacent tissue reconstruction. Flaps based on the random circulation of the subdermal capillary plexus under the skin allows for undermining and advancement or flap creation and rotation of skin and subcutaneous tissues (Figure 6).

Random flaps are useful in any portion of the body from scalp to toes where redundancy of tissue in one direction will allow for linear closure of the donor site and advancement or rotation of tissues to fill the defect needs. Due to the random nature of the circulation, areas of greater vascularity such as the face and neck will allow for more disproportionate length and width dimensions of the flap. Generally on the trunk and lower extremities, length of the flap and base–width of the flap must be equal in order to achieve circulation to the tip of the random flap.[6-8] (Plates 33 and 34).

Axial Flaps

More complex on the reconstructive ladder are the axial flaps (Figure 7). When larger or deeper defects such as Stage IV, "V" (injury including bone) and "VI" (open joints) wounds occur, thicker, better vascularized and more durable flaps will be necessary (Plates 35–37). Transferring a "tongue" of tissue based on its own blood supply yet leashed to its origin is the concept of transferring skin, subcutaneous tissue, fascia, muscle and bone as a flap. These myo–fascio–osseo–cutaneous flaps are useful in reconstruction of oral, face and neck cancers and traumatic extremity injuries.

Free Tissue Transfer Flaps

State–of–the–art techniques including micro–revascularization have allowed for composite tissues to be transferred from one body area such as the face or back to the defect site. Supple well vascularized fascia or muscle tissue may be transferred as a "free–flap" (Figure 7) to defects in the leg which would have otherwise progressed to limb loss (Plates 38–40). These free tissue transfers are more technically challenging but are now the basis for complex oral and maxillo–facial reconstructions from cancer. Traumatic reconstructions of the legs and dynamic reconstructions for patients with nerve injuries or hand dysfunctions are other examples of the use of free tissue transfers.

Postoperative Surgical Care

Common sense should be our guide regarding postoperative wound care. Understanding the concepts of the "wound healing curve"[9] (Figure 3) will provide the basis of wound healing dynamics.

While skin graft take is occurring, immobilization of the wound site is mandatory to allow for adherence and neovascularization. Disruption of the partial or full thickness skin graft due to sliding or direct pressure forces will cause separation of the graft from its vascularized bed with seroma, hematoma, fibrin or purulent secondary effects. Immobilization with the use of splinting, restricted motion and at times pinning or external fixation across joints may be necessary. A sterilized wound bed and antibiotics should be maintained to reduce skin graft loss due to infection. At approximately 5 to 7 days when the first dressings are removed, reassessment is made and topical dressings applied according to wound matching schemes.[10] Considering the need for collagen anchoring of the skin graft to its bed, 3 to 6 weeks of protected care may be necessary until the tensile strength between the skin graft and its bed will prevent further disruption. Lower extremity surgery will necessitate longer immobility and greater protection using firm compressive dressings and continuous elevation of the site. Other skin grafted wounds closer to and including the head region without pressure, dependency, or movement will require less immobility and are usually already elevated.

Pressure ulcer reconstructions and large flaps require 6 weeks of protection including the use of pressure reducing specialty beds, turning schedules, proper nutrition and hydration.

Should partial epidermolysis occur, then cleansing, occlusive style moist environment dressings would be needed. On occasion, these dressings create an erythematous dermatitis possibly due to candida but easily treated with antifungal creams applied 2 to 3 times daily.

Random adjacent tissue transfers and all flaps require elevation, pressure relief, immobilization and reduction of shearing forces. These "round" wounds have been reconstructed in "linear" fashion. While these flaps are vascularized, they also develop neovascularization from their wound bed. Any disruption between the overlying flap and underlying wound bed will cause similar problems including seroma, hematoma, fibrin separation and purulent consequences endangering the flap viability. While linear wound healing is certainly faster than round wound healing, the incision line should be protected from infection, incontinence of urine and stool and tension. Suture selection is imperative to provide the appropriate time for collagen deposition and remodeling of the scar to reduce wound dehiscence. Suture or staple removal timing is dependent upon their site. Pressure bearing areas and sites of dependency such as pressure ulcer flap reconstructions or lower extremity wound flap reconstructions necessitate 6 weeks of wound approximation to approximate 60 percent tensile strength before attempting to stress the incision line. Three weeks, approximating 30 percent tensile strength of suture or staple reinforcement, is provided for major trunk and upper extremity flap reconstructions. When consideration is made regarding the aesthetic appearance of the scar in the less stressed regions of the face and neck or in smaller reconstructive sites, sutures may be removed at 5 to 7 days when layered dermal closure has also been performed.

Prevention of shearing or pressure at the site of wound reconstruction follows all prior recommendations including the use of static and dynamic splints, static and dynamic support surfaces as well as local care.

Reassessment for reconstructive wound healing failure is timed according to the risk of its occurrence as well as the magnitude of the problem that such a complication might create. A small random flap reconstruction of a basal cell cancer excision on the cheek may need re–evaluation at 5 days when sutures are to be removed, but a free flap to a large leg reconstruction may need hourly reassessment in the intensive care unit.

Should wound disruption, infection, underlying collection of fluids or vascular compromise occur during the early wound healing phases, these grafts and flaps may be rescued by directing medical or surgical attention to the adverse problem.

Summary

Current goals for wound care include the reversal of wound progression in order to save limb and life. Thereafter, healing, function and aesthetics are desired outcomes.

Many present day patients with chronic, debilitating neurologic maladies, malnutrition and immobility may never heal a chronic wound, nor are they suitable candidates for reconstruction. For these patients, compassionate local management and dignified holistic care are reasonable alternatives that should be provided.

For selected patients whose length of healing would be extraordinarily long in months or years and whose health status is appropriate for rapid healing, surgical reconstructive options are considered.

References

1. Agency for Health Care Policy and Research. Clinical Practice Guideline, Numbers, *Treatment of Pressure Ulcers.* Public Health Service, U.S. Department of Health and Human Services; 1994 Dec. AHCPR Publication No. 95–0652.
2. McCraw JB, Dibbell DG. Experimental definition of independent myocutaneous vascular territories. *Plat Reconstr Surg* 1977;60:212.
3. McCraw JB, Dibbell DG. Clinical definition of independent myocutaneous vascular territories. *Plast Reconstr Surg* 1977;60:341.
4. McCraw JB. The recent history of myocutaneous flaps. *Clin Plast Surg* 1980;7:3.
5. Mathes SJ, Nahai F. *Clinical Application for Muscle and Myocutaneous Flaps.* St. Louis, MO, C.V. Mosby, 1982.
6. Gillies HD. The tubed pedicle in plastic surgery. *NY Med J III* 1920;1.
7. Milton SH. Pedicled skin flaps: The fallacy of length: width ratio. *Br J Surg* 1970;57:502.
8. Gillies HD. The design of directed pedicle flaps. *Br Med J* 1932;2:1008.
9. Schilling J. Wound healing. *Surgical Rounds* 1983;Jul:46–62.
10. Krasner D. Dressing decisions for the twenty–first century: On the cusp of a paradigm shift. In: Krasner D, Kane D, *Chronic Wound Care, Second Edition: A Clinical Source Book for Healthcare Professionals.* Wayne, PA, Health Management Publications, Inc., 1996, pp 139–151.

31

Postoperative Care of Skin Grafts, Donor Sites and Myocutaneous Flaps

Cecilia Rund, RN, CETN

Rund C. Postoperative care of skin grafts, donor sites and myocutaneous flaps. In: Krasner D, Kane D. *Chronic Wound Care, Second Edition*. Wayne, PA, Health Management Publications, Inc., 1997, pp 245–250.

Introduction

Management of postoperative wounds, such as skin grafts and myocutaneous flaps, has evolved over the years as patient care has become more complex and responsibilities of healthcare professional have increased. Patients are either being discharged very quickly following surgical procedures or having same day procedures and returning to the home care environment with home care visits. Other patients are having surgical procedures and returning to long term care environments where nursing care will be needed.

Whether the patient is in an acute care, a long term care or a home care environment, it behooves healthcare professionals to have the necessary skills to properly care for and manage a postoperative skin graft or flap procedure. Despite having a vast amount of information available to clinicians regarding various wound care dressings, persons are often confused about how to manage wounds, especially when they may be complicated surgical procedures that necessitate specific postoperative management. Research has shown that even qualified nurses practice by tradition rather than science, may be resistant to change or even allow power and authority issues to influence their choices in wound management.[1] Other studies have revealed that healthcare professionals lack sufficient knowledge regarding appropriate wound care, thereby choosing inappropriate wound dressings which lead to wastage, delay in healing and increased length of stay.[2]

Having protocols for care and management of the postoperative skin graft patient and the myocutaneous flap patient will provide the healthcare professional with guidelines for appropriate patient management and will prevent general confusion. The protocols that follow take into consideration a broad range of patient issues, as patients should be treated with a holistic approach.[3]

Wound management is a complex issue. Each wound is as individual as its host. There are many factors, such as medical condition, diet, mobility, psychosocial issues, and environment, which will influence the management of wounds.[3,4] Postoperative wound management actually begins preoperatively, as thorough patient assessment and careful patient selection will affect surgical outcomes.[5] Additional research is needed to identify criteria for selecting patients who will benefit from skin grafting and myocutaneous flap repair procedures. However, the following criteria are outlined by the AHCPR guidelines for the treatment of pressure ulcers: medically stable patients, adequately nourished patients, patients who can tolerate the surgical procedure, and patients who can tolerate the postoperative restrictions such as bed rest and immobility.[3,4,6]

In order to achieve surgical success and optimum wound healing, healthcare professionals will need to consider the following issues: quality of life, patient preferences, patient compliance,[7] treatment goals, risk of recurrence of original problem, anticipated rehabilitative outcomes, ability to provide and create an adequate postoperative environment which is conducive to wound healing and patient well–being, overall patient prognosis, general risk factors, and the risk/benefit ratio.

The ability to create an environment conducive to wound healing and patient well–being can be an immense (if not impossible) task. Such an environment may include a proper bedding surface, physical therapy, nursing care, proper hygiene and proper nutrition. All of these factors are dependent upon the patient and the patient's support system: the family situation, abilities and support of a significant other or caregiver, financial position, insurance benefits, and the patient's living condition.[4,8,9]

for infection is increased.[4] Following surgery, one tends to be hypotensive and hypothermic, thus, blood supply to the postoperative site is decreased. Many clinicians believe that administering nasal oxygen following surgery is imperative to increase oxygen tension.[4,9] Dehydration can also affect tissue perfusion; surgical patients will need to be adequately hydrated.[9]

Nutrition (vitamins and minerals). Nutrition has been discussed thoroughly in other chapters in this source book. It is well documented that a starving postoperative patient will not heal.[9]

...persons who smoke are at risk for wound hypoxia.[9,10]

Factors Affecting Wound Healing

Many factors can impair the healing process of surgical wounds. Some of these factors include smoking, oxygen demands, nutrition, diabetes, alcohol intake, medications, patient compliance, and local surgical factors. A brief discussion of these factors is valuable since understanding them will enable the clinician to provide sound pre– and postoperative education and to use prudent judgement when assessing wound healing and when choosing wound dressings.

Smoking. Skin grafts and flaps depend upon blood supply and oxygenation to survive.[9] Heavy smoking has been associated with facelift skin flap necrosis.[9] Nicotine has a vasoconstrictive effect and can produce vasoconstriction up to 50 minutes following administration. Cigarette smoke also contains levels of carbon monoxide (3 to 6 percent) which binds to hemoglobin in the pulmonary capillaries and forms carboxyhemoglobin, thus limiting blood oxygen–carrying capability. Carboxyhemoglobin levels have also been associated with platelet adhesiveness that can lead to additional limitation of local blood flow. Chronic cigarette smoking is also associated with higher rates of atherosclerosis. And, finally, smokers are prone to pulmonary problems such as asthma, emphysema, and bronchitis. Therefore, persons who smoke are at risk for wound hypoxia.[9,10] Smoking also robs the body of vitamin C stores.[11]

Oxygen demands. Wounds need oxygen to repair themselves. Without oxygen, collagen synthesis is impaired, new vessel formation is compromised, epithelialization is slowed and the potential

Patients taking vitamins and mineral supplements prior to surgery will need to reassess their needs preoperatively, especially if one foresees being NPO or on a restricted diet following surgery. Various vitamins and minerals can have a positive effect on wound healing, but too much of a good thing can also be harmful.

If a person is deficient in zinc, zinc supplementation can be beneficial.[9] Conversely, too much zinc can be toxic, having adverse effects on the immune system.[11]

Also, one should discontinue vitamin E for 2 to 3 weeks prior to surgery,[7] as vitamin E decreases platelet aggregation. Mega–doses of vitamin E can lead to delayed wound healing and prolonged bleeding.[11]

Adequate levels of vitamin C are necessary for wound healing. Vitamin C toxicity is rare since it is excreted via the kidneys. However, persons with renal impairment will need special evaluation of their vitamin C needs. Large doses of vitamin C can interfere with the accuracy of both occult blood monitoring and blood glucose monitoring,[11] so that persons taking high doses of vitamin C should discontinue this drug 24 to 48 hours prior to having such tests.

Decreases in serum vitamin A levels have been noted in patients following surgery or serious injury. Rettura and associates found that immobilization of rats led to a decrease of vitamin A levels in the serum, liver, testes and kidney.[10]

Administering large doses of cortisone also resulted in depletion of vitamin A from the rat liver and kidneys.[10,11] Nutritional deficiencies in vitamin A can also increase the incidence of infection. So, supplementing with vitamin A may be necessary to influence wound healing and improve host defense response.[10,11]

Requirements for vitamins and minerals in general will generally be increased in the aged population, in patients having surgery and in those who have followed a diet deficient in vitamins and minerals. Supplementing these persons, following a thorough assessment of their needs, seems to be prudent prior to performing graft or flap procedures.[10]

Diabetes. Diabetics have many problems that predispose them to poor wound healing: neuropathy, atherosclerosis and increased incidence of infection.[4,12] The blood glucose levels in diabetes must be controlled both pre– and postoperatively for successful wound healing. Maintaining a blood glucose level of less than 200 mg/dL is considered by most experts to be "the single most advantageous action clinicians can take to normalize healing in these persons."[4]

Alcohol intake. Excessive alcohol intake can impair the immune system, lead to malnourishment and cause liver damage. Alcoholics may also suffer from gastritis, pancreatitis, and diarrhea. All of these factors can lead to a high risk surgical candidate and a patient that will heal poorly following surgery.[10,12]

Medications. It suffices to say that, although overlooked by many clinicians, discovering what medications a patient is taking (both prescription and OTC) is a necessary step in thorough patient assessment. One should investigate what vitamins are being taken, how much, and for how long. What OTC nonsteroidal anti–inflammatory drugs (NSAIDs) are being consumed on a daily basis? Velasco and Guaitero propose that these agents can have a negative effect upon wound healing.[13] And, of course, the negative effects of steroids on wound healing have been well documented.[10,13]

Patient compliance. Dr. Ralph Millard, Jr. summarizes the importance of patient compliance quite eloquently in the following quote:

"...disaster can be traced back to the patient. This is particularly well exemplified by any patient with a flap or graft, and certainly one after an extensive face lift with tight postauricular flaps, who sits up in bed several hours postoperatively, in spite of warnings, puffing on a cigarette and causing necrosis at the periphery of the flaps."[7]

Local surgical factors. There are many local factors, such as infection, edema, hematoma formation, and seroma, that will impede healing of a surgical wound. Other factors include increased wound tension, excessive pressure over the operative site, muscle spasms and incontinence contamination. All

of these injurious factors should be eliminated and/or prevented, whether through surgical technique or through preoperative planning and postoperative management.

Generally, wound infection prolongs the inflammatory response and retards the healing process. Wounds will not heal until infection is controlled. The human body has several protective mechanisms against infection. However, when these mechanisms are altered, bacteria can invade. Keeping the skin intact and dry can limit bacterial invasion and staphylococcal proliferation. However, excessively dry skin can crack and fissure, allowing bacteria to enter. Wet or macerated skin can allow staphylococcus to grow. Sebum, from the sebaceous glands, produces bactericidal and fungicidal fatty acids. However, when these fatty acids are removed through harsh cleansing agents, or when they are diluted with edema, the patient is more susceptible to infection.[10]

Slight edema and hematoma formation will occur immediately postoperatively. Excessive fluid and blood accumulation is usually removed via special drains that must be kept patent. Patent drains will prevent the pooling of blood and fluids within the surgical site. If fluid or blood is allowed to accumulate beneath a flap, a seroma or hematoma will form. Both place undue pressure and tension on the tissues and suture lines, compromising blood flow. Hematomas also serve as an excellent medium for bacterial growth, releasing toxic substances and precipitating infection.[12,14]

Surgical procedures can result in excessive amounts of wound tension. Other causes of tension include seroma or hematoma formation and even the dressing technique itself. Every effort must be made to reduce excessive flap and graft tension. Blood vessels can be stretched or twisted, and blood clots can form.[14] Clinicians should avoid stretching and pulling of the suture line, the flap or the graft when applying dressings. Dressings that are too tight may also compromise flap circulation.[5]

Direct pressure over the postoperative site can lead to blood flow problems, hematoma formation, and ischemia. Correct patient positioning is critical.[5] The AHCPR guidelines for the treatment of pressure ulcers recommend minimizing pressure to postoperative sites by placing the patient on an air–fluidized bed, a low air–loss bed or a Stryker frame for a minimum of 2 weeks.[6] Hester and Schneider recommend special bed therapies for 2 to 3 weeks.[5]

Muscle spasticity can be a challenge to wound healing. Muscle spasms can cause suture line tension, can interrupt collagen deposition and can interfere with wound healing in general. Control of these spasms, through either medication or surgery, is necessary.[6]

- Observe for clinical signs of infection and report to surgeon immediately.
- Gently dry periwound skin.

A surgical wound that has not been protected from incontinence gets repeatedly insulted with bacteria, wetness and chemical trauma.[6]

A surgical wound that has not been protected from incontinence gets repeatedly insulted with bacteria, wetness and chemical trauma.[6] Unscheduled dressing changes due to fecal/urinary contamination can also lead to mechanical trauma. Flap or graft failure and/or infection can be a result of uncontrolled incontinence.[15]

All of the aforementioned information should be considered when developing protocols for postoperative care of the skin graft or myocutaneous flap patient. Patient education is a key element in this development process. The material previously discussed gives the healthcare provider sufficient information to develop an individualized patient education program. Following are examples of protocols for patients who have had skin grafts or myocutaneous flaps. General wound care is detailed; however, the educational component must be tailored to the individual patient.

Postoperative Care of the Split Thickness Skin Graft: Donor Site

Goals of Care:
- to promote a moist wound environment,
- to absorb and contain excessive amounts of drainage,[16]
- to protect area from trauma,
- to insulate wounded site,
- to promote epithelialization,
- to prevent external contamination, and
- to promote patient comfort and ADLs.

Procedure:
- Assess patient's continence status and prevent incontinence contamination to wounded site. (This may be done by using absorbent products, collection devices or a waterproof dressing.)
- Remove all old dressings in an atraumatic fashion and dispose of properly. (The initial dressing is usually removed by the surgeon.)
- Cleanse entire wounded area and surrounding skin with an appropriate wound cleanser or normal saline solution to remove exudate and dressing residue.[10,13]

- If periwound skin is dry or fragile, place a liquid skin film and allow to dry (This will protect the skin from any adhesives).

Option A:
- Apply a waterproof, bacteria proof foam dressing if wound is heavily exudating.
- Change dressing when it has exhausted its absorbing capacity.[17]

Option B:
- Apply a zinc or petrolatum based impregnated gauze if the wound is lightly to moderately exudating.[10]
- Cover with a nonadherent, absorbent dressing. (Use a dressing with an adhesive border or tape dressing in place.)
- Change daily.

Option C:
- Apply a hydrocolloid dressing or a transparent dressing if the wound is dry or very lightly exudating. Hydrocolloid dressings will absorb drainage and should be changed when the dressing has exhausted its absorbing capacities.
- Change the transparent dressing when excessive amounts of wound drainage have accumulated beneath dressing or whenever leakage occurs.[17]

Postoperative Care of the Skin Graft

Goals of care:
- to protect from trauma,
- to protect from outside contaminants,
- to absorb excessive exudate,[13]
- to insulate area, and
- to immobilize the grafted area immediately postoperatively.[5,18]

Special notes: Postoperatively, there will be a bulky, compression dressing in place along with a splint (if the grafted area is on a limb). The surgeon will usually remove the initial dressing, examine the graft and provide instructions regarding care and removal of the splint. The initial dressing usually stays on 5 to 7 days following surgery.[8] An affected limb will usually be immobilized, requiring that the patient learn to walk with crutches or even stay in bed. (This period of immobilization may be as long as 3 to 6 weeks.) During this time, the patient is usually instructed to elevate the extremity to decrease edema in the operative site. If a compression dressing is to be reapplied, the surgeon should perform this procedure and leave explicit instructions for the caregiver. Once the compression dressings have been removed, a non–compression dressing can be applied, and the caregiver can proceed as follows.

Procedure:
- Assess the patient's continence status and prevent incontinence contamination to the wounded site. (This can be done by using absorbent products, collection devices or a waterproof dressing.)
- Remove dressing in an atraumatic fashion and dispose of properly.
- Gently cleanse graft site of old dressing residue and drainage using an appropriate wound cleanser or normal saline solution. Cleansing must not be so forceful as to disrupt the graft.[13]
- Gently dry the periwound skin.
- Report any clinical signs of infection, graft sloughing, graft tears, or suture line separation to surgeon immediately. Also, report any periwound rash/dermatitis.
- Apply a thick layer of a petrolatum/paraffin impregnated dressing.[10]
- Cover with a nonadherent dressing.
- Tape, wrap, or use a bordered dressing to hold impregnated gauze in place. If wrapping is done, a figure of eight pattern should be used and care should be taken not to apply excessive compression that could compromise blood flow to the graft.
- Change as directed by surgeon, or if dressing becomes soiled.
- Discontinue dressings once all suture material has been removed and the graft has healed.
- After healing is complete, patient may use moisturizing creams to the grafted site.

Postoperative Care of the Myocutaneous Flap

Goals of care
- to protect operative sites from trauma,
- to keep the suture line clean,
- to eliminate pressure over the myocutaneous flap, the donor site, suture lines and drains,[5,8]
- to protect postoperative sites from external contamination (i.e. incontinence), and

- to keep all drains patent[3] to allow suctioning of all excessive blood and fluids.[5,8,12]

Special notes: Postoperative care includes observing the flap site for signs of a seroma and wound infection.[5]

Signs of a seroma are moderate to large amounts of serous and/or serosanguinous drainage leaking from the suture line or from around the drain site; fluctuation of the flap site when compressed with the hand; and a bulging flap site.

Signs and symptoms of a wound site infection are induration of the suture line; increased pain of the operative site; fever; drainage of frank pus from either the suture line or the drain sites; and wound dehiscence with foul drainage.

The initial dressing following surgery will be removed and the area evaluated by the surgeon. Drains are usually left in place for 5 days and then removed when serous drainage has stopped. Bedrest is essential; the patient should be positioned so that excessive pressure over the operative site is avoided for 2 to 3 weeks. Turn sheets should be used to minimize suture line and flap tension. The head of the bed should be elevated no more than 15 to 30 degrees to decrease shear and pressure at the surgical site. The patient may be on antibiotics for 7 days postoperatively. Sutures are usually left in place for 21 days and then should be removed carefully, avoiding tearing of the skin.[19] Incontinence will need to be contained to prevent contamination of the operative site. A bowel/bladder program may be instituted or one may consider the use of collection devices (fecal incontinence collectors, external condom catheters). Waterproof dressings can be used to protect the area from external contaminants.

Procedure:
- Carefully remove all dressings from the operative site without placing undo tension on the flap and suture lines.
- Cleanse all suture lines and drain sites thoroughly with a wound cleanser or normal saline solution to remove excess dressing debris and wound drainage.
- Gently dry areas.
- Optional: Apply a liquid skin protectant to protect skin against adhesives and allow to dry.
- Apply appropriate solutions, ointments or impregnated gauzes to drain sites as ordered by the surgeon.

Option A:
- Apply a transparent, semipermeable film dressing to all surgical sites except drain sites.

- Remove only if wound fluid collects beneath the dressing or if the dressing wears off.
- Gently remove the transparent dressing at time of suture removal.[17,19]

Option B:
- Apply a nonadherent, absorbent composite dressing.
- Change when excessive drainage is noted on the absorbent pad.[8]
- Remove dressings at time of suture removal.

Care of the Drains and Reservoirs

Special notes: A closed, suction drainage system is preferable to an open system.[5,8,10] Dressings around drain sites may include absorbent, nonadherent dressings or impregnated gauze dressings. These dressings should be changed whenever wound drainage is noted.

Procedure:
- Milk drains BID or more frequently as needed to keep drains patent.
- Keep all reservoirs compressed to promote wound drainage and empty when the reservoir is half full.
- If drainage systems are obstructed, notify the surgeon for follow–up instructions.

Conclusion

Postoperative management of skin grafts and flap procedures is complex, involving a multidisciplinary team approach. This chapter focused upon the care of both patient and surgical wound. The protocols provided are an attempt to provide the healthcare professional with enough information to prevent confusion in care. Of course, patient education is an essential part of any protocol; therefore, any patient should have all of this information condensed and presented in an understandable fashion. And, since each patient and wound is unique, there will be deviations in this protocol. However, the general principles of care are the same. With this in mind, clinicians can utilize these guidelines for their surgical patients who have undergone such procedures.

References

1. Flanagan M. Variables influencing nurses' selection of wound dressings, from the Proceedings of the Second European Conference on Advances in Wound Management, Oct. 20–23, 1992, Harrogate, UK, pp. 119–122.
2. Bux M. Assessing the use of dressings in practice. *WOUNDS* 1996;5(7):305–308.
3. Muter P: Surgical management of pressure sores in a specialized nursing environment, from the Proceedings of the Third European Conference on Advances in Wound Management, Oct. 19–22, 1993, Harrogate, UK, pp. 20–21.
4. Cooper DM. Acute surgical wounds. In: Bryant R (ed). *Acute and Chronic Wounds: Nursing Management*. St. Louis, MO, Mosby Yearbook, Inc., 1992, pp. 91–104.
5. Mathes SJ, Nahai F. *Clinical Applications for Muscle and Musculocutaneous Flaps*. St. Louis, MO, CV Mosby Co, 1982, pp. 154, 455, 532–3, 634–5, 695–6.
6. Bergstrom N, Bennett MA, Carlson CE, et al. *Treatment of Pressure Ulcers*. Clinical Practice Guideline, No. 15. Rockville, MD: U.S. Department of Health and Human Services. Public Health Service, Agency for Health Care Policy and Research. AHCPR Publication No. 95–0652. December 1994.
7. Millard DR Jr. *Principlization of Plastic Surgery*. Boston, MA, Little, Brown and Co., 1986, pp. 139–141.
8. Gottrup F. Setting standards for the management of surgical wounds, from the Proceedings of the Fourth European Conferences on Advances in Wound Management, Sept. 6–9, 1994, Copenhagen, Denmark, pp. 10–14.
9. Miller SH, Rudolph R. *Clinics in Plastic Surgery*. Philadelphia, PA, WB Saunders Co., 1990, pp. 463–469, 557.
10. Cohen K, Diegelmann RF, Lindblad WJ. *Wound Healing: Biochemical & Clinical Aspects*. Philadelphia, PA, WB Saunders Co, 1992, pp. 110–112, 248–268, 544–551, 567–576, 584–6, 587–9, 590–3.
11. Sheldon SH. *The Doctor's Vitamin and Mineral Encyclopedia*. New York, NY, Simon and Schuster, 1990.
12. David J. *Wound Management: A Comprehensive Guide to Dressing and Healing*. London, England, Martin Dunitz Ltd., London, 1987.
13. Bryant RA (ed). *Acute and Chronic Wounds: Nursing Management*. St. Louis, MO, Mosby Yearbook, 1992.
14. Black JM, Matrassarin–Jacobs E. *Luckman and Sorenson's Medical–Surgical Nursing, Fourth Edition*. Philadelphia, PA, WB Saunders & Co, 1993.
15. Wornum IL. Surgical intervention: Grafts and flaps. In: Krasner D (ed). *Chronic Wound Care: A Clinical Source Book for Healthcare Professionals*. King of Prussia, PA, Health Management Publications, Inc., 1990, pp. 378–389.
16. Winter GD. Healing of skin wounds and the influence of dressings on the repair process. In: Harkiss KJ (ed). *Surgical Dressings and Wound Healing*. Middlesex, England, Bradford University Press, 1971.
17. Thomas S. *Handbook of Wound Dressings*. London, England, Macmillian Magazines, Ltd., 1994.
18. Gogia P. *Clinical Wound Management*. Thorofare, NJ, SLACK Inc., 1995.
19. Harding K, Jones V. Wound management: Good practice guidelines. *Journal of Wound Care* 1996:4–5.

32

Physical Therapy Intervention in Wound Management

Prem P. Gogia, PhD, PT

Gogia PP. Physical therapy intervention in wound management. In: Krasner D, Kane D. *Chronic Wound Care, Second Edition*. Wayne, PA, Health Management Publications, Inc., 1997, pp 251–259.

Introduction

Effective management of chronic wounds requires dedicated efforts of the wound management team which generally consists of physicians, nurses, dieticians, social workers, and physical therapists. Physical therapists (PTs) play an important role as a part of the wound management team. Most clinicians have difficulty understanding the role of PTs in wound management. Historically, management of tissue injury is not new to PTs. For years, PTs have been treating soft tissue injuries. The healing process of soft tissue is quite similar to open wound healing with the exception that the wounds are at high risk of developing infection whereas the risk of infection is relatively low in closed injuries.

PTs can help improve patient mobility as well as assist in patient positioning, which may reduce the risk of developing pressure ulcers. PTs can fit patients with splints to eliminate or reduce the pressure over bony prominences, thereby again minimizing the risk of developing pressure ulcers. In most states, PTs are allowed to perform sharp debridement of wounds. Besides assisting in improving patient mobility, positioning patients, and fitting patients with splints, PTs can perform a number of adjunct modalities such as hydrotherapy, electrical stimulation, ultrasound, low–energy laser, ultraviolet–C, and compression therapy which may enhance the healing process.

Hydrotherapy

Hydrotherapy is one of the most commonly used modalities in physical therapy for the management of chronic wounds. Hydrotherapy encompasses use of water and other liquids delivered via whirlpool and other irrigation systems. Although the effects of whirlpool on healing have not been studied, whirlpool has been commonly used to promote wound cleansing for decades. Whirlpool removes cellular debris, foreign contaminants, and loosely attached necrotic tissue from the wound bed, which may reduce the risk of infection. It breaks up blood coagulum and accelerates the debridement process by softening thick, hard necrotic tissue. Whirlpool removes toxic residues which may be left behind by various topical agents and produces a moist environment for wound healing. Whirlpool agitation produces a massaging effect on tissues which promotes reduction of edema and inflammation. The use of whirlpool for ischemic extremities can promote circulation. For wound management, whirlpool should be used at a neutral temperature between 92 and 96 degrees F, for 10 to 15 minutes (Figure 1).

Antimicrobial solutions are frequently added to whirlpool water to kill bacteria present in the infected wounds. Careful selection of these antimicrobial solutions should be made since a number of them have been known to have cytotoxic effects on the cells which are actively engaged in the healing process. Precaution should also be taken in cleaning the tanks after each use to prevent cross–contamination. Clinicians are encouraged to follow the guidelines established by the Center for Disease Control (CDC) while cleaning and disinfecting whirlpool tanks after each use. Periodic cultures of the whirlpool tanks may also eliminate the risk of cross–contamination.

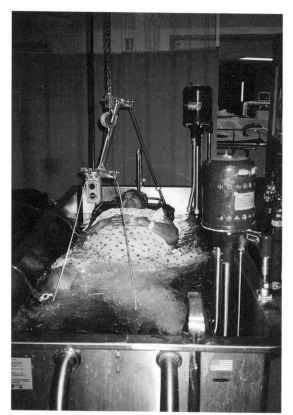

Figure 1. Patient in full–body whirlpool.

The most common contraindications and precautions of whirlpool are listed in Table 1. Precautions should also be taken when treating patients with high fever. Furthermore, if whirlpool is considered as a choice of treatment for a patient with a venous ulcer, a specially designed seat is placed in the whirlpool tank to enable the patient to maintain the leg in a horizontal position, and the water temperature is also kept low.

According to the AHCPR (Agency for Health Care Policy and Research) guideline for pressure ulcers, whirlpool treatment should be discontinued when the ulcer is considered clean.[1] If whirlpool is considered as a choice of treatment for clean wounds, the tanks designed on hydrosound systems should be used to avoid the risk of damaging healthy granulation tissue and newly formed epithelial layers.

Other irrigation systems, such as jet lavage, are also effective for treating chronic wounds, particularly for patients with decreased medical condition. Care must be taken to avoid high irrigation pressure while using the lavage system.

Table 1
Contraindications/Precautions of Whirlpool

Congestive heart failure
Pulmonary disease
Upper respiratory infection
Acute phlebitis
Venous ulcers
Severe neuropathy
Clean and well granulated wounds
Recent skin grafts and flaps

Electrical Stimulation

Use of electrical stimulation (ES) for wound management has gained significant popularity in the past few years. There is now a substantial body of experimental and clinical research to support the use of ES for wound healing. Now there is adequate support in the literature to prove that high voltage pulsed current (HVPC) is more effective than low voltage direct current. Both experimental and clinical research have shown that HVPC is an effective adjunct modality to enhance the healing process. The HVPC improves blood flow to the tissues, decreases edema, decreases number of mast cells, and inhibits bacterial growth.[2–5] It also accelerates the rate of wound contraction and epithelialization as well as increases the tensile strength of collagen.[6,7] A number of controlled clinical studies have shown increased rates of healing in pressure ulcers.[8–10]

It is important to note that treatment protocols, intensities, voltages, pulse rates, polarities, and electrode placements vary considerably from one study to another. More research is needed regarding these parameters and controlled studies. Current density of 0.1 to 2.0 mA/cm^2 is considered to be effective by most experts. Literature also clearly suggests that polarity is an important consideration with ES. For treatment of chronic wounds which are infected or inflamed, negative polarity is recommended, whereas for chronic wounds that are neither infected nor inflamed, positive polarity is recommended. For chronically infected and inflamed wounds, use of negative polarity for the first three to four days alternating to positive polarity has also been found to be effective. The active electrode needs to be cut to the size of the wound and covered with either saline–moist gauze or hydrogel impregnated gauze and directly placed over the wound bed. The dispersive electrode is typically four times as large as

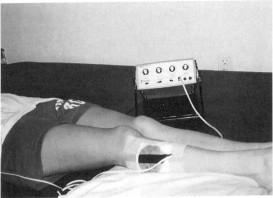

Figure 2. Set–up for electrical stimulation.

Table 2
Contraindications/Precautions of Electrial Stimulation

Wounds with osteomyelitis
Wounds with cancerous tissue
Patients with demand type cardiac
   pacemakers
Patients with a history of dysrhythmia
Electrode placement over cartoid sinuses
During pregnancy
Wounds containing heavy metal residue

the active electrode. Based on Becker's theory of "current of injury," some researchers recommend the placement of the positive electrode proximally close to the origin of the spinal nerve root. Therefore, when treating wounds with negative polarity, the positive or dispersive electrode should be placed cephalically close to the spinal cord in relation to the negative electrode whenever possible, whereas while treating wounds with positive polarity, the dispersive or the negative electrode should be placed caudally further away from the spinal cord in relation to the positive electrode whenever possible. The intensity of the ES needs to be set at a subthreshold muscle contraction. The recommended duration of treatment is 45 to 60 minutes five days a week (Figure 2).

The AHCPR clinical practice guideline on pressure ulcer treatment recommends that a course of treatment with electrotherapy (electrical stimulation) may be considered if a pressure ulcer has been found to be unresponsive to conservative treatment.[1] The guideline also emphasize the importance of having proper equipment and trained personnel to follow the protocols that have been shown to be effective and safe. Table 2 lists the most common contraindications and precautions related to ES. For wounds receiving topical application containing heavy metal ions, the clinicians should make sure that the wounds have been thoroughly irrigated and the topical residues have been removed from the wound bed before applying the electrodes to avoid concentration of the electric current over the ions.

Ultrasound

During recent years, use of ultrasound therapy for wound management has gained more acceptance. Ultrasound is high frequency mechanical vibration transmitted at a frequency above the range of human hearing which can be used therapeutically to accelerate wound healing.

There is now considerable evidence that suggests that therapeutic ultrasound can produce changes at the cellular level resulting in increased cell membrane permeability. When used therapeutically, ultrasound can result in mast cell degranulation; increased vascular permeability; increased calcium uptake in fibroblast cells; increased collagen synthesis; increased release of mitogenic growth factors; rapid migration of macrophages, fibroblasts, and endothiocytes; and increased tensile strength and elasticity.[11–14] Although ultrasound therapy accelerates wound healing in all phases, it is most effective when used during the inflammatory phase of wound healing.

When treating wounds with ultrasound, non–thermal forms which can be produced at a frequency of 3 MHz should be used. Also, ultrasound intensities for wound management are to be kept at a low level, typically 0.1 to 0.3 W/cm^2, since high intensities are associated with excessive edema and tissue destruction. Recently, Brown and associates found increased inflammation when full–thickness wounds in guinea pigs were sonated with 3 MHz frequency at 1.0 W/cm^2 intensity.[15] Since ultrasound is most effective during the inflammatory phase, the acute conditions are treated once or twice a day and eventually reduced to every other day. A direct technique is preferred when using ultrasound for wound management. This technique can be accomplished by applying an aqueous gel–based sterile dressing over the wound bed after the wound has been thoroughly irrigated. A thin layer of coupling gel/lotion is then applied over the dressing and the wound bed is sonated with ultrasound (Figure 3). Another direct technique used to treat wounds over irregular surfaces and bony prominences consists of immersing the wound area and ultrasound applicator in water.

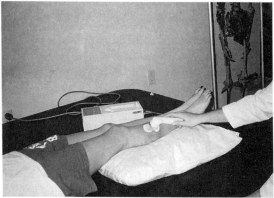

Figure 3. Ultrasound for wound management.

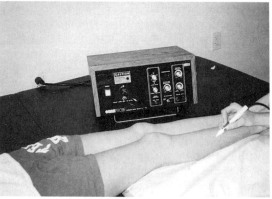

Figure 4. Administration of low–intensity laser.

Table 4
Contraindications/Precautions of Low–Intensity Laser
Over tumorous tissues
Over fontanelles of growing children
Patients with photosensitive skin
Patients taking photosensitive drugs
During pregnancy
Note: Do not stare directly into the laser beam.

Although ultrasound therapy has an impressive record of safety and efficacy when used in a correct manner, it can be potentially dangerous when used inappropriately. The most common contraindications and precautions are listed in Table 3.

Low–Intensity Laser

Laser is an acronym for light amplification by stimulated emission of radiation. Low–intensity lasers (LILs) for wound management have only been used in the United States for over a decade, whereas LILs have been successfully used in Eastern Europe and Russia for nearly three decades. The United States Food & Drug Administration (USFDA) still considers a LIL an investigational device. Use of LIL is limited to research purpose only and needs to be approved by the Institutional Review Board (IRB).

The effects of LIL on biological systems are best understood at the cellular level. The interactions of LIL at the cellular level provide the underlying rational for clinical use. Decreased edema, reduced inflammation, increased phagocytosis and collagen synthesis, and accelerated epithelialization are a few of the physiological effects which have been reported with LIL.[16–18]

Although LIL research at the cellular level has been the most convincing evidence, the clinical safety and efficacy of LIL has not been established. Obviously, further controlled clinical studies on large numbers of patients are needed to confirm the clinical efficacy of LILs on wound healing. The most common contraindications and precautions of LIL have been listed in Table 4.

Treatment guidelines associated with LIL are based on the amount of energy density delivered to a square centimeter of tissue surface. The quantity of laser is calculated in Joules per square centimeter (J/cm^2). Care must be taken when selecting energy density for treating wounds with LIL. Generally, energy densities of 0.05 to 4.0 J/cm^2 are safe and produce biostimulatory effects, whereas higher energy densities may produce inhibitory effects. Clean wounds with viable tissue are treated with the "grid" technique. The wound bed is visually divided into square centimeter grids and each grid is treated by holding the laser probe perpendicular to the wound bed at a distance of 0.5 to 1.0 cm. Each square is treated by sweeping the probe in a circular motion (Figure 4). For wounds which are covered with eschar, the periphery of the wound is treated.

Ultraviolet "C"

The natural source of ultraviolet (UV) is sunlight. However, there are a number of generators (lamps) which provide UV energy that are used clinically. UV radiation has been used in the past to treat a variety of dermatological conditions such as boils, carbuncles and psoriasis. The literature addressing the effectiveness of UV radiation, particularly on wound healing, is scarce.

Biological changes in the tissues irradiated with UV energy differ at different wavelengths. Wavelengths from 315 to 400 nm (UVA) can produce pigmentation of the skin and a weak erythema which is less effective in producing desired physiological changes in the tissue. Wavelengths from 280 to 315 nm (UVB) may produce intense erythema resulting in possible blistering and tissue damage. Wavelengths from 200 to 280 nm (UVC) are safe and more effective in producing biological changes in the tissue. UVC radiation is therapeutically used to treat chronic wounds which fail to respond to conventional treatment. Erythemal effectiveness from UVC peaks at 250 nm and rarely causes an intense erythema or blistering. In addition, cell inactivation as well as nucleic acid absorption also peaks at 250 nm wavelength.

UVC radiation has been reported to enhance epithelialization by increasing epithelial cell turnover followed by epidermal thickness (hyperplasia).[19,20] It is believed that hyperplasia may result from release of prostaglandin precursors which contribute to UV induced erythema and may mediate cell proliferation.[21] UVC is reported to enhance nucleic acid absorption resulting in an accelerated rate of DNA synthesis in fibroblasts.[22] UVC radiation also produces bactericidal and virucidal effects on wound pathogens. In addition, UVC irradiation causes increased blood flow in cutaneous capillaries and improved oxygenation in tissue, enhancing the formation of granulation tissue. UVC irradiation can also promote sloughing of necrotic tissue and eschar.

UVC (250 nm wavelength) radiation can be provided by holding a cold–quartz lamp centered over the wound either at a distance of 2.5 cm from the skin or in close contact with the skin. The treatment guidelines associated with UVC are based on the exposure time to produce a light pink erythema of

the skin. Since skin pigmentation has negligible effects on absorption of UVC, this dose may be used as a baseline dose to calculate longer duration doses to produce desquamation or debridement effects. For a fully granulated wound with clear exudate, exposure time is 15 seconds (E1 dose) with the lamp held at a distance of 2.5 cm from the skin. For a wound with a pale/grayish base which is not fully granulated and has cloudy or purulent exudate, exposure time is increased to 90 seconds (E3 dose) with the lamp held at a distance of 2.5 cm from the skin. For a wound with adherent yellow necrotic and/or pale base with or without undermining, exposure time is further increased to 120 seconds (E4 dose) with the lamp held in contact with the skin. For a wound with eschar, exposure time is 240 seconds (2E4 dose) with the lamp held in contact with the skin. If the appearance of the wound base is not consistent, each different area can be exposed at different dosages. This can be accomplished by covering the area which is not being treated with either petrolatum or a paper towel. The recommended frequency of treatment is three times a week. The most common contraindications and precautions are listed in Table 5.

Intermittent Compression Therapy

Intermittent compression therapy (ICT) has been used for many years to reduce lymphedema. ICT is thought to promote healing of venous ulcers by enhancing venous blood flow and systemic fibrinolytic activity. Recently, several controlled clinical studies have reported improved rates of healing of chronic venous ulcers with sequential ICT.[23–25] A significant increase in transcutaneous oxygen after the application of sequential ICT has been found in post–thrombotic leg ulcers.[26] Venous ulcers are reported to heal faster when ICT is used along with Unna Boot therapy.

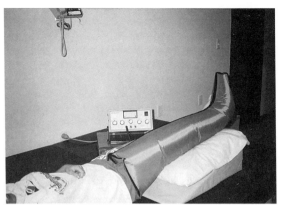

Figure 5. Set–up for sequential compression therapy.

Table 6
Contraindications/Precautions of Intermittent Compression Therapy

Deep vein thrombosis
Acute phlebitis
Venous ulcers associated with arterial occlusion

Once the wound is cleaned, the extremity is wrapped in a plastic bag to keep the compression sleeve from being soaked with wound exudate. The patient is placed in the supine position (Figure 5), the extremity is elevated, and a properly fitting compression sleeve is applied. The duration of treatment is set for 30 minutes to an hour at a pressure below the diastolic pressure. Generally, 50 to 60 mm Hg is effective. The ICT is set at an intermittent compression cycle of 90 seconds of compression and 30 seconds of relaxation. In conjunction with ICT, application of either an elastic or nonelastic wrap is usually required in order to provide compression to the extremity when the patient is in upright position and ambulatory. The most common contraindications and precautions of ICT are listed in Table 6.

Summary

Physical therapists play an important role as a part of the wound care team. Use of physical modalities may enhance the wound healing process, thereby shortening the length of hospitalization and reducing patient suffering. This chapter has focused on a brief description of various physical modalities frequently used for the management of chronic wounds. Clinical safety and efficacy of a few of these modalities have been studied; however, more controlled clinical studies are needed to establish a solid research base for practice. Additionally, clinicians need to keep in mind that these modalities should be used as adjunct treatments. Conventional wound care remains of utmost importance.

References

1. Bergstrom N, Bennett MA, Carbon CE, et al. *Treatment of Pressure Ulcers.* Clinical Practice Guideline #15. Rockville, MD: U.S. Dept. of Health and Human Services. Public Health Service. AHCPR. AHCPR Publ. #95–0652. December 1994.

2. Mohr T, Akers TM, Landry RL. Effect of high voltage stimulation on edema reduction in the rat hind limb. *Phys Ther* 1987;67:1703–1708.
3. Reed BV. Effect of high voltage pulsed electrical stimulation on microvascular permeability to plasma protein: A possible mechanism in minimizing edema. *Phys Ther* 1988;68:491–495.
4. Reich JD, Cazzaniga AL, Mertz PM, et al. The effect of electrical stimulation on the number of mast cells in healing wounds. *J Am Acad Dermatol* 1991;25:40–46.
5. Kincaid CB, Lavoie KH. Inhibition of bacterial growth in vitro following stimulation with high voltage, monophasic, pulsed current. *Phys Ther* 1989;69:651–655.
6. Cruz NI, Bayron FE, Saurez AJ. Accelerated healing of full–thickness burns by the use of high–voltage pulsed galvanic stimulation in the pig. *Ann Plast Surg* 1989;23:49–54.
7. Brown M, McDonnell MK, Menton DN. Polarity effects on wound healing using electrical stimulation in rabbits. *Arch Phys Med Rehabil* 1989;70:624–627.
8. Feeder J, Kloth L. Chronic dermal ulcer healing enhanced with monophasic pulsed electrical stimulation. *Phys Ther* 1991;70:639–649.
9. Griffin JW, Tooms RE, Mendius RA, et al. Efficacy of high voltage pulsed current for healing of pressure ulcers in patients with spinal cord injury. *Phys Ther* 1991;71:433–442.
10. Kloth LC, Feedar JA. Acceleration of wound healing with high voltage, monophasic, pulsed current. *Phys Ther* 1988;68:503–508.
11. Byl NN, McKenzie AL, West JM, et al. Low–dose ultrasound effects on wound healing: A controlled study with yucatan pigs. *Arch Phys Med Rehab* 1992;73:656–664.
12. Harvey W, Dyson M, Pond J, et al. The *in vitro* stimulation of protein synthesis in human fibroblasts by therapeutic levels of ultrasound. *Proceedings of the Second European Congress on Ultrasonics in Medicine, Excerpta Medica.* Amsterdam. 1975, pp 10–21.
13. Webster D. The effect of ultrasound on wound healing. Thesis, University of London, 1980.
14. Young SR, Dyson M. Macrophage responsiveness to therapeutic ultrasound. *Ultrasound Med Biol* 1990;16:809–816.
15. Brown M, Gogia PP, Sinacore DR, et al. Effects of ultrasound on wound healing in guinea pigs. (unpublished).
16. Lam TS, Abergel RP, Castel JC, et al. Laser stimulation of collagen synthesis in human skin fibroblast cultures. *Lasers Life Sci* 1986;1:61–77.
17. Haina D, Brunner R, Landthaler M, et al. Animal experiments in light–induced wound healing. *Laser Basic Biomed Res* 1982;22:1–3.
18. Lyons RF, Abergel RP, White RA, et al. Biostimulation of wound healing *in vivo* by a helium–neon laser. *Ann Plast Surg* 1987;18:47–50.
19. Sams W. Inflammatory mediators in ultra–violet erythema. In: Pathak M (ed). *Sunlight and Man.* Tokyo, Japan, University of Tokyo Press, 1974.
20. Agin P, Rose A, Lane C, et al. Changes in epidermal forward scattering absorption after UVA or UVB irradiation. *J Invest Dermatol* 1981;76:174–177.

21. Eaglstein W, Weinstein G. Prostaglandin and DNA synthesis in human skin: Possible relationship to ultraviolet effects. *J Invest Dermatol* 1975;64:386–396.

22. Parrish J, Jaenicke K, Anderson R. Erythema and melanogenesis action spectra of normal human skin. *Photochem Photobiol* 1982;36:187–191.

23. Coleridge–Smith P, Sarin S, Hasty J, et al. Sequential gradient pneumatic compression enhances venous ulcer healing: A randomized trial. *Surgery* 1990;108:871–875.

24. McCulloch JM, Marler KC, Neal MB, et al. Intermittent pneumatic compression improves venous ulcer healing. *Advance Wound Care* 1994;7:22–26.

25. Mulder G, Robinson J, Seeley J. Study of sequential compression therapy in the treatment of non–healing chronic venous ulcers. *WOUNDS* 1990;3:111–115.

26. Pekanmaki K, Kolari PJ, Kiistala U. Intermittent pneumatic compression treatment for post–thrombotic leg ulcers. *Clin Exp Dermatol* 1987;12:350–353.

27. Brown M, Gogia PP, Sinacore DR, et al. High voltage galvanic stimulation on wound healing in guinea pigs: Longer–term effects. *Arch Phys Med Rehabil* 1995;76:1134–1137.

28. Brown M, Gogia PP. Effects of high voltage stimulation on cutaneous wound healing in rabbits. *Phys Ther* 1987;67:662–667.

29. Brown M, McDonnell MK, Menton DN. Electrical stimulation effects on cutaneous wound healing in rabbits: A follow–up study. *Phys Ther* 1988;68:955–960.

30. Mulder GD. Treatment of open–skin wounds with electrical stimulation. *Arch Phys Med Rehabil* 1991;72:375–377.

31. Unger PG. Wound healing using high voltage galvanic stimulation. *Stimulus* 1985;10:8–10.

32. Edmonds PD, Sancier KM. Evidence of free radical production by ultrasonic cavitation in biological media. *Ultrasound Med Biol* 1983;9:635–639.

33. Fyfe M, Chahl LA. Mast cell degranulation and increased vascular permeability induced by therapeutic ultrasound in the rat ankle joint. *Br J Exp Pathol* 1984;65:671–676.

34. Mortimer AJ, Dyson M. The effect of therapeutic ultrasound on calcium uptake in fibroblasts. *Ultrasound Med Biol* 1988;14:499–506.

35. Mummery CL. The effect of ultrasound on fibroblasts *in vitro*. University of London, 1978. Thesis.

36. Hart J. The effect of therapeutic ultrasound on dermal wound repair with emphasis on fibroblast activity. University of London, 1993. Thesis.

37. Hogan RD, Franklin TD, Fry FT, et al. The effects of ultrasound on microvascular hemodynamics in skeletal muscle: Effects on arterioles. *Ultrasound Med Biol* 1982;8: 45–55.

38. Hogan RD, Burke KM, Franklin TD. The effect of ultrasound on hemodynamics in skeletal muscle: Effects during ischemia. *Microvas Res* 1982;23:370–379.

39. Young SR. The effect of therapeutic ultrasound on the biological mechanisms involved in dermal repair. University of London, 1988. Thesis.

40. Byl NN, McKenzie A, Wong T, et al. Incisional wound healing: a controlled study of low and high dose ultrasound. *J Ortho Sports Phys Ther* 1993;18:619–628.

41. Webster D. The effect of ultrasound on wound healing. University of London, 1980. Thesis.

42. El Batouty MF, El Gindy I, El Shawaf I, et al: A comparative evaluation of the effects of ultrasonic and ultraviolet irradiation on tissue regeneration. *Scand J Rheumatol* 1986;15:381–386.

43. McDiarmid T, Burns PN, Lewith GT, el al. Ultrasound and the treatment of pressure sores. *Physiotherapy* 1985;71:66–70.

44. Nussbaum EL, Biemann I, Mustard B. Comparison of ultrasound/ultraviolet–C and laser for treatment of pressure ulcers in patients with spinal cord injury. *Phys Ther* 1994;74:812–825.

45. Dyson M, Franks, C, Suckling J. Stimulation of healing of varicose ulcers by ultrasound. *Ultrasonics* 1976;14:232–236.

46. Dyson M, Suckling J. Stimulation of tissue repair by ultrasound: A survey of the mechanisms involved. *Physiotherapy* 1978;64:105–108.

47. Roche C, West J. A controlled trial investigating the effect of ultrasound on venous ulcers referred from general practitioners. *Physiotherapy* 1984;70:475–477.

48. Callam MJ, Harper DR, Dale JJ, et al. A controlled trial of weekly ultrasound therapy in chronic leg ulceration. *Lancet* 1987;2:204–206.

49. Eriksson SV, Lundeberg T, Malm M. A placebo controlled trial of ultrasound therapy in chronic leg ulcers. *Scand J Rehab Med* 1991; 23:211–213.

50. Kana JS, Hutschenreiter G, Haina D. Effect of low–power density laser radiation on healing of open skin wounds in rats. *Arch Surg* 1981;116:293–296.

51. Mester E, Jaszagi–Nagy E. The effect of laser radiation on wound healing and collagen synthesis. *Stud Biophys* 1973;35:227–230.

52. Abergel RP, Lyons RF, Caster JC, et al. Biostimulation of wound healing by lasers: experimental approaches in animal and in fibroblast cultures. *J Dermatol Surg Oncol* 1987;13:127–133.

53. Hardy LB, Hardy FS, Fine S, et al. Effect of ruby laser radiation on mouse fibroblast culture. *Fed Proc* 1967;26:668.

54. Hallman HO, Basford JR, O'Brien JF, et al. Does low–energy helium–neon laser irradiation alter *in vitro* replication of human fibroblast. *Lasers Surg Med* 1988;8: 125–129.

55. Kubasova T. Kovacs L, Somosy Z, et al. Biological effect of He-Ne laser: Investigations on functional and micromorphological alterations of cell membranes, *in vitro*. *Lasers Surg Med* 1984;4:382–388.

56. Passarella S, Casamassima E, Molinari S, et al. Increase of proton electrochemical potential and ATP synthesis in rat liver mitochondria irradiated *in vitro* by helium–neon laser. *FEBS Lett* 1984;175:95–99.

57. Haas AF, Isseroff RR, Wheeland RG, et al. Low–energy helium– neon laser irradiation increases the motility of cultured human keratinocytes. *J Invest Dermatol* 1990;94:822–826.

58. Rood PA, Haas AF, Graves PJ, et al. Low–energy helium–neon laser irradiation does not alter human keratinocytes differentiation. *J Invest Dermatol* 1992;99:445–458.

59. Mester E, Spiry T, Szende B, et al. Effect of laser rays on wound healing. *Am J Surg* 1971;122:532–535.

60. Braverman B, McCarthy RJ, Ivankovich AD, et al. Effect of helium–neon and infrared laser irradiation on wound healing in rabbits. *Laser Surg Med* 1989;9: 50–58.

61. Kovacs IB, Mester E, Gorog P. Stimulation of wound healing with laser beam in rat. *Experientia* 1974;30:1275–1276.

62. Surinchak JS, Alago ML, Bellamy RF, et al. Effects of low–level energy lasers on the healing of full–thickness skin defects. *Lasers Surg Med* 1983;2:267–274.

63. Basford JR, Hallman HO, Sheffield CG, et al. Comparison of cold–quartz ultraviolet, low–energy laser and occlusion in wound healing in a swine model. *Arch Phys Med Rehabil* 1986;67:151–154.

64. Hunter J, Leonard L, Wilson R, et al. Effects of low energy laser on wound healing in a porcine model. *Lasers Surg Med* 1984;3: 285–290.

65. McCaughan JS, Bethel BH, Johnston T, et al. Effect of low–dose argon irradiation on rate of wound closure. *Laser Surg Med* 1985;5:607–614.

66. Kami T, Yoshimura Y, Nakajima T, et al. Effects of low–power diode lasers on flap survival. *Ann Plast Surg* 1985;14:278–283.

67. Namenyi J, Mester E, Folder I, Tisza S. Effect of laser irradiation and immunosuppressive treatment on survival of mouse skin allotransplant. *Act Chir Acad Sci Hung* 1975;16:327–335.

68. Santoianni P, Monfrecola G, Martellotta D, et al. Inadequate effect of helium–neon laser on venous leg ulcers. *Photodermatology* 1984;1:245–249.

69. Gogia PP, Marquez RR. Effects of helium–neon laser on wound healing. *Ostomy/Wound Management* 1992;38:33–41.

Appendix 1
Summary of High Voltage Pulsed Stimulation Wound Healing Studies

Findings	Type of study
Increased blood flow[2]	In vivo
Decreased edema[3]	In vivo
Reduced number of mast cells[4]	In vitro
Inhibitory effects of growth of microorganisms[5]	In vitro
Faster rate of wound contraction and higher fibroblast responses[6]	In vivo
Increased tensile strength[7,27]	In vivo
Better organization of collagen tissue[28,29]	In vivo
Enhanced rate of epithelialization[7,29]	In vivo
Increased healing in pressure ulcers[8–10,30,31]	Clinical

Reprinted with permission from Ostomy/Wound Management 1996;42(1):47. Health Management Publications, Inc.

Appendix 2
Summary of ultrasound therapy wound healing studies

Findings	Type of study
Production of free radicals[32]	In vitro
Mast cell degranulation and increased vascular permeability[11,33]	In vitro/In vivo
Increased calcium uptake in fibroblasts[34,35]	In vitro
Increased collagen synthesis[11,12]	In vitro/In vivo
Increased release of mitogenic growth factors[14,36]	In vitro
Vasoconstriction of small arterioles[37]	In vivo
Increased capillary density[38]	In vivo
Rapid migration of macrophages, fibroblasts, and endothiocytes[39]	In vivo
Increased tensile strength and elasticity[11,40,41]	In vitro
Increased healing[11,42]	In vivo
Increased healing in infected pressure ulcers[43]	Clinical
Increased healing in pressure ulcers[44]	Clinical
Increased healing in venous stasis ulcers[45–47]	Clinical
Increased healing in chronic leg ulcers[48]	Clinical
No increased healing in chronic leg ulcers[49]	Clinical

Reprinted with permission from Ostomy/Wound Management 1996;42(1):48. © Health Management Publications, Inc.

Appendix 3
Summary of low–energy laser wound healing studies

Findings	Type of study
Increased collagen production[16,18,50,51]	*In vitro/In vivo*
Increased mRNA procollagen synthesis[52]	*In vitro*
Increased fibroblasts cells[53]	*In vitro*
No fibroblast proliferation[54]	*In vitro*
Increased binding ability of the fibroblast cells to lectin[55]	*In vitro*
Increased membrane potential, proton gradient, and ATP synthesis[56]	*In vitro*
Increased keratinocyte migration[57]	*In vitro*
No increased keratinocyte migration[58]	*In vitro*
Enhanced healing[50,59]	*In vivo*
Increased tensile strength[18,60–62]	*In vivo*
Increased granulation tissue and enhanced epidermal regeneration[17]	*In vivo*
No increased healing[63–65]	*In vivo*
Increased vascularization and improved graft/flap survival[66,67]	*In vivo*
No increased healing in chronic venous stasis ulcers[68]	Clinical
No increased healing in leg ulcers[69]	Clinical

Reprinted with permission from Ostomy/Wound Management 1996;42(1):50. © Health Management Publications, Inc.

33

Systemic Hyperbaric Oxygen Therapy as an Aid in Resolution of Selected Chronic Problem Wounds

Keith Van Meter, MD, FACEP

Van Meter K. Systemic hyperbaric oxygen therapy as an aid in resolution of selected chronic problem wounds. In: Krasner D, Kane D. *Chronic Wound Care, Second Edition*. Wayne, PA, Health Management Publications, Inc., 1997, pp 260–275.

Introduction

Systemically administered hyperbaric oxygen therapy has been found to be clinically useful in selected cases in healing chronic problem wounds including diabetic extremity wounds, venous insufficiency ulcers, pressure ulcers, and arterial insufficiency ulcers.[1] Systemic hyperbaric oxygen therapy is defined as the pressurization of an entire patient in a chamber to a pressure greater than one atmosphere while the patient breathes surface equivalent breathing mixtures in excess of 100 percent oxygen. Topical hyperbaric oxygen therapy is defined as the application of more than 100 percent surface equivalency of oxygen applied by pressure in a closed container sealed to a body part, either while the patient is maintained in a one atmosphere environment or while the total patient is pressurized in a hyperbaric chamber, in which case both topical and systemic administration of hyperbaric oxygen may be accomplished. This chapter will discuss the use of only systemically administered hyperbaric oxygen.

In the physiology of the above examples of chronic wounding, tissue hypoxia is both an aid and a deterrent to chronic wound resolution.[2] Systemic hyperbaric oxygen therapy, because of potential oxygen toxicity to the patient, can only be administered intermittently. Intermittency of patient exposure is best for patient tolerance. Non–healing wounds are often under–perfused by physiologic tissue oxygen supply from capillary blood flow. Rapid wound healing relies on both hypoxic and normoxic/hyperoxic tissue environments for most effective wound resolution, as will be discussed later in this chapter.

Basic Physiology of Hyperbaric Oxygen Therapy Applicable to Improving Host Response in Resolving Problem Chronic Wounds

In diving medicine, one atmosphere of pressure absolute (ATA/Abs) is equated to 33 feet of sea water (fsw), 14.7 pounds per square inch (psi), 760 mmHg, or 1034 cm water. Calculation of the surface equivalency of oxygen in the hyperbaric environment includes "counting in" the atmosphere of pressure that envelopes the earth and its human inhabitants, plus the additional atmosphere (or fraction thereof) to which the patient is pressurized. Adding up the atmospheres of total exposure and multiplying this number by the percent of oxygen inhaled results in the SEF_{IO_2} (surface equivalent fraction of inhaled oxygen). For example, breathing 100 percent oxygen at sea level or F_{IO_2} 100%) can be improved upon by "descending" the patient in a hyperbaric chamber to one additional atmosphere pressure (33 fsw or 14.7 psi) to give a total pressure exposure of two atmospheres. What happens, in essence, is that the one atmosphere pressure provided by the gaseous envelope

Table 1
SEFI0$_2$ and approximate arterial oxygen partial pressures (paO$_2$s)

Hyperbaric Pressure Exposure	SEFI0$_2$	paO$_2$
2.0 ATA/Abs	200%	1433 mmHg
2.5 ATA/Abs	250%	1753 mmHg
3.0 ATA/Abs	300%	2193 mmHg

Table 2
Human Organ Oxygen Extraction Rates

Brain	6.1 vol%
Kidney	1.5 vol%
Heart	11.0 vol%
Muscle	5.0 vol %
Skin	2.0 vol%

surrounding the earth adds to the increased pressure provided by pressurizing the patient in a hyperbaric chamber to compress the 100 percent inhaled oxygen mix to twice as rich an oxygen concentration or SEFI0$_2$ 200 percent.

Table 1 equates SEFI0$_2$ and approximate arterial oxygen partial pressures (paO$_2$s) achievable by breathing 100% oxygen at various hyperbaric oxygen treatment depths. Patients with varying pulmonary functions and ventilation/perfusion characteristics often produce paO$_2$s slightly less than predicted (an arterial pCO$_2$ of 40 mmHg plus a water vapor pressure at 98.6° F of 47 mmHg equals 87 mm Hg and must be subtracted from the total atmospheric pressure to which the patient is exposed).

Another important consideration in hyperbaric oxygen inhalation is the increased dissolved oxygen content achievable in the plasma fraction of blood. For an average patient, each gram of hemoglobin carries 1.34 ml of bound gaseous oxygen. Each atmosphere of inhaled air adds just 0.3 cc of dissolved oxygen per 100 cc of blood. The carriage of oxygen in a one atmosphere air breathing patient with a hemoglobin of 15 is 20.10 cc (1.34 x 15 g/100 cc) plus 0.3 cc, which equals 20.4 cc per 100 cc of blood or 20.4 vol% (one vol% = one cc per 100 cc).[3] In a hyperbaric oxygen environment, each atmosphere of pure oxygen adds 2.2 cc of dissolved oxygen per 100 cc of blood. Hyperbaric oxygen exposure to SEFI0$_2$ 200%, 250%, and 300% produces a dissolved oxygen content of plasma of 2.2 vol%, 4.4 vol%, and 6.6 vol%, respectively.

As early as 1960, a Dutch cardiovascular surgeon, I. Boerema, took advantage of the increased dissolved oxygen content achievable by hyperbaric oxygen inhalation for an experiment in piglets (exsanguinated to hemoglobins of 0.4 g/100 cc and intravenously volume reloaded with dextran, D5W,

and Ringer's Lactate). Boerema demonstrated that he could keep the piglets alive at 3 ATA with SEFI0$_2$ 300% for at least 15 minutes; 6.6 vol% of dissolved oxygen alone was possible in these hyperbarically exposed subjects.[4]

Human organ oxygen extraction rates (amount of oxygen in milliliters extracted for each 100 mL of blood flowing through the organ) are detailed in the Table 2.[5]

In hyperbaric oxygen inhalation exposure, the dissolved oxygen alone can meet most of the reparative tissue needs in organ injury or wounding. The capillary beds in periwound and wound tissue are often partially occluded by microthrombi to passage of red blood cells. Biglow demonstrated that plasma flow still exists in the microthrombosed capillary beds of injured tissue.[6] In hyperbaric oxygen therapy, "plasma skimming" as characterized by Biglow, brings plasma with enough dissolved oxygen to oxygenate wounded tissue supplied by only partially patent capillary beds.

Hyperbaric oxygen inhalation therapy affords high enough dissolved plasma oxygen levels to allow for effective oxygen diffusion through tissue edema, hematoma, and devitalized tissue. In fact, the calculated diffusion of oxygen through tissue supplied by the last "plasma patent" capillary bed is four-fold at the arterial end and two-fold greater at the venous end when comparing inhalation of F$_{102}$ 20% to the SEFI0$_2$ 200% afforded by hyperbaric oxygen therapy.[7]

Dependence of Wound Healing Physiology on Tissue Normoxia and Hypoxia

The following are oxygen dependent tissue reparative processes:
1. Leukocyte bacterial killing (of both aerobic and anaerobic microbes)[8]

2. Effective proteolysis of necrotic wound tissue by macrophages and polymorphonuclear leukocytes[9]
3. Thrombolysis of wound and periwound capillary bed microthrombi[10]
4. Fibroblastic proliferation with collagen matrix elaboration with endothelial ingrowth by capillary budding (i.e., formation of granulation tissue)[11,12]
5. Osteoclastic and osteoblastic bone repair[13]
6. Advance of epithelialization of the wound margin over a well–granulated open wound.[14]

Phagocytic leukocytes (macrophages, polymorphonuclear leukocytes, and osteoclasts) have NADPH oxidase in their cytoplasmic membrane to include the invaginated cytoplasmic membranes that wall off into phagosomes. NADPH oxidase with ultimate production of superoxide (O_2^-), peroxide (H_2O_2), and hydroxyl (OH^-) free radicals, which in part assist in leukocyte bacterial killing. Polymorphonuclear leukocytes, which have five percent by dry weight of myeloperoxidase, convert these oxygen–free radicals into chlorinated oxidants (hypochlorous acid) utilizing the normal saline abundantly available in tissue. This "endogenous Dakin's solution" therein produced preferentially combines with the methionine moiety specific to the leukocyte protease shield (endogenous leukocyte protease inhibitor in tissue) and becomes inactivated. This inactivation allows leukocyte protease, which is without a methionine moiety, to digest wound debris unchecked.[9]

In a similar manner, the endogenous tissue plasminogen activator inhibitor, in thrombosed capillary beds at the margins of a chronic wound, contains a methionine moiety that combines with hypochlorous acid to become inactivated. This combination then allows endogenous tissue plasminogen activator to thrombolyse capillary bed microthrombosis in an unchecked fashion and may thereby help to keep capillaries patent at the base of a chronic wound.[10] Through patent capillaries, oxygen–dependent fibroblasts marginate into the wound to proliferate and to lay down collagen. Collagen requires oxygen for the hydroxylation of lysine and proline for the crosslinking to form a matrix for capillary ingrowth into the avascular base of the wound.[11,12]

The proteolytic destruction of connective tissue slows as fibroblasts replace leukocytes in the wound and as the new blood supply to the wound delivers in the plasma flow, the antiprotease shield mentioned previously.

Bone is repaired by oxygen–dependent osteoclastic and osteoblastic activity. In necrotic bone, the bone is removed and new bone is built up.[12] While both osteoclastic and osteoblastic cellular tissue repair processes are oxygen dependent, the osteoclastic process requires approximately 100 times more oxygen than osteoblastic bone activity.[13]

Epithelialization from the wound margin is oxygen dependent. Both proliferation and migration of epithelial cells have been shown to be accelerated by hyperbaric oxygen therapy in the select problem chronic wounds discussed in this chapter.[14]

Hypoxia–Dependent Tissue Reparative Process

The elaboration of macrophage angiogenic stimulating factor is dependent on tissue hypoxia.[15] Wound healing will only progress as long as a sharp tissue oxygen gradient exists between the viable wound margin, the hypoxia of the devitalized tissue, and the dead space in the center of the wound.[16] In essence, endogenous wound healing factors are elicited by wound hypoxia, while the actual cellular repair process of wound healing factor–stimulated cells is largely oxygen dependent.[17]

Management of Refractory or Limb Threatening Diabetic Wounds, Venous Insufficiency Ulcers, Pressure Ulcers and Arterial Insufficiency Ulcers

The managed resolution of chronic wounds is truly an application of baromedicine (medicine of changing pressure environments). An important challenge for baromedicine is improvement in weight unloading dressings to prevent wounding from pressure points which compress capillary and lymphatic vessels supplying ischemic wounds. Another challenge for baromedicine is control and improvement in patient nutrition. For example, maintenance of adequate serum albumin levels alters oncotic pressure in capillary and lymphatic vessels supplying chronic wounds.

Application of baromedicine to chronic wound healing by intermittent hyperbaric oxygen therapy is not the only way to increase arterial oxygen partial pressure, which in turn increases wound tissue oxygen partial pressures. There is a place for intermittent, one atmosphere oxygen inhalation, topical hyperbaric oxygen administration, and one atmosphere oxygen administration by occlusive bag or by 10% to 20% benzoyl peroxide cream topically under semi–occlusive dressings.

Venous insufficiency ulcers, pressure ulcers, and arterial insufficiency ulcers vary in pathophysiology and medical therapeutic approach. However, in both pathophysiology and medical therapeutic approach all three of these chronic wound categories are represented in part by chronic wounding common in the extremities of diabetic patients.

Until recently, no prospective, double–blinded, randomized clinical human study existed for any successful conventional or unconventional therapeutic approach for treatment of all four chronic wound categories detailed in this chapter.[17] Exceptions are a controlled non–blinded application of hyperbaric oxygen therapy (HBOT) to resolve diabetic foot wounds,[18] a controlled blinded application of HBOT to venous leg ulcers,[19] and a controlled double–blinded topical application of platelet–derived growth factors to treat problem wounds.[20,21]

An ample body of medical literature exists to support use of many of the conventional medical, surgical, and baromedical approaches to wound healing. No one can dispute the therapeutic efficacy of immediate resolution of a chronic wound by amputating the body part on which the chronic wound resides. However, even this surgical approach has not been subjected to a prospective randomized double–blinded trial.

Multidisciplinary approaches utilizing orthopedic and podiatric surgery, vascular surgery, infectious disease medicine, endocrinology, physical medicine, nutritional medicine, baromedicine, and plastic and general surgical care will continually strive for wound resolution, first by body part salvage for function, and then for cosmetics.

Recently, coverage of a non healing open dermal wound with cultured epithelial autografts (CEA's) appears to confer quicker resolution of the dermal defect.[22] Despite the advantages of any one approach, a coordinated multidisciplinary approach to even the simplest chronic refractory wound will leave the patient with the best outcome. The era of the sophisticated wound care team is here to stay, even in the current emphasis on primary care medicine in patient management.

Diabetic Extremity Wounding

Case Presentation. The following is a case report of a 45–year–old black female with a recognized 12–year history of insulin dependent diabetes mellitus. Five months earlier than her presentation to our facility, she stepped on a coat hanger, puncturing her right great toe on the plantar surface. The patient had proprioceptive and pain sensation deficits in both lower extremities. With conservative management, using antibiotic and topical

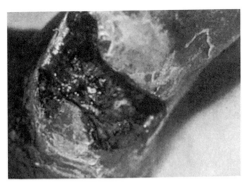

Figure 1a.

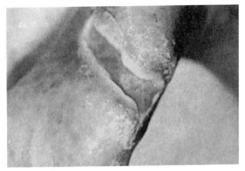

Figure 1b.

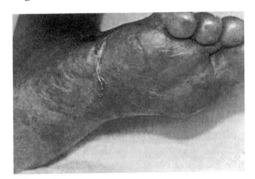

Figure 1c.

wound care, this wound resolved. Initially, the patient's small toe became inflamed after she picked at a small callus. Shortly thereafter, she was admitted to the hospital. Five days later she had a fifth ray amputation in the metatarsal/midshaft region. The open wound became gangrenous and was cultured for a polymicrobial infection. *Bacteroides melaninogenicus, Streptococcus viridans, Pseudomonas aeruginosa, Enterobacter aerogenes,* and *Staphylococcus epidermidis* were isolated. The patient was placed on mexlocillin, metronidazole, and gentamycin by IV piggyback administration. The patient's brachial/ankle pulse index was 1.0. The open wound appeared gangrenous and the patient was taken back to the operating room 14 days later for a plantar space debridement. The gangrenous process

Table 3
Multifaceted Etiology in Part of Diabetic Extremity Wounding[24,25]

1. Increased prevalence of distal segmental atherosclerotic peripheral vascular disease
2. Changes in capillary membrane to include increased thickness with impaired nutrient and oxygen diffusion through the same
3. Peripheral motor, sensory, and autonomic neuropathy
   a. Sudomotor dysfunction with "cracking" of the cutaneous envelope
   b. Vasomotor dysfunction with A/V shunting between the arterioles and the veins with capillary bed hypoxemia; development of neuropathic tissue edema by hydrostatic pressure of the lower extremity vascular column transmitted to dilated capillary beds
   c. Motor dysfunction with flattening of foot with claw-toe deformity
   d. Pain and proprioceptive sensory dysfunction with unprotected mechanical wounding to soft tissue and bone
4. Rheologic changes with impaired RBC deformability for passing through capillary bed
5. Impaired leukocyte phagocytosis.

Table 4
Grading of Diabetic Foot Wounds by Severity and Extent (Wagner)[26]

0. foot deformity without cutaneous breakdown
1. cutaneous break or partial–thickness cutaneous wound
2. confined full–thickness cutaneous wound
3. full–thickness wound with involvement or exposure of subcutaneous tissue, fat, muscle, fascia, tendons, or bone
4. local gangrenous change of soft tissue with or without underlying osteomyelitis
5. extensive gangrenous change of the entire foot.

Table 5
Diabetic Foot Wound Categorization Based on the Etiologic Components of Infection, Ischemia, and Neuropathy (Jeffcoate)[27]

I. Infection
  A. Cellulitis
    1. Complicating an obvious ulcer
    2. No obvious associated ulcer
    3. Associated with pre-existing gangrene
    4. Caused by trauma
  B. Osteomyelitis
    1. Complicating an obvious ulcer
    2. No obvious precipitating ulcer
    3. Associated with gangrene

II. Ischemia
  A. Symptomatic ischemia without an ulcer
    1. Claudication
    2. Rest pain
  B. Painless scabbed lesions of the skin
    1. Single
    2. Multiple
  C. Gangrene
    1. of a digit or digits
    2. of a forefoot
  D. Persistent unhealing ischemic lesions
    1. Neuroischemic ulcers
    2. Following surgery
    3. Following other trauma
    4. With no known cause
  E. Ischemic heel ulcers
    1. Small
    2. Large
    3. Painful cracks
  F. Blisters (epidermis intact)
    1. Caused by definable trauma
    2. No known cause

III. Neuropathy
  A. Ulcers with surrounding callus over an area of increased pressure
    1. Under metatarsal head
    2. On toe
    3. Complicating Charcot deformity
    4. Complicating surgery
    5. Complicating other deformity
  B. Neuropathic ulcers under the calcaneus
  C. Ulcers caused by unnoticed trauma

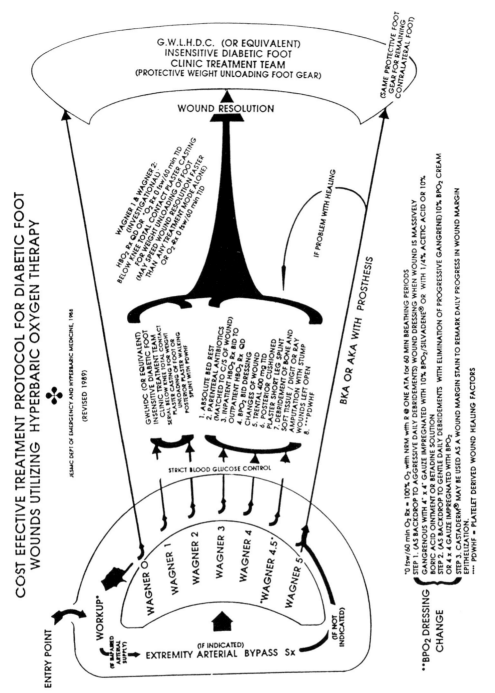

Figure 2.

continued in the open wound and hyperbaric medicine was consulted nine days later. Ten percent benzoyl peroxide cream impregnated gauze packing was placed into the patient's wound in daily dressing changes. The patient had 45/90 (2.4 ATA/Abs pressurization in the chamber for 90 treatment minutes) HBOT treatment, BID initially, tapered to QD. The patient was discharged in one month from the hospital and went to the United States Public Health Hospital in Carville, Louisiana for outpatient total contact plaster casting to weight unload her foot. She returned to work two weeks later, continuing HBOT as an outpatient for a total of 80 treatments, completing the entire course two months later.

Initially, clinicians at the United States Public Health Hospital suggested that a Syme's amputation

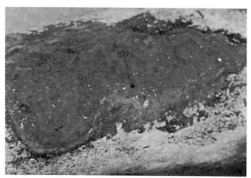

Figure 3a.

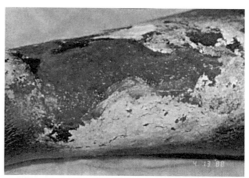

Figure 3b.

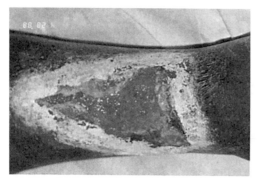

Figure 3c.

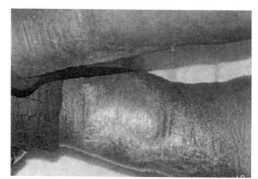

Figure 3d.

be performed on the patient. The total contact plaster cast was removed weekly, showing improvement with combined HBOT and topical wound management. The plaster cast was bivalved and used as a splint so that daily benzoyl peroxide dressings could be changed. As the wound improved, the clinicians at the United States Public Health Hospital advised free muscle flap and split–thickness skin graft. However, the wound was well resolved by secondary intention healing to include complete, durable epithelialization one month after completion of HBOT.

As a precaution against rewounding, the patient was given healing sandals with plastazote molded insole, rigid sole, and rocker bottom. She has had no recurrent wound breakdown upon follow–up. (Figures 1a–1c)

Case Discussion. In the United States, 11.5 to 12 million people are affected with diabetes; approximately eighty per ten thousand patients require an amputation each year.[23] Table 3 depicts the multifaceted etiology in part of diabetic extremity wounding.[24,25]

Diabetic foot wounds have been graded by severity and extent by Wagner (Table 4).[26] More recently, Jeffcoate has suggested an alternative diabetic foot wound categorization based on the etiologic

components of infection, ischemia, and neuropathy (Table 5).[27]

Figure 2 is a multidisciplinary treatment algorithm for managed care of foot wounds that attempts to modify the many facets of pathophysiology detailed above.

Important to the treatment of the chronic diabetic extremity wound is ascertainment of the arterial supply to the extremity with correction by arterial bypass graft surgery or by percutaneous balloon angioplasty if indicated. Wounds should have daily debridements with forceps and sharp scissors to remove necrotic debris well as periwound callus. A callus often acts as a space–occupying material in foot gear to further compress and injure precariously perfused tissue at the margin of the wound.

Topical use of 10 to 20 percent benzoyl peroxide cream mixed 50/50 with silver sulfadiazine cream in relatively clean wounds additionally mixed with mupericin and/or metronidazole gel in necrotic wounds under semi–occlusive Telfa® pad cover has proven to be a valuable approach to debride a necrotic wound at the Hyperbaric Medicine Unit at Jo Ellen Smith Medical Center in New Orleans, Louisiana.

One gram of benzoyl peroxide gradually releases 4 ml of nascent oxygen into the wound topically per 24 hours.[28] Therefore, 10cc of 10% benzoyl peroxide cream kneaded into a gauze 4x4 pad gently packed into an open wound will provide this constant topical dose of oxygen. Semi–occlusive Telfa pads overlying the packed open wound prevent undue drying of the dressing while still preventing maceration of the cutaneous borders of the wound. Op–site® can replace a Telfa pad cover if more wound dressing occlusion is needed initially. These benzoyl peroxide cream dressings should be changed only once a day. If after 24 hours, one takes a smear of the copious green–yellow exudate from under the dressing, a full field of WBCs is seen by microscope with few to no microbes in sight. The green discoloration of the exudate is from myeloperoxidase mentioned earlier in the chapter. Pseudomonas species colonization in the wet aerobic environment provided by this dressing can be minimized by mixing the benzoyl peroxide cream with silver sulfadiazine cream (or if necrotic wound debris penetration is needed, then with mupericin and metronidazole cream).

The selection of an antibiotic for the invariably polymicrobially infected chronic diabetic foot wound is important. Osteomyelitis is discoverable in the floor of an open diabetic foot wound by a probe being able to grate on bone surface.[29] This makes an economic diagnosis of osteomyelitis in diabetic foot wounding, where otherwise bone scans and X–rays for diabetic osteolysis and osteomyelitis often look alike.[30] If osteomyelitis is felt to be present, then a culture–guided ten week course of oral antibiotics can be given in a cost effective approach.[31]

Weight unloading or pressure injury protection of the diabetic wound extremity is essential. Dressings that distribute externally applied pressure evenly over a broad adjacent unwounded area of the extremity are necessary. An elegant weight distribution dressing for the chronic diabetic foot wound is a total contact plaster cast or posterior plaster walking splint and plastazote healing sandal (plastazote insole with rigid sole rocker bottom after P. Brandt and W. Coleman of the United States Public Health Hospital (Gillis W. Long Hansen's Disease Center in Carville, Louisiana). The casting or splinting foot gear evenly distributes weight away from the wounded foot areas to take concentrated weight off pressure points and to prevent the milking of bacteria up and down soft tissue planes of the wounded foot by normal foot motion.[32] Inhalation hyperbaric oxygen therapy assists wound oxygenation by plasma delivery of oxygen to the wound.

In serious wound infection, while topical antibiotics might be helpful, parenterally administered antibiotics are most often needed. A corollary exists for the pharmaceutical use of oxygen in wound healing. While topical oxygen is useful as applied by oxygen releasing benzoyl peroxide cream or Topox units, systemically administered oxygen by inhalation of hyperbaric oxygen is often required.

Dosing the patient with hyperbaric oxygen therapy must be considered in the same way as dosing with other pharmacologic agents. In severe necrotizing infection or wet gangrenous progression of a wound, QID treatment tapering to BID treatment frequency may be needed to check the forward destructive advance of the wound.

Under hyperbaric oxygen inhalation, oxygen loads into tissue much like inert gases do in diving. The tissue is decompressed of dissolved oxygen in part by the "oxygen window"[33] (or, more simply, by the metabolic consumption of the oxygen) as well as by the actual unloading of oxygen from tissue on decompression. Still, oxygen has been demonstrated to be elevated in muscle compartments for one–hour, post–hyperbaric oxygen therapy treatment and for up to four hours in subcutaneous tissue.[34]

The advantage of using the above treatment algorithm is that the majority of patients can be managed as outpatients or, after shortened hospital stays, can be converted to outpatient care. Most often, Wagner I and II wounded feet heal with the application of weight unloading orthotics (total contact plaster cast, posterior short leg splint, or plastazote molded insole foot gear with rigid rocker bottom sole) and good topical wound care. Hyperbaric oxygen therapy is usually reserved for Wagner III or greater grade of foot wounding. There is, however, a strong indication that combined hyperbaric oxygen therapy and conventional orthotic weight unloading therapy markedly shorten wound healing in Wagner I and II foot wounding. Hyperbaric oxygen, compared to foot amputation, has been demonstrated to be cost effective while salvaging the foot.[35]

Venous Insufficiency Ulceration

Case Presentation. A 63–year–old black male scraped the anterior tibial surface of his left lower leg on a door frame after coming in from working in the fields on a farm. The wound slowly expanded to a 13 by 7.5 cm wound. The patient sought medical care and was recognized as a non–insulin dependent diabetic. He had a brachial/ankle index of 0.8. The patient was placed on glyburide 5 mg QD. He had proprioceptive and pain sensation deficits in both lower extremities. The patient's wound was cultured for Group D *Enterococcus* and

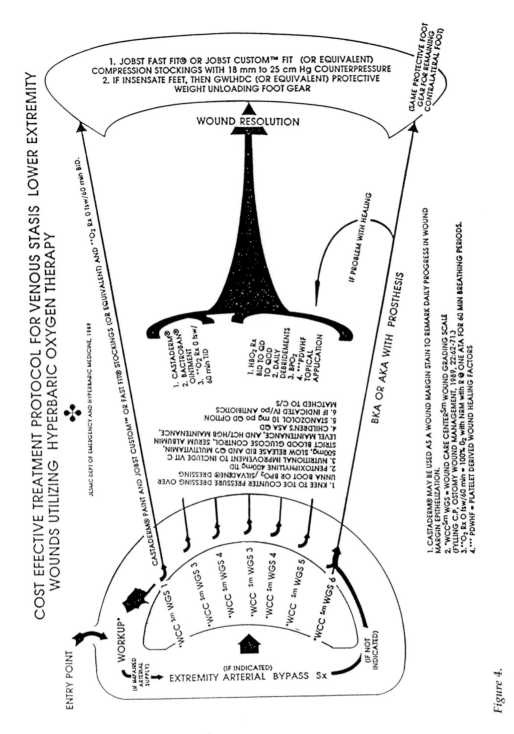

Figure 4.

Pseudomonas aeruginosa. The patient's wound was dressed with topical benzoyl peroxide cream 10 percent mixed 50/50 with silver sulfadiazine cream impregnated in gauze 4 by 4 pads changed once daily. The patient had Sof Roll® with Ace® overwrap compressive dressings from his knee to his toe. He was treated for a four month period with a total of 79 hyperbaric oxygen therapy treatments on a daily 45/90 multiplace table. The patient's wound completely epithelialized and he was given a prescription for Jobst Form Fit® stockings, which exerted an 18 to 25 mmHg counterpressure. The patient has had no breakdown to date (Figures 3a–3d).

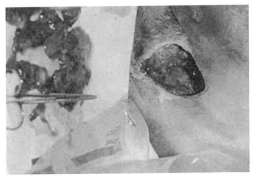

Figure 5a.

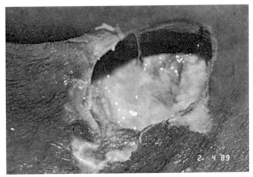

Figure 5b.

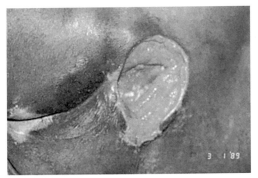

Figure 5c.

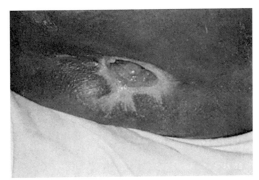

Figure 5d.

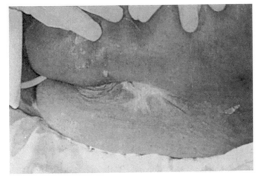

Figure 5e.

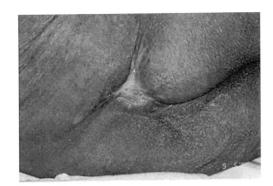

Figure 5f.

Case Discussion. Topical counterpressure provided by either Unna's® boot, Duke's® boot (occlusive dressings like DuoDerm® with Unna's boot and Ace® overlap from the infrapatellar notch to the metatarsal head have been reported to resolve large venous dermal ulcerations by secondary intention healing in time periods of six months to a year or more depending on the size of the wound.[36,37] The calf muscle in the leg acts as a pump in exercise, but requires intact venous valves to assure active venous drainage from the leg. Valvular insufficiency allows the hydrostatic pressure of the veins to transmit injury to the dermal capillary beds.[38]

Venous insufficiency has been theorized to produce tissue hypoxia under the assumption that if blood cannot get our of dermal structures by venous drainage, then blood cannot get into dermal structures by arteriolar supply.[39] It has also been speculated that pre–capillary bed A/V shunting with dermal capillary bed steal may be a cause of venous insufficiency ulceration.[40] Currently, both of these explanations have been felt to be innacurate or incomplete. Blood flow in the skin of recumbent patients with venous insufficiency of their legs has been discovered to be increased with increased skin oxygen tension. Accordingly, the

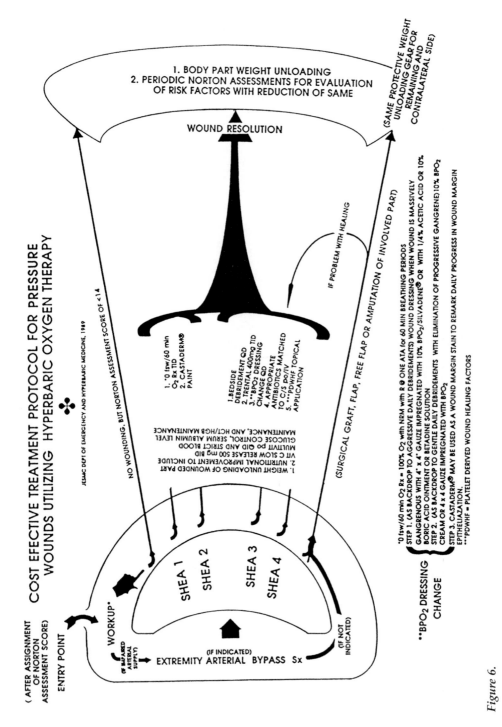

Figure 6.

old designation "venous stasis ulcer" has been changed to be venous ulcer or venous insufficiency ulcer.[41] Venous ulcers do heal even with persistence of pericapillary fibrin cuffs.[42] In the past, it had been suggested that capillary bed hypertension in venous disease forces open endothelial pores to let fibrinogen leak out of capillaries. This fibrinogen,

by polymerization, forms a pericapillary fibrin deposition, which was felt to block oxygen and nutrient entry into dermal tissue. The hypothesis corresponds with the observation that both blood and tissue fibrinolytic activity were significantly depressed as sampled from patients with venous ulceration.[43] More recently, the fibrin cuff has been

VAN METER

felt not to be a barrier to oxygen and nutrient diffusion, but instead a trap for needed tissue growth factors.[44]

In venous insufficiency wounding, hyperbaric oxygen therapy provides oxygen which may block tissue plasminogen activator inhibitor, allowing leukocyte and plasma plasminogen activator to resolve the pericapillary fibrin buildup from fibrinogen endothelial pore leak. Diminishment of the pericapillary[13] fibrin buildup wound would resolve the fibrin growth factor trap and allow venous dermal ulcer resolution. The dermal capillary bed hydrostatically injured by venous insufficiency is a leukocyte trap.[45] HBOT and not normobaric oxygen reversibly blocks leukocyte adhesion, lessening white cell accumulation against endothelial surface.[46] Figure 4 is a flow chart utilized by the Department of Emergency and Hyperbaric Medicine at Jo Ellen Smith Medical Center for a protocol of care of patients with venous insufficiency ulcers refractory to conventional management. The Wound Care Center[SM] grading system was used.[47]

Problem Pressure Wounds or Decubitus Wounds

Case Presentation. A 60–year–old black female with a 30–year history of deforming and debilitating rheumatoid arthritis (having had a total knee prosthetic replacement on the right eleven years before, ten years before on the left and nine years before a left hip replacement), presented with a two–week history of dermal breakdown on her sacral skin. The patient was living at home with her daughter, who was caring for the wound with topical Betadine and with attempts at weight unloading. The wound was 6 by 5 cm with a gangrenous change to the sacral periosteal surface. The wound cultured *Proteus mirabilis, Morganella morganii, Group B Streptococcus*, and *Enterococcus faecalis*. The patient had daily bedside debridements performed with forceps and scissors. The would was packed with 4 by 4 gauze impregnated with benzoyl peroxide 10 percent cream and silver sulfadiazine cream mixed in equal proportion. The patient had 32 inpatient hyperbaric oxygen treatments while she was hospitalized for 20 days. She had 51 follow–up treatments on an outpatient basis for a month, for a total of 83 treatments. The patient's wounds closed completely by secondary intention healing. The patient was placed on a prophylactic mattress when in the hospital and when discharged to a nursing home (Figures 5a–5f).

Case Discussion. A flow chart (Figure 6) for the protocol of wound management was applied to the patient.

Pressure ulcers occur in three to seven percent of hospitalized patients and in 15 to 20 percent of nursing home residents.[48] The incidence of pressure ulcers is 43 to 100,000 population, with a median cost of $27,000 per patient to care for each wound.[49] Rating of risk factors for pressure ulcers has ben proposed by Norton[50] and Braden[51] and grading of pressure ulcers has been proposed by Shea[52] and updated by the National Pressure Ulcer Advisory Panel.[53]

When external pressure exceeds arteriolar pressure (32 mmHg), capillary pressure (20 mmHg), and venous pressure (12 mmHg), venous and lymphatic obstruction follow, resulting in ischemia and tissue necrosis.[54] Directly applied pressure or sheer stress over bony prominences (including the sacrum, ischial tuberosities, trochanters, heels, and lateral malleoli) produce microthrombosis in the microvasculature adjacent to the pressure ulcer with a decrease in fibrinolytic activity.[55] The provision by hyperbaric oxygen therapy of oxygen to the ischemic base of pressure ulcers may provide for fibrinolysis and prevention of leukocyte endothelial adherence as discussed earlier in the chapter.

Attention to nutritional status is also crucial. Taylor demonstrated in a randomized placebo–controlled trial that ascorbic acid at 500 mg PO BID reduced the surface area of pressure ulceration by 84 percent, whereas placebo treatment reduced surface area by only 43 percent (p<0.005).[56] Agarwal suggested that malnutrition was second only to pressure as a precipitator of pressure ulcers, with every decrease by gram of serum albumin enhancing the odds of developing the pressure ulcer three–fold.[57]

Arterial Insufficiency Ulcers

Case Presentation. A 39–year–old white male had been discovered to have Wright's Disease at age six, which led to hypertension and renal failure. He had been on dialysis since age 21 and had a renal transplant from a cadaver, which lasted eight years. At age 29, he had parathyroidectomy for secondary hyperparathyrodism. Ten years later, the patient had an amputation of his fourth and fifth digits with the development of an ulcer over his third proximal interphalangeal joint. He developed a 2 cm left heel wound. Four months later, the toe wounds on his left foot required a transmetatarsal amputation of the same. The open wounds were cultured for *Staphylococcus epidermidis, Candida albicans, Staphylococcus aureus, Enterococcus faecalis, Pseudomonas aeruginosa*, and *Enterobacter cloacae*. The patient was placed on oral

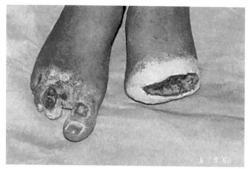

Figure 7a.

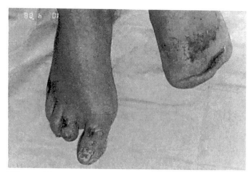

Figure 7b.

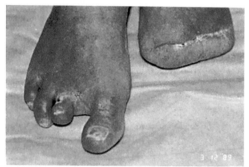

Figure 7c.

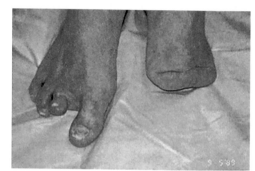

Figure 7d.

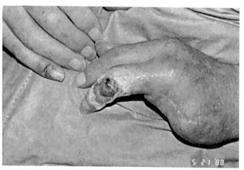

Figure 8a.

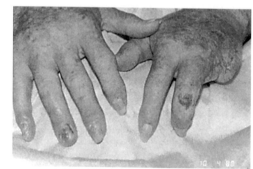

Figure 8b.

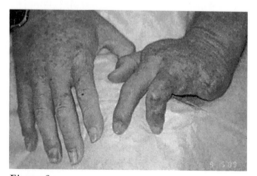

Figure 8c.

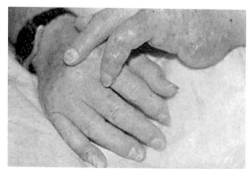

Figure 8d.

VAN METER

ciprofloxacin and underwent a series of hyperbaric oxygen treatments for a total of 66 45/90 tables over a three month period. His wounds resolved entirely by secondary intention healing.

Because of intensive calcific changes in his extremity arteries, the patient was considered inoperable for vascular reconstruction. His wounds healed by secondary intention and have remained healed to date. He has worn protective plastazote molded insole, rigid sole, rocker bottom healing sandals (Figures 7a–7d, 8a–8d).

Case Discussion. In attempting to salvage wounded extremities in patients with peripheral vascular disease, arterial reconstruction, if possible, must be performed. Hyperbaric oxygen therapy increases blood flow and oxygenation of the soft tissue envelope in wounded extremities of peripheral vascular disease patients.[58,59] Hyperbaric oxygen therapy provides improved tissue oxygenation in the afflicted ischemic peripheral vascular diseased extremity by vasoconstriction of less diseased arterial supply in other parts of the body, producing reflex vasodilation of the ischemic wounded extremity. Such an increase in blood flow and the resulting tissue oxygenation is attributable to the opening of non–functional capillaries, which enhances the oxygen diffusion area.[60]

In individuals with significant limb ischemia, auto–regulating vasoconstriction does not occur, allowing benefits of hydrostatic pressure to improve tissue perfusion.[61] In fact, dependency of ischemic limbs can increase transcutaneous pO_2 by 22 mmHg and concomitant administration of nasal oxygen adds an additional 12 mmHg and has been used as an adjunct to wound healing in peripheral vascular disease extremity wounds.[62]

Transcutaneous pO_2 maps of skin oxygen tension have been used to prognosticate unsuccessful amputation levels in peripheral vascular disease patients with extremity wounds.[63]

Perhaps in a combined therapeutic approach to include hyperbaric oxygen therapy in the treatment of patients with occlusive arterial disease with lower extremity wounds, dependent lower leg transcutaneous pO_2 determinations at depth in a hyperbaric chamber while the patient is inhaling O_2 would prognosticate and allow better success in the wound healing rate and in extremity salvage. Figure 9 is a flow chart used at the Jo Ellen Smith Medical Center Department of Emergency and Hyperbaric Medicine for protocol use of hyperbaric oxygen therapy in resolution of problem arterial insufficiency ulcerations or wounds. Minimization of reperfusion injury afforded by hyperbaric oxygen is making its use in the peri–operative setting of vascular reconstruction of an ischemic limb

encouraging, and the near future may hold its routine use.

Summary

In summary, baromedicine attempts to lessen pressure insult in injury by weight unloading plantar prominences on insensate feet and bony prominences on bedridden patients with nutritional and central nervous system deficits. Baromedicine uses pressure constructively in compressive bandaging to apply counterpressure to the soft tissue envelope in venous insufficiency ulcers of the lower extremities. Baromedicine addresses nutritional impairment to change the oncotic pressure of intravascular plasma to keep interstitial tissue spaces unburdened with edema.

By oxygen inhalation in hyperbaric environment locally ischemic wounds with still reasonable large vessel blood supply can be induced to normal or supra–normal physiologic tissue oxygen tensions to support a myriad of oxygen–dependent cellular wound repair processes. By the same token, intermittency of hyperbaric oxygen exposure allows the few important hypoxically driven cellular repair processes in wound healing to effectively prevail for part of the time.

Perhaps chronic refractory wounds (diabetic extremity wounds, venous insufficiency ulcers, pressure ulcers, and arterial insufficiency ulcers) persist by being a type of chronic subclinical reperfusion injury of the soft tissue envelope of the body. The diabetic neuropathic foot allows the patient to repeatedly occlude and open pedal microvasculature by exposure of the dermal surface to increased blunt microtrauma of unprotected gait. Venous insufficiency in the leg allows the hydraulic pressure of the accumulating venous blood return to alter dermal perfusion based on leg posture. The patient with a disability that impairs movement runs the risk of exposing the microvasculature of the body's soft tissue envelope to periods of intermittent occlusion. The extremity with arterial insufficiency faces swings in perfusion of dermal microvasculature induced by change in posture. More indirectly, the metabolism of exercise of an extremity with arterial insufficiency imposes an oxygen demand which outstrips supply. This mismatched functionally induces episodes of ischemia followed by reperfusion.

Hyperbaric oxygen therapy is a strong modifier of endothelial leukocyte adherence[64] and of free radical injury.[65] Hyperbaric oxygen therapy has very few side effects compared to conventional, equally potent pharmaceuticals which alter these pathophysiologic processes equivalently.[66]

Perhaps the future holds volatile or gaseous pharmaceuticals to include antibiotics, which can be administered "parenterally" to patients without pain and in meaningful doses through hyperbaric inhalation therapy.

References

1. Myers RAM: Hyperbaric oxygen therapy, a committee report. *Undersea and Hyperbaric Medical Society*, Bethesda, MD 1989; 44–48.
2. Sheffield PJ: Problem wounds, the role of oxygen (Davis JC, Hunt TK, eds). Elsevier, NY 1988; 17–51.
3. Davenport HW: *The ABC's of Acid Base Chemistry*. University of Chicago Press, Chicago, IL 1958; 7–8.
4. Boerema I, Meijne NG, Brummelkamp WK, et al: Life without blood. *J Cardiovascular Surgery* 1: 133–146, 1960.
5. Smith JJ, Kampeine JP: *Circulatory Physiology—Essentials*. Williams and Wilkins, Baltimore, MD 1984; 139.
6. Biglow WG: The microcirculation. *Canadian J Surgery* 7: 237–249, 1964.
7. Krogh A: The number and distribution of capillaries in muscle with calculations of the oxygen pressure head necessary for supplying the tissue. *J Physiology* 52: 409–415, 1919.
8. Han DC, MacKay RD, Halliday B, Hunt TK: Effective O2 tension on microbial functions of leukocytes in wounds and in vitro. *Surgery Forum* 27: 18–20, 1976.
9. Travis J, Salvesen GS: Human plasma proteinase inhibitors. *Ann Rev Biochem* 52: 655–709, 1985.
10. Lawrence DA, Loskutoff DJ: Inactivation of plasminogen activator inhibitor by oxidants. *Biochemistry* 1986; 25: 6351–5
11. Hunt TK, Pai MP: The effect of varying oxygen tensions on wound metabolism and collagen synthesis. *Surgery, Gynecology, and Obstetrics* 135: 561–567, 1975.
12. Silver IA: Local systemic factors which affect the proliferation of fibroblasts. In: *Biology of the Fibroblasts* (Kulomen E, ed). Academic Press, New York 1973; 507–520.
13. Mader JT, Gukian JC, McGoss DL, Reiniarz JA: Therapy with hyperbaric oxygen for experimental osteomyelitis due to staph aureus in rabbits. *J Infectious Diseases* 138: 312–318, 1978.
14. Kivissari J, Niinikioski J: Effects of hyperbaric oxygenation and prolonged hypoxia on healing of open wounds. *Acta Chir Scand* 141: 14–19, 1976.
15. Knighton D, Hunt TK, Schouenstuhl H, et al: Oxygen tension regulates the expression of angiogenesis factor by macrophages. *Science* 221: 1283–1285, 1983.
16. Hunt TK, Twomey P, Zederfeldt B, et al: Respiratory gas tension and pH in healing wounds. *Am J Surgery* 114: 302–308, 1967.
17. Davis JC, Buckley CJ, Barr PO: Compromised soft tissue wounds: Correction of wound hypoxia. In: *Problem Wounds: The Role of Oxygen* (Davis JC, Hunt TK, eds). Elsevier, NY 1988; 143–144.
18. Baroni G, Porro T, Faglia E, et al: Hyperbaric oxygen in diabetic gangrene treatment. *Diabetes Care* 19(1): 81–86, 1987.
19. Hammarlund C, Sundberg T: Hyperbaric oxygen reduced size of chronic leg ulcers: a randomized double–blind study. *Plast Reconstr Surg* 93(4): 829–833, 1994.
20. Knighton DR, Ciresi K, Fiegel VD, et al: Stimulation of repair in chronic nonhealing cutaneous ulcers: a prospectively randomized blinded trial using platelet–derived wound healing formula. *Surg Gynecol Obst*, 170: 56–60, 1990.
21. Brown GL, Nanney LB, Griffen J, et al: Enhancement of wound healing by topical treatment with epidermal growth factor. *New Eng J Med* 321(2): 76–79, 1989.
22. Limova M, Mauro T: Treatment of leg ulcers with cultured epithelial autografts: treatment protocol and five year experience. *Wounds* 7(5): 170–180, 1995.
23. Ross H, Rifkin H: Diabetes mellitus: An overview, management of the diabetic foot. (Brennan MA, ed) Williams and Wilkins, Baltimore, MD 1987; 3–7.
24. Levin ME: The diabetic foot: Pathophysiology, evaluation and treatment. In: *The Diabetic Foot* (Levin ME, O'Neal LW, eds). C.V. Mosby Co., St. Louis 1988; 1–50.
25. McMillan DE: The blood viscosity problem. *Clinical Diabetes* 7(4): 61–71, 1989.
26. Wagner FW: A classification and treatment program for diabetic neuropathic and dysvascular foot problems. In: *American Academy of Orthopedic Surgeons: Instructional Course Lectures*, Volume 28. C.V. Mosby Co., St. Louis, 1979.
27. Jeffcoate WJ, MacFarlane RM, Fletcher EM: The description and classification of diabetic foot lesions. *Diabetic Medicine*. 10: 676–679, 1993.
28. Pace WE: Treatment of cutaneous ulcers with benzoyl peroxide. *CMA Journal* 115: 1101–1106, 1976.
29. Grayson MC, Giffons GW, Balagh K, et al: Probing bone in infected pedal ulcers, a clinical sign of underlying osteomyelitis in diabetic patients. *JAMA* 273(9): 721–723, 1995.
30. Lipsky B, Pecoraro R, Hurley J: Diagnosis of bone lesions in diabetic feet: osteomyelitis or osteorthropathy. In: *Program and Abstracts of the 29th Interscience Conference on Antimicrobial Agents and Chemotherapy*. Houston, TX. American Society for Microbiology, 1989; Abstract 913.
31. Eckman MH, Greenfield S, MacKey WC et al: Foot infections in diabetic patients: decision and cost–effectiveness analyses. *JAMA*, 273(9): 712–720, 1995.
32. Brand PW: Repetitive stress in the development of diabetic foot ulcers. In: *The Diabetic Foot* (Levin ME, O'Neal LW, eds). C.V. Mosby Co., St. Louis 1988; 90.
33. Buhlmann AA: *Decompression Sickness*. Springer–Verlag, Berlin, Germany 1984; 17.
34. Wells CH, Goodpasture JE, Horrigan DJ, et al: Tissue gas measurements during hyperbaric oxygen exposure. In: *Proceedings of the Sixth International Congress on Hyperbaric Medicine* (Smith G, ed). Aberdeen University Press, Aberdeen 1977; 118–124.
35. Cianci P: Adjunctive hyperbaric oxygen therapy in the treatment of the diabetic foot. *J Am Pod Med Assoc*, 84(9): 448–455, 1994.
36. Koone MD, Burton CS: Conservative management of a long–standing venous stasis ulcer. *Wounds* 1(2): 90–94, 1989.
37. Kitahama A, Elliot LF, Kerstein MD, Menendez CV: Leg Ulcer, conservative management or surgical treatment? *JAMA* 247(2): 197–199, 1982.
38. Burnard KG, Whimster LW, Clemenson G, et al: The relationship between the number of capillaries in the skin of venous ulcer bearing area of the lower leg and the fall in foot vein pressure in exercise. *BR J Surg* 68: 297, 1981.
39. Homans J: The etiology and treatment of varicose ulcers of the leg. *Surg Gynecol Obstet* 24: 300–311, 1917.
40. Piulacks P, Vidal–Barroquer F: Pathogenic study of vericose veins. *Angiology* 4:59–100, 1953.
41. Dodd HJ, Galyarde PM, Sarkany I: Skin oxygen tension in venous insufficiency of the lower leg. *J R Soc Med* 78: 373–376, 1985.
42. Falanga V, Kirsnor R, Katz MH, et al: Pericapillary fibrin cuffs in venous ulceration: persistence with treatment and during ulcer healing. *J Dermatol Surg Oncol* 18: 409–414, 1992.
43. Browse NL, Burnand KG: The cause of venous ulceration. Lancet 2(8292): 243–245, 1982.
44. Falanga V, Eaglstein WH: The "trap" hypothesis of venous ulceration. *Lancet* 341: 1006–1008, 1993.
45. Shami SK, Shields DA, Scurr JH, Smith C: Leg ulceration in venous disease. *Postgrad Med J* 68: 779–785, 1992.
46. Zamboni WA, Roth AC, Russell RC, et al: Morphologic analysis of the microcirculation during reperfusion of ischemic skeletal muscle and the effect of hyperbaric oxygen. *Plast Reconstr Surg* 91: 1110–1123, 1993.

47. Fylling CP: Comprehensive wound management with topical growth factors. Ostomy/Wound Management 22: 62–71, 1989.

48. Cowart V: Pressure ulcers preventable, say many clinicians. *JAMA* 257(S): 589, 1987.

49. Melcher RF, Longe RL, Gelbert AO: Pressure sores in the elderly: A systemic approach to management. *Post Grad Med* 83(1): 299–308, 1988.

50. Norton D, McLaren R, Exton–Smith AU: An investigation of geriatric nursing problems in hospital. (1962) Reissue 1975. Elinburgh, Churchill, Livingston, 193–238, 1975.

51. Bergstrom N, Braden BJ, Laguzza A, Holman V: The Braden scale for predicting pressure sore risk. *Nurs Res* 36(4): 205–210, 1987.

52. Shea JD: Pressure sores: Classification and management. *Clinical Orthopedics* 112: 89–100, 1975.

53. National Pressure Advisory Panel: Pressure Ulcers: Incidence, economics, risk assessment. Consensus Development Statement. *Decubitus* 2(2): 24–8, 1989.

54. Rousseau MD: Pressure ulcers in an aging society. *Wounds* 1(2): 135–141, 1989.

55. Burnand K, Clemenson G, Morland M, Jarrett PEM, Browse NL: Venous lipodermatosclerosis: Treatment by fibrinolytic enhancement and elastic compression. *British Med J* 280: 7–11, 1980.

56. Taylor TV, Rimmer S, Pay B, Butcher J, Dymark JW: Ascorbic acid supplementation of pressure sores. *Lancet* 2: 544–546, 1974.

57. Agarwal N, DelGuericio LRM, Lee B: The role of nutrition in the management of pressure sores. In: *Chronic Ulcers of the Skin* (Lee BY, ed). McGraw Hill, New York 1985.

58. Fredenucci P: Oxygenotherapie hyperbare et arteriopathies. *J Mal Vasc* 10: 166–172, 1985.

59. Yephuny SN, Lyskin SI, Fakina TS: Hyperbaric oxygenation in the treatment of peripheral vascular disorders. *Inter Angio* 4:207–209, 1985.

60. Visona A, Lusni L, Rusca F: Hyperbaric oxygenation in the treatment of peripheral vascular disease. *J Hyper Med* 2(4): 223–227, 1985.

61. Eskloff JH, Henrickson O: Local regulation of subcutaneous forefoot blood flow during orthostatic changes in normal subjects in sympathetically denervated patients and in patients with occlusive arterial disease. *Cardiovascular Res* 19: 219–227, 1985.

62. Johnson WC, Grant HI, Baldwin RN, Hamilton JV, Dion JM: Supplemental oxygen and dependent positioning as adjunctive measures to improve forefoot tissue oxygenation. *Arch Surg* 123: 1227–1230, 1988.

63. Kalsamouris A, Brewster DC, Megarman J, Cina C, Darling RC, Abbott WM: Transcutaneous oxygen in selection of amputation level. *Am J Surg* 147: 510–517, 1984.

64. Zamboni WA, Roth AC, Russell RC, Smoot EC: Effect of hyperbaric oxygen on reperfusion of ischemic axial skin flaps: a laser doppler analysis. *Ann Plast Surg* 28(4): 339–341, 1992.

65. Thom SR, Elbuken ME: Oxygen dependent antagonism of lipid peroxidation. *Free Radical Biol Med* 10(6): 413–426, 1991.

66. Youngberg JT: Complications from hyperbaric oxygen therapy. *Ann Emerg Med* 19(11): 1356–1357, 1990.

34

Selecting Support Surfaces

Janice C. Colwell, RN, MS, CETN

Colwell JC. Selecting support surfaces. In: Krasner D, Kane D. *Chronic Wound Care, Second Edition.* Wayne, PA, Health Management Publications, Inc., 1997, pp 276–283.

Introduction

Support surfaces, an important component of prevention and management of skin breakdown, vary in their capacity to counteract the forces contributing to skin breakdown. Support surfaces can be defined as devices that reduce or relieve pressure while a patient is sitting or lying. They may have additional characteristics which contribute to the reduction of shear, friction and moisture. The reduction and/or relief of interface pressure (force per unit area that acts perpendicularly between the body and support surface)[1] can be achieved by utilizing a surface that maximizes body surface contact and distributes the body weight over the support surface allowing the pressure to be distributed more evenly.

The challenge in the clinical arena is to match the patient to the most efficacious surface. Prior to beginning an evaluation, available support surfaces must be organized into descriptive categories. Then the patient population that will utilize the support surfaces must be assessed to determine needs. Product selection for the healthcare setting will consider the patient population, caregiver abilities, product performance, cost issues and company performance. Criteria can then be developed that will assist in selecting the appropriate product for the individual patient.

Product Characterization

Product characterization is best organized by defining the therapeutic effects of the support surface, either pressure reduction or pressure relief.

Therapeutic effect: Pressure reduction. Pressure reduction products reduce interface pressure, but not necessarily below the level required to close capillaries.[2] If interface pressure exceeds capillary pressure for a prolonged period of time, ischemia results leading to tissue destruction. Capillary closing pressure is at best an average measure and can vary from patient to patient. It is therefore difficult to utilize capillary closing pressure as the sole determinant to assess a support surface for pressure reduction. An important criterion of a pressure reduction support surface is that it should become deformed by bony prominences, allowing the body to sink and displace the body weight. Pressure reduction devices must always be used in conjunction with a repositioning schedule.

Pressure reduction surfaces are available in overlays and therapeutic mattresses. An overlay, which is placed on top of a mattress, is available in various foam configurations, air, gel or water–filled products. A therapeutic mattress, which replaces a standard mattress, is usually constructed of foam, gel, or air.

Foam overlays. Several characteristics of foam are important for effective pressure reduction: base height, density and indentation load deflection.

Foam overlays are available in a variety of heights. Height should be measured from the bottom of the foam overlay to the lowest point of the convolution. A foam overlay with a 2 inch base does not significantly reduce pressure when compared with a standard hospital mattress.[3] Krouskop has determined adequate thickness for pressure reduction to be 3 to 4 inches.[4]

Density of foam is a measure of the amount of foam in the product: the higher the density, the lower the pressure. The minimum density of the foam pad should be 1.3 to 1.6 pd. per cubic foot.[4]

Indentation load deflection (ILD) is a measurement of the firmness of the foam and describes the foam's ability to conform. The ILD gives indication of the ability of the foam to distribute the mechanical load (the weight of the patient's body). It is recommended that a therapeutic foam overlay feature a 25 percent ILD of about 30 pounds.[3]

Advantages of foam overlays:
• Available in different sizes (an important consideration with cribs and isolettes in the pediatric population);
• Easy to transport and install, can be transported to home if indicated;
• Minimal maintenance;
• Low cost and onetime charge.

Disadvantages of foam overlays:
• Easily soiled by incontinence;
• Environmental concerns about disposal;
• Safety issues related to increase of mattress height by 4 inches.

Clinical considerations for foam overlays:
• Utilize a cover over the foam overlay (generally available with each manufacturer's product) to decrease soiling of the product;
• When using a flat top sheet, tuck sheet under the foam overlay to prevent the top sheet from being pulled tight (a tight top sheet will prevent the patient from sinking into the foam surface and displacing body weight).

Air Overlays. Air overlays are available in a static configuration (in which there is no active air movement) or in a dynamic configuration (in which the air is in motion).

Static air mattresses are designed with interlocking air cells that allow air to conform to the patient's body. The surface redistributes the body weight to take the extra weight or load from the bony prominences and place more load on the regions that are under lower pressures.[5]

Dynamic air overlays consist of rows of air cells arranged length wise that are alternately inflated and deflated by an air pump. The air pressure in one row increases while it decreases in another row. This alternating process allows the relieved site to recover while a new region is under compression.[6]

Advantages of air overlays:
• Ease of cleaning;
• Durable for long term use;
• Economical;
• Low maintenance.
 Disadvantages of air overlays:
• Set up required and ongoing monitoring: static devices must be "hand checked" to determine effectiveness;

• Electricity required (on the dynamic models);
• Can be damaged by sharp objects;
• Air alteration may be upsetting to patients.

Clinical considerations for air overlays:
• If skin moisture is a patient issue, choose a system that has a constant low volume air flow.

Gel overlays. Gel overlays are filled with silicon elastomer, silicon, polyvinyl chloride or similar gel materials. The gel is displaced by the patient's body weight and provides floatation.

Advantages of gel overlays:
• Ease of cleaning;
• Requires limited maintenance;
• Durable/appropriate for multi–patient use.

Disadvantages of gel overlays:
• Weight of product;
• When used for extended periods of time in a Fowler position the gel has a potential to form a hard area at folds or creases.

Clinical considerations for gel overlays:
• Keep product stored in flat position to prevent pooling of gel in creases/folds.

Water overlays. Water overlays are water–filled vinyl mattress systems. When a water overlay is filled appropriately, the patient should displace the water without bottoming out.

Advantages of water overlays:
• Ease of cleaning;
• Low cost.

Disadvantages of water overlays:
• Weight of product;
• Overlay must be filled with the correct amount of water for the patient; too much water does not allow pressure reduction, too little water will allow the patient to bottom out, i.e. to flatten the overlay at pressure points and make contact with the mattress.
• If overlay does not have compartments, when head of bed is raised, gravity displacement of water away from upper portion of body occurs, increasing interface pressures.

Clinical considerations for water overlays:
• Choose a product with a thermometer as the water can cool when patient is off overlay for an extended period of time (some products have a water heater).

Therapeutic mattresses. Therapeutic mattresses are designed to replace standard hospital mattresses and provide pressure reduction. Therapeutic mattresses are constructed with a combination of foam and/or gel products, utilizing high density and low ILD foam. Most therapeutic mattresses have top coverings (the side in contact with the patient) manufactured to reduce friction and shear and have some degree of vapor permeability to reduce moisture.

Advantages of therapeutic mattresses:
• Pressure reduction built into patient's plan of care without the need for individual patient evaluation and staff time to obtain a pressure reduction device and place under patient;
• Cost savings: elimination of pressure reduction overlays, overall reduction in expenditures related to prevention and management of skin breakdown.[7]

Disadvantages of therapeutic mattresses:
• Initial up–front cost of purchasing mattresses;
• Over reliance of product to assist in pressure ulcer prevention, when other pressure reduction products might be more appropriate.

Clinical considerations of therapeutic mattresses:
• Most therapeutic mattresses are available with a warranty period of 2 to 5 years. Schedule a yearly mattress check day, (some manufacturers offer assistance with this process). All mattresses should be evaluated for integrity of exterior cover, if accessible check integrity of inside components (many of the therapeutic mattresses have outside zippers). To facilitate the maintenance of the warranty agreement, date all new mattresses upon delivery to the patient care units;
• If the top covering of the therapeutic mattress is made to reduce friction/shear, a flat top sheet may not stay tucked under the mattress; fitted sheets may need to be considered

Therapeutic effect: Pressure relief. Pressure relief products reduce interface pressure below capillary closing pressure.[2] These surfaces will become deformed by the bony prominences, allowing maximum contact of the body into the support surface. Pressure relief products are adjusted to individual patients to maintain capillary blood flow and eliminate shear and friction and reduce moisture.[3]

Pressure relief surfaces are available in two types of dynamic air therapy: low air loss and air fluidized. These therapies are available as overlays (air support placed on top of a standard hospital mattress); mattress replacement systems (air support placed on the bed frame, takes the place of the standard mattress); and air support systems (all inclusive systems, the bed frame and the support system integrated).

Low air loss therapy. Low air loss therapy is provided with a series of connected air filled pillows. The air filled pillows are supplied with a predetermined amount of air continuously in movement from an attached motor. Each pillow or section is inflated with air to specific pressures on the basis of each patient's weight, height and body shape. The cover material of each pillow reduces friction and shear; some moisture should be reduced because of the low air loss from the pillow material. Most low air loss systems have incorporated an adjustment factor into the inflation/deflation of the pillow when the head of the bed is elevated or flattened (usually a microchip system). Low air loss therapy is available as an overlay (usually 4 inches in depth), a mattress replacement system (institutional mattress is removed, the low air loss system is placed on the bed frame and the motor is attached to the foot of the bed frame) or as an air support system (the low air loss therapy comes attached to a bed frame). Low air loss therapy is available as a purchase or rental item.

Advantages of low air loss therapy:
• Provides pressure reduction for patients of varying sizes and shapes, as each section can be custom "pressurized" to the individual patient;
• Clinical documentation that supports the use of low air loss therapy is available;[9]
• Set up, service (on–call personnel, problem solving) and pickup are handled by the contracting company if the product is rented. This convenience can decrease the load on the patient care, supply and mechanical staffs;
• Use of institutional owned bed frame (when utilizing the overlay or mattress replacement system) decreases costs and increases staff comfort with the bed frame controls. Using the air support system means the institutional bed frame is put in storage, and the patient care staff must be educated to utilize a new frame with new controls.

Disadvantages of low air loss therapy:
• Electricity is required;
• Cost considerations: if rented must have an ongoing evaluation of appropriateness, including indications for start up of therapy as well as continuation and discontinuation of therapy; must have system developed with rental company to determine weekly therapy activity (patients on/off therapy with dates and type of therapy) to provide accounting of monies/outcomes spent/obtained utilizing low air loss therapy;

- If determined to be a daily patient charge, charge must be entered into financial system;
- Motor may be noisy;
- A four inch low air loss overlay may introduce safety issues of the patient being too high as related to the bed side rails;
- When using a mattress replace system, a system must be developed where the institutional mattresses are stored. The storage of the mattress may or may not include healthcare staff (may encounter "lost" mattresses);
- If therapy is rented, may encounter a delay in the start up because of lag time between order and delivery of product.

Clinical considerations of low air loss therapy:
- If therapy is rented, consider the following in a rental agreement: initial and ongoing inservicing of staff or product utilization; collection of data on each patient placed on therapy (indications for placement, type of skin impairment if present, risk assessment score every 7 days, demographic data, length of time on therapy, etc.); weekly reports: on/off dates of each patient's therapy, type of therapy, location of each patient, and other support activities as each institution requires;
- For patients requiring low air loss therapy making frequent in bed "trips" (to radiology, to physical therapy, etc.), consider utilizing a transport pack on the mattress replacement or low air loss therapy bed to prevent patient contact with the bed frame while in transit. The low air loss overlay will deflate upon transport; however, the patient will be on the mattress, which should be tolerable for short periods of time;
- If rental therapy is utilized on an ongoing basis, may consider purchase of the therapy if institutional support systems are available (product maintenance and cleaning).

Air fluidized therapy. Air fluidized therapy uses a high rate of air flow to fluidize fine particulate material to produce a support medium that has characteristics similar to liquid.[2] The air fluidized support surface deforms to the body contours, relieving the interface pressure to below capillary closure. An air fluidized support system does not use a mattress, but consists of small beads in a tank covered by an air permeable sheet. The beads are put in motion by air forced through the beads and the patient floats on the sheet with one third of the body above the surface and the rest of the body immersed in the beads.[3] Air fluidized therapy is available as a purchase or rental item.

Advantages of air fluidized therapy:
- May facilitate management of excessive skin and wound moisture because of high rate of air flow around the patient's body;
- May be treatment of choice for patients with surgical flaps and grafts because of the pressure relief, decreased moisture and maintenance of a supine position, which reduces edema in the graft site;[7]
- May provide pain relief for some patients;[8]
- May decrease need to change a patient's position.[9]

Disadvantages of air fluidized therapy:
- Potential for dehydration related to the circulation of warm, dry air;
- Pulmonary complications related to ineffective mobilization of secretions (lack of support for patient to cough effectively);
- Difficulty in transporting patient in and out of bed because of tank edge (edge is higher than patient level, making it difficult to transfer patient out of bed; patient must be lifted over edge);
- Very heavy bed; cannot be easily transfered from room to room; may not be suitable for home use because of excessive weight.

Clinical considerations of air fluidized therapy:
- Continuous circulation of air may dry moist wound dressings and/or desiccate wound bed: if identified as a problem consider utilizing underpads under patient's wound dressing which prevent air flow;
- The bed system circulates room air and warms the room air considerably; set thermostat to control this issue;
- Patients with severe debilitating pain may be good candidates for this system because of the decreased need to turn the patient;
- Monitor drainage from catheters and drains that are usually managed by dependent drainage. Because the patient is supported below the bed edge, the drainage tubes may be higher than the area to be drained.

Bariatric system. Patients weighing over 500 lbs. or having a body mass index above 40 or patients who carry the bulk of their weight in one area of the body should be considered for placement on a bariatric system. The needs of the obese patient vary, but safety is the primary consideration. Bariatric systems utilize a reinforced frame to support the body mass and should include a chair feature. The chair feature allows the bed to be put in a chair position, the head of the product at a 45 degree angle and the feet in a downward position.

This feature will allow the patient to easily leave the bed surface if he/she is able to walk. Other features that some systems include are wider than normal beds, side rails that tilt out to each side to allow the patient more room, built in scales, anti–shear surface and pressure reduction surfaces. A recent development has been the inclusion of a low air loss mattress on some bariatric systems. This will address the skin care issues of obese patients.

Advantages of the bariatric system:
• Provides a safe support for obese patients;
• Wider than normal bed surface will facilitate repositioning of patient;
• Chair function allows patient to become mobile and to acquire a high fowler's position if necessary.

When air fluidized and low air loss therapies are combined, air fluidized therapy is featured in the lower two thirds of the support system, and low air loss therapy is featured in the upper section.

Advantage of hybrid system:
• Air fluidized and low air loss therapy supports the patient to effectively cough and sit up in bed for activities.

Disadvantages of hybrid system:
• Kinetic therapy may be upsetting to patient;
• Kinetic therapy appears to be effective for a short window of time; monitoring the patient's ventilatory status is a must.

It is advisable to limit products to an amount that will allow the staff to become familiar with the surfaces and comfortable making clinical usage decisions.

Disadvantage of the bariatric system:
• If a wider than normal bed frame is utilized, the bed may not fit through standard door frames or elevated door.

Clinical considerations of the bariatric system:
• In acutely ill, obese, respiratory patients, the chair function may assist in ventilatory status;
• Low air loss overlays on the bariatric system that has a chair function can cause a problem when the chair function is utilized. Because the surface "breaks" in two areas: the head to be in a high fowler's position and the area under the knees, some overlays can not bend adequately to the chair surface. A static air overlay that is available in sections can accommodate the bariatric chair function.

Hybrid support system. Hybrid support systems are available as combinations of low air loss and kinetic therapies or of air fluidized and low air loss therapies. When low air loss and kinetic therapies are combined, the surface provides the low air loss therapy as described above and continuous movement of patient from side to side. The continuous patient movement can contribute to the mobilization of respiratory secretions, decreasing the risk of atelectasis and pneumonia. When the scope of the immobile patient's problems moves beyond the skin, kinetic therapy may be considered.[7]

Clinical considerations of the hybrid system:
• Determine criteria to support the use of kinetic therapy; include skin and pulmonary considerations.

Practice Setting: Product Selection

Product selection for the healthcare setting will consider the patient population, caregiver abilities, product and company performance, and cost issues. It is advisable to limit products to an amount that will allow the staff to become familiar with the surfaces and comfortable making clinical usage decisions. When beginning the product selection process, a committee of key people should be developed. Committee membership should include staff nurses (include several disciplines, pediatric, adult, critical care), an infection control expert (to advise on issues of cleaning, cross contamination), materials management staff (may be in charge of product distribution, or receiving it on the dock), financial department agent (can be instrumental in setting up charge codes, will be able to advise in reimbursement matters, may play a role in the purchase of capital purchase items), a housekeeping staff member (to advise on cleaning issues, practical concerns on storage), and clinical nurse specialists (generally represent a wide scope of patient concerns/issues). If institutional based, include home care staff, discharge planners and case managers. The committee leader should be a clinical expert who can provide the clinical reality along with the expertise in the field of wound and skin care.

Patient population needs must be identified. One method for obtaining a snapshot of skin care issues is to conduct a prevalence study. One day is chosen in which all patients in a setting are examined. Skin is pressures. Note the population studied on the support surfaces, check comparability with the setting's patient population. Determine if research on the support system has been published in a scientific journal. If limited research is available on products of interest, it is advisable to conduct a test to evaluate the product's effectiveness.[3]

Each patient must be assessed to determine needs, and the goal of skin/wound care interventions should be identified, including prevention versus intervention issues.

---

assessed for integrity issues. Once impairment in skin integrity is found, further investigation is done to determine if the skin breakdown is related to pressure, shear, friction or moisture. Information can also be collected on the support surfaces currently used and the appropriateness of usage. By tabulating the number of patients examined, the amount and etiology of skin breakdown encountered, and product utilization, a descriptive picture of the patients and their needs develops. Healthcare settings that have a population of high risk patients may need to consider the use of therapeutic mattresses for every patient. An acute care setting that has a patient population that ranges from ambulatory patients to critically ill patients (patients with mobility issues) will want to consider stocking a variety of surfaces to meet the needs of such a diverse group. Settings that are determined to have patients who have skin breakdown related to shear or friction may need to consider the surface of the support surfaces and the use of assistive devices such as overhead trapezes. Pediatric populations should not be excluded from examination. Acutely ill pediatric patients from neonates to adolescents may require support surfaces.

While examining support surfaces, consider the staff that will choose, set up and maintain the surfaces. Criteria for usage will need to be developed, and the caregivers will need to be able to operate the device. Some thought should be given to the option of rental versus purchase of low air loss therapy. Some institutions have found that owning low air loss beds can be a cost effective alternative to renting.[10] If used at home and the primary caregiver is not a healthcare provider, the product should be simple to operate, not excessively heavy (some air fluidized beds can weigh well over 800 lbs.), and the caregiver should have access to personnel for problem solving.

When assessing product effectiveness, check for independent written literature that reports interface

Whether purchasing or renting support systems, gather information on the company manufacturing, selling or renting the products. When purchasing a support system, note the warranty, check what is covered and for how long and what the company will provide to help check product performance while covered under warranty. Determine if a maintenance contract is available and what is included. For rental items note the set–up fee, time between placing an order and delivery (same with discontinue services), availability of problem solving 24 hours/day with use of an 800 number to reach the company representative. As an evaluation process is planned, check with the companies involved regarding a trial procedure. Education of the users of the product is key to a successful program. Company supplied education should be available 24 hours and on an ongoing basis (don't forget orientation of new employees). It is advisable to talk with other institutions/healthcare settings who have used the support system to find out how long they have used the product and how they feel about the outcomes.

The cost of support systems should be considered. Many pressure reduction surfaces are purchased. Therapeutic mattresses are generally a capital purchase and may need to be phased into the healthcare setting. Indirect costs of support surfaces such as set up, cleaning, and repair should be considered. If an institution's bed frame is not being utilized and a company's bed frame and support surface is being rented, the non–used institution's bed frame can be considered a liability.

Patient Assessment: Product Selection

Many factors need to be considered when choosing a support system. Each patient must be assessed to determine needs, and the goal of skin/wound care interventions should be identified, including

Table 1
A Comparison of Support Surfaces

Support Surface	Pressure Effect	Treatment Therapy	Intervention
Overlays			
Foam	reduction	prevention	
Air	reduction	prevention	
	relief	intervention	
Gel	reduction	prevention	
Water	reduction	prevention	
Therapeutic mattresses	reduction	prevention	
Low air loss therapy	relief	prevention	
		intervention	
Air fluidized therapy	relief	intervention	post surgical flap protection
Hybrid services	reduction	prevention	decrease resp.
		intervention	complications
Bariatric product	reduction	prevention	patient safety
	relief	intervention	issues

prevention versus intervention issues. This assessment must be ongoing, insuring that the therapy will meet the patient requirements. Some healthcare settings utilize decision trees, guidelines or algorithms to assist staff in decision making;[2,11,12] others identify a clinical expert. Criteria for support surface placement and termination should be developed and made available to staff members.

Factors that should guide decision making:

Mobility. Is the patient immobile, can the person make changes in body position without assistance? Can the patient be turned easily from side to side, and once positioned can or will the patient stay comfortably on his/her side? When turned does the patient demonstrate pain or significant discomfort? How long can the patient tolerate various positions? If at home are the family members able to adequately position patient (will the patient allow the family to correctly position the him/her?). A high risk patient who cannot be repositioned needs pressure relief.

Sensory perception. Can the patient perceive discomfort and communicate the need to be repositioned to caregivers? Does the patient have limited capacity to feel pain over part of his/her body?

Existing skin integrity. Does the patient have existing skin breakdown? What is the goal in treating the skin breakdown? If healing is not the goal

but maintenance of the intact skin is, can the patient be positioned off the affected surface? How many unaffected surface are available? Patients with existing pressure ulcers may still be at risk for additional pressure ulcers and may therefore need the protection provided by a pressure reducing surface.[2] It is also important to note past problems with tissue integrity.

Moisture issues. Is skin moisture a problem? How often are linens changed? Moisture issues can often be managed with careful selection of low air loss and air fluidized systems.

Patient's current medical status. Does repositioning contribute to respiratory distress? What is the tissue fluid level of the patient? Is dependent edema an issue contributing to skin breakdown? What is the shape and size of the patient? Obese patients may need pressure relief that is customized to their weight distribution, for example, sections in low air loss systems can be adjusted to conform to patients who carry most of their body weight in the center portion of their bodies.

Recent flap or graft surgery. The objective will be to alleviate pressure, shear and friction when the patient must be positioned over the area. Air fluidized therapy would help meet these objectives.

Cost and availability. Is the product financially feasible? Does it meet the criteria for the patient's

COLWELL

reimbursement? Will the product be available for the patient in the next healthcare setting? Is electricity available? Is the surface of choice covered by the reimbursement source? In many situations, documentation must be very specific to meet the reimbursement agency's criteria.

It is necessary to consider the clinical condition of the patient, the surroundings of the patient, the factors listed above as well as the therapeutic benefit of the pressure reducing and relief products. Ongoing reassessment must be built into the treatment plan to insure utilization of the appropriate support surface.

issue, but must be written into the usage criteria for pressure relief and reduction support surfaces.

Conclusion

Support surface selection remains a challenge for the clinician. There are currently no universally set criteria for product selection that demonstrate that one product category performs better than any other. Therefore, it is imperative that the clinician be familiar with the categories of support surfaces and with the factors that need to be considered when selecting one of these surfaces for an individual

---

Documentation of the factors utilized to determine the choice of a support surface is an important component of the plan of care.

Documentation of the factors utilized to determine the choice of a support surface is an important component of the plan of care. Documentation communicates the factors considered in patient placement and may for some patients provide the basis for reimbursement of the product. Reimbursement issues for support surfaces continue to change; however, the entire plan of care will always need to be communicated, and the support surface is an important component of the plan of care, either a prevention or intervention plan.

Other issues to consider when examining support systems include pressure relief and reduction devices for chairs and the "layering" issues.

The issue of pressure relief and reduction devices for chairs has only recently received attention from manufacturers, yet it is a major issue in many healthcare settings. A plan of care may call for increasing patient mobility by utilizing chair surfaces, yet very few products have been shown to address the issues of pressure reduction/relief, shear and friction in a chair product. It is a challenge to construct a product that can achieve the necessary benefits, yet conform to the healthcare setting (be reusable, able to be cleaned, provide therapeutic benefits). This is an area that needs further attention.

Regarding the "layering" issue, a pressure reduction relief support surface should become deformed by bony prominences, allowing the body to sink and displace body weight. By placing several layers of sheeting between the patient and the support surface, it becomes difficult for the patient to sink into the support surface. This is an educational

patient. See Table 1 for a matrix comparing types of support surfaces.

References

1. Panel for the Prediction and Prevention of Pressure Ulcers in Adults. *Pressure Ulcers in Adults: Pressure Ulcers in Adults: Prediction and Prevention. Clinical Practice Guideline, Number 3*. AHCPR Publication No. 92–0047. Rockville, MD: Agency for Health Care Policy and Research, Public Health Service, U.S. Department of Health and Human Services. May 1992.
2. Bergstrom N, Bennett MA, Carlson CE, et al. *Treatment of Pressure Ulcers. Clinical Practice Guideline, No. 15*. Rockville, MD: U.S. Department of Health and Human Services. Public Health Service, Agency for Health Care Policy and Research. AHCPR Publication No. 95–0652. December 1994.
3. Bryant R, Shannon M, Pieper B, Braden B, Morris D. Pressure ulcers. In: Bryant R (ed). *Acute and Chronic Wounds: Nursing Management*. St. Louis, MO, Mosby Year Book, 1992, pp 105–163.
4. Krouskop T. Scientific aspects of pressure relief. Lecture presented at the 1989 IAET Annual Conference. Washington, DC, June 8, 1989.
5. Flam E. Dynamics of pressure ulcer management: interaction of load and duration. *Journal of Enterostomal Therapy Nursing* 1991;18(6):194–189.
6. Holzapfel SK. Support surfaces and their use in the prevention and treatment of pressure ulcers. *Journal of Enterostomal Therapy Nursing* 1993;20(6):251–260.
7. Doughty D, Fairchild P, Stogis S. Your patient: which therapy? *Journal of Enterostomal Therapy Nursing* 1990;17(4):154–159.
8. Lekander B, Hoyman K. Improved care of critically ill patients: contributions of therapeutic beds and mattresses. *Perspectives in Critical Care* 1988;1(2);49–67.
9. Pieper B, Mikols C, Adams W, Mance B. Low and high air loss beds in acute care hospitals. *Journal of Enterostomal Therapy Nursing* 1990;17(3):131–136.
10. Swope C. The team approach: using hospital owned low air loss beds. *Ostomy/Wound Management* 1994;40(6):40–47.
11. Thomas C. Specialty beds: decision making made easy. *Ostomy/Wound Management* 1989;23(3):51–59.
12. Cuzzell JZ, Willey T. Pressure relief perennials. *American Journal of Nursing* 1987;87(9):1157–1160.

35

The Role of Technology in Pressure Ulcer Prevention

Susan L. Garber, MA, OTR, FAOTA and Thomas A. Krouskop, PhD, PE

Garber SL, Krouskop TA. The role of technology in pressure ulcer prevention. In: Krasner D, Kane D. *Chronic Wound Care, Second Edition*. Wayne, PA, Health Management Publications, Inc., 1996, pp 284–292.

Introduction

The prevention of pressure ulcers and the treatment of the early stages of pressure–induced tissue damage can be extremely difficult for even the most conscientious patients and caregivers. Although the etiology of pressure ulcers has been well documented in the literature,[1-4] this knowledge is incomplete and has not been translated into effective strategies for prevention and treatment. Practical solutions that accommodate daily activity patterns and many of the technological advances that reduce the individual's risk of developing ulcers are not widely disseminated and utilized.

The normal structure of the skin and the physiological processes involved in maintaining healthy tissue are fairly well understood. During normal activities, such as sitting, lying, and leaning against another surface, relatively small volumes of flesh are compressed between the internal bony skeleton and the external surface. Since most of the body weight is carried by the skeleton, extremely high tissue stresses can be generated. Classically, pressure ulcers are assumed to be caused by pressure–induced vascular ischemia resulting in tissues deprived of oxygen and nutrients as the non–rigid walls of blood and lymph vessels collapse under pressures higher than the fluids inside. Also, mechanical deformations of flesh due to high levels of sustained load (or more moderate, repetitive forces) greatly contribute to tissue damage.

During the past twenty–five years, a number of scientific studies have provided substantial information about the factors involved in the formation of pressure ulcers, creating a basis for improving preventive techniques. Most of these studies have focused on the biomechanical aspects of pressure ulcer formation and, therefore, emphasized the effects of support surfaces on pressure. However, more than a decade ago, investigators began to appreciate that tissue breakdown was a multi–dimensional process and, hence, a number of other variables also were identified. They comprise two major categories: factors that are intrinsic to the patient and those that are extrinsic to the patient.

Intrinsic factors include diagnosis, absent or diminished sensation, tissue history (previous breakdown, surgical repair), body build, and magnitude and distribution of interface pressures. Extrinsic factors are number of hours of sitting or lying on a particular support surface (bed, wheelchair or chair); types of activities performed especially during sitting; psycho–social factors (living arrangements, family/caregiver support mechanisms, finances); usage environment (climate, continence) ; level of functional independence; type of wheelchair, cushion and bed surface; and ease of patient follow–up.

While these considerations applied in varying degrees to all persons who were immobilized as a result of disability or disease, the traditional acute–care model of pressure ulcer management did not use much of this information to ameliorate the problem. Historically, the approach to pressure ulcer management consisted of medical and surgical treatment once the ulcer became clinically significant. Moreover, the concept of an individualized pressure management program was virtually non–existent due to the lack of technical expertise necessary to assess patient needs and to prescribe equipment consistent with the individual's lifestyle. Consequently, the acute–care model of service delivery was associated with a remarkably high recurrence rate of pressure ulcers within the populations at risk.

Alarm systems. In the 1970s, a number of researchers developed alarm systems that reminded persons sitting in their wheelchairs to shift their weight on a regular basis in order to prevent pressure ulcers. These devices were developed and tested primarily for populations of persons with spinal

---

In order for a technological device to be valuable to physically impaired persons or their caregivers, it must be reliable, have a defined and useful life, and be compatible with other technological aids needed to maximize patient autonomy.

Effective pressure ulcer prevention depends upon the coordinated efforts of healthcare professionals both within hospital and rehabilitation settings and, when possible, carried over into the home by patients and their families.[5] These efforts have been described within the context of multidisciplinary teams and include organized and consistent programs of education and clinical practice.[6–8] Pressure ulcer prevention programs established in spinal cord injury centers often served as models for approaches developed in other healthcare environments.[9–12] In fact, many of the advances in technology relevant to pressure ulcer prevention and management have been derived from the efforts of researchers and clinicians working with persons with spinal cord injury. Central to this approach is the integration of research into service and educational activities that result in effective patient assessment, individualized equipment prescriptions, and increased awareness by the patient and family of their responsibilities for pressure ulcer prevention.

Types of Technology

Over the past decade, the many advances in electronics and computer technology have resulted in a myriad of systems to assist the patient, the therapist, and the caregiver in preventing pressure ulcers. Unfortunately, many of the devices developed have not fulfilled their designer's expectations because some of the variables controlling the systems were not considered. In order for a technological device to be valuable to physically impaired persons or their caregivers, it must be reliable, have a defined and useful life, and be compatible with other technological aids needed to maximize patient autonomy. The current array of technological contributions to pressure ulcer prevention and management can be classified as 1) alarm systems, 2) evaluation tools, 3) support products, and 4) educational materials.

cord injury who had impaired or absent sensation.[13–17] They were designed to record the number of weight shifts and the number of times the patient was reminded by the alarm to shift positions.[18] Although these devices were cleverly designed from an electronics standpoint and were found to be useful training tools during hospitalization, they were unsuccessful in preventing pressure ulcers long–term for several reasons. First, it was not possible to determine what sitting interval was "safe" for a given patient. Second, users of this equipment became annoyed with the attention–drawing characteristics of the alarm. Finally, the systems were limited by timing parameters and data storage.

In 1986, researchers reported that they had developed a microprocessor–based wheelchair patient training monitor that overcame the problems of versatility in varying timing parameters and in data storage.[18] As stated by these investigators, the system had application in hospital rehabilitation programs. Although this device seemed to be technologically sophisticated, it is not known to what extent the system was further developed for use by patients who have left the hospital and returned to their communities, nor is it known to what extent it was successful with persons with physical and sensory impairments since it was tested on only one non–physically impaired individual.

In 1986, Grip and Merbitz developed a wheelchair–based mobile measurement device that monitored the pressure relief performance of persons confined to wheelchairs.[19] Data were recorded on a custom portable computer and then transferred for analysis to an Apple IIe. The mobile computer signaled the patient to perform a weight shift on the basis of preset criteria and the patient's ability. This system, like the one reported by Cumming, et al., underwent several technological improvements,

---

but it is unclear how or when it was integrated into the pressure ulcer prevention program at their facility.

White, Mathews, and Fawcett extended the work of earlier investigators by developing a device called "Beep 'n Lift" which consisted of instructions, prompting with a watch beeper and alarm avoidance.[20] It was evaluated clinically with two eleven year old boys with spina bifida. Although both participants indicated that the device was useful, they found the alarm to be embarrassing and intrusive.

any point on the body contact area as well as the overall distribution of pressure under the seated or recumbent patient. Among the more practical and clinically useful pressure evaluation systems are the Texas Interface Pressure Evaluator (Teekay Applied Technology, Stafford, TX), the Talley Pressure Monitor (Talley Inc., Ramsey, England), the QA Pressure Measurement System (Gabel Medical Instruments, Ltd., Victoria, BC, Canada), and the Force Sensing Array (Vistamed, Winnipeg, Canada). Other systems such as the Tekscan System (Cambridge, MA) and the Next Generation

---

...comparative evaluations of interface pressure permit the clinician to select the support surface that provides the lowest peak pressures as well as the best pressure distribution over the supporting tissue.

The above studies reflect the difficulty in transferring technology from the laboratory or hospital environment to practical solutions that are effective in the daily lives of persons vulnerable to the effects of pressure. Today, many very good alarm systems remain on laboratory shelves because they are not applicable to the life–styles of the persons for whom they were designed.

Evaluation tools. Currently, there are no clinically measurable tissue viability factors that evaluate the status of the tissue and predict when the tissue is in danger of dying. The most reliable and easily used element in the clinical environment has been interface pressure, the pressure exerted between a person's body and another surface. While not perfect predictors of tissue damage, comparative evaluations of interface pressure permit the clinician to select the support surface that provides the lowest peak pressures as well as the best pressure distribution over the supporting tissue. Interface pressures provide "snapshot" data and can be used to compare the relative effectiveness of different products from the vast selection that are on the market today.[21]

A number of interface pressure evaluation systems are currently available. They provide information that is useful in evaluating differences in the pressure reducing and supportive properties of mattresses, beds, and wheelchair cushions. The large matrix systems, which allow the clinician to observe the pressure distribution over areas that approximate either the wheelchair seat or mattress surface, identify the maximum pressure situated at

Company's (Temecula, CA) digital interface pressure evaluator have been developed, but information about them is not widely disseminated. Babbs, et al. developed a pressure–sensitive mat for measuring the contact pressure distribution of patients lying on hospital beds.[22] However, this system was created as a research tool and was not intended to be marketed.

When interface pressure is used as a screening tool for product selection, care must be taken to assure that the data being used for the comparison are actually comparable. Generally, interface pressure data collected using different instrumentation or even collected by different investigators often are not comparable. The instrumentation used to measure interface pressures affects the readings; the size, shape, and positioning of the pressure sensors affect the absolute value of the pressure being monitored. When comparing differences between sensors, Ferguson–Pell and Cardi found that similar results could not be obtained for each subject–cushion combination.[23] They attributed these discrepancies to a number of interacting factors such as effects of flexion on the sensors, hammocking, and the way the sensor mechanically couples with the body support interface. One method to make the data collected by different groups comparable is to have the data presented, not as absolute pressure readings, but rather as percentages of the interface pressures that are generated when the subjects are supported on a standard surface such as a new hospital mattress or the unpadded sling seat of a wheelchair. This technique greatly reduces

GARBER AND KROUSKOP

the differences in the readings that are due to the operating characteristics of the instrumentation used to make the measurements.

Further complicating the issue of selecting a support surface is the continuing confusion and controversy about the importance of maintaining interface pressure below 32 mm Hg. It must be remembered that 32 mm Hg is an average value for the capillary pressure in the fingertips of young healthy male volunteers; the range of capillary pressure is from less than 20 mm Hg to more than 40 mm Hg. In the literature, capillary pressures as low as 12 mm Hg have been reported in geriatric patients. Moreover, interface pressure measurements do not necessarily reflect the actual pressures acting on the capillaries. Therefore, although maintaining interface pressures below 32 mm Hg may be a useful guideline, it does not assure that flow in the capillaries will be uninterrupted. Interface pressure readings, therefore, should be used only to make relative judgments about the effectiveness of various products. By choosing from products that produce the lowest interface pressures, the clinician can eliminate products that are ineffective for a particular user.

Once several products have been selected on the basis of lower interface pressures, there are other factors that should be considered before the selection is finalized. These factors include cost effectiveness, compatibility of the product with the overall patient management plan and lifestyle, and service provided by the supplier (e.g., warranty).

Although pressure evaluators provide the clinician with objective information from which to decide on a particular support surface, the computer–based systems are generally very expensive and not portable. Furthermore, they do not replace the clinical judgment of the therapist who must integrate the data from the evaluator with knowledge about the patient's lifestyle and habits.

Support surfaces. Although support surfaces are covered in detail in Chapter 34, their role in pressure ulcer management is included in this chapter on technology because of their significant impact on patient care.

Beds, mattresses, and overlays. Support of the recumbent body should provide stability for the skeleton, distribute body weight over the maximum area to reduce tissue pressure, and control shear forces that are generated on the skin surface. These conditions require ingenuity and judicious use of materials. In recumbent positions, it is important to maintain low tissue pressure since the hydrostatic head (a pressure measurement equal to the height of the person's torso and head), present when a person is no longer sitting, assists in maintaining flow of blood and lymph in the tissue. Moreover, the variability of tissue shape is more exaggerated when a person is in a recumbent position as opposed to the sitting position. This phenomenon leads to the need for a support surface capable of large deformations without large restoring forces or shears.

Although not always practical in a hospital or other healthcare institution, ideally, the support surface should be individualized to the person using it. Therefore, it is essential that attention be given to products that produce the lowest interface pressures for the majority of the populations served within a particular facility. When these products are being considered, it is advisable to ask the distributors for data on the standard deviation associated with the mean peak pressures that are often recorded in the marketing literature. A small standard deviation means that the average value, quite often, will represent the pressures that will be generated under the individual using the product. Conversely, a large standard deviation means that the range of the data is great and that the average value is probably a poor indicator of the product performance.[24]

In recent years, many hospitals have been replacing their standard mattresses with pressure–reducing foam mattresses to eliminate the costly overlays that were used for comfort and to protect patients at risk for the development of pressure ulcers. However, little information has been forthcoming on the pressure–reducing capabilities of the used mattresses. In 1994, a study was conducted to determine how well a foam replacement mattress retained its pressure–reducing and supportive characteristics when used in an acute care hospital.[25] The results of this study indicate that, over time, the stiffness of the foam in the mattresses decreased slowly. This softening, therefore, is a long–term process most notable when patients report "sinking" into the mattress or when it becomes difficult to transfer patients onto and off of the mattress. This phenomenon, as described in an earlier study,[26] is related to decreases in the foam's ability to carry loads and to increases in interface pressures. When the stiffness of the foam significantly decreases, as with extended use of three years or more, the foam no longer can carry the load. The weight is then transferred to the underlying structure used to support the foam. In other words, the mattress "bottoms out." In addition to stiffness, the foam must also have a high enough compression resistance to support the load fully. The ideal combination is a mattress with low stiffness under small compression forces and a high resistance to compression under large loads.[25] However, these characteristics change with time. A new product may approximate the ideal, but as its properties change

Table 1
Types of Air Flotation Beds

Air –fluidized bed

Advantages: Ease of operation
                Fail safely
                Control of skin maceration

Disadvantages: Requires foam for positioning
                Heavy weight

Low–air–loss bed

Advantages: Comfortable
                Control of skin maceration
                Positioning for posture control

Disadvantages: Requires skilled set up
                Fail safety

with use, it may no longer be effective in either redistributing loads or in providing comfort. Therefore, institutions need to have a mechanism to evaluate the long–term ability of a mattress to provide support and protection from the effects of pressure.

In an ongoing evaluation of foam core hospital replacement mattresses in an acute care hospital, it has been found that differences between the stiffness of the foam at various sites were critical to comfort. When there was a difference of more than fifty percent between the highest and lowest readings of stiffness, patients consistently reported the mattress to be uncomfortable, and when the readings decreased by more than 30 percent as the result of use, the mattress became uncomfortable and unusable.

These findings are based on data collected on 200 mattresses using a portable indentor and force gauge system. In the study, a flat circular plate 8 inches in diameter was pressed into the foam to a given depth, e.g. 25 percent of the foam's original height (if the foam is originally 6 inches high, the indentor is pressed into the foam 1.25 inches), and the force required to cause the deformation was recorded. This process was repeated at three different locations along the axis of the mattress, i.e., at the head, at the middle, and at the foot of the bed and the differences were computed for the stiffness at these locations.

This information may be useful when establishing contracts between an institution and a mattress

supplier to determine when a mattress should be replaced under the warranty.[27]

Although the literature is replete with numerous studies on support surfaces for the bed, there is a paucity of prospective, controlled, clinical studies on the efficacy of these products. Additionally, there is a lack of standardized information on them.[28] It has been suggested that standardization would assist the healthcare professional in making more informed decisions about the use of support surfaces. It would also help researchers to design and implement controlled, clinical studies by defining the characteristics of surface evaluation. Performance–based criteria, non–invasively measured, constitute the parameters of standardization and include 1) life–expectancy of the surface; 2) skin moisture control; 3) skin temperature control; 4) redistribution of pressure; 5) product service requirements; 6) fail safety; 7) infection control; 8) flammability; and 9) patient/product friction. This model will accomplish a number of clinically relevant outcomes. Among these are facilitating the development of new, effective support surfaces and enabling the clinician to select a support surface to meet patient needs based on product performance. Standardization also will facilitate the design of better controlled clinical studies and enhance the clinician's ability to make decisions about support surfaces based on outcomes and the results of well–designed controlled clinical studies.[28] Multi–site clinical trials with appropriate matching of patient needs and produt support characteristics would provide important information on the effectiveness of products to either reduce the risk of developing pressure ulcers or facilitate their healing.

Specialty beds. In some cases, a simple mattress overlay or mattress may not be the most appropriate support surface. An air flotation bed should be considered under the following conditions: 1) the patient has contractures that prohibit supine lying; 2) the patient is at very high risk for pressure ulcers (based on one of the risk assessment scales); 3) there is limited access to skilled nursing care; and 4) the patient has complications that prohibit repositioning.

The current technology in air flotation beds is reflected in two major categories of these devices: the air–fluidized bed and the low air–loss–bed (Table 1). There have been no controlled studies that compare air–fluidized with low–air–loss beds. However, according to the AHCPR's Clinical Practice Guideline, *Treatment of Pressure Ulcers*,[29] clinicians generally prefer the low–air–loss bed for three primary reasons: 1) it can be raised and lowered; 2) the head of the bed can be elevated; and 3)

GARBER AND KROUSKOP

transferring patients in or out of bed is easier. When an institution is choosing a product line, the supplier of the product is another critical variable since the product's performance depends on how well it is serviced and how well the sales/service representatives interact with the clinical staff at the institution.

Wheelchair cushions. Prior to 1970, the selection of a wheelchair cushion usually was an arbitrary decision based on the rehabilitation or medical team's familiarity with and the availability of these devices.[30] In hospitals, patients often could be seen sitting on their bed pillows that had been placed in their wheelchairs or in the chairs next to their beds. In many hospitals, patients were seated on air rings or "doughnuts" with the hope that they would be comfortable and that their skin would not be compromised. Very little was known about the usefulness or effectiveness of these devices because there were no clinically practical methods of evaluating them. Furthermore, few clinicians correlated the occurrence of skin problems with the cushion itself.

The primary purpose of a wheelchair cushion is to reduce the risk of pressure ulcers in persons who are mobility and/or sensory impaired. Secondarily, wheelchair cushions enhance posture and balance, endurance, and, ultimately, functional independence. An effective wheelchair cushion reduces interface pressure, promotes sitting balance and stability, and provides comfort. However, wheelchair cushions neither prevent nor heal pressure ulcers despite the claims of some of the manufacturers of these products. The wheelchair cushion can be only as effective as the surface on which it is placed. Therefore, the wheelchair itself must be appropriate for the mobility needs and life–style of the patient and accurately measured to insure both safety and function. In addition, the wheelchair cushion must be compatible with the wheelchair and any accessory equipment attached to it such as back cushions or custom designed contoured or molded back systems. Many new wheelchair cushions have been developed and marketed. However, a cushion that serves all potential users for an indefinite length of time has yet to be introduced. While most cushions serve a specific group of people quite effectively, clinicians are still limited in their ability to decide which cushion should be used with which patient.

Wheelchair cushion prescriptions in pressure management clinics have been examined to establish a correlation between characteristic variables of wheelchair users (body weight and build, gender, level of spinal cord lesion, etc.). No significant correlations have been found between any single patient variable and the wheelchair cushion ultimately prescribed in the clinic. Based upon this

---

Table 2
Classes of Static Support Surfaces Used in Wheelchairs and Beds

<u>Air –filled products</u>

Advantages:	Lightweight
	Easy to clean
	Effective with many people

Disadvantages:	Subject to puncture
	Repair process may be difficult
	Inflation must be frequently checked
	User stability

<u>Liquid–filled flotation devices</u>

| Advantages: | Cleanable |
| | Effective |

| Disadvantages: | Subject to puncture |
| | Weight |

<u>Gel–filled devices</u>

| Advantages: | Adjusts to body movement |
| | Cleanable |

Disadvantages:	Weight
	Cost
	Storage space

<u>Foam Products</u>

Advantages:	Availability
	Many variations
	Inexpensive
	Lightweight
	Can easily be modified

Disadvantages:	Wear out more rapidly
	Not cleanable
	Properties change with time
	Can support combustion

---

analysis, however, the range of cushions considered for an individual has been narrowed. The final selection is based now on a pressure evaluation and consideration of lifestyle factors, postural stability, continence of bladder and bowel, and cost of alternative cushions.

In the 1960s and 1970s, a number of investigators began to explore ways in which pressure at the interface of the body and another surface could be quantifiably measured.[2,31,32] However, most of these devices were impractical for use in monitoring persons with physical impairments or they were not developed beyond the testing laboratory. Other investigators evaluated the pressure distribution characteristics of commercially available cushions in an attempt to identify the most effective cushion for reducing the risk of pressure ulcers.[33–36] In none of these studies did any one cushion significantly out–perform the others in reducing pressure. Despite the efforts of these investigators to quantitatively and objectively measure pressure and its distribution under the seated wheelchair patient, there remains today controversy and disagreement concerning the validity, reliability, and clinical usefulness of these measurements. For all of its problems, however, the evaluation of interface pressure remains the most reliable factor utilized in the clinical environment. Although not a perfect predictor of wheelchair cushion efficacy, it enables the clinician to select a support surface which provides the lowest peak pressures on the supported tissue as well as the best pressure distribution over the supporting tissue.

In recent years, computer technology has provided the most sophisticated means of objectively evaluating interface pressures. Several systems have been developed in Canada and England that have enhanced the ease and accuracy of evaluating pressure for the purpose of selecting a pressure reducing device for the wheelchair or bed. Although these systems are expensive, they provide the type of measureable outcome information that supports reimbursement from third party payors. Despite these advances in both wheelchair cushion and evaluation technology, the prescription of a wheelchair cushion is not determined by pressure measurements alone.[37–38] A number of other factors must be considered. Of particular note are the following: 1) patient's diagnosis; 2) upper extremity function; 3) postural problems such as scoliosis, lordosis, and kyphosis; 4) number of hours spent on the cushion each day; 5) usage environment such as climate, pollution, humidity, temperature, and terrain; 6) patient's continence; 7) living arrangements; 8) tissue history including past pressure ulcers and their treatment; 9) decreased sitting tolerance secondary to medical or social factors; 10) patient's body build; 11) wheelchair style (manual or motorized, lightweight or standard); and 12) psychosocial factors such as attitude, interest, and motivation. It must be remembered also that the support surface prescribed during the early phases of rehabilitation or hospitalization may not be the device of choice when the person returns home.[30]

Static wheelchair cushions make up the largest category of wheelchair cushions (ahead of dynamic cushions and molded or contoured seating systems) and serve the widest range of potential users. The three major types of static wheelchair cushions are fluid (air, water, etc.), gels, and foams (Table 2).

Technology in Pressure Ulcer Education

The primary purpose of hospital or institutional based education programs is to produce knowledgeable competent caregivers as well as informed consumers.[39] The primary purpose of pressure ulcer prevention educational programs is to reduce the occurrence of pressure ulcers. Many educational programs designed to teach pressure ulcer prevention have been established and are reported in the literature. However, the effectiveness of these programs over long periods of time has not been established. The development and consistent implementation of structured, comprehensive, multidisciplinary programs of pressure ulcer prevention are successful in reducing the occurrence of pressure ulcers in a variety of healthcare settings. These programs use education as the mechanism for translating knowledge about pressure ulcers into effective strategies for prevention and treatment. Unfortunately, traditional approaches to education have not been successful in significantly reducing the incidence of pressure ulcers in hospitals, nursing homes, or rehabilitation facilities today.

Within the last twenty years, healthcare educators have developed a variety of programs designed to teach pressure ulcer prevention and management. Most of these programs have been in written form, but more recently have included the slide–sound and video media. Within the last decade, healthcare educators have been introduced to computer technology.[40] Basically, this technology has taken two major forms: computer–assisted instruction (CAI) and interactive videodisc (IVD). The CAI program allows interaction with the program by use of the computer's keyboard whereas interaction with most IVD programs is accomplished by touching designated spots on the computer monitor's special touch–screen or by pointing and clicking a computer mouse. The addition of motion video and sound with IVD makes it possible to display on the computer screen the same real–life examples enjoyed on videotape. The advantages of these instructional technologies

GARBER AND KROUSKOP

include reduced learning time, round–the–clock access, and cost–effectiveness. These advantages, however, do not preclude the educator from such tasks as assessing the need for specific information, prescribing the appropriate learning strategy, preparing the learner, and, most importantly, providing follow–up.[40] Despite these advantages, instructional technology also presents several disadvantages including the initial cost of hardware and software, security problems, and lack of familiarity and comfort with computer use. These disadvantages have been overcome to some degree by the marketing of purchase plans that include free computers with the purchase of a specific number of programs and by the recent computer price wars. Finally, healthcare professionals entering their fields

---

...technology must be used judiciously as part of an overall management program individualized for each patient.

---

today are more computer–literate than their predecessors and, therefore, are capable of incorporating the use of computers into the many tasks for which they are responsible.

Summary

Technology contributes significantly to understanding the scope of the pressure ulcer problem. However, it must be emphasized that technology can provide only the tools that people themselves must use to solve the problem because the use of "high tech" equipment will not independently answer all patient needs. Technology can provide cost–effective devices that can reduce dependence on other assistive systems such as personal care attendants, but technology does not eliminate the need for such assistance. In order to reduce the impact of pressure–induced tissue damage on a person's life, technology must be used judiciously as part of an overall management program individualized for each patient.

References

1. Kosiak M. Etiology and pathology of ischemic ulcers. *Arch Phys Med Rehabil* 1959;40(2):62–69.
2. Lindan O. Etiology of decubitus ulcers: An experimental study. *Arch Phys Med Rehabil* 1961;42(11):774–783.
3. Bennet L, Kavner D, Lee BY, Trainor FA. Shear vs pressure as causative factors in skin blood flow occlusion. *Arch Phys Med Rehabil* 1979;60(7):309–314.
4. Krouskop TA. A synthesis of the factors that contribute to pressure sore formation. *Medical Hypothesis* 1983; 11: 255–267.
5. Dimant J, Francis ME. Pressure sore prevention and management. *J Geron Nurs* 1988;14(8):18–25.
6. Khun JK, Wygonoski C: A multidisciplinary team approach to decubitus ulcer care. *Nursing Homes* 1984;33(1):29–33.
7. Levine JM, Simpson M, McDonald RJ. Pressure sores: A plan for primary care prevention. *Geriatrics* 1989;44(4):75–76,83–87,90.
8. Nickel LD, Waters RL, Klein NE. Pressure ulcerations: A philosophy of management. *Modes of Systems Spinal Cord Injury Digest* 1982;4(1):36–48.
9. Krouskop TA, Noble PE, Garber SL, Spencer WA: The effectiveness of preventive management in reducing the occurrence of pressure sores. *J Rehab R & D* 1983;22(3):10–38.
10. Andberg MM, Rudolph A, Anderson TP. Improving skin care through patient and family training. *Topics in Clinical Nursing* 1983;5(2): 45–54.
11. Noble PC. The prevention of pressure sores in persons with spinal cord injuries. *World Rehabilitation Fund, Inc.* 1975: Monograph #11.
12. King RB, Boyink M, Keenan M (eds). *Rehabilitation Guide.* Chicago, IL, The Rehabilitation Institute of Chicago, 1977, pp 62–80.
13. Ananthan PR, Srinivasan TM, Antia NH, Ghista DN. Pressure warning system for patients with insensitive feet to avoid ulceration. In: Kenedi RM, Cowden JM, Scales JT (eds). *Bedsore Biomechanics.* Baltimore, MD, University Park Press, 1975, pp 207–210.
14. Ferguson–Pell MW, Wilkie IC, Reswick JB, Barbenel JC. Pressure sore prevention for wheelchair–bound spinal injury patients. *Paraplegia* 1980;18:42–51.
15. Fordyce WE, Simons BC. Automated training system for wheelchair pushups. US Public Health Service, Public Health Report 83, 1968;527–528.
16. Malament IB, Dunn ME, Davis R. Pressure sores: Operant conditioning approach to prevention. *Arch Phys Med Rehabil* 1975; 56: 161–165.
17. Temes WC, Harder P. Pressure relief training device. *Phys Ther* 1977;57:1152–1153.
18. Cumming WT, Tompkins WJ, Jones RM, Margolis SA. Microprocessor–based weight shift monitors for paraplegic patients. *Arch Phys Med Rehabil* 1986;67:172–174.
19. Grip JC, Merbitz CT. Wheelchair–based mobile measurement of behavior for pressure sore prevention. *Computer Methods and Programs in Biomedicine* 1986;22:137–144.
20. White GW, Mathews RM, Fawcett SB. Reducing risk of pressure sores: Effects of watch prompts and alarm avoidance on wheelchair push–ups. *Journal of APplied Behavior Analysis* 1989;22(3):287–295.
21. Krouskop TA, Garber SL, Cullen B. Patient support surfaces and other issues in pressure sore prevention. *Transplantation / Implantation Today* 1989;6:43–47.
22. Babbs CF, Bourland JD, Graber GP, Jones JT, Schoenlein WE. A pressure–sensitive mat for measuring contact pressure distributions of patients lying on hospital beds. *Biomedical Instrumentation and Technology* 1990;September/October:363–370.
23. Ferguson–Pell M, Cardi M. Pressure mapping systems. *Team Rehab Report* 1992;October:28–32.

24. Krouskop TA, Williams R, Herszkowicz I, Garber S. Evaluating the effectiveness of mattress overlays. *Rx Home Care* 1985;7:97–103.
25. Krouskop TA, Randall CJ, Davis J, Garber S, Williams S, Callaghan R. Evaluating the long–term performance of a foam–core hospital replacement mattress. *J WOCN* 1994;21(6):241–246.
26. Noble PC, Goode B, Krouskop TA, Crisp B. The influence of environmental aging upon the load–bearing properties of polyurethane foams. *J Rehabil R & D* 1984;21:31–38.
27. Randall C, Davis J, Krouskop TA. Unpublished data. 1995.
28. Krouskop TA, van Rijswijk L. Standardizing performance–based criteria for support surfaces. *Ostomy/Wound Management* 1995;41(1):34–45.
29. Bergstrom N, Bennett MA, Carlson CE, Frantz RA, Garber SL, et al. *Treatment of Pressure Ulcers*. Clinical Practice Guideline No. 15. Rockville, MD: U.S. Department of Health and Human Services. Public Health Service, Agency for Health Care Policy and Research. AHCPR Publication No. 95–0652. December 1994.
30. Garber SL. Wheelchair cushions: A historical review. *American Journal of Occupational Therapy* 1985;39:453–459.
31. Bush CA. Study of pressure on skin under ischial tuberosities and thighs during sitting. *Arch Phys Med Rehabil* 1969; 46: 202–213.
32. Mooney V, Einbund MJ, Rogers JE, Stouffer ES. Comparison of pressure distribution qualities in seat cushions. *Bulletin of Prosthetics Research* 1971;10:129–143.
33. Garber SL, Krouskop TA, Carter RE. A system for clinically evaluating wheelchair pressure relief cushions. *Amercian Journal of Occupational Therapy* 1978;32:565–570.
34. Cochran GVB, Slater G. Experimental evaluation of wheelchair cushions: Report of a pilot study. *Bulletin of Prosthetic Research* 1973;10:29–61.
35. Souther SG, Carr SD, Vistnes LM. Wheelchair cushions to reduce pressure under bony prominences. *Arch Phys Med Rehabil* 1974;55:460–464.
36. DeLateur BJ, Berni R, Hangladarom T, Giaconi R. Wheelchair cushions designed to prevent pressure sores: An evaluation. *Arch Phys Med Rehabil* 1976;57:129–135.
37. Nelham RL. Seating for the chair–bound disabled person: A survey of seating equipment in the United Kingdom. *Journal of Biomedical Engineering* 1981;3:267–274.
38. Garber SL, Krouskop TA. Body build and its relationship to pressure distribution in the seated wheelchair patient. *Arch Phys Med Rehabil* 1982;63:17–20.
39. Bergstrom N, Allman RM, Carlson CE, Eaglstein W, Frantz RA, Garber SL, et al. *Pressure Ulcers in Adults: Prediction and Prevention*. Clinical Practice Guideline No. 3. Rockville, MD. U.S. Department of Health and Human Services, Public Health Service, Agency for Health Care Policy and Research. AHCPR Publication No. 92–0047, May 1992.
40. Bolwell C. Using computers as instructional technology in the pressure ulcer field. *Decubitus* 1993;6(4):20–25.

36

Teaching Wound Care to Patients, Families, and Healthcare Providers

Paula Erwin–Toth, MSN, RN, CETN and Brenda P. Stenger, MEd, RN, CETN

Erwin–Toth P, Stenger B. In: Krasner D, Kane D. *Chronic Wound Care, Second Edition*. Wayne, PA, Health Management Publications, Inc., 1997, pp 293–297.

Introduction

Effective patient/caregiver education is an essential component of successful wound management. In order for successful learning to take place, healthcare personnel providing patient/caregiver education must have knowledge and skills in wound care and adult education.

Decreasing lengths of stay in acute care institutions has given further impetus to healthcare personnel to provide meaningful patient/caregiver education in a variety of settings. Interventions derived from research–based outcome criteria will further standardize care. The Joint Commission on the Accreditation of Healthcare Organizations (JCAHO) and the Agency for Healthcare Policy and Research (AHCPR) have identified patient/caregiver education as a critical component of care.[1,2]

Work redesign efforts directed at decreasing healthcare costs may result in both licensed and unlicensed healthcare personnel participating in chronic wound management. It is imperative that all healthcare providers acting in this capacity are well rounded in chronic wound management. Skills in patient/caregiver education should be nurtured in these individuals as well. The ability of healthcare providers to facilitate patient/caregiver competency in chronic wound care is essential to the success of the management plan.

Principles of Adult Learning

Adult Learning Theory. Knowles in 1984 stated that "learning is an elusive phenomenon."[3]

Educational activities are designed to initiate a change in behavior, knowledge, and skill. Whether learning has actually taken place can be difficult to assess.

Has the learner truly manifested a change in behavior, knowledge, and skill? Will this change endure across time and place? How do you accurately assess and document these findings? How do you modify your education plan if effective learning is not taking place?

Androgogy, as defined by Knowles is the "art and science of helping adults learn."[3] Knowles' androgogical model is based on six major assumptions:

1. *The need to know.* Adults need to know why they need to learn something before undertaking to learn it.
2. *The learner's self–concept.* Adults have a self–concept of being responsible for their own decisions, for their own lives. They resent and resist situations in which they feel others are imposing their wills on them.
3. *The role of the learner's experience.* In any group of adults there will be a wider range of individual differences than in a group of youths. Any group of adults will be more heterogeneous in terms of background, learning style, motivation, needs, interests, and goals than is true of a group of youths. Hence, the great emphasis in adult education is on individualization of teaching and learning strategies.
4. *Readiness to learn.* Adults become ready to learn those things they need to know and be able to do in order to cope effectively with their real life situations.

5. *Orientation to learning.* Adults are life–centered (or task–centered or problem–centered) in their orientation to learning. They learn new knowledge, understanding, skills, values, and attitudes most effectively when they are presented in the context of application to real life situations.

6. *Motivation.* While adults are responsive to some external motivations (better job, promotions, higher salaries and the like), the most potent motivators are internal pressures (the desire for increased job satisfaction, self–esteem, quality of life and the like).[3]

While androgogy is appropriate for most types of adult learning situations, Knowles recognized that occasionally pedagogical strategies used in teaching children may be selectively applied to adult learners.[3] In the pedagogical model the teacher assumes "full responsibility for making all decisions about what is learned, how it will be learned, when it will be learned, and if it has been learned."[3]

Learners that need to be taught by the pedagogical model characteristically are dependent, have no experience with the content area, do not perceive the relevance of the content, need to accomplish a required performance, or feel no internal need to learn the content.[3]

However, for learning to develop and endure it is important to apply androgogical strategies once the initial learning has taken place.

Adult education. In a prospective study of pressure ulcer risk in spinal cord injury patients the researchers discussed the importance of discerning health beliefs and ongoing educational programs to reinforce learning related to pressure ulcer prevention.[4] They discovered that little or no education was provided following the initial acute care and rehabilitation phase for spinal cord injured patients.

Despite the high prevalence of pressure ulcers in the 60 study participants (25 percent control group and 28 percent experimental group) none of them requested "additional information about skin care or to be re–evaluated for pressure related problems." Even though the subjects recognized the importance of skin care and pressure ulcer prevention, they neither requested nor were provided with information.

When planning an adult education program the following components should be included:
1. Needs assessment (e.g. What does the learner perceive to be important?),
2. Context analysis (e.g. What does the content mean to the overall or long term plan?),
3. Objectives (e.g. What will the learner be expected to do at the completion of the program?),
4. Learning/content (e.g. What is the content and how will it be presented?),
5. Evaluation (e.g. How will the learner's knowledge be assessed and how will he/she evaluate the education?), and
6. Related arrangements (e.g. Where will the teaching take place, what audiovisual aids or materials will be used?).[5]

Brookfield has identified 6 principles of adult education: 1) Participation is voluntary; 2) Respect for self–worth is fostered; 3) Adult learning is collaborative; 4) Ongoing evaluation is critical for success of the endeavor; 5) Adult education fosters a spirit of critical reflection; and 6) The aim of adult education is the nurturing of self–directed, empowered adults.[6]

Other influences. Consideration of familial and cultural influences is important in adult learning as well. Current and past interactions of families and significant others with the patient will influence the effectiveness of education. Knowledge of the learner's ethnic and cultural background can provide valuable insight into identifying learning needs and developing effective teaching strategies. One must be cautious to avoid stereotyping learners based on family relationships and ethnic backgrounds.[7]

Consideration of the chronological ages and developmental stages of the patient and caregivers can assist the educator in identifying special considerations to be included in the teaching plan. Older adults are capable of learning new tasks,[3] but the educator must consider the effects of concomitant medical and social conditions which can influence the patient's/caregiver's ability to learn.

Attention to pain management should be addressed along with self–care activities.[8] Patients who are in pain will not be capable of learning a new behavior. Caregivers may be reluctant to participate in activities which they perceive as being hurtful to the patient. See Chapter 43 on pain.

Body image in patients with chronic wounds is not well researched. Since positive self–esteem has been identified as an important component of adult learning it is logical to assume that a negative body image may contribute to low self–esteem and may have a negative impact on learning. Willis in 1994 observed that "Since appearance and self–esteem usually go hand in hand, what happens to our self–esteem when negative changes occur in our appearance?"[9] Patients with chronic wounds should be encouraged to maintain good physical hygiene and an optimal physical appearance.

People who feel good about themselves are more likely to feel motivated in their care.[9]

Literacy of the patient/caregiver should be considered as a teaching plan is developed. Sensitivity by the healthcare provider must be used during this portion of the assessment. Asking for an individual's highest level of education is rarely sufficient. There are several standardized tests available to determine reading level; however, use of these instruments is rarely practical in a clinical setting. Yasenchak and Bridle in 1993 recommended asking patients/caregivers "Do you like to read?" instead of the more threatening "How well do you read?"[10] Before beginning to teach, have the patient/caregiver read aloud a section of the written instructions. Reading ability and comprehension can then be assessed.

Boyd in 1987 reported that in a review of the literature a majority of the people in the United States have a reading level at or below the eighth grade level, while 60 to 92 percent of patient education material requires a reading level of eighth grade or higher.[11]

Nursing theories. Numerous nursing models and theories can be applied to enhance patient/family education. Dorthea Orem's "Self Care Deficit Theory"[12] and Calista Roy's "Adaptation Model"[13] can provide theoretical frameworks to assist the clinician in developing an effective teaching plan.

Orem in 1980 stated that "self–care is a conscious deliberate series of actions in response to an objectively demonstrable need."[12] The requirement for dependent care emerges when an individual on either a temporary or permanent basis is unable to master or perform all or selective self–care activities. Based on the self–care deficits manifested by the patient the nurses' interventions will be wholly compensatory, partly compensatory, or supportive.[12] Teaching strategies can then be directed at encouraging a patient's/caregiver's progression from dependence to independence.

Roy's Adaptation Model of 1971 is another approach that may be useful to the clinician teaching wound care.[13] Roy's model views a person as an adaptive system. A response is considered adaptive when it contributes positively to the general goals and development of the person.

This model is especially appropriate when interacting with patients/caregivers who are experiencing difficulty adjusting to the chronic wound experience. Roy describes a series of four adaptive modes.[13] The physiological mode, self–concept mode, role function mode, and interdependence mode. Nursing activities are directed at assisting the patient/caregiver in identifying and working toward eliminating ineffective behaviors and promoting positive adaptive behaviors which will maximize their health and well–being.

Reimbursement Issues

In this era of cost containment and shrinking health care dollars, there may be pressure to reduce educational activities. In the 1960s and 1970s the fee for service system expanded to include education and other services since costs could be directly or indirectly absorbed into an institution or agency's operating budget.

The advent of DRGs (Diagnostic Related groups) in the 1980s set a global fee an institution would receive for a particular patient diagnosis or surgical procedure. This resulted in health care providers and reimbursement specialists to thoroughly examine what ought to be considered essential versus non–essential services.[14]

A further impetus to change was stimulated by the emergence of a managed care model. Under this system, primary care providers act as the gate keepers for a group of patients enrolled in a particular managed care plan. In most cases the primary care provider is in private practice. In this system there is generally a disincentive for the primary care physician to either admit patients to hospital or refer to specialists.[15] An emphasis should be placed on preventative care and a required referral for specialty or hospital services.

An HMO (Health Maintenance Organization) primary health care providers may be employees of the HMO. There is usually an emphasis on preventative care as well as strict guidelines regarding services provided. All services must be pre–approved by the primary care provider and those individuals are carefully monitored regarding their referral patterns. In some managed care and HMO plans, cost referrals will directly reduce the income or bonus received by the primary care provider.

The next system to emerge is capitation. A capitated system covers an individual for life and not per episode. There is a definite incentive to provide preventative care, education, and health promotion as these activities will reduce the long term costs to the plan. Providers of care may also serve as the insurers, therefore in order to remain solvent they must provide care to the maximum number of clients for the least amount of dollars in the least expensive setting.

Integrated delivery systems (IDS) are emerging as reimbursement and care patterns evolve. Local, regional and national not–for–profit and for–profit IDS are forming alliances to streamline services and reduce costs. In addition further reduction of health care costs is achieved by controlling utilization as well as reduction of operating costs.[14] Wound care providers may be required to standardize protocols, products, and education within the IDS network.

Factors influencing health care include shrinking resources, competition for market share, and regulatory and payor constraints. These relatively rapid changes have left many patients, families, providers, and insurers scrambling to form a new paradigm of health care.[14] It is vital for wound care providers to be aware of the financial issues at stake and promote the role of education as a key to reducing health care costs.

Education of patients, families, caregivers, and health care providers is the key to a proactive program of prevention, and timely, appropriate interventions. Not only will this approach improve the quality of life for clients it will reduce the amount of health care dollars spent caring for wounds.

This approach is best served by a multidisciplinary team. The care goal should be to provide seamless care of the client regardless of the setting. Often a case manager or social worker can be the key in coordinating this continuum of care. In this system ideally the care is patient focused. All disciplines concentrate on improving outcomes for clients. At times case mapping or critical pathways can facilitate this process. Variance analysis can reveal where clients are not following the expected pattern and the team can modify the plan of care to address these variances. The key to success in this approach and all education activities is the active role played by the client/family and the interdisciplinary, interdepartmental and interagency cooperation evidenced by the health care team.

Teaching Healthcare Providers

Education of licensed and unlicensed healthcare providers should be an ongoing process. Although educational preparation and responsibilities among healthcare providers may vary, optimum wound management is dependent upon knowledge of and compliance with the wound care plan.

A needs assessment should be conducted prior to planning wound care education programs. The majority of healthcare providers, both licensed and unlicensed, are motivated by the desire to provide quality care. Heavy patient assignments may result in the healthcare provider feeling overwhelmed and under–appreciated. Focusing on methods of wound prevention and management techniques that can be completed effectively and efficiently will enhance the education experience of the healthcare providers. (See Chapter 3 on prevention.)

The content of an educational program will be dependent upon the type of healthcare provider to be taught. A nursing assistant may need to know both the rationale and techniques for proper positioning, turning, and skin care. He/she needs to know how to identify changes in the patient's skin and overall condition. Their knowledge of basic nutrition and hydration is important as well. It is not enough to just tell unlicensed personnel what to do; they are adult learners and need to know why something is important. Educational programs should be directed at building on and developing wound care knowledge. This approach will help facilitate the nursing assistant's internal motivation to learn and to perform the learned activities.

Licensed healthcare personnel should be provided with the scientific rationale for wound prevention and management techniques based on their scope of practice. Educational programs relating to anatomy and physiology, nutrition, topical therapies, positioning techniques and support surfaces, psychosocial issues and patient/caregiver education are only a few of the areas that licensed personnel may require to provide optimum care. As with unlicensed healthcare providers licensed individuals need to have educational programs based on information and techniques that will directly affect their practices.

Needs assessment surveys should be conducted regularly with all levels of healthcare providers. The location, duration and timing of educational programs will vary. Clinicians practicing at the bedside may benefit from educational experiences with a simulation, workshop, and/or practice component. Before effective patient/caregiver education can take place all levels of healthcare providers need to be well–versed in chronic wound management.

Teaching the Patient/Caregiver

A patient/caregiver needs assessment should be performed and documented. Baseline information relating to knowledge, belief, and health practices as well as the learner's perceived educational needs should be obtained. Information pertaining to psychosocial and cultural variables should be obtained as these issues may influence teaching strategies. And finally are the patient/caregiver ready to learn? The healthcare provider needs to identify barriers to learning. These barriers may be environmental, physiological, or psychological. Lack of privacy, limited space, poor lighting and frequent interruptions can all have a negative impact on learning. For example, finding a private room or at least pulling the curtain, turning off the television, providing adequate lighting and turning off pagers can enhance the learning environment.

ERWIN–TOTH AND STENGER

Efforts should be made to optimize the patient's physical condition. Pain is a barrier to learning. Effective pain management through pharmacological, electrical stimulation, positioning, and/or biofeedback techniques may be beneficial to both the patient and caregiver. (See Chapter 43 on pain.) Timing of these interventions should be done to elicit maximum relief with minimal affect on cognitive abilities.

Identification of psychological, social, and cultural barriers is an important part of a comprehensive assessment. Techniques to promote effective coping skills and to facilitate open communication, and efforts to acknowledge and work within cultural and religious values should be undertaken by the healthcare provider. Economic barriers to effective wound management should be considered as well. The inability to purchase proper food or nutritional supplements, medications, topical therapies, and/or assistive devices will have a negative impact on healing. If any of these barriers are present, consultation with a social worker may benefit the patient/caregiver.

In the acute care environment it may be necessary for the healthcare provider to focus on survival issues: the need to know versus nice to know. Reinforcement of teaching and expansion of the breadth and depth of patient/caregiver education can be conducted at an extended care facility, home, or ambulatory care setting.

Healthcare providers should collaborate with the patient/caregiver to identify the overall learning goal and specific learning objectives. The method, timing and venue of the teaching should be clearly described. Evaluation of the effectiveness of patient/caregiver learning should be conducted. Specific outcome–based criteria should be listed and notations made as to whether the patient/caregiver successfully demonstrated understanding and competence. If ineffective learning has taken place, reassessment and revision of the teaching plan should be instituted by the healthcare provider.

On–going reassessment, reinforcement of previous instruction and addition of new material should continue during and after wound healing has occurred. Finally, patients/caregivers should have the opportunity to evaluate the quantity and quality of the education they have received.

Conclusion

Education is an essential component of successful chronic wound management. Knowledgeable healthcare providers will be better prepared to facilitate learning through patients/caregivers. Principles of adult learning, adult education and nursing theory can be applied to enhance the effectiveness of educational endeavors. Identification of specific learning goals, objectives, methods, and evaluation will help to create an effective wound management education plan.

References

1. Joint Commission on the Accreditation of Hospitals. *1996 Comprehensive Accreditation Manual for Hospitals.* Chicago, IL, JCAHO, 1996.
2. Panel for the Prediction and Prevention of Pressure Ulcers in Adults. *Pressure Ulcers in Adults: Prediction and Prevention. Clinical Practice Guideline, Number 3.* AHCPR Publication No. 92–0047. Rockville, MD: Agency for Health Care Policy and Research, Public Health Service, U.S. Department of Health and Human Services. May 1992.
3. Knowles M. *The Adult Learner, A Neglected Species.* Houston, TX, Gulf Publishing Co., 1984.
4. Rodriguez G, Garber S. Prospective study of pressure ulcer risk in spinal cord injury patients. *International Medical Society of Paraplegia* 1994;32(3):150–8.
5. Knox AB. *Helping Adults Learn.* San Francisco, CA, Jossey–Bass, 1987.
6. Brookfield S. *Understanding and Facilitating Adult Learning.* San Francisco, CA, Jossey–Bass, 1986.
7. Leahe, M, Wright L. *Families and Psychosocial Problems.* Springhouse, PA, Springhouse Corporation, 1987.
8. Krasner D. The chronic wound pain experience. A conceptual model. *Ostomy/Wound Management* 1995;41(3):20–25.
9. Willis J. *Beautiful Again, Restoring Your Image and Enhancing Body Changes.* Santa Fe, NM, Health Press, 1994.
10. Yasenchak PA, Bridle MJ. A low literacy skin care manual for spinal cord injury patients. *Patient Education & Counseling* 1993;22(1):1–5.
11. Boyd MD. A guide to writing effective patient education materials. *Nursing Management* 1987;18(7):56–57.
12. Orem D. *Nursing, Concepts of Practice, Second Edition.* NY, NY, McGraw–Hill, 1980.
13. Roy C. Adaptation, A basis for nursing practice. *Nursing Outlook* 1971;19:254–257.
14. Coleman J. MCO trends. *The Case Manager* 1996;7(3):44–47.
15. Banja J. Ethics: Conflicts of interest and the health provider's role as a "fuduciary." *The Case Manager* 1996;7(3):40–43.

37

Designing and Developing Healthcare Educational Programs

Sharon Baranoski, MSN, RN, CETN

Baranoski S. Designing and developing healthcare educational programs. In: Krasner D, Kane D. *Chronic Wound Care, Second Edition.* Wayne, PA, Health Management Publications, Inc., 1997, pp 298–302.

"May there never develop in me the notion that my education is complete but give me the strength and leisure and zeal continually to enlarge my knowledge."– unknown

Introduction

Chronic Wound Care: A Clinical Source Book for Healthcare Professionals, Second Edition is a multidisciplinary book written by experts in the field of wound management. This book is filled with chapters of knowledge that healthcare professionals can benefit from. The educational needs and concerns are expressed throughout the many chapters.

"Without the education of healthcare professionals, any attempt to improve wound care for patients is likely to be frustrated. Educational requirements is an area that merits urgent attention."[1]

This chapter provides the essential strategies needed to ensure successful program development. It is not meant to be all encompassing but a blueprint for a strong program foundation (Figure 1). The discussion begins with an explanation of learning needs and program design and concludes with promotional strategies.

Learning Needs Assessment

A "learning needs" assessment is the infrastructure of the program. It will guide you to set activities appropriate to the expected outcomes and experiences of the audience. A common mistake of program planning is to assume that you know what adult healthcare professionals need to learn. It behooves the program chair/planner to take the time to assess the targeted audience's needs. A variety of data gathering techniques can be utilized: surveys, questionnaires, literature reviews, new trends/technology, peers in profession, past evaluation forms and expert opinion/faculty.

Creating a planning or advisory committee can be an invaluable asset for validating the needs of the target audience as well as for future assistance with other elements of planning.

Developing programs for a multidisciplinary audience that brings diverse experience and knowledge must also be addressed when assessing the needs of the group. Audiences, such as that of *Chronic Wound Care*, cross many continuums of care and represent many areas of practice, creating an added venture for the planning committee. The results of a learning needs assessment can then be utilized to explore which needs may be amenable to educational programming. Once completed, you will then be ready to design a program that addresses the audience's readiness to learn and willingness to participate in a learning experience relevant to their perceived needs and interest. A needs assessment cannot guarantee a successful program, but it certainly improves the odds.

Designing the Program

Once needs have been identified, the next step is to translate them into appropriate topics and content for the program. The development of topics and content is usually a major step in designing a program. This challenging task is best accomplished with a group discussion of a planning committee or selected panel of people whose input is respected in the field being addressed. If no planning committee is available, collaborate with peers, faculty, and administration. Remember, programs should reflect the needs and interests of the participants, not the planner or the planning committee.

Topics and titles. The breakdown or number of topics selected obviously depends on the length of the program being planned. Topics should fall into a logical sequence for short programs. Longer programs may present a myriad of topics and have many themes to cover. "Once topics have been selected the committee focuses on how to work the topics into the titles for the activity. A general suggestion is to use simple, down–to–earth titles, avoiding 'cute' ones, those that are in vogue, or those that include jargon that may be comprehensible only to persons in the "in–group."[2]

Titles should have a focal–point of interest to the participants. A title is the program's "drawing card;" it piques interest and therefore attendance. Multidisciplinary attendance is often "turned–off" by a title that refers to one discipline and excludes others. This is an important part of the designing efforts and should not be taken lightly.

The actual time it takes to plan a program depends on the complexity of the educational offering. According to Miller, "short learning activities that are one to two hours in length, take two to five weeks for planning. For longer programs, lasting one or two days, more lead time is needed. In general, fourteen to sixteen weeks is needed."[2] This is a significant part of planning; therefore, allowing enough time to develop the program should not be downsized. It is better to change the planning date than to go ahead and be disappointed with the results.

Objectives/Content. The objectives of the program are often another "selling point" for participants or those approving their attendance. Objectives need to be specific, not vague, and a benefit to the learner, institution or professional practice. Every effort needs to be taken to express the expected outcomes in measurable, behavioral objective terms. Participants want to know what they will get out of a session, what they will be able to do as a result, and/or how this program will impact their professional practice.

Puetz and Peters define an *objective* as a behavior desired as a result of the learning process.[3] They also define a *behavior* as a visible activity displayed by the learner (demonstrated, written, or verbal). Each objective should begin with a verb that describes the behavior; be stated in terms of the learner, not the person presenting; state only one expected behavior action (i.e. "define" and "describe" are two actions); involve a single sub-

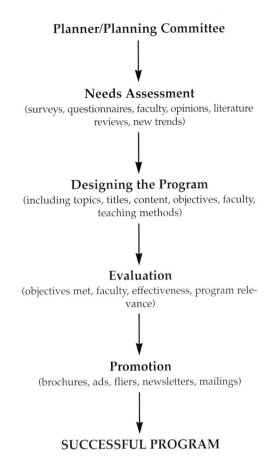

Planner/Planning Committee

↓

Needs Assessment
(surveys, questionnaires, faculty, opinions, literature reviews, new trends)

↓

Designing the Program
(including topics, titles, content, objectives, faculty, teaching methods)

↓

Evaluation
(objectives met, faculty, effectiveness, program relevance)

↓

Promotion
(brochures, ads, fliers, newsletters, mailings)

↓

SUCCESSFUL PROGRAM

Figure 1. Planning blueprint

ject, not state, three signs and symptoms of wound infection and the nursing interventions (this is two subjects); and be stated clearly so the reader will know what outcome is expected.

Bloom's Taxonomy is considered the "tried and true" approach in the development of learning objectives.[4] This approach divides learning into three parts: 1) cognitive domain, 2) affective domain, and 3) psychomotor domain.

"The first domain, *cognitive*, identifies needs that are met through knowledge, understanding, or thinking skills. The second, *affective*, deals with feelings, attitudes, and values. The final, *psychomotor*, deals with motor skills needed to perform a certain activity."[4] By using this classification system, the planners can determine that objectives are comprehensible to the identified learning needs. Objectives are the guidelines for determining appropriate content for each topic selected.

Faculty/Presenters/Speakers. The next step is to select faculty, presenters, or speakers that are experts in the topics chosen. Selecting faculty to present at a program can be very challenging and rewarding. Faculty are the "heart" of the program.

	S. Baranoski	J. Jones	B. Smith	D. White
Confirmation letter	✓	✓	✓	✓
Agreement letter	✓	✓	✓	✓
Objectives	✓		✓	
Content outlines	✓		✓	
Curriculum vitae				✓
Audiovisual needs	✓			
Handouts		✓	✓	
Travel arrangements	✓	✓	✓	✓
Hotel	✓	✓	✓	✓
Honoraria	✓		✓	
Social Security Number	✓	✓	✓	✓

Figure 2. *Faculty checklist*

Their ability to meet the needs of the audience will make or break the success of the program. Take time to investigate the "who's–who" of the topic and get the best qualified presenter(s) for the program. Attendees expect to be educated and informed and/or to enhance their practice by learning from presenters who have a strong reputation in the field, have experience that is current or advanced and have good presentation skills. Many of us have sat through a presentation only to be bored because the speaker read to the audience, had poor audiovisuals, or did not stick to the topic. It is wise to have heard speakers present first hand or to have knowledge of their style from respected peers before inviting them to participate.

Inviting faculty to speak means that the program planner has educated the faculty on topic, expected content, objectives, audience, and available audiovisuals. Any specific needs that the planning committee has suggested for a particular topic should be mentioned to the presenter. A commitment in writing is usually sent to the faculty members outlining the program expectations and his/her role. If the planner has not adequately informed the presenter, then the audience and program may not get what they expected.

Another point that needs to be mentioned to the presenter, especially in multidisciplinary programs, is the knowledge level of attendees. Programs that involve many disciplines, i.e. wound care conferences, have participants of varying levels of expertise in attendance. It is of benefit to the presenter to understand the makeup of the audience so that the lecture includes something for everyone. It may also be helpful to use a legend to rate the lecture expectation, such as basic, intermediate or advanced knowledge. This approach will assure that attendees have selected the level of knowledge they are seeking.

After all faculty have been determined, it is customary to send out a letter of agreement. This letter should cover all elements of the program. Include title of presentation, date, time presenting, social security number (needed if paying honoraria) audiovisual needs, biographical form (needed for continuing education hours), handout requests, duplication needs, and a deadline for returning this information. It is suggested that you call all faculty several weeks before the deadline submission. This allows those who have left things to the last minute to be courteously reminded. (A sample checklist of faculty needs is included in Figure 2.)

Biographical data or curriculum vitae (C–V) requests of faculty are needed if applying for continuing education hours. They are also useful for verifying the credentials of faculty. The detail of a biographical or C–V request varies with individual accrediting bodies. Usually a one page biographical history is adequate. Accrediting associations, i.e. ANCC, APTA, etc., will provide you with the necessary formats.

A program that provides continuing education (C.E.) hours is an added benefit to the attendee. Many states require a certain number of C.E. hours for licensure. It is recommended that all programs for healthcare professionals apply for appropriate C.E. hours. Any enhancement that encourages participation should be utilized.

Teaching methods/Materials. Teaching methods and materials should enhance the overall program. A joint decision by the planning committee and the faculty should be understood. The most common form of presentation is the basic lecture format followed by a question and answer period. Other options to consider are group breakout discussions, skill labs, case presentations, poster presentations, short abstract presentations and study guides.

Audiovisual needs must be considered in relationship to the size of the audience. Large groups often prefer slides or video enhancement instead of overhead projection which can be hard to read. Smaller groups can use workbooks, overheads, group discussions, or slides. Computer visualization is an excellent format, but it is quite costly and not available at all programs. Audiovisual needs, whatever they may be, are a very important part of the presentation to the audience. Give considerable thought to planning this element of the program.

Participants find it very helpful to have an outline of the program for each presented topic. Detailed outlines are preferred. Attendees then can concentrate on listening instead of writing notes. Many presenters will share a copy of their lecture presentation with the audience. Handouts and bibliographical references from the faculty are always an added plus for the program. Be sure to include extra paper for those who want to take detailed notes.

Participants need recognition, which can be accomplished by use of name tags that list name, credentials, position, institution, and city and state if out of town attendees are expected. Placement of the name tag is critical if it is to be useful. If placed on a belt loop it is useless. Consider what the armed services do: pin the name tag to the right lapel so it is easily read when shaking hands.

A list of attendees is beneficial; it allows continued networking to occur after the program. Other materials that can enhance the program are maps, location, directions, exhibitor information (if present), local restaurants, parking and taxi costs, and mention of food provided or on their own. (This same information should be part of the brochure or flier or advertisement process for marketing the program.)

Program Evaluation

The evaluation process is an important part of all educational offerings. It is designed to demonstrate that the participants have achieved the objectives they personally set as well as the objectives of the program. It should also be utilized to evaluate the effectiveness of faculty and the relevance of content to the overall program. Various standards or criteria must be evaluated if providing a C.E. program utilizing an "approved provider" status (ie. ANCC, APTA, etc.). These standards are part of the application process for continuing education hours.

Evaluation	Label Explanations
1 = Poor	**Speaker expertise:** Was the speaker knowledgeable in this area?
2 = Fair	
3 = Good	
4 = Excellent	**Content organization:** Was the content of the presentation easy to follow?

Speaker effectiveness: Did the speaker hold your attention, use methods to convey the content effectively?

Materials used: Did the materials used (slides, handouts, etc.) add to your understanding of the presentation?

Objectives met: How well did the session meet the stated objectives?

Relevance to practice: Can you use the information from this session in your practice?

Speaker Name: _____

Speaker expertise	1	2	3	4
Content organization	1	2	3	4
Speaker effectiveness	1	2	3	4
Materials used	1	2	3	4
Objectives met	1	2	3	4
Relevance to practice	1	2	3	4

Figure 3. Sample evaluation form, four point Likert scale

Objectives of the program become the criteria against which individuals conduct their evaluations. The program evaluation form should include a question asking individuals to rate the extent to which objectives were met, faculty effectiveness, and overall relevance of the program. A four or five point Likert scale is most often used (Figure 3). Additional questions, such as overall quality of program, physical facility appropriateness, suggestions for future topics, and locations are also beneficial to the evaluation process.

An evaluation provides the planner and/or committee with the opportunity to see the strengths and weaknesses of the program. It also allows them to improve their developmental skills for future endeavors. And most importantly, it provides the answer to the question, "Were objectives met?" An overview of the evaluations should be sent to the faculty presenters so that they may improve by way of feedback. Evaluations are an invaluable contribution to program planning and development.

Program Promotion

The final and integral step of program development is marketing. Most healthcare agencies have a marketing, media, or public relations department. Hopefully someone from this department has been involved with the planner and/or committee. If not, it is crucial that this person become involved and brought up to date with the program plans. His/her expertise is invaluable at getting a successful marketing plan set up.

Many factors go into marketing a successful program. One factor is the development of a time–line for promotional activities. There are standards in the world of advertising about "timely–appropriateness" of running ads and sending out brochures. Generally, "the timeline should include an eight to twelve week notice for participants. This means program information and brochures should be developed sixteen weeks before the program and mailed twelve to fourteen weeks in advance of the program."[2] Internal or community–based programs may require much less time.

Additional factors to consider are budget limitations, available resources, mailing lists, and whose responsibility it is to do all of the above. Again, the planning committee should be involved and have pieces of the marketing plan assigned. It is easier and less resource–intensive when a team approach is utilized.

Brochure development, design, color, logo, and layout can be handled by the marketing department or external resource. Remember, learner needs, objectives, and content are the deciding factors in participants selecting your program. Make sure they are clearly spelled out in the brochure, ads, fliers, or any media communications.

Mailing lists can be purchased through local, regional, or national associations. Utilize any previous program attendance lists and association directories.

The type and volume of promotional activities chosen should be gauged by the size of the program, the targeted audience, space limitations, budget limitations, and the overall purpose of the program.

Conclusion

This chapter has presented the knowledge, skills, and steps needed to succeed in planning professional programs. Included in this process are the essential steps of using a needs assessment and of designing content, topics, titles, objectives, faculty decisions, teaching methods, materials, the evaluation process, and basic marketing needs. The steps used should be viewed as a framework or guide for developing a chronic wound care program or any health related program.

It is my hope that by providing you, the reader, with practical information, you will find the road a bit easier to travel.

References

1. Harding KG. Wound care: Putting theory into clinical practice. In: Krasner D (ed). *Chronic Wound Care: A Clinical Source Book for Healthcare Professionals, First Edition*. King of Prussia, PA, Health Management Publications, Inc., 1990, p 29.
2. Miller PJ. Planning programs: Strategies for success. In: Kelly K (ed). *Nursing Staff Development Current Competence, Future Focus*. Philadelphia, PA, JB Lippincott Company, 1992, pp 117–154.
3. Puetz BE, Peters FL. *Continuing Education for Nurses, A Complete Guide to Effective Programs*. Aspen Publications, Rockville, MD, 1981.
4. Krathwol DR, Bloom BS, Masia B. *Taxonomy of Educational Objectives, Handbook*. David McKay, New York, NY, 1964.

38

Wound Care in Alternative Settings

Jan Cuzzell, MA, RN

Cuzzell J. Wound care in alternative settings. In: Krasner D, Kane D. *Chronic Wound Care, Second Edition.* Wayne, PA, Health Management Publications, Inc., 1997, pp 303–308.

Introduction

In order to fully appreciate the impact of wound care and delayed healing on patient outcomes and healthcare costs, treatment issues must be considered within the larger context of the U.S. healthcare delivery system. Wound care issues are common to all age groups and patient care settings: hospitals (including emergency rooms and burn centers), subacute and transitional care facilities, rehabilitation facilities, long term care facilities and retirement communities, home care, hospice care, and individual and group physician practices.

There is considerable cost associated with treating wounds.[1–3] In 1992 alone, nosocomial infections cost the healthcare system an estimated 4.5 billion dollars. Additional costs per patient were almost double for surgical wound infections ($3,152) compared to other types of infection ($1,617), and inpatient stay was extended by an average of 4.8 days. The cost of caring for chronic wounds is also a need for concern. In addition to an estimated 1992 expenditure of $570 million on wound care products, the intangible costs in labor, resources, and lost productivity are more difficult to quantify. A retrospective study by Frantz of pressure ulcer management in a long term care facility revealed nursing costs to be as much as three to ten times higher than the cost of supplies, regardless of ulcer severity. Similarly, the average cost to heal one venous leg ulcer is estimated by Wood to be $1,951, with costs of labor far exceeding that of supplies.

Although trends toward less invasive surgeries will decrease the potential for certain postoperative wound complications, changes in demography will significantly impact future wound care needs.[4] The elderly population is the fastest growing segment of our population, with those 85 years and older the fastest growing cohort of all. Between 1995 and 2075, the 65 and older age bracket is expected to increase by 145 percent, the 75 and older age bracket by 205 percent, and the 85 and older bracket by 345 percent. The implications inherent in these projections are significant, especially when considering the potential impact on wound care trends. An aging population is at much higher risk for undergoing surgical procedures and, more importantly, experiencing problems with delayed healing. In addition, the elderly are more prone to developing chronic wound problems such as leg ulcers due to poor circulation and pressure ulcers from immobility.

Hospitals

The old paradigm of healthcare is failing, primarily because of spiraling healthcare costs.[5] In the 19th Century, the Diagnostic Related Group (DRG) was introduced as a mechanism to manage reimbursement and better control the costs associated with hospitalization. However, ushering in the 21st Century are healthcare reform mandates that call for even more drastic measures to increase the efficiency of healthcare delivery systems while further reducing spending. The impact on hospitals will not only be in terms of decreased length of stay, but also in overall utilization of inpatient services. With current trends moving in the direction of managed competition and capitated payments, it is predicted that inpatient utilization may decrease as much as 50 percent in the coming years. As a result, wound diagnostic procedures, complex wound treatments, and related surgeries will increasingly be performed in less–costly outpatient settings such as wound clinics.

With decreased inpatient utilization, progressive downsizing of hospital administrative and professional staff and redesign of work processes are also likely to occur.[6] Nonprofessional staff will be trained to perform tasks such as simple dressing changes, and professional nurses will assume a less "hands–on" role. Highly specialized caregiver roles, such as Wound Specialists, will most likely be merged into fewer, more general roles with increased fiscal responsibilities for the care delivered.

Delayed healing and risk for nosocomial complications, such as wound infections and pressure ulcers, have the potential to negatively impact both the length of stay and the hospital readmission rate. For this reason one might expect a renewed interest in prevention and early detection of nosocomial skin and wound complications, an increased emphasis on staff education, and introduction of innovative methods to move patients safely and efficiently from inpatient to outpatient settings without sacrificing continuity of care. Multi–disciplinary clinical pathways or "maps" are one answer to streamlining patient care across the continuum of healing.[7] However, "user friendly" wound pathways are difficult to design and implement due to the multiplicity of diagnoses and variances that can occur with individual patients. The first conceptual model for a wound care clinical pathway that can be adapted to multiple wound types and patient care settings was introduced in 1996 by Barr and Cuzzell.[8] While the validity and reliability of this tool is yet to be proven, this model provides a practical alternative to managing the outcomes of complex wounds across the healing continuum.

A variety of traumatic injuries such as abrasions, lacerations, puncture wounds, animal bites and minor burns are commonly treated in the hospital emergency room (ER). Hospitals lacking ambulatory care services for follow–up treatment commonly have these patients return to the ER for dressing changes and suture removal. While use of the ER for nonemergent care can be revenue–producing, it contributes to inefficient use of space, equipment, and staff. Customer complaints are common and usually a result of long waiting periods to receive care while staff attend to more urgent problems. In addition, patient outcomes may be adversely affected by a lack of wound care expertise and caregiver continuity. This is especially true in patients at high risk for wound–related complications. In the future, hospitals can be predicted to seek alternative settings to off–set inappropriate utilization of ER services. Opening or aligning with outpatient wound clinics is one solution to this problem.

Burn Centers are by far the most specialized inpatient wound treatment facilities. The prolonged recovery time associated with catastrophic burn injury has traditionally required lengthy hospitalization. Likewise, the unique psychosocial and rehabilitative problems of the burn victim discourage early discharge, primarily because of the lack of coordinated outpatient services and expertise needed to provide adequate care. On the other hand, minor burns can easily be managed on an outpatient basis. Most minor burns are treated in the ER and released. Because of the complex nature of burn injuries compared to other traumatic wounds, even minor burns can result in scarring, loss of function, and permanent disability if mismanaged. As economic pressures continue to result in selective admissions and earlier discharge, providing quality burn care in outpatient settings will prove especially challenging to the healthcare system.

Subacute and Transitional Care Facilities

Subacute and Transitional Care Facilities are increasing in number in response to the need to decrease length of stay in acute care facilities. Interestingly, many subacute facilities are incorporating a "Wound Care" unit or floor. This approach suggests that wound–related problems are more often than not associated with prolonged hospitalization and require specialized treatment to obtain optimal outcomes. However, wound care specialization is in its infancy in this setting. The patient population in general is at high risk for skin breakdown and delayed healing. In the future, optimal and cost–effective patient outcomes may depend largely on the availability of "expert" resources to assist with care planning, as well as educational preparation of the staff in wound prevention and treatment.

Rehabilitation Facilities

While rehabilitation is a specialty in and of its own, the future survival of rehabilitation facilities is dependent on alignment with acute care and other settings so that rehab services can be provided across the continuum of recovery.[9] A large population of patients treated in rehabilitation facilities have diagnoses associated with chronic, slow–healing wounds. Victims of spinal cord injury, stroke and major burns, to name a few, require ongoing intervention to prevent and treat skin complications. Some physical and occupational therapists have limited education in the pathophysiology of wound healing. Consequently, some complex wound problems have the potential to be managed with less than optimal results. An increased focus on education and the availability of highly specialized wound consultants to serve as a resource for protocol development and care management would greatly enhance the quality of service provided in most rehabilitation settings.

Long Term Care Facilities

Nursing homes have long been plagued with wound care problems. Either patients are admitted from the acute or home care setting with open wounds, or a lack of emphasis on prevention results in a high incidence of skin breakdown and pressure ulcers. The problem is compounded by a lack of "on–site" professional staff to manage care as well as by limited availability of skin care equipment and supplies. The average incidence of pressure–related complications in long term care is estimated at 20 percent.[10] Of the patients that develop skin breakdown, many require readmission to acute care facilities for septicemia and other wound–related complications. In fact, the problem of pressure ulcers has become so great that in 1990 the Agency for Health Care Policy and Research (AHCPR) reported that costs associated with the treatment of pressure ulcers ranked as one of the top seven conditions initially targeted by the U.S. Department of Health and Human Services for the development of clinical practice guidelines. Federal guidelines for pressure ulcer prevention and treatment have recently been published. (See Chapter 5) Unfortunately, compliance with these guidelines currently remains at the discretion of the facility. As federal and state regulation of this problem gains momentum, nursing homes will be incentivised to comply with accepted standards of care.

Home and Hospice Care

Home care remains one of the fastest–growing and most economical settings in which to render wound care. A study of four healthcare agencies in Florida in 1991 showed that patients with wounds accounted for 31 percent of the admissions to all four agencies combined.[11] Of that 31 percent, over half the wounds were pressure ulcers (30.2 percent) or draining surgical wounds (31.2 percent). The average cost of healing a wound, including supplies, averaged $13,120 compared to a previously estimated $40,000 in other settings. Although this study supports economical care in the home, it is important to note that only 36.3 percent of all wounds treated were healed during the period of time skilled nursing care was delivered. This fact suggests that wound care expertise is also lacking in home care, and that increased emphasis needs to be placed on standardization of treatment protocols and problem–specific patient outcomes.

The status of wound management among home health agencies is further supported by a 1993 study that showed of 296 agencies responding to a survey,

a majority (56 percent) did not have written policies and procedures specific to wound management.[12] What is needed is a standardized program of education and skills certification in wound management that prepares all professional and nonprofessional staff to deliver a higher level of care. With standardization of specialty–related policies and procedures, the availability of wound care specialists to help with problem–solving, and increased emphasis on educating the client and caregiver in wound prevention, better outcomes can be expected in fewer visits.

Independent and Group Physician Practices

Wound care is one of the few problems that is common to all medical and surgical specialties — family practice, endocrinology, infectious disease medicine, gerontology, plastic surgery, dermatology, obstetrics, orthopedics, vascular surgery, pediatrics, and general surgery. With the exception of surgeons, most physicians have traditionally preferred to treat primary medical problems and leave wound care decisions to nursing. Reluctance on the part of physicians to aggressively treat wounds is explained in part by the fact that wound healing has only recently emerged as a science. Many of these clinicians still practice outdated treatment modalities with the expectation that slow–to–heal or non–healing wounds are acceptable complications of certain disease processes. In addition, many physicians have been reluctant to refer a patient to a specialist for evaluation for fear of losing the patient to another doctor.

In the managed care environment, the need for specialized wound care becomes an even greater issue. Avoiding unnecessary complications and hospitalization is key to controlling healthcare costs. Both the failure of traditional medicine to address wound care needs and the increasing demand for better outcomes are reflected in the recent emergence of specialized wound care clinics.

While the concept of specialized wound clinics is a sound one, clinics that focus on a limited wound type or therapy fail to meet the wound care needs of the larger population. A successful managed care system requires treatment options for all wound types, both acute and chronic, as well as a range of therapies to address individual patient needs in all settings.

Wound Care Solutions in a Managed Care Environment

Non–healing wounds and wound care are a common denominator to patient outcomes in all

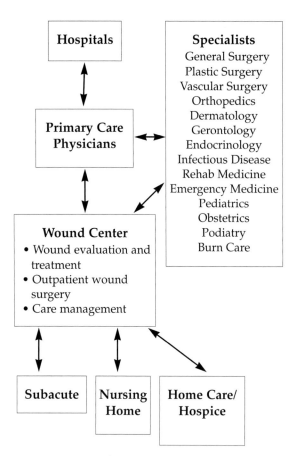

	Specialists
Hospitals	**Specialists** General Surgery Plastic Surgery Vascular Surgery Orthopedics Dermatology Gerontology Endocrinology Infectious Disease Rehab Medicine Emergency Medicine Pediatrics Obstetrics Podiatry Burn Care

Primary Care Physicians

Wound Center
- Wound evaluation and treatment
- Outpatient wound surgery
- Care management

Subacute   **Nursing Home**   **Home Care/ Hospice**

Figure 1. Integrated wound management services

healthcare settings. In the managed care environment, optimal and cost–effective care depends on integration of patient care services across the continuum of healing.[13] Service integration requires several components: 1) an information system that facilitates communication of wound care services within multiple settings; 2) access to a comprehensive, outpatient wound center or clinic; 3) educational programs designed to maintain wound care knowledge and skills at all levels; 4) standardized prevention programs specific to each setting; 5) standardized wound assessment and treatment plans that provide for a continuum of care between settings; 6) coordination of care by wound specialists; and 7) ongoing evaluation of patient outcome based on wound type.

In most systems, implementation of this concept is most easily accomplished through reorganization and integration of existing services, and introduction of standardized methodologies (Figure 1).

Information System

A key component to the success of an integrated model is a state–of–the–art information system that allows healthcare providers in different settings to have ready access to patient information. Theoretically, patients with more complex wounds, such as major burns or dehisced surgical wounds, could be discharged to a subacute unit or home much earlier if up–to–date information regarding wound progress was available at the punch of a button. As new technology emerges, the potential for monitoring wounds from a central location using computer–generated images becomes more likely. With an effective information system, not only is productivity and quality of care enhanced, but the cost and inconvenience of unnecessary hospitalization can be minimized.

Wound Centers

While oversight of patients with wounds can be centralized to any location, the ideal location is an outpatient wound clinic. There are many advantages to this approach, but the major objective is to centralize wound expertise in a setting that provides "one–stop–shopping" for patients that require on–site evaluation and intervention.

With the exception of major surgeries such as vascular reconstruction, amputations and tissue flaps, most wound care procedures can be easily and safely accomplished in an outpatient setting. In addition, the full range of services necessary for comprehensive wound care (including treatment plan management) are far more convenient to the patient and easier to coordinate in a single location. Ideally, clinic services should include wound–specific treatment plan management, outpatient surgery, vascular assessment, nutritional consultation, orthotics evaluation and fitting, podiatry consultation and services, medical equipment and supplies, rehabilitation consultation and services, IV infusion capabilities, and access to transportation services.

Unlike current trends in outpatient wound clinics, a full scope of services must be made available for all wound types, both acute and chronic. A different approach to organization of services and a higher level of medical and nursing expertise than are currently available in most wound clinics today are thus required.

Model A: Physician–Run Center

With this model, the center is run by one or more physicians who have chosen to specialize specifically in wound care. Experience has shown that finding dedicated physicians that are willing to devote their practice to the wound care specialty is difficult if not impossible. Most physicians interested in wounds, e.g. vascular surgeons or plastic surgeons, have experience with only one or two wound types. They are not always comfortable treating the range of complex problems and chronic complications encountered in an integrated delivery system. However, with the availability of standardized "problem–specific" medical protocols and a state–of–the–art information system to facilitate the consultation process, this obstacle can be overcome. In addition, Model A is easily adaptable to university–affiliated hospitals where a residency program provides the physician support needed as the practice grows.

Centralized management of patient care within the integrated system is ideally conducted by nursing experts in wound care, such as Enterostomal Therapy Nurses, Clinical Specialists, and Nurse Practitioners. These nurses use standardized clinical pathways as guidelines to move patients safely through the system and to coordinate outpatient follow–up. They also serve as nursing resources to assist with problem–solving wound management issues in acute care, subacute facilities, nursing homes, and home care. To preserve the "one–stop–shopping" concept, additional services such as nutritional counseling, rehabilitation, and orthotics evaluation may either be housed on–site or scheduled on–site at prearranged times.

It is also recommended that home care nurses be available to accompany their patients to the wound center when possible. The advantage of this approach is that it allows home care nurses to communicate directly with the physician in the patient's presence and to participate actively in multi–disciplinary care planning. Home care provided by skilled nurses who understand the care plan and treatment goals not only promotes increased continuity and better outcomes, but also decreases the number of clinic visits required. Also, home care nurses can be easily cross–trained to perform clinic responsibilities as well as wound care services in other settings. This cross– training promotes more cost–effective utilization of staff while at the same time helping the home care nurse maintain a high skill level (Figure 2).

Model B: Nurse–Managed Center

In this model, physician support is provided by a group of specialists with "on–site" practices similar to a group practice. Wound patients are referred to the appropriate medical specialist for initial evaluation and treatment based on wound type. Coordination of referrals, follow–up care, and ongoing management of the treatment plan is performed by a Nurse Practitioner with specialized training in wound care. Depending on the size of the system and patient volume, additional staffing is provided by enterostomal therapists or professional nurses with specialized training.

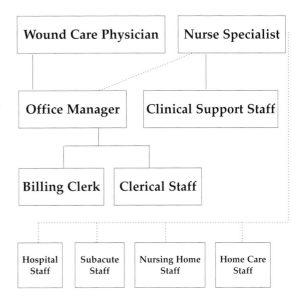

Figure 2. Model A

A major advantage of this model is that outpatient follow–up for routine dressing changes and post–op evaluation can be conducted by the Nurse Practitioner (or a Physician's Assistant). These routine visits are time–consuming and primarily focused on patient education, better utilization of a nurses's time as compared to a physician's. Again, standardized wound care protocols and clinical pathways are used to guide intervention and insure optimal outcomes. As with Model A, additional services such as dietary consultation, rehabilitation, and orthotics evaluation as well as home care may either be housed on–site or available on–site at prearranged times (Figure 3).

Standardization and Education

Care delivery is facilitated through standardization of educational programs, prevention strategies, and wound treatment protocols. Protocols can be customized based on physician preference. However, optimal patient outcomes require input from national wound care experts with routine protocol revisions based on the most current research findings. In addition, educational programs and quality improvement activities, planned and conducted by national experts, enhance program credibility.

Outcome Evaluation

The ability to track the outcomes of patients with complex wounds is key to the successful integration

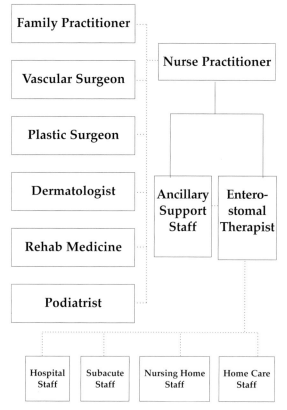

| Family Practitioner |
| Vascular Surgeon |
| Plastic Surgeon |
| Dermatologist |
| Rehab Medicine |
| Podiatrist |

| Nurse Practitioner |

| Ancillary Support Staff | Entero-stomal Therapist |

| Hospital Staff | Subacute Staff | Nursing Home Staff | Home Care Staff |

Figure 3. Model B

of multiple disciplines, a necessary component to marketing services in a managed care environment. This ability also provides a mechanism for continuous improvement of care rendered. One assessment tool has recently been introduced for monitoring pressure ulcer progress and further adapted for computer application.[14,15] (See Barbara Bates–Jensens' Chapter 6 on pressure ulcer assessment and documentation.) Using this system, wound assessment information is collected, quantified, and stored in a central data base. Outcome tracking for participating facilities can be performed on a routine basis, directing changes in therapy and providing essential documentation of patient care. Application of such a system to multiple wound types would greatly facilitate outcome measurement in the clinical setting. Generation of a national "wound care" data base with which to perform comparative analysis could enhance communication between clinicians, and potentially advance the practice of wound care in all settings. However, the validity and reliability of such data needs to be considered carefully as does the ease with which such a tool can be implemented in the clinical arena and across multiple settings.

Conclusion

With the advent of managed care, management of patients with acute and chronic wounds will change dramatically. To provide quality care across the continuum of healing, the traditional boundaries that have segregated care in alternative settings will need to dissolve. The result will be a seamless wound care delivery system with common goals and focused outcomes. Only through a pooling of resources, shared expertise, improved communication, and standardization of treatment modalities can wound care advocates hope to meet the challenges of healthcare reform in the 21st Century.

References

1. MMWR. Public Health Focus: Surveillance, prevention, and control of nosocomial infections. *MMWR* 1992;41:783–787.
2. Frantz RA. Pressure ulcer costs in long–term care. *Decubitus* 1989;2:56–57.
3. Wood CR, Margolis DJ. The cost of treating venous leg ulcers to complete healing using an occlusive dressing and a compression bandage. *Wounds* 1992;4:138–141.
4. Health Care Financing Administration; Social Security Administration, Office of Programs: 1993 Data from the Office of the Actuary.
5. Blancett SS, Flarey DL. Changing paradigms: The impetus to reengineer healthcare. In: Blancett SS, Flarey DL (eds). *Reengineering Nursing and Healthcare: The Handbook for Organizational Transformation.* Gaithersburg, MD, Aspen Publishers, Inc., 1995, pp 3–14.
6. Hansen RB, Sayers B. *Work and Role Redesign: Tools and Techniques for the Healthcare Setting.* Chicago, IL, American Hospital Publishing Company, Inc., 1995.
7. Zander K. Caremap systems and case management: Creating waves of restructured care. In: Blancett SS, Flarey DL (eds). *Reengineering Nursing and Healthcare: The Handbook for Organizational Transformation.* Gaithersburg, MD, Aspen Publishers, Inc., 1995, 203–222.
8. Barr JE, Cuzzell J. Wound care clinical pathway: A conceptual model. *Ostomy/Wound Management* 1996;42(7):18–26.
9. Wolf M. Surviving in healthcare. *Rehabilitation* 1995;4(2):11–13.
10. Panel for the Prediction and Prevention of Pressure Ulcers in Adults: *Treatment of Pressure Ulcers.* Clinical Practice Guideline, Number 15. AHCPR Publication No. 95–0652. Rockville, MD: Agency for Health Care Policy and Research, Public Health Service, U.S. Department of Health and Human Services, December 1994.
11. Arnold N. A study of wound healing in home care. *Ostomy/Wound Management* 1992;38(7):38–44.
12. Goldrick B, Larson E. Wound management in home care: An assessment. *Journal of Community Health Nursing* 1993;10(1):23–29.
13. Porter–O'Grady T. Reengineering in a reformed health care system. In: Blancett SS, Flarey DL (eds). *Reengineering Nursing and Healthcare: The Handbook for Organizational Transformation.* Gaithersburg, MD, Aspen Publishers, Inc., 1995, pp 47–49.
14. New Products. *Ostomy/Wound Management* 1995;41(5):72.
15. Bates–Jensen BM. Indices to include in wound healing assessment. *Advances in Wound Care* 1995;8(4):25–33.

Section III

THE CUTTING EDGE

39

Running an Outpatient Wound Center

Laurel A. Wiersema–Bryant, MSN, RN, CS, ANP

Author. Chapter title. In: Krasner D, Kane D. *Chronic Wound Care, Second Edition*. Wayne, PA, Health Management Publications, Inc., 1997, pp 309–320.

Introduction

In this chapter, the development of an outpatient wound center for the care and management of non–healing and chronic wounds is discussed. Providing for the coordinated management of patients with wounds is the focus of an outpatient wound center.

The concept of a multidisciplinary team approach to the care of patients with wounds is not new. Utilization of the team approach in the care and management of wounds has been encouraged in acute care and long–term care for some time. Data exist to support the influence of the team approach in achieving cost–effective outcomes. An increasing number of patients with wounds are being cared for in the outpatient arena.[1] A quick look at where these patients are being managed reveals home care, general practitioner offices, the offices of general surgery, dermatology, rheumatology, hematology/oncology, internal medicine, plastic surgery, orthopedic surgery, cardiology and vascular surgery. Management of these patients is as varied as the settings, so coordination of care can be difficult.

In response to the increasing number of patients with non–healing and chronic wounds, more and more wound care clinics are being developed. A well–planned, well–coordinated wound care clinic provides for comprehensive assessment, medical and surgical management, state–of– the–art treatment and follow–up care. The clinic should not be conceived as a place of last resort for treatment failures, but as a central place for the management of wounds.

This chapter will discuss the process of establishing a wound care center and ongoing management of the clinic.

Identification of the Need

The initial step in the development of a wound care clinic is the identification of the need for such a service. Market research must provide clear, concise information about the need for the clinic. Utilize a marketing department, if available, to assist in the needs assessment process. Information regarding the demographics of the population served by your facility, referral patterns and networks, the proximity of similar services and willingness of other providers to refer patients is information which should be included in the market research.

Demographic data is necessary for the ultimate volume forecast: (1) What is the specific geographic and clinical population to be served by the program? (2) What are the demographics of the population to be served? Demographic data should also include population age, mobility, transportation type and needs, physical needs, and the types of wounds to be seen. This information is critical in planning for the type of space needed for the center and the necessary support services. (3) Where is the care of these patients currently provided? It is important here to evaluate both internal and external competitors to the proposed clinic. Competition for patients may be detrimental to the success of the clinic. Therefore, the proximity of other similar clinics or centers offering similar services must be assessed. (4) What is the reimbursement pattern for the expected patient volume? Important to assess here is the probable mix of private pay, private insurance, Medicare, Medicaid, and healthcare contracts. If your outpatient facility depends heavily on negotiated contracts it is critical that those in the position of negotiating the contracts be aware of the service.

From the geographic and demographic information, assumptions need to be made regarding the

Table 1
Patient characteristics and potential needs to be considered

Patient Characteristic	Special Needs	Access Required
Ambulatory	– None required	– Routine – Easy access to parking is helpful – Valet parking is helpful
Wheelchair bound	– Disability access – May need lift assistance to examine – Examination rooms which accommodate wheelchair	– Located with ready access from disabled parking – Valet parking is helpful. – Wheelchairs available near facility entrance for patients
Stretcher bound	– Ready access for transport/ambulance to deliver patient for the visit – Lift assistance may be required. – Examination rooms which accommodate stretcher/bed	– Movement of stretcher-boundpatients may be restricted to area of access – evaluate routes when selecting clinic location – A hospital bed or stretche may need to be available
Other Special Needs Patients	– The weight–challengedpatient may require the availability of furniture throughout the clinic which will accommodate weight in excess of 400 pounds	– Patient scales which range from 0 to 750 pounds – Waiting room furniture which is rated to 750 pounds – Lift assistance may be required – Examination table/chair which will accommodate to 750 pounds – Assorted sizes of BP cuffs – Patient gowns in size 5X to 8X

anticipated volume of patients to be seen during years one to five. The projected volume of service should be described by visit type, procedures, and. Another aspect of volume projection is the opportunity for secondary inpatient admissions, surgical procedures and referrals to other ancillary services as a result of the clinic volume. Will inpatient days be reduced by offering the program and can resource utilization be contained, further showing cost justification for the service? Finally, one needs to take a critical look at commitment by the physician community to refer patients to the center. Can you obtain physician commitment to the volume assumptions? Are there physician leaders who can be identified as supporters and potential partners in the wound clinic venture?

Other potential influences on the success of the clinic require one to take a critical look at environmental trends which may impact the future of the clinic. These trends may include, but are not limited to, political, legal, economic and social arenas.

Once the need for the clinic has been identified and supported with research based facts, the next step is to write the proposal for the service.

Planning for Success

The business plan should be written to incorporate the data obtained during the market research phase of the project. Key elements of the business plan include introduction, description of the business, market and competition analysis, product

Table 2
Equipment to be considered when setting up a wound care center

General	Specific
	Wound care supplies:
Reception area	Dressings which meet protocols
MD office	Diagnostic testing facilities (Vascular)
Storage space	35 mm Camera with macro lens and ring flash
4 to 6 exam rooms with:	Wound measuring guides (clear with mm grid)
Exam table	Transcutaneous Oxygen monitor
Good lighting	Documentation system (computer based?)
Stretcher/bed access (?)	Tape measuring device
Sphygmomanometer with cuffs in a variety of	Transparency film, or other clear film for wound
sizes	tracing
Linen	Digitizing palette
Oxygen access (if plan includes TCO2 monitoring)	
Vacuum access (if plan includes wound cleansing	
devices which require suction)	
Doppler(s)	

(Equipment needed will vary based on the type of patients expected in the clinic)

development, marketing and distribution plan, organizational plan, development schedule, financial plan, executive summary.[2]

In determining the direction and focus of the wound clinic, it is important to write a Mission Statement. This statement should be global in scope and provide a shared sense of purpose, direction and achievement.[3] Once written, the Mission Statement will help to define and focus the remainder of the plan. The plan should include both short term (1 year) and long term (3 to 5 year) goals. The goals should include, but not be limited to, patient/visit volume projections, growth in the type of services provided, research opportunities, monitors for success of the clinic, and cost savings to the institution (if hospital based).

Assuming the research phase has supported the need for the wound clinic, there are a few additional operational issues which need to be assessed. These issues include the size and type of space needed by the population expected to be served, any special equipment which will be needed, and staffing needs. These issues tie directly into the financial plan.

Location . The space needed requires a careful, thorough evaluation of the patient population expected (Table 1). This information should be available as a result of the market research data. The following questions must be explored: Is existing space available for the clinic? Where is the space located? If the space available is a multifunction area, is the time slot open that is needed to run the clinic efficiently? How

and by whom are the staff to be trained? How accessible is the location to patients? Do you anticipate patients arriving by ambulance, wheelchair, ambulatory? Should the patients be wheelchair or bed–bound, are stretchers/beds available for them in the facility? Is there space to accommodate stretcher/bed–bound patients? Should the patient require lift or transfer assistance, is the appropriate lift equipment available, or are other means of assisting with patient lifting utilized in your setting? If the space available does not accommodate stretcher patients, the type of patient seen may need to be restricted to those who are ambulatory or wheelchair bound. Also, if the appropriate lift equipment is not available, this equipment will need to be added to the start–up costs.

Equipment. Equipment needs will be determined by the type of services to be provided by the clinic. When setting up one clinic a few years ago, it was determined that existing space could be utilized; therefore, all traditional examination room equipment was already available. The clinic referred patients to the vascular laboratory when vascular testing was required and referrals were made to orthotics/prosthetics when indicated. The only major purchase needed was a good 35 mm camera with a macro lens and a ring flash for wound photography. As the clinic has grown, the services added include the presence of an orthotist during clinic hours and the presence of a vendor representative for durable medical equipment. These additions allow patients to obtain

Table 3
An example of an organizational structure for a wound center

Medical Director

Clinic Services		Ancillary Services	
Physicians	Nurses and Allied Health	Office Staff	Other
Vascular Surgeon	Program Director (CNS/ET)	Secretary/Receptionist	Housekeeping
Plastic Surgeon	Staff Nurses	Billing Coordinator	Materials Mgmt
Internist	Techs	Marketing	Lift orderlies
Orthopedic Surgeon	Diabetes CNS		
Pain Management	Dietician		
Behavioral Medicine	Physical Therapist		
	Social Services		

wound care supplies and any support equipment at the time of the visit and minimize the need for them to go shopping after they leave the office (Table 2).

Personnel. Methods of staffing the wound clinic and the organizational structure of the staff may take any of a variety of forms. Generally, staffing requires a Medical Director and a program manager (a clinical nurse specialist, ET nurse, or another nurse knowledgeable in the management of non–healing and chronic wounds), nurses skilled in performing wound care, and a secretary and/or receptionist. Larger clinics may include additional staff (for example, additional physicians representing specialties not represented by the Medical Director, physical therapists, dietician, orthotist, social worker, home health nurses, or a combination of these). As these patients tend to require more nursing time in care and teaching, it may be beneficial to staff the clinic with technical persons who are trained to perform the basics, such as vital signs, dressing removal and basic wound care. Ancillary staff include laboratory technicians, financial, legal, supply, and housekeeping personnel.

The organizational structure establishes the chain of command, and the authority ascribed to the members of the structure can be delineated in the job descriptions (Table 3). The job descriptions should provide minimum preparation for the position as well as detailed responsibilities for each member of the team. Expectations should be clear and accepted by both the employer and employee. Intervals for performance appraisal should also be identified.

Daily Operations

Scheduling. The actual daily operations of the wound clinic will depend on a number of factors. If the clinic is set up as a part–time service in a multi–function area, the time of actual patient visits will be confined to designated hours and day(s) of the week. The opportunity afforded by initially opening as a part–time service takes advantage of existing space, and to some degree, existing staff. This scenario provides low start–up cost relative to hiring staff and renting space for a full–time service. A part–time service also allows for patient volume to build gradually, which is especially important if the volume data gathered during the assessment phase was largely theoretical. One difficulty with a part–time service is providing patients with access to the staff in order to have questions or problems managed after clinic hours. This problem can be easily handled with appropriate telephone triage, but needs to be planned prior to the first patient visit. Problems or concerns rarely seem to occur during clinic hours.

The number of patients scheduled during a given time will depend on the type of visit and the level of acuity. Scheduling is a challenge, as patient visits generally require a disproportionate amount of nursing to physician time. This difficulty can result in lack of efficiency, especially for the physicians. The amount of time needed for direct care, for teaching and support, and for assessment needs to be carefully accounted. It may be helpful to have a schedule which allows for patient support and teaching after evaluation by the physician(s) and after physician hours in the clinic. It is helpful to be generous when initially scheduling patients as well as allowing a greater amount of time for initial visits than for follow–up visits.

If testing is required, it is wise to schedule this test to allow time for the results to be obtained by the clinic staff prior to the patient's next appointment. Ideally, non–invasive testing can be performed at the time of the initial visit. Patients referring to the wound clinic may arrive with test results from their referral source,

WOUND CARE CENTER
PATIENT HEALTH HISTORY

Name: _____ Date: _____
Primary Physician: _____
Physician Address: _____
Physician Phone Number: _____
Referred by: _____
Significant other/Relationship: _____
                    Phone Number: _____
Home Health Agency/Phone Number: _____
Home Health Nurse: _____

Wound History:
Reason for your visit to the Wound Care Center: _____
_____
_____
Please describe your symptoms and when they began: _____
_____
_____
Have you been treated for this in the past? **Yes   No**
   If yes, when: _____
   If yes, by whom: _____
What has been tried? _____
_____
What are you doing presently? _____
Do you currently do your own wound care? **Yes   No**
   If no, who assists you? _____

Medical History:
Allergies: _____
_____
Previous Surgeries:
(please list)

Surgery/Hospitalization	Year

Current Medications: (please list)

Medication	Dosage/Frequency	How long

Figure 1a.

Please circle those health problems that apply to you:

HEAD	NEUROMUSCULAR	RHEUMATOLOGIC
Dizziness	Stroke	Arthritis
Frequent Headache	Contractures	Joint pain/swelling
Head injury	Spinal Cord injury	Redness of joints
Eye Problems	Loss of feeling in legs	Vasculitis
Seizures		Lupus

LUNGS	CARDIOVASCULAR	HEMATOLOGIC
Asthma	Angina	Blood thinning
Bronchitis	Blood clots	medications
Chronic Cough	Heart Attack	Sickle Cell Disease
Emphysema	Heart Failure	Easy Bruising
Short of breath	High Blood Pressure	Phlebitis
TB	Irregular Heart beat	Anemia
	Pacemaker	

DERMATOLOGIC	Palpitations	GI
Skin allergies	Swelling of feet/legs	Colitis
Dermatitis	Varicose Veins	Inflammatory bowel
Eczema		disease
Rashes		Hepatitis
Itching/Pruritus	ONCOLOGIC	Jaundice
Scleroderma	Cancer:	Liver Disease
	Type: _____	Bowel Incontinence
	Location: _____	
KIDNEY/BLADDER	Received Chemotherapy	MISCELLANEOUS
Kidney Disease	Received Radiation	Diabetes
Hemodialysis		Thyroid Problems
Urinary incontinence		

FAMILY HISTORY:
Cancer   Diabetes   High Blood Pressure   TB   Heart Disease

Do you smoke? **Yes**   **No**
  If yes, for how long: _____ how much? _____
  If you stopped smoking, how long has it been since you last smoked? _____

Do you drink alcohol? **Yes**   **No**
  If yes, how often? **Daily**   **Weekly**   **Occasionally**   **Socially**

Do you exercise? **Yes**   **No**
  If yes, describe: _____
  If no, what limits you: _____

Figure 1b.

which further facilitate the visit. When testing is required, the patient may require an appointment of several hours in duration; this needs to be considered in the schedule.

The patient visit will be further expedited if additional information is available prior to the visit. For example, when a patient arriving on a stretcher may require a specific exam room, this information should be communicated and the appropriate room reserved. Perhaps a patient is bed–bound and needs to be weighed. With appropriate planning, an appropriate bed scale can be available, as well as the staff to perform the weighing procedure. Patients requiring special assistance may be coded on the schedule to allow

NUTRITION QUESTIONNAIRE

Name: _____   Date: _____

Age: _____   Height: _____   Weight: _____

(please circle your answer)

1.   Have you had any weight change over the past 6 months?
      Yes   **No**

      If so, how much? _____ Gain   _____ Loss
      Was the weight change **planned or unintentional?**

2.   How would you describe your appetite?
      Excellent   Good   Fair   Poor

3.   Do you have difficulty chewing or swallowing?
      Yes   No

4.   Is there anything that interferes with your ability to eat well balanced meals?
      Yes   No

      If yes, what? _____
      _____
      _____

5.   Do you have any **nausea, vomiting, constipation or diarrhea?**

6.   Are you taking any vitamin or mineral supplements?
      Yes   No

      If yes, what? _____

7.   Are you taking any high calorie high protein oral supplement?
      Yes _____   **No**

8.   Are you restricting anything in your diet?
      Yes _____   **No**
      _____

9.   Have you seen a dietitian in the past year?
      Yes   No

      If yes, when? _____
      why? _____
      where? _____

Figure 1c.

for further efficiency in, for example, lift assistance, specific exam room, testing, and procedures.

Assessment. Patient assessment and, specifically, wound assessment can take many forms. In general, a careful medical history and physical exam should be performed. Laboratory studies may be ordered which should include a complete blood count, a blood sugar count, and, if needed, a hemoglobin

BACKGROUND
Primary Med. Dx. _____
Primary Nurse Dx. _____
Wound Duration _____
Current Tx. _____
Contr. Med. Dx. _____
Braden Risk Score _____
Wound Type _____
Race _____ Pigmentation:__Dark ___Medium ___Light

Location: Anatomic site. Identify right(R) or left(L); number if multiple and mark diagram accordingly:

_____ Sacrum and coccyx	_____ Lateral ankle	
_____ Trochanter	_____ Medial ankle	
_____ Ischial tuberosity	_____ Heel	Other site _____

Shape: Overall wound pattern; assess by observing perimeter and depth. Check appropriate description: (number as in location if necessary)

_____ Irregular	_____ Linear or elongated	
_____ Round/oval	_____ bowl/boat	
_____ Square/rectangle	_____ Butterfly	Other shape_____

ITEM	ASSESSMENT	DATE:	DATE:
Vital Signs			
1. Size	1 = Length x Width x Depth		
2. Depth (If wound is healing with granulation tissue, must select #3 or higher.)	1 = Non-blanchable erythema on intact skin 2 = Partial-thickness skin loss involving epidermis and/or dermis 3 = Full-thickness skin loss involving damage or necrosis of subcutaneous tissue; may extend down to but not through underlying fascia; and/or mixed partial or full-thickness and/or tissue layers obscured by granulation tissue 4 = Obscured by necrosis 5 = Full-thickness skin loss with extensive destruction, tissue necrosis or damage to muscle, bone, or supporting structures		
3. Edges	1 = Indistinct, diffuse, none clearly visible 2 = Distinct, outline clearly visible, attached, even with wound base 3 = Well-defined, not attached to wound base 4 = Well-defined, not attached to base, rolled under, thickened 5 = Well-defined, fibrotic, scarred, or hyperkeratotic		
4. Under-mining	1 = Undermining < 2 cm in any area 2 = Undermining 2 to 4 cm involving < 50% wound margins 3 = Undermining 2 to 4 cm involving > 50% wound margins 4 = Undermining > 4 cm in any area 5 = Tunneling and/or sinus tract formation		

Figure 2a.

A1C, nutritional indices, and wound culture. A nutritional history is also helpful, as is assessment for familial medical history. During the initial interview, it is helpful to obtain social information with respect to smoking, alcohol consumption, exercise regimen, and the availability of support persons. Finally, it is suggested to take an inventory of past and current wound care. When eliciting this information, it is most helpful to identify actual wound care being performed, as this may differ considerably from the current order.

An example of an initial patient questionnaire is included in this chapter as a reference tool. The facility may have a standard questionnaire already in place (Figures 1a, 1b, 1c).

The wound profile should be carefully documented. Both quantitative and qualitative information should be gathered. Quantitative information includes wound size and depth, surface area, a photograph of the wound and surrounding skin, possibly wound volume and, if venous in nature, ankle

5. Necrotic Tissue Type	1 = None visible 2 = White/gray non-viable tissue and/or non-adherent yellow slough 3 = Loosely adherent yellow slough 4 = Adherent, soft black eschar 5 = Firmly adherent, hard black eschar		
6. Necrotic Tissue Amount	1 = None visible 2 = < 25% of wound bed covered 3 = 25% to 50% of wound covered 4 = > 50% and < 75% of wound covered 5 = 75% to 100% of wound covered		
7. Exudate Type	1 = None 2 = Serosanguineous: thin, watery, pale red/pink 3 = Serous: thin, watery, clear 4 = Purulent: thin or thick, opaque, tan/yellow 5 = Foul purulent: thick, opaque, yellow/green with odor		
8. Exudate Amount	1 = None 4. Moderate 2 = Scant 5. Large 3 = Small		
9. Skin Color Surrounding Wound	1 = Pink or normal for ethnic group 2 = Bright red and/or blanches to touch 3 = White or gray pallor or hypopigmented 4 = Dark red or purple and/or non-blanchable 5 = Black or hyperpigmented		
10. Peripheral Tissue Edema	1 = Minimal firmness around wound 2 = Non-pitting edema extends < 4 cm around wound 3 = Non-pitting edema extends $\geq$ 4 cm around wound 4 = Pitting edema extends <4 cm around wound 5 = Crepitus and/or pitting edema extends $\geq$ 4 cm		
11. Peripheral Tissue Induration	1 = Minimal firmness around wound 2 = Induration < 2 cm around wound 3 = Induration 2 to 4 cm extending < 50% around wound 4 = Induration 2 to 4 cm extending $\geq$ 50% around wound 5 = Induration > 4 cm in any area		
12. Granulation Tissue (If Depth is 1 or 2, must select "1")	1 = Skin intact or partial-thickness wound 2 = Bright, beefy red; 75% to 100% of wound filled and/or tissue overgrowth 3 = Bright, beefy red; < 75% and > 25% of wound filled 4 = Pink, and/or dull, dusky red and/or fills $\leq$ 25% of wound 5 = No granulation tissue present		

Figure 2b.

and calf circumference measurements. Qualitative information includes wound description, description of peri–wound skin, odor, exudate, edema, anatomic location, pain (quantify with self–report using pain scale if possible), type of tissue exposed and color. An example of a wound documentation form follows. Another option is to utilize one of the computerized tools such as the Bates–Jensen PSST[4] or the Pressure Sore Status Tool. Figure 2a through 2d represent a sample of a documentation tool which incorporates the Bates–Jensen tool.

Depending on the differentiation of wound by type, other testing may be required. Wounds with a potential vascular origin may require vascular testing. Vascular testing generally involves non–invasive testing of assessment of pulses, doppler wave form, ankle/brachial doppler pressure and transcutaneous oxygen analysis. Invasive vascular testing may involve arteriography. Other vascular testing may be indicated based on assessment. Diagnostic radiography may be indicated to rule out the presence of osteomyelitis. This testing may require plain films,

13. Epi-theliali-zation	1 = 100% of wound covered, surface intact 2 = 75% to < 100% of wound covered and/or epithelial tissue 3 = 50% to < 75% of wound covered and/or epithelial tissue extends to < 0.5 cm into wound bed 4 = 25% to < 50% of wound covered 5 = < 25% of wound covered		
14. Pressure Sore Pain	1 = No response at all during sore care 2 = No verbal or non-verbal evidence of pain in the sore, responds to touch and can feel care procedures 3 = Minimal pain at the sore site, attempts to move away from caregiver, verbalizes discomfort during care 4 = Moderate pain at the sore site, withdraws during care procedure, moans or verbalizes pain, moans, or cries 5 = Severe pain at the sore site, attempts to push caregiver away, strongly withdraws from care procedure or verbalizes pain, moans, cries and demands procedure stop.		
15. Nutrition	1 = Normal well balanced diet or on TPN 2 = Normal diet, consumer 75%, requires prompt 3 = Tube feeding or poor oral intake with no attempts to supplement 4 = Oral diet consumes 50% on supplement 5 = Poor oral diet, consumes <50%, refuses supplement, refuses tube feeding		
16. Functional Ability	1 = No change, able to perform ADLs 2 = Slightly diminished, must decrease time up in chair by less than 2 hours 3 = Decreased, must decrease activity by 50% compared to before sore occurrence 4 = Impaired, must decrease activity level by > 50%, remains in bed 5 = Markedly impaired, bedridden, signs of disuse atrophy, activity < 25% of what it was prior to sore development		
17. Adherence to Therapy	1 = Highly motivated. Allows or performs 100% of all care procedures. 2 = Motivated and committed to healing ulcer. Allows or performs > 75% of direct care procedures, some aspects of care not done. 3 = Committed to healing ulcer. Allows or performs 75% of direct care procedures. 4 = Not committed to healing ulcer. Allows or performs 50% of direct care procedures. 5 = Not motivated and not committed to healing ulcer. Allows or performs < 50% of direct care procedures.		

Figure 2c.

bone scan, or MRI. If the area is suspicious for infection, a wound/bone biopsy may be indicated.

Policy and procedure. Applicable institutional policies and procedures may be utilized to the extent to which they fit the needs of the clinic. Applicable general policies may include policies regarding patient scheduling, staffing, medical authority, documentation and infection control. The team involved in the wound clinic will want to develop policies specific to the service. These policies may include wound cleansing and debridement policies, a wound cultur-

ing policy, topical wound care policies and policies for adjuvant management such as sequential compression therapy, orthotic devices and pressure relief. Any protocols which are developed subsequent to the policies and procedures should be compatible with the same. An example of a flow chart for the management of lower extremity edema is provided in Figure 3.

Management of referrals. The management of patient referrals to the wound center depends on timely communication with the referring source. The

Treatments:
Pressure relief (bed)_____
Pressure relief (chair)_____
Dressing: Gauze_____
          Transparent_____
          Hydrocolloid: Sweep_____
                   Aquacel_____
          Hydrogel sheet_____
          Hydrogel amorphous_____
          Alginate dressing_____
          Alginate packing_____
          Foam - Mitraflex_____
                Allevyn_____
          Exu-Dry_____
          Collagen: Fibracol_____
                Medifil_____
          Paste boot_____
          Other:_____

Topicals: Silvadene_____ Triple anti____
        Gentamicin_____ Other_____
        Bactroban_____
        Dakins_____

Moisturizer: Elta_____ LacHydrin_____   Other_____
           Curel_____ Lubriderm_____
           Eucerin_____ Neutrogena_____

Treatment frequency:_____

Compression garment/wraps:_____

Consults: Dietician:_____   Orthotics:_____
           Vascular:_____   Dermatology:_____
           Orthopedics:_____   Social Work:_____
           Physical Therapy:_____ Occupational Therapy:_____
           Home Health:_____
           Other:_____

EDEMA MEASUREMENTS:

LEFT	RIGHT
Ankle_____	Ankle_____
Calf_____	Calf_____

DEBRIDEMENT:
_____
_____
_____

Goals:(progress of)_____
_____
_____

Comments:_____
_____
_____
_____
_____
_____
_____

Return to Clinic:_____ Signature:_____

Return to Clinic:_____ Signature:_____

Figure 2d.

referral source may be a self–referral, but more likely it is from a physician or other healthcare provider. One complaint about specialty type clinics is that of inadequate communication with referral sources. A plan to provide such communication should be in place before the first patient is seen. Another method of minimizing "referral anxiety" is to establish the wound center as a "consult" service by stressing that it does not intend to take over primary care of the patient, but to assist with the management of the patient only with respect to wound care. It is important that all patients seen in the wound center have a primary care physician/provider.

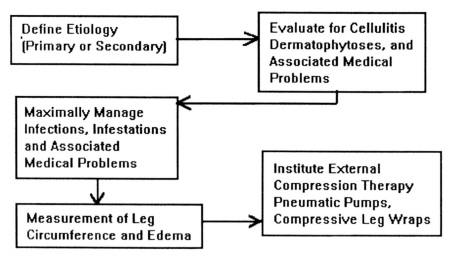

Figure 3. *Management of lower extremity edema.*

Evaluation of Program

A plan for evaluating the program should be in place from the inception and planning phases. The goal of the evaluation process is to measure progress, monitor outcomes, and evaluate established goals and objectives. Program evaluation may include such issues as infection rate, time to wound closure, recidivism rate and others. Another aspect of the program to monitor is in the area of demographics. How closely does the actual patient population match the projected statistics? This information is useful for concurrent planning and for the marketing department that may have facilitated the research during the planning phase. Finally, it is helpful to have periodic team meetings to discuss the evaluation findings. Meetings provide all staff with the opportunity to hear the data, comment on the results and formulate ideas for future research.

Summary

Running an outpatient wound center can be an exciting process. The concept is relatively new and the vitality which can be brought to such a setting will make a difference for both staff and patient. A center focused on the care and management of non–healing and chronic wounds brings together interested professionals who are willing to learn, to teach and to share with the patient a coordinated approach to management of an often difficult problem.

This chapter has focused on the process of formalizing an idea and bringing it to reality with careful research and planning. It is my hope that the concepts presented in this chapter will facilitate the process of opening a wound center for those

individuals contemplating such a service. Certainly there are additional areas which could be covered, including the development and use of protocols for both diagnosis and topical wound care. For additional information with these aspects of operating a wound clinic, I recommend other chapters of this source book and other articles on selecting treatment modalities and wound healing and repair.

Conclusion

It should be stressed that there are many methods for achieving organized treatment of non–healing and chronic wounds. Establishing an outpatient wound center is simply one of these ways. Even with respect to the wound center, the structure may take many forms from the model presented or from any of a number of variations. The center, if it is to be successful, needs to meet the needs of the population expected to be served. Therefore, careful analysis of that population cannot be underestimated. Likewise, a careful, realistic appraisal of potential referral sources and competitors needs to be completed. The best designed, best planned clinic will not survive without patients.

References

1. Baxter CR. Wound care clinics – a need? *Scars and Stripes* 1993;3(2):5.
2. Johnson JE. Developing an effective business plan. *Nursing Economics* 1990;8(3):152–154.
3. Shipes E. Continence clinics. In: Doughty DB (ed). *Urinary and Fecal Incontinence: Nursing Management.* Mosby Year Book, 1991, pp 151–165.
4. Bates–Jensen, B: Pressure Sore Status Tool: Wound Intelligence System, 1995.

WIERSEMA

40

Building a Wound Care Healing Team

Dale Buchbinder, MD, FACS; Clifford F. Melick, PhD;
Mary M. Hilton, RN, BSN, CDE; and Gloria J. Huber, RN

Buchbinder D, Melick CF, Hilton MM, Huber GJ. Building a wound care healing team. In: Krasner D, Kane D. *Chronic Wound Care, Second Edition*. Wayne, PA, Health Management Publications, Inc., 1997, pp 321–324.

Introduction

The community is replete with patients who have chronic non–healing wounds. Frequently, chronic wound patients are passed from one practitioner to another, no one understanding the patient, the disease or the principles required to bring about healing. While many practitioners understand either the disease mechanisms or the appropriate diagnostic modalities, more often than not they lack the knowledge required to manage the chronic non–healing wound. Most practitioners view chronic non–healing wounds with frustration or disinterest, and consequently treat the wound with antiquated methods. Optimal treatment of chronic non–healing wounds crosses multiple healthcare specialties, including primary care, general surgery, endocrinology, vascular surgery, orthopedic surgery, plastic surgery, podiatry, nursing, physical therapy, pharmacy, dietary, social work, discharge planning and suppliers. But because wound healing is only a minor part of any of these specialties, and because most practitioners enjoy treating the usual problems of their specialty, the chronic non–healing wound is variously viewed as a complication or annoyance.

Comprehensive wound management programs have been established to provide an optimal environment for the care of the chronic non–healing wound patient. These programs require a team of dedicated individuals who have specialized training in the diagnosis and management of chronic non–healing wounds. The team should consist of committed physicians, nurses, technicians, social workers, and others who operate together to provide the patient with appropriate comprehensive care.

In 1991, we established a wound treatment center at our institution in association with a nationally recognized wound management corporation. Since that time, we have seen an average of 700 new patients per year, and currently have in excess of 7,000 patient visits per year to our center. The center's success is based in large measure on the building of an efficient, cohesive and multi–disciplinary wound healing team. The remainder of this chapter will share some of the insights that were gained while building the team of the Baltimore center.

Physical Plant and Equipment

Ideally, a wound healing center is a separate, identifiable entity where patients can be evaluated by the team, and appropriate diagnostic testing can be accomplished or easily obtained. An adequate number of treatment rooms, used for minor surgical debridement, application of casts, and physical assessment of patients, is required. At our center, eight examination rooms are clustered around a central work station. Each examination room is equipped with an electronic podiatric chair that can be converted to a stretcher. These chairs are specially designed to allow easy ingress/egress for the patient and optimum positioning facilitating provider access to the patient's wound. In addition to the standard equipment required in any examination room (e.g., blood pressure cuffs), these treatment rooms must be outfitted with sets of conventional surgical instruments, wound–related supplies and good lighting.

The wound center should stock a variety of off–loading devices, such as surgical shoes, and have the ability to customize these devices. There should be equipment for the application and removal of casts, as well as doppler devices for measuring blood flow. A full vascular laboratory and radiology facilities should be readily available for patient referrals. Easy access to the facility for patients in wheel chairs or on stretchers is a critical consideration. Our facility has a conference room where patients can view videos or receive comprehensive training in the care and management of their wounds with team members.

Members of the Wound Healing Team

Administrative:

Program Director. This individual is responsible for the day–to–day operation of the wound center. Wound center employees should report directly to the Program Director, who is responsible for all operational issues. The Program Director needs to work closely with the nurses, physicians and technical personnel to ensure the orderly and smooth operation of the facility. The Program Director, in concert with the center's medical director, is responsible for all major policy decisions affecting patient care. The Program Director oversees marketing strategies and public relations, and should be highly knowledgeable in the hands–on treatment of patients with chronic wounds. Our Program Director has a B.S.N. and functioned as a diabetes educator for many years prior to assuming her current position.

Administrative staff. The administrative staff consists of trained medical secretaries who are familiar with patients and able to take care of patient scheduling needs, as well as keep patient records up–to–date. Members of the administrative staff with specific training in financial matters are required to accomplish accurate and efficient patient billing, especially within the ever–changing environment of healthcare finance. It is important that these staff members develop the ability to relate to wound center patients in an understanding and compassionate manner, promoting an environment of good will and contributing to the patient's desire to continue treatment and adhere to the treatment protocol.

Nursing:

Nurse manager. It is necessary to have a nurse manager who assumes leadership in research utilization and research implementation in the clinical setting. This person is responsible for assisting staff in development, facilitating problem solving and monitoring patient progress through the system.

Quality assurance is coordinated by the nurse manager who assigns physicians and their follow–up of patients to staff nurses on a monthly basis. He or she is a resource for all staff and clearly needs to be a leader whose expertise can be respected by the entire nursing staff. Our nurse manager has seventeen years of nursing experience with five years dedicated solely to healing chronic wounds.

Staff nurses. Registered Nurses and Licensed Practical Nurses can be used as case managers or as primary care nurses for wound care patients. Regardless of certification, the staff nurse must be knowledgeable in the concepts of wound healing and treatment. At our center, each patient is initially assessed by a staff nurse. The staff nurse charts the wound healing progress and physical descriptions of each wound. In order to provide optimal care, the staff nurse forms a collaborative relationship with the patient's team of doctors. Each staff nurse is required to participate in continuing education which emphasizes the topics of wound care management and related fields.

Staff nurses can be specially trained in wound management, enterostomal therapy, or nutrition or may have experience as medical or surgical nurses. It is essential that staff nurses display an interest in wound healing and be able to closely relate to the patients and their needs. At our center, many of the nurses have established close relationships with the patients and their families. Many times they have made house calls or delivered supplies to patients' residences. They have conversations with and lend support to family members. They teach patients, family members and care givers the techniques for properly applying dressings, bandages, compression stockings and other devices, and often the staff nurses are the first to know when chronic wound patients are non–compliant. Good relationships between the nursing staff and chronic wound patients bring about better patient compliance to the treatment regimen and significantly contribute to the success of our healing programs.

Ancillary and Technical Staff. Vascular and x–ray technologists may be needed to perform routine diagnostic studies on site. However, these services can also be contracted from free–standing, or hospital–based facilities. It is important that the technologists performing these studies have an appreciation for the chronic wound patient, at least ensuring that appropriate studies are carried out.

The wound center should be able to provide a compression therapist. This person can be either employed directly by the wound center or associated with the center through an outside vender. At our wound center, approximately 50 percent of patients require some form of compression, be it stockings, pumps or compression dressings. It is imperative that compression devices are correctly fitted to ensure maximal patient compliance. The compression therapists at our center have developed long–term relationships with the patients, ensuring that patients are wearing and using well–fitting devices which are designed to remain intact.

Because many of its patients are confined to bed or wheelchair, the wound center may utilize contracts with transportation companies to transport chronic wound patients from their homes to the center, allowing the patient to receive specialized care in a setting that is specifically designed for its delivery.

Mental healthcare:

Social workers/Psychotherapists/Home health providers. The wound center needs to establish close working relationships with both social workers and psychotherapists. Many chronic wound patients require complicated arrangements in order to adequately care for their wounds in an outpatient setting. Social workers are critical in helping these patients arrange for the delivery of the appropriate services. Also, the chronic wound patient may have complex family and inter–personal relationships that the social worker or psychotherapist may be useful in aiding the patient to resolve. A large proportion of chronic wound patients have been on pain medications that are addictive and may require substantial psychotherapy in order to ameliorate the addiction. Psychotherapists are especially helpful with compliance issues related to pain control. The ability to use both social workers and psychotherapists as a resource for the wound center is an integral part of overall patient care.

A large percentage of chronic wound patients require home health services. Our wound center works directly with the home healthcare agency run by our hospital. Working together enables us to provide patients with easy access to nursing services, physical and occupational therapy, nutritional assessment and dietary education.

The wound center may also be affiliated with a durable medical equipment company that provides specialty beds, wheelchair or chair cushions and off–loading appliances to its patients.

Physicians:

Physician team. It is essential to recruit a team of physicians who are interested in caring for patients with chronic wounds. It is also desirable to recruit physicians with diverse medical backgrounds so that they may complement each other in caring for the patients.

Medical Director. A Medical Director should be appointed. This person is responsible for maintaining an appropriate quality assurance program, oversees all medical protocols, and works in partnership with the facility's Program Director to ensure that proper care is delivered to all patients at the wound center. The Medical Director deals with physician–related problems and is responsible for appropriate disciplinary actions as well. The Medical Director oversees all aspects of medical care and treatment at the wound center.

Physicians can be recruited from a variety of sub–specialties, including family practice, internal medicine, endocrinology, general surgery, vascular surgery, plastic surgery, orthopedic surgery and podiatry. Regardless of specialty, the physicians at our wound center are required to attend a course on the treatment of chronic wounds, as well as a clinical workshop prior to beginning practice at the center. Our wound center is staffed by 4 vascular surgeons, 2 general surgeons, 5 plastic surgeons, 3 podiatrists, 1 endocrinologist, and 1 internist. The wound center schedules physicians of different specialties to practice simultaneously, thus allowing instantaneous consultation or brain–storming between specialties. Additionally, all problem cases are presented monthly at a multi–disciplinary conference. There have been algorithms established for evaluating and caring for patients, coupled with a quality assurance plan that sorts out difficult wounds and ensures that they are reviewed by the medical director and possibly presented at the conference.

While all of the treating physicians are trained in the general principles of wound management, sub–specialists bring added expertise to wound care management. The general surgeon is skilled in debriding large abdominal or thoracic wounds and treating surgical complications in the chronic wound patient. The podiatrist is skilled in the management of complex foot disease where partial foot and toe amputations may be required, as well as in creating methods for off–loading foot wounds. The plastic surgeon is trained in multiple surgical procedures which allow direct tissue coverage for healing wounds. Internists, endocrinologists, and other medical specialists can optimize the chronic wound patient's medical conditions which will promote wound healing (e.g., maintenance of stable diabetic control). Vascular surgeons have the skills necessary to revascularize ischemic extremities or to correct severe venous disease.

Upon admission to care, the chronic wound patient is triaged to an appropriate specialist. All general wounds can be treated by any of the treating physicians in accordance with the guidelines of their specialty. Patients with complex problems should be triaged to a physician in an appropriate specialty, or a physician of the appropriate specialty should be consulted during the patient's course of treatment. In order for the center to be successful, treating physicians need to be aware of their limitations and should refer patients to appropriate specialists. Along with this cadre of treating physicians, we have a consulting panel where chronic wound patients can be referred for any other concomitant medical problem. It is important to remember that many chronic wound patients are referred to the center by their primary care physicians, and these physicians must be kept appraised of their patients' progress. It is also imperative that these patients be returned to their primary care providers for follow–up and necessary medical management whenever possible.

The key component to building a physician team for the treatment of chronic wounds is to have diverse specialization in a group of physicians with a common interest in healing chronic wounds. Our center has an open staff policy which only requires that an interested physician be on the staff of our associated hospital.

Conclusion

Building a wound care program is a difficult process that requires strong cooperative and collaborative efforts between administrative, nursing, technical, home support and physician personnel, and the chronic wound patient. It is critical that chronic wound patients be quickly diagnosed and that an effective treatment plan is devised and implemented in a well–designed, well–equipped, well–staffed setting. The wound care team must assure compliance to the specialized treatment protocol, not only by the patient, but also by healthcare providers. It is important that obstacles to wound healing be recognized and removed by this multi–disciplined team. Treating patients who have complex problems causing their chronic non–healing wounds is truly a team effort. A successful wound center requires assemblance of a compatible, cooperative and collaborative staff as a strong foundation.

41

Technologies for Wound Assessment

William J. Ennis, DO and Patricio Meneses, PhD

Ennis WJ, Meneses P. Technologies for wound assessment. In: Krasner D, Kane D. *Chronic Wound Care, Second Edition*. Wayne, PA, Health Management Publications, Inc., 1997, pp 325–332.

Introduction

In all science, form and function are interwoven concepts. Advertisements promoting everything from automobiles to housewares stress ergonomics and describe how the product was "formed to our needs." The complete development of an individual mirrors the development of the species as described by the theory "Ontogeny recapitulates Phylogeny." The skin of an individual developed its basic functions of protection, thermoregulation, metabolism and communication as a result of the biological needs of the species over time.

Our quest for knowledge to understand the form and function of various organ systems has led to an explosion of invasive and non–invasive diagnostic techniques and imaging devices. Until recently, the same could not be said for new developments to assess the skin. The fact that we could simply "look" at a patient and arrive at a preliminary dermatological working diagnosis significantly delayed the field. Techniques such as biopsy, photography, computer wound analysis and high frequency ultrasound have been developed to analyze dermal form and structure. The measurement of the functional status of skin, however, has been somewhat more elusive. Techniques aimed at functional parameters include thermographic imaging[1] and evaporimetry.[2] The status of the microcirculation is another functional parameter worthy of measurement.

In addition to adequate nutrition, immunocompetency and a plethora of local wound and systemic influencing factors, the micro–circulation is of paramount importance to wound healing. Vascular surgeons and internists have perfected assessment, diagnosis and treatment, both surgical and interventional, for many macrovascular diseases. The macrovascular system refers to those blood vessels large enough to be named, and visualized by the unaided eye. The microcirculation describes the enormous "web" of microscopic vessels and their communications which the skin and other tissues are dependent upon for nutrients and oxygen. It is a commonly held belief that adequate provision of macrovascular flow is enough for successful wound healing to occur. The focus of many wound healing research groups, however, has turned towards the microcirculation. Although there is an obvious anatomic connection between the macro and micro–vascular beds, the patency of the former does not ensure adequate flow in the latter. It is now known that the microvascular response can not be extrapolated from current macrovascular measurement techniques.

For clarification, here is a clinical scenario which explains the above concept. If you were given a normal ankle–brachial index and doppler waveform result from your local vascular lab, you would be inclined to assume that the circulation was adequate for wound healing to occur, for example, in a leg ulcer. The patient might, however, have long standing venous hypertension with subsequent lipodermatosclerosis (subcutaneous scarring) and have a transcutaneous oxygen measurement that indicates relative hypoxemia at the skin surface. This type of information might lead you down a different therpeutic pathway. In our clinic, we have just begun to incorporate this type of data into our overall wound assessment process, and envision this type of information will be critical to both wound product and treatment modality (i.e. hyperbaric oxygen, electrical stimulation) selection.

Several tools such as capillary and fluorescence microscopy, isotope washout techniques, and remittance spectroscopy have been developed to study

Table 1
The Diameters of the Micro–Vessels and the Larger Arteries

Microcirculation	Diameter (mm)	Macrocirculation	Diameter (mm)
Terminal Arteriole	0.017–0.026	Posterior Tibial Artery	1.5–3
Capillary	0.010–0.012	Popliteal Artery	4–6
Post–Capillary Venule	0.018–0.035	Common Iliac	6–13
Capillary Intra–Papillary Loop	0.008–0.010	Aorta	17–25

the dermal microcirculation; however, these technologies for the most part have remained in the research arena.[3] This chapter will review three other analytical techniques to assess the microcirculation, metabolism, and functional status of granulation tissue and skin. Transcutaneous oxygen monitoring and laser doppler imaging are two non–invasive techniques used today by many wound care practitioners to assess wound healing potentials. ^{31}P–NMR spectroscopy is an invasive research tool currently under investigation by the authors which is now being developed by other dermatology groups as a non–invasive tool. These techniques will be discussed following a brief review of the anatomy of the micro–circulation.

Microcirculation

The circulation of the skin arises from cutaneous branches off subcutaneously located musculocutaneous arteries. Table 1 lists the diameters of the micro–vessels and the larger arteries for comparison. A single artery pierces the dermis and divides into smaller arterioles.[4] A superficial and deep plexus of arterioles and venules is present within the dermis, connected by multiple communicating vessels.[5] The deep plexus is parallel to the skin surface and is located deep in the reticular dermis (Figure 1). The superficial plexus also lies parallel to the skin surface just below the papillary dermis (sub–papillary plexus). The majority of microcirculatory flow occurs in the superficial plexus. The vessels located at the plexus level include end arterioles, capillaries, and post–capillary venules. The venules are more numerous and can be recognized histologically by their multilaminated basement membranes in contrast to the homogeneous membrane seen in the arteriole.[6] Many of the physiological events in the microcirculation, including changes in permeability, WBC diapedesis, and vasculitis as a result of immune–complex deposition on the vessel wall, occur at the venule.[7] It is the superficial plexus that gives rise to the "capillary loop." Projections of the

dermis, along with accompanying blood vessels and nervous tissue into the epidermis, make up the papillary system. Each papillae usually contains one capillary loop, consisting of an intra and extrapapillary segment.[6]

The RBC moves through the capillary with a velocity of 0.4 mm to 0.8 mm/second, and remains in the capillary for several seconds allowing for exchange of gases and fluids. Cardiac pulsations, autoregulation, and intrinsic vasomotion are all factors in capillary flow.[8] Filtration is favored at the arteriolar limb of the capillary loop and absorption at the venular limb. Increases in pressure at either end of the capillary loop will lead to increased interstitial edema formation as capillary pressure exceeds plasma oncotic pressure. Clinically this process occurs in chronic venous insufficiency. The venous pressure is elevated, leading to a capillary pressure which exceeds plasma oncotic pressure, and the patient ends up with lower extremity edema. The body has a built–in protective mechanism for capillary hypertension known as the veno–arteriolar reflex. As the increased pressure in the capillary is sensed, a reflex sympathetic response leads to a constriction on the arterial side, thereby decreasing overall flow to the capillary and indirectly lowering the pressure. This mechanism is defective in the patient with diabetes. This defect, along with microsclerosis, which can occur in the microcirculation of the diabetic patient, leads to abnormal responses to inflammation, infection, and wound healing. The hypertensive patient demonstrates narrow arterioles and dilated venules due to the smooth muscle hypertrophy in the vessel wall from the constant assault of elevated pressures. The hypertensive patient also demonstrates fewer capillary loops in the dermis than normal. This again emphasizes the importance of the microcirculation, as the hypertensive patient may have bounding pulses and normal dopplers but demonstrates abnormalities on testing for the microcirculation.

There are specialized arteriovenous shunts (Glomus bodies) which allow blood to bypass the

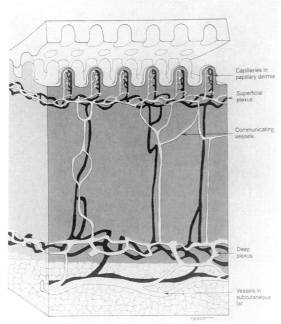

Figure 1. *The dermal vasculature consists of a three–dimensional network of two plexuses that parallel the skin surface: one in the lower part of the reticular dermis (deep plexus), the other beneath the papillary dermis (superficial plexus). Perpendicularly oriented communicating blood vessels connect the deep and the superficial plexuses. The rich capillary supply of the adventitial dermis constitutes a microcirculation, in contrast to the relatively straight, large conduits of the two parallel plexuses and their communicating vessels.*

Reprinted with permission from Jakubovic H, Ackerman B. Structure and function of skin: Development, morphology, and physiology. In: Moschella S, Hurley H (eds). Dermatology, Third Edition. W.B. Saunders Company, Philadelphia, PA, p 40.

capillary bed and are important in thermoregulation. This parallel circulation can provide much greater blood flow than is metabolically required. The distinction between nutritive and non–nutritive flow is difficult to assess with indirect techniques.[9] For example, an indirect measurement of a near normal perfusion may be the result of shunted (non–nutritive flow) perfusion and not reflect "nutritive" (cutaneous) flow. It is therefore critical to assess not only flow (oxygen transport), but cellular metabolism (oxygen utilization and energy production). The three techniques discussed in this chapter taken together illustrate the point clinically. The laser doppler can tell us about the microcirculatory flow, but one would need to add a transcutaneous oxygen measurement to understand if the oxygen delivered to the tissue was utilized. As noted above, high levels of either shunted (non–nutritive flow) or

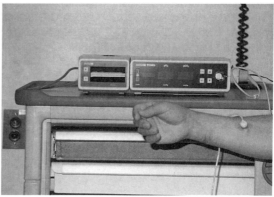

Figure 2. *Transcutaneous oxygen monitoring being used to assess transcutaneous oxygen tension.*

dermal (nutritive) blood flow would be detected but not differentiated by laser doppler. The ^{31}P–NMR spectroscopy data could then reveal at a cellular level that the oxygen was in fact consumed by the cell and that energy requiring processes (i.e. healing) might be able to proceed.

Trancutaneous Oxygen Monitoring

Since the supply of oxygen to the tissue is critical for survival and the microcirculation is the conduit by which it is transported, measuring tisue oxygen is an indirect monitor of the microcirculation. Ninety–five percent of the energy generated in the body normally originates from aerobic pathways.[10] The measurement of tissue oxygen provides information concerning the amount of O_2 that is available to the tissue and is influenced by arterial pO_2 concentration and blood flow rates.[11] The tissue O_2 level reflects the degree to which the metabolic requirements of the tissues have been nourished, especially when overall flow rates are slow as opposed to high blood flow rates (when the $tcpO_2$ can approach that of arterial pO_2). The tissue perfusion state is therefore indirectly obtained via $tcpO_2$ measurements.

Lavoisier performed the first measurement of oxygen in 1779.[10] Tissue oxygen can be analyzed via direct or indirect techniques (probe placed inside of or on top of the tissue surface). Mass spectrometry and optical fluorescence technologies have been used, but the indirect polarographic electrode has become the most popular for wound care applications.[10] A dime–sized Clarke type solid state polarographic electrode (E5280) containing a platinum cathode with a reference electrode of silver–chloride is housed in a probe tip along with a heater and thermistor. The tip of the probe is covered with a permeable membrane. An electrolyte solution fills the reservoir inside the probe. The reduction of oxygen at the cathode generates a current which is then fed into the pO_2 channel of a monitor and converted into a voltage and digitized.

The electrode is attached via a fixation device to the immediate peri–wound skin and heated to 43 to 45° C, which induces hyperemia, and the dissolution of keratin lipids thereby increasing gas permeability (Figure 2). The examination takes 20 minutes and should be repeated at the same tissue site at each examination. The final $tcpO_2$ result may be influenced by capillary temperature, blood flow and metabolic O_2 consumption. Although there is a short distance from the probe tip to the capillary (0.3 mm), the oxygen has to pass through metabolically active tissue and is therefore partially consumed. The $tcpO_2$ value therefore does not directly correlate to the arterial blood gas, often causing for confusion among healthcare providers working with this equipment. The technique generates a value that is more a reflection of the difference between oxygen delivery and utilization than an approximation of arterial pO_2.

Various researchers have attempted to utilize the technique to help in the clinical selection of appropriate amputation levels.[12,13] Clyne, et al. studied the $tcpO_2$ values in the gaiter distribution (medial lower leg) of patients with chronic venous insufficiency and found very low levels.[14] This technique can and should be used in patients with diabetes because the doppler derived ankle pressures are frequently falsely elevated secondary to calcified vessels. This problem can be overcome with the adjunctive use of the $tcpO_2$ monitor because the technique is not influenced by this process, thereby giving the investigator a more representative picture of the circulatory status of the patient.[15] Recently, Colin, et al. described the use of $tcpO_2$ monitoring in the evaluation of support surfaces and the prevention of pressure ulcers.[16]

Laser Doppler Flowmetry (LDF) and Laser Doppler Imaging (LDI)

Continuous recording of microvascular perfusion is possible when utilizing laser light and the doppler phenomenon. Light particles (photons) enter the tissue and collide with stationary tissues and the moving cells. Moving particles cause the backscattering of light at a spectrally–broadened frequency different from the original source (doppler shift). The fact that laser light is a highly stable, monochromatic light source makes it ideal for this application. Some of the light is absorbed and various tissue characteristics, such as melanin or callus, may interfere with the quantity of light reflected and therefore the laser

doppler values.[17] Laser light sources can penetrate a prescribed tissue depth, which is important when trying to separate "nutritive" blood flow in the superficial dermal plexus and capillary loops from the "non–nutritive" blood flow found in the deeper plexus.[18]

Laser doppler flowmetry (LDF) is a non–invasive tool for the microcirculation with results comparable to xenon–clearance techniques.[19,20] The technique requires the attachment of a probe to a specific skin site for measurement. One of the main problems with the technique is the tremendous amount of spatial variations in tissue blood flow between adjacent measurement positions and even within the same position over time.[21,22] Despite these problems LDF has been compared favorably with other non–invasive methods of skin perfusion pressure measurement and has been utilized to help select amputation levels.[23] The problem of variable intra–site perfusion values can be partially overcome with laser doppler imaging (LDI).

LDI corrects for spatial variations by imaging a larger surface area and calculating average perfusion values. Two mirrors guide a He–Ne laser beam sequentially over the skin surface. At each measurement site (4096 maximum) a tissue volume of a few hundred micrometers is illuminated. A photodetector records backscattered doppler–broadened light which is created by the interaction of the beam with the moving blood cells. The light signal is converted into an electrical signal and transferred to a signal processor and stored in computer memory. An image matrix is created by dividing the full range of values into six color coded intervals. This process results (using a color printer) in a multicolored picture which represents the microvascular perfusion at the scanned region. By converting the image matrix to ASCII format, the data may be analyzed by any spread–sheet or statistical software package.[24] The process is therefore painless and quick, with scan times under eight minutes. Two caveats are that ambient lighting will interfere with the results and that the patient must remain motionless for the exam.

Laser doppler flowmetry has been utilized for several years in wound care. The addition of the laser doppler imaging technique has allowed for an even wider user base. The following clinical applications for laser doppler testing were highlighted from a clear, succinct chapter by E. Tur, MD in *Bioengineering of the Skin*.[25] The technique demonstrated an increase in dermal flow with p.o. nifedipine use in hypertensive patients (microvascular pathology in hypertension previously discussed). Pentoxifylline (p.o.) therapy has been shown to increase skin blood flow in the lower extremity of diabetic patients as measured by laser doppler. Intravenous insulin infusions have

ENNIS AND MENESES

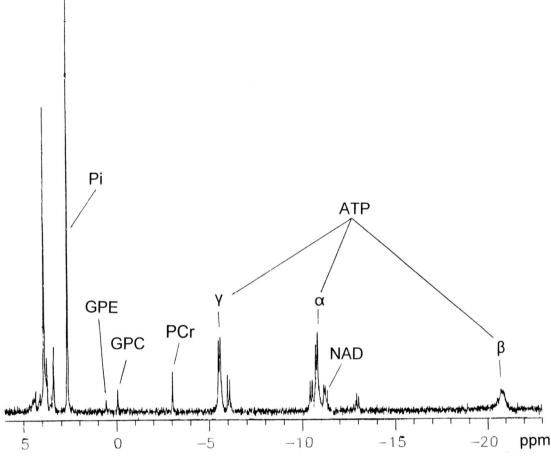

Figure 3. ^{31}P *NMR spectrum of granulation tissue. Each signal represents a single phosphate group attached to a specific metabolite, with the exception of Pi, which is the free phosphate molecule. Pi: inorganic phosphate; GPE: glycerophosphoethanolamine; GPC: glycerophosphocholine; Pcr: Phosphocreatine; ATP: adenosinetriphosphate; Y: end group phosphate; α: middle–group phosphate; ß: phosphate esterified to the ribose molecule (first phosphate); NAD: nicotinamide adenide dinucleotide; ppm: parts per million.*

had the effect of redistributing dermal flow towards the capillary loop (nutritive flow) and away from the A–V shunt (non–nutritive flow) when assessed by laser doppler. Laser doppler studies have also shown that compression stockings and experimental medications such as defibrotides (pro–fibrinolytic agent) have impacted the veno–arteriolar reflex and slowed the progression of microcirculatory deterioration in diabetic patients. Laser dopler imaging and flowmetry provides a non–invasive method of assessing the dermal effects of systemic pharmacologic therapy. This type of data is paramount for the wound care clinician. Diabetic foot ulcers are difficult to treat in the best situations and many of the above mentioned therapies would not impact the results of non–invasive vascular tests aimed at the macro–vascular circulation (i.e. segmental pressures, arterial doppler signals, ankle index etc).

Quantifiable measurements in dermal flow could be used to assess wound care product performance and wound healing potentials.

Magnetic Resonance

Nuclear Magnetic Resonance (NMR) is a science that was developed in the late 1940's as a spectroscopic analytical tool for the characterization of molecules in their natural environment.[26,27] The first magnetic resonance image of a human tumor was obtained in 1971.[28] Since then two distinct technologies utilizing the same principles of magnetic resonance have been used in research. Nuclear Magnetic Resonance (NMR) has functioned as a chemical and physical tool, where Magnetic Resonance Imaging (MRI) has established itself as a premier radiological tool. Recently the

Table 2
Results of two patients with chronic venous insufficiency and ulceration on the lower extremity

		Patient #1	Patient #2
tcpO$_2$ *(mm Hg)*			
	Baseline	52.00	31.00
	After one week	69.00	32.00
Perfusion Imaging** *(Perfusion Units)*			
	Baseline	324.17	358.01
	After one week	615.74	388.16
ATP *(Percent of total phosphorous detected by NMR)*			
	Baseline	17.76	14.26
	After one week	38.44	21.60
Energy Charge *(Ratio of ATP, ADP, and AMP (no unit)*			
	Baseline	0.75	0.63
	After one week	0.75	0.78

incorporation of NMR spectroscopy with Magnetic Resonance Imaging (Magnetic Resonance Spectroscopy–MRS) has allowed the study of not only the anatomical structure, but also the *in vivo* metabolism, giving us a potential tool for analysis of both form and function in one.

Proton (^{1}H), carbon (^{13}C), and phosphorus (^{31}P) are the most common nuclei studied in biological chemistry and medicine.The organic chemical composition of the cell gives the carbon and proton studies their importance. Phosphorous, which is an important metabolic marker, makes it useful as an indicator of cellular metabolism. Both MRI and NMR assess biochemical problems. Utilizing the NMR spectrum or MR image one can visualize the biological environment through biomolecular interactions. Using these techniques, the interaction of molecules in metabolic pathways, membrane dynamics, and the flux of metabolites and their interaction with water can be analyzed. In essence, the overall cell energy status can be measured.

Magnetic resonance spectroscopy (MRS) has been applied to a variety of tissues with variable success. The main problem with this technique is identification and delineation of the tissue studied *in vivo*. The development of specific MRS coils for different regions of the body are being developed but as yet are not perfected to the same degree as MRI coils.

Other problems with the MRS technique include high cost and time consuming studies.

NMR, on the other hand, has been used extensively in the *in vitro* study of cellular metabolism. The perchloric acid (PCA) extract technique from tissue biopsies has demonstrated spectroscopic profiles of small phosphorylated metabolites, which include phosphocreatine (energy storage molecule) and ATP (the source of chemical energy). Figure 3 shows a typical ^{31}P NMR spectrum of a PCA extracted sample from granulation tissue in a chronic leg ulcer. To calculate the relative concentrations of these molecules in the spectrum, the integral value of each signal must be measured. The sum of all represents 100 percent of the phosphorus detected, and each resonance signal represents a percentage of that total. The energy charge[29] describes the equilibrium between the ATP–generating reactions and the ATP–requiring processes by using the following equation:$(0.5 [ADP] + [ATP]) / [AMP] + [ADP] + [ATP]$. Metabolically active tissues, like muscle, have an energy charge of 0.85.

In recent years, the skin has been studied via MRS and NMR. In 1989 Zemtsov and colleagues reported for the first time the use of phosphorus MRS in human wounds.[30] Since then, several other researchers have used the technique to analyze the viability of skin flaps in plastic surgery[31,32] and the depth of dermal injury after burns.[33,34] MRS has also been used in animal models to help explain the pathophysiology of venous ulcerations.[35] These findings were corroborated by Ennis, et al.[36] analyzing PCA extracts of human venous ulcer bed biopsies via ^{31}P–NMR spectroscopy.

Other potential ^{31}P–NMR sources of study involving skin and dermal ulcers include phospholipid analysis which has been carried out in other human tissues.[37] These dermal studies, not yet published by the authors, demonstrate that skin contains phosphatidylcholine (PC), alkylacylyglycero–phosphoholine (AAPC), phosphatidylinositol (PI), sphingomyelin (SM), phosphatidylserine (PS), phosphatidylethanolamine (PE), ethanolamineplasmalogen (Eplas), dihydrosphingomyelin (DHSM), an ethanolamine derivative not yet identified, and diphosphatidylglycerol (DPG).

Although this technique offers the unique advantage of assessing form and function, it also has several limitations. The equipment is costly and not found in most hospitals. The heterogeneous pattern of micro–perfusion and therefore oxygen delivery, previously mentioned, makes focal "biochemical" biopsy site NMR analysis difficult to interpret.

Clinical Experience

As a means for clinical comparisons between these techniques, the authors have included the clinical information from two patients (previously unpublished) in which all of these tests were performed. Two patients with chronic venous insufficiency and ulceration on the lower extremity were studied.

Patient # 1 was a 65 year–old caucasian male with a 40 year history of a non–healing leg ulcer. The wound was evaluated, measured (6.0 cm^2) and biopsied (benign). The patient's wound was assessed via transcutaneous oxygen monitoring, laser doppler imaging, and ^{31}P–NMR spectroscopy, both before and after 1 week of therapy including compression and a hydrocolloid dressing.

Patient # 2 was a 64 year old caucasian female with a 2 year old non–healing wound. This patient was treated in a similar fashion. Table 2 displays the results for these 2 patients. Plates 41 and 42 represent the color images obtained via laser doppler imaging before and after 1 week of treatment in patient #1.

Transcutaneous oxygen monitoring was performed on the immediate peri–wound skin utilizing the TINA™ (Radiometer) system. The first patient demonstrated an improvement from 52 mm Hg to 69 mm Hg; however, no change was seen for patient #2. Patient #2 however, originally had a tcPO$_2$ of 8 mm Hg four weeks prior. The patient had received compression therapy for the 4 weeks prior to enrolling in this project. Laser doppler imaging was performed on both patients by the protocol outlined above (laser doppler imager 3.0 LISCA). The average laser perfusion values increased for both patients but more dramatically in case # 1. A portion of the biopsy sample was processed via the perchloric acid extraction technique for ^{31}P–NMR spectroscopy and the values are noted in Table 2. The spectrometer employed was a General Electric 500NB NMR instrument with an 11.75T Oxford superconducting magnet.

Although strong statistical inferences cannot be made from two patients treated for only one week, a comment concerning the interpretation of the data might be entertained. Patient #1 was able to increase perfusion not only to the wound bed and the delivery of oxygen to the tissue, but also in its utilization as reflected by the increase in ATP. Patient #2 had already achieved improved perfusion and O$_2$ delivery, most likely secondary to prior elimination of micro–edema via compression therapy. The week of hydrocolloid therapy and compression, however, resulted in the improved cellular metabolism as noted by increases in both the ATP and energy charge values. Patient #2 went on to heal in 12 weeks, while patient #1 healed in 20 weeks.

Summary

The concept of form and function is demonstrated at the cellular level when analyzing the microcirculation. The skin is bountifully supplied with collateral flow and when the A–V shunted flow is taken into account, this flow far exceeds the metabolic demands of normal skin function. However, in time of stress (i.e. ischemia), this flow becomes vital and more importantly the "nutritive component" of the flow is critical to the ultimate survival of the tissue. The authors have previously shown that ischemic, intact skin stores high levels of phosphocreatine (an energy storage molecule) when compared to non–ischemic skin.[36] The skin and dermal wounds therefore require both perfusion (delivery of blood and oxygen) and appropriate utilization of those vital nutrients. Hopkins, et al. demonstrated a mismatch in oxygen delivery and fractional extraction using oxygen–15 inhalation in patients with venous ulcerations.[38] The exciting technologies mentioned in this chapter are helping piece together the puzzle of dermal microcirculatory flow and wound healing. The wound care clinician needs to become familiar with the concept of microcirculation and the techniques by which it can be measured. As noted, many therapeutic interventions, both systemic and local, may have a profound effect at the microcirculatory level while not dramatically affecting the macrovascular circulation. The interesting results of ^{31}P–NMR Spectroscopy studies may in the future take wound care clinicians to a new frontier in which the cellular function of a wound can be monitored non–invasively. As practicing clinicians we need to continuously question what we are currently doing and always ask, could it be done better, quicker, and more cost effectively?

References

1. Black CM, Clark RP, Darton K, et al. A pyroelectric thermal imaging system for use in medical diagnosis. *J Biomed Engineering* 1990;12:281–286.
2. Nilsson GE. Measurement of water exchange through skin. *Med Biol Eng Comput* 1977;15:209–218.
3. Wahlberg JE, Lindberg M. Assessment of skin blood flow: An overview. In: Beradesca E, Elsner P, Maibaich HI (eds). *Bioengineering of the Skin: Cutaneous Blood Flow and Erythema*. Ann Arbor, MI, CRC Press, 1995, pp 23–27.
4. Ryan T. Cutaneous circulation. In: Goldsmith LA (ed). *Physiology, Biochemistry, and Molecular Biology of the Skin, Second Edition*. Oxford, UK, Oxford Univ Press, 1991, pp 1019–1064.
5. Jakubovic HR, Ackerman B. Structure and function of skin: Development, morphology and physiology. In: Moschella, Hurley (eds). *Dermatology, Third Edition*. Philadelphia, PA, WB Saunders, 1992, pp 3–79.
6. Braverman IM, Yen A. Capillary loops of the dermal papillae. *Journ Invest Derm* 1977;68:44–52.
7. Yen A, Braverman IM. Ultrastructure of the human dermal microcirculation: The horizontal plexus of the papillary dermis. *Journ Invest Derm* 1976;66:131–142.
8. Wilkin JK. Poiseville, periodicity and perfusion: Rhythmic oscillatory vasomotion in the skin. *Journ Invest Derm* 1989;93:113S–118S.
9. Tooke JE, Fagrell B. The human microcirculation. In: Janssen H, Rooman R, Robertson JIS (eds). *Wound Healing*. Petersfield UK,Wrightson Biomed Pub, 1991, pp 137–155.
10. Gottrup F, Niinikoski J, Hunt TK. Measurement of tissue oxygen tension. In: Janssen H, Tooman R, Robertson JIS (eds). *Wound Healing*. Petersfield, UK, Wrightson Biomed Pub, 1991, pp 155–164.
11. Rooke TW, Hollier LH, Osmundson PJ. The influence of sympathetic nerves on transcutaneous oxygen tension in normal and ischemic lower extremities. *Angiology* 1987;38:400–410.
12. Bacharach JM, Tooke TW, Osmundson PJ, et al. Predictive value of transcutaneous oxygen pressure and amputation success by use of supine and elevation measurement. *J Vasc Surg* 1992;15:558–563.
13. Ameli FM, Byrne PB, Provan JL. Selection of amputation level and predicting healing using transcutaneous tissue oxygen tension. *J Cardiovasc Surg* 1989;30:22–224.
14. Clyne CAC, Ransen WH, Chant ADB, et al. Oxygen tension on the skin of the gaiter area of limbs with venous disease. *Br J Surg* 1985;72:644–647.
15. Lyons DM, Morse MJ. Transcutaneous oxygen measurement in peripheral vascular disease. *Cont Pod Physician* 1992;8(92):35–36.
16. Colin D, Loyant R, Abraham P, Saumet JL. Changes in sacral transcutaneous oxygen tension in the evaluation of different mattresses in the prevention of pressure ulcers. *Adv Wound Care* 1996;9(1):25–28.
17. Bernardi L, Leuzzi S. Laser doppler flowmetry and pho-tophlethsymography. In: Berardesca E, Elsner P, Maibaich HI (eds). *Bioengineering of Skin: Cutaneous Blood Flow and Erythema*. Ann Arbor, Mi, CRC Press, 1995, pp 31–56.
18. Marks N, Trachy RE, Cummings CW. Dynamic variations in blood flow as measured by laser doppler velocimetry: A study in rat skin flaps. *Plastic Recon Surg* 1984;73:804–810.
19. Engelhart M, Kristensen JK. Evaluation of cutaneous blood flow response by 133 Xenon washout and a laser doppler flowmeter. *Journ Invest Derm* 1983;80:12–15.
20. Malvezzi L, Castronuovo JJ,Wayne S, et al. The correlation between 3 methods of skin perfusion measurements: Radionucleide washout, laser doppler flow and photophlethysmography. *Journ Vasc Surg* 1992;15:823–830.
21. Tenland T, Salervd G, Nilsson GE, et al. Spatial and temporal variations in human skin blood flow. *Int J Microcirc* 1983;2:81–90.
22. Braverman IM, Keh A, Goldminz D. Correlation of laser doppler wave patterns with underlying microvascular anatomy. *Journ Invest Derm* 1990;95:283–286.
23. Adera HM, James K, Castronuovo JJ, et al. Prediction of amputation wound healing with skin perfusion pressure. *J Vasc Surg* 1995;21:823–829.
24. Wardell K. *Laser Doppler Perfusion Imaging*. Linkoping, Sweden, L.J. Foto and Montage/Samhall Klintland, 1994.
25. Tur E. Cutaneous laser doppler flowmetry in general medicine. In: Berardesca E, Elsner P, Maibach HI (eds). *Bioengineering of Skin: Cutaneous Blood Flow and Erythema*. Ann Arbor, MI, CRC Press, 1995, pp 133–154.
26. Block F, Hansen WW, Packard M. The nuclear induction experiment. *Phys Rev* 1946;70:474–485.
27. Purcell EM, Torey HC, Pound RV. Resonance absorption by nuclear magnetic moments in solids. *Phys Rev* 1946;69:37–38.
28. Damadian R. Tumor detection by nuclear magnetic resonance. *Science* 1973;171:1151–1153.
29. Atkinson DE. Adenosine nucleotide as stoichiometric coupling aents in metabolism and as regulatory modifiers: The adenylate energy charge. *Metabol* 1977;5:1–21.
30. Zemtsov A, NG TC, Xue M. Human in–vivo P–31 spectroscopy of skin: Potentially a powerful tool for non–invasive study of metabolism in cutaneous tissue. *J Derm Surg Onc* 1989;15:1207–1211.
31. Chen Y, Richards TL, Izemberg S, et al. In vivo phosphorous NMR spectroscopy of skin using cross over coil. *Mag Res in Med* 1992;23:46–54.
32. Kanno K, Hirakawa K. Chronological observations on the energy mtabolism of skin flaps by 31–P NMR MRS: A novel approach to evaluate the state of a flap. *Plast Recon Surg* 1993;91:322–328.
33. Nagel TL, Alderman DW, Schoeborn RR, et al. The slotted cross over coil: a detector for in vivo NMR of skin. *Mag Res in Med* 1990;16:252–268.
34. Schweitzer MP, Olsen JL, Shelby, et al. Non–invasive assessment of metabolism in wounded skin by 31–P NMR in vivo. *J Trauma* 1992;33:828–833.
35. Zemtsov A, Dixon L. Monitoring wound healing of venous stasis leg ulcers by in vivo 31 P magnetic resonance spectroscopy. *Skin Res and Tech* 1995;1:36–40.
36. Ennis WJ, Driscoll DM, Meneses P. A preliminary study on 31 P NMR spectroscopy: A powerful tool for wound analysis using high energy phosphates. *WOUNDS* 1994;6:166–173.
37. Driscoll DM, Ennis WJ, Meneses P. Human sciatic nerve phospholipid profiles from non–diabetes mellitus, non–insulin dependent diabetes mellitus and insulin dependent diabetes mellitus individuals. A 31 P–NMR spectroscopy study. *Int J Biochem* 1994;26:759–767.
38. Hopkins NF, Spinks TJ, Rhodes CG, Ranicar ASO, Jamieson CW. Positron emission tomography in venous ulceration and liposclerosis: a study of regional tissue function. *Br Med J* 1983;286:333–336.

42

Palliative Care: A Wound Care Option

Judy L. Gates, RN, C

Gates JL. Palliative care: A wound care option. In: Krasner D, Kane D. *Chronic Wound Care, Second Edition*. Wayne, PA, Health Management Publications, Inc., 1997, pp 333–335.

Introduction

In the world of healthcare, it is an unspoken assumption that palliative care is for the terminally ill. It is most often associated with the cancer patient or with the immunosuppressed. It is considered to be the "end" measure. Palliative care, however, is often an acceptable and appropriate approach for other situations, including wound care.

The definition of palliative care is "affording relief, to relieve symptoms."[1] It does not suggest that it is a measure for terminal care only or that it is less than acceptable care. It does imply that the direction of care should make things easy, simple and pain free. Palliative care has been practiced across the spectrum of healthcare. The terminal patient comes to mind with programs directed at comfort and pain management such as hospice. Hospice programs usually include the family in the treatment process, assuring that family and patient goals are headed in the same direction.[2] Pain management programs for those patients with chronic surgical pain or pain related to chronic disease processes, such as rheumatoid arthritis, often focus on management of the problem, not resolution.[3]

As the population of chronic wound patients increases, recognition of the "terminal" wound care problem must be addressed. It must be understood and accepted that not every wound will heal. Despite 3000 wound care products and 35+ years of research, the answer for some patients will be a life-long plan to manage the wound.

Nonhealing Wounds

In evaluating each patient, the most important assessment will be to determine the reason for a nonhealing wound. Some well documented causes for nonhealing include disease processes such as peripheral vascular disease, pulmonary disease and diabetes. Other factors that are becoming more common include noncompliance (whether intentional or environmental), lifestyle decisions and self–inflicted reinjury. Patients who have one or a combination of these problems are naturally going to have decreased healing potential.

Establishing the Need for Palliative Care

There are several areas which need to be assessed in order to determine what will be the best plan of care for a long term care program.

Goals. The initial assessment must focus directly on the patient's goals or expectations. The patient should be interviewed to determine specific expectations, i.e. wound closure, elimination of odor, management of drainage, or the ability to return to normal daily routine. Inquiry should be made as to what the patient is able and/or willing to do. It should be determined if the patient is homebound, in what type of residence he/she abides, and what his/her general lifestyle habits include.

Next, it will be important to establish what the household or family members are expecting. They may or may not share the goals and expectations of the patient. If goals and expectations are different, a plan of care may fail, or the outcome may be significantly impaired. If the support system is weak or nonexistent, the plan of care may need alteration to accommodate the patient's abilities.

Finally, the physician and clinician must evaluate their goals.[4] The practitioner may not be comfortable with less aggressive care, even though it may be the patient's choice. Despite years of education and practice, practitioners should not make the patient choose more aggressive care, nor should they make the patient change lifestyle. To avoid frustration, education which allows the patient to decide on the outcome is the best measure.

Environment. The length of exposure a patient has to a setting will affect the short and long term goals for the patient. Acute care settings have very brief, one time encounters with the patient. The goals are to initiate care and then discharge. The specified care may be appropriate in a clinical setting, but upon discharge the care may not be best suited to the patient or his/her environment. Discharge planning has begun to incorporate post hospital needs into the care process.

Long term care settings have a long relationship with the patient and family. Practitioners in this setting can acquire a more realistic picture of the patient's goals, tolerance of care and family interaction. This environment allows for frequent educational opportunities.[5]

In home healthcare there is usually a long term relationship and excellent exposure to the patient's environment, lifestyle and family interaction. It may enlighten healthcare professionals as to why a patient is noncompliant or chooses to live with a chronic wound, for example, a patient may decide that school or work is more important than wound healing. Or some patients may have poor environmental amenities such as a lack of running water, electricity or adequate ventilation. All of these factors can affect the patient's overall decision making process.

The clinic is probably where the longest medical relationship will be established. Long after the hospital, nursing home and home healthcare are out of the picture, the primary physician will still be there. When wound healing is not being appreciated, the physician will need to determine if the situation is correctable or if it has occurred by patient choice, and then must plan accordingly.

Developing a Palliative Care Plan

Once it is established that progressive/aggressive care is not appropriate, a palliative care plan will need to be developed. It must be sensitive to the lifestyle, environment, family support and ability of the patient. Other factors, such as pain and nutrition, must also be considered.[6]

Wound care. It will be important to determine who will be performing the wound care. If it is the patient, what physical limitations are involved? Can the wound be reached? Keeping the dressing simple and cost effective is critical. Since wound healing is not the goal, these patients are not candidates for expensive dressing components. Ideally,

dressings that manage exudate and protect the wound from contaminants are best.

If the patient is experiencing significant pain from the wound or from wound care, a gentle or non-stick dressing will encourage compliance.

Environment. Determine where the patient will be spending time. When at home, to what is that environment conducive? It may require a home evaluation to assess if the care will fit the living situation, for example, protect the wound from pet hair or pests. If the environment has many pets or is not sanitary, a semi-occlusive or occlusive dressing may better protect the wound from contaminants. If the patient is working or going to school, will the dressing tolerate transfers or long hours sitting? Finally, it is necessary to determine what resources the patient has readily available for performing care, i.e. running water.

Cost. Since treatment will be long term, it will also need to be a cost effective option. Evaluation of the family finances may need to be considered as some insurance plans will not cover supplies for palliative care. It does not mean that the cheapest dressing is necessarily the best, but it does mean that dressings that decrease frequency and manage the wound exudate will often end up being the most cost effective and the easiest to manage.[7]

Nutrition. Nutrition is an important factor in preventing the patient from becoming weak or susceptible to infection. Education on adequate calorie and protein intake will be valuable.[7] A vitamin supplement may also be helpful, again an area of patient choice. If the patient is a smoker or takes alcohol in excess, he/she will certainly be at higher risk for complications as his/her immune system will be weakened. It will be impossible to prevent a determined patient from choosing certain lifestyles.

When to Initiate a Palliative Care Plan

In light of patient assessment, environment, prognosis and goals, the question is when is it appropriate to stop aggressive treatment and initiate palliative care? Certainly in terminal or end stage disease processes, palliative care is an appropriate option. Other transition points will be patients who become noncompliant because of choice, and when there are no determinable end points (despite all possible measures the wound has not progressed or continues to fail). In these situations, adopting a simple, easy to follow long term program is a pragmatic solution.

Changing to a palliative care plan. When the decision is made to change treatment goals, the associated care may also need adjustment. Home healthcare will not be appropriate for patients in this mode of care, so the patient or family members will need to be instructed on wound care. Clinic appointments will need to decrease in frequency as well. Periodic appointments to assess for infection or complications will be sufficient. The patient can be instructed on signs and symptoms of infection, and necessary actions. A decision concerning wound care and attaining supplies should be made. If finances are limited, and insurance will not cover the necessities, inquiries should be made about free medical clinics or charitable medical facilities, as they often have access to donated supplies. If the patient has a disease such as cancer or bowel disease, the corresponding organization or support group may also have access to supplies.

Using as few steps as possible in the wound care will enhance compliance. It is essential to educate the patient on what to expect in the daily care of the wound.[8] And it should be made very clear that this care may be necessary for years.

Summary

While wound healing has been the focus of research for many years, the need for alternative objectives and outcomes is becoming clear. Many patients with wounds, whether they be leg ulcers, foot ulcers or pressure ulcers, find that aggressive wound care requires too great a sacrifice of time, energy, or money. The request to stop the patient's daily activities is not a reasonable option and, therefore, the patient will become noncompliant with care.

Palliative care is an acceptable plan for many terminal processes and should be considered for those patients who simply do not share the healthcare practitioner goals. A patient's decision to follow a less aggressive plan of care should be accepted, and a plan should be designed that will allow the patient and practitioner to experience success. This decision may mean the primary goal will be to prevent infection or manage exudate, not to contract or heal the wound. If palliative care allows the patient to have more control and improved quality of life, it is a much better solution for everyone involved.

When performing follow up visits, outcomes will best be measured by evaluating patient wound care performance, wound appearance (has it remained stable and free of infection?), pain management, exudate management and patient ability to perform daily activities.

This chapter has focused on alternatives to aggressive wound care, assessment of goals, the environment and development of plans of palliative care. Much more must be written on palliative

wound care. The 2000 titles reviewed on palliative care, all focused on hospice, cancer or immunosuppressed patients. It is my hope that this chapter will provide insight and consideration of some palliative care options for wound care. It is also my hope that clinicians will find satisfaction in providing good, cost efficient care to patients who do not have healing as a goal. The impact on each patient's quality of life will be great as we learn to work within individual expectations.

Conclusion

A well designed palliative care plan for wound care will have many benefits. Patient satisfaction and compliance can be enhanced by an individually tailored plan.

Other benefits include cost effective wound management; appropriate management of exudate and odor; minimal pain with wound care; simple, easy to follow instructions with few steps; improved quality of life for the patient; development of common goals between practitioners and patients; and educated patient decisions.

When everyone respects the goals chosen by the wound care patient, frustration is minimized. Realistic, measurable outcomes can provide satisfaction with a palliative plan of care for the patient with a chronic wound.

References

1. Miller B, Keane C. *Encyclopedia and Dictionary of Medicine, Nursing, and Allied Health*. Philadelphia, PA, W.B. Saunders Co., 1978, pg 743.
2. Morrison RS, Morris J. When there is no cure: Palliative care For The dying patient. *Geriatrics* 1995;50(7):45–51.
3. Carr DB, Jacox AK, Chapman CR, et al. *Acute Pain Management: Operative or Medical Procedures and Trauma*. Clinical Practice Guideline No. 1. AHCPR Pub. No. 92–0032. Rockville, MD: Agency for Health Care Policy and Research, U.S Department of Health and Human Services, Feb. 1992.
4. Darkovich SL. Essay: When is no treatment the right treatment. *Advances in Wound Care* 1996;Jan/Feb.
5. Rutman D, Parke B: Palliative Care Needs of Residents, Families, and Staff in Long–Term Care Facilities. *Journal of Palliative Care* 1992;8(2):23–9.
6. Hiqqinson I. Palliative care: A review of past changes and future trends. *Journal of Public Health Medicine* 1993;15(1):3–8.
7. Bergstrom N, Bennett MA, Carlson CE, et al. *Treatment of Pressure Ulcers*. Clinical Practice Guideline No. 15. Rockville, MD: U.S. Department of Health and Human Services. Public Health Service, Agency for Health Care and Policy and Research. AHCPR Pub. No. 950652. December 1994, pg 45–57, 27–28.
8. Papantonio CT. Home healthcare management of chronic wounds, In: Krasner D (ed). *Chronic Wound Care: A Clinical Source Book for Healthcare Professionals*. King Of Prussia, PA, Health Management Publications, Inc., 1990, pp 318–326.

43

Chronic Wound Pain

Diane Krasner, MS, RN, CETN

Krasner D. Dressing decisions for the twenty–first century: On the cusp of a paradigm shift. In: Krasner D, Kane D. *Chronic Wound Care, Second Edition*. Wayne, PA, Health Management Publications, Inc., 1997, pp 336–343.

Abstract

Chronic wound pain, a phenomenon accompanying the presence of many chronic wounds, has only recently begun to receive the attention and study that it warrants. For many patients the problem is a very serious concern, affecting quality of life and general well–being. Interdisciplinary efforts to develop a comprehensive plan of wound care for such patients, that includes adequate measures to control pain, is essential. This paper reviews recent research on chronic wound pain and on pain assessment and presents the Chronic Wound Pain Experience Model that I developed. Results of my hermeneutic study on nurses' reflections on patients with pressure ulcer pain are discussed. Pragmatic suggestions for the clinical management of chronic wound pain are addressed.

Introduction

Chronic wounds are challenging for patient and caregiver alike. Add the dimension of chronic wound pain and we are faced with a problem of enormous proportions. Given the significance of the chronic wound pain problem, it is astonishing that so little attention has been paid to this phenomenon until relatively recently.

In today's climate of outcome focused healthcare, clinicians should consider the use of "no–pain" or "reduced pain" outcome measures. They can be highly measurable target goals or they can serve as intermediate goals on the way to healing outcomes. Furthermore, in the case of palliative care where healing may not be a realistic outcome measure, reduction in pain may be an appropriate long–term goal.

It is important to remember that from the suffering patient's perspective, chronic wound pain can be a significant problem, impacting on quality of life and general well–being. The words of an ancient Greek epigrapher come to mind:

To cure – occasionally.
To relieve – often.
To comfort – always.

Review of the Literature

Historically, research on chronic pain has tended to focus on such illnesses as low back pain,[1–3] headache pain[4,5] and arthritis pain.[6,7] The research that has been published on wound pain has generally involved acute wounds or burns.[8,9]

Given the recent explosion of general interest in pain and the proliferation of algological literature, it is no surprise that there has also been a growing interest in the issue of chronic wound pain.[10–17] Interest in the subject has also been stimulated by the publication, *Treatment of Pressure Ulcers, Clinical Practice Guideline #15* (Agency for Health Care Policy and Research,U.S. Department of Health and Human Services), which addresses pressure ulcer pain particularly as it relates to wound dressings and debridement.[18] The panel notes that while there is only cursory mention of pressure ulcer pain in the literature, clinicians report anecdotally that pressure ulcer–related pain is experienced by patients. Clinicians are urged to assess pain, not to assume that pain does not exist in nonverbal or unresponsive patients, and to undertake the clinical research that is needed in this area. The panel recommends three specific guidelines related to pressure ulcer pain: 1) Assess all patients for pain related to the pressure ulcer or its treatment (p. 30). 2) Manage pain by eliminating or controlling the source of pain (e.g. covering wounds, adjusting support surfaces, repositioning). Provide analgesia as needed and appropriate (p. 31). 3) Prevent or manage pain associated with debridement as needed (p. 49).

The *Treatment of Pressure Ulcers* document is recommended for further details on these guideline recommendations as are the other AHCPR Clinical Practice Guidelines related to pain which will be discussed in the next section of this chapter.[19,20]

Two recent studies show that wound pain deserves closer scrutiny. Using a qualitative case–study approach, Hollinworth in 1995 found that nurses' assessment, management and documentation of pain at wound dressing changes was most often inadequate and uninformed.[14] She observed nurses' failure to assess pain verbally or to use pain assessment tools. Instead, there was reliance on nursing experience or non–verbal patient indicators to assess pain. Hollinworth found inadequate pain management and poor accountability. Pain assessment and management efforts were not documented, leading the researcher to conclude that "the future management of patients' pain at dressing changes may be compromised owing to impaired communication between healthcare professionals."[14]

Dallam, et al. in 1995 in a cross–sectional quantitative study of one hundred thirty–two patients with pressure ulcer pain, found that 59 percent reported having pain of some type, however, only 2 percent were given analgesics for the pain (within four hours of interview).[10] The researchers recommend that "the domain of pain must be added to the assessment of pressure ulcers. Further investigation should be completed to identify and quantify pain associated with pressure ulcers. Additional research is also needed to identify which combinations of interventions will most effectively relieve the pain associated with pressure ulcers. Educational programs should be developed to sensitize healthcare providers to the association of pain with pressure ulcers and to increase timely and appropriate assessment and treatment" (p. 216).

Assessment of Pain

Given the subjective nature of pain and in light of McCaffery's widely accepted definition of pain ("Pain is whatever the experiencing person says it is and exists whenever he says it does,"[21] (p. 8), it is no surprise that the tools and procedures developed over the last thirty–five years for pain assessment have been based on or have incorporated patient self–report. The AHCPR Acute Pain Management

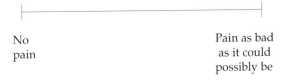

Figure 1. Visual Analogue Scale from the AHCPR Clinical Practice Guideline #1. (A 10 cm baseline is recommended for VAS scales.)

Guideline Panel endorses, in the strongest terms, this approach to pain assessment stating, "The single most reliable indicator of the existence and intensity of acute pain – and any resultant affective discomfort or distress – is the patient's self–report."[19] (p. 11).

The pain assessment tools in general use today range from simple visual analogue scales to complex multidimensional, multi–page instruments. They all have their purpose and place. For example, the visual analogue scale (Figure 1) measures only one dimension of the pain phenomenon at a time (e.g. intensity – from "no pain" to "worst possible pain"), using words, numbers, faces or other culturally congruent objects (e.g. coins, poker chips). Visual analogue scales are particularly useful in clinical practice for patients who are actively in pain and do not have the capacity to complete a long, arduous questionnaire. Visual analogue scales may also be used to measure pain distress and have been shown to be highly reliable instruments, even with the elderly.[22] More complex pain assessment tools, such as the McGill Pain Questionnaire[23,24] and its modifications like the Dartmouth Pain Questionnaire[25] are used primarily in specialized pain centers and for clinical research.

Many pain history–taking tools have also been developed (See AHCPR Clinical Practice Guidelines #1 and #9 for further specifics on pain history–taking and examples).[19,20] Nurses will want to include relevant NANDA nursing diagnoses in their assessments, such as "Alteration in Comfort: Pain" and "Alteration in Comfort: Chronic Pain." There is no question that the assessment and management of pain in patients with severe wounds, in the elderly or in nonverbal or unresponsive patients, presents very special challenges[26–28] and that more research in this area is needed.

The Chronic Wound Pain Experience Model

Scientists and researchers have traditionally classified pain as either acute (defined as pain lasting for less than six months), or chronic (defined as pain lasting for greater than six months). At the 1986

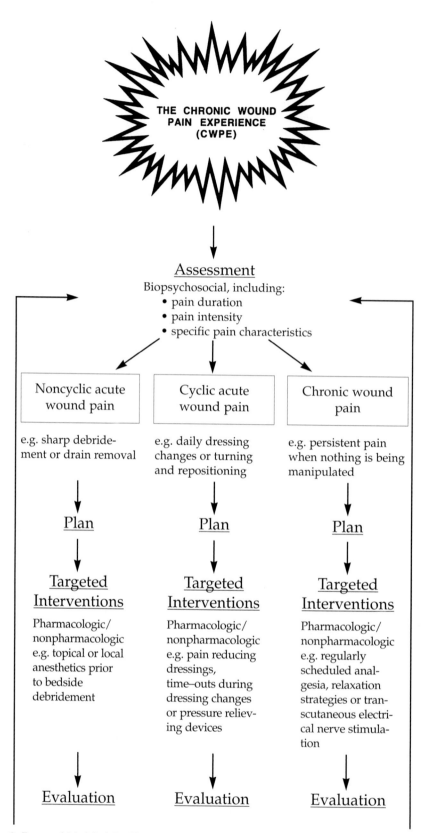

**THE CHRONIC WOUND
PAIN EXPERIENCE
(CWPE)**

Assessment
Biopsychosocial, including:
- pain duration
- pain intensity
- specific pain characteristics

Noncyclic acute wound pain	Cyclic acute wound pain	Chronic wound pain

e.g. sharp debride-
ment or drain removal

e.g. daily dressing
changes or turning
and repositioning

e.g. persistent pain
when nothing is being
manipulated

Plan

Plan

Plan

Targeted Interventions

Pharmacologic/
nonpharmacologic
e.g. topical or local
anesthetics prior
to bedside
debridement

Targeted Interventions

Pharmacologic/
nonpharmacologic
e.g. pain reducing
dressings,
time–outs during
dressing changes
or pressure reliev-
ing devices

Targeted Interventions

Pharmacologic/
nonpharmacologic
e.g. regularly
scheduled anal-
gesia, relaxation
strategies or tran-
scutaneous electri-
cal nerve stimula-
tion

Evaluation

Evaluation

Evaluation

Figure 2. Proposed Model of the Chronic Wound Pain Experience © Copyright 1995 Diane Krasner

KRASNER

National Institutes of Health Consensus Development Conference on pain, a different pain classification with three pain categories was proposed: acute, chronic malignant and chronic non–malignant.[29] Neither classification system adequately reflects the complex pain experience of most patients with chronic wound pain. The chronic wound pain experience does not fit neatly into any one of these proposed categories. Furthermore, the cut–off point of six months seems arbitrary and inconsistent with definitions of chronic wounds.

I underwent surgeries in 1991, 1993 and 1995, first experiencing an open wound, then an infected wound and finally, hypertrophic scarring. These experiences,[30,31] in addition to my previous experience in caring for patients with chronic wounds for over ten years, stimulated me to consider a different conceptual model with definitions that would be more congruent with the experience of patients with chronic wound pain. Ultimately, I developed and proposed the Chronic Wound Pain Experience (CWPE) Model (Figure 2) with theoretical definitions (Table 1).[15] The model was empirically and inductively derived. It relates the CWPE to the nursing process and to NANDA nursing diagnoses.

The model divides the CWPE into three distinct pain categories: noncyclic acute wound pain, cyclic acute wound pain and chronic wound pain. One can assume that most chronic wound patients will experience all three types of pain at some time, although not necessarily simultaneously. It is also recognized that some patients may not experience or be able to indicate pain at all. Others may not experience one of the pain types due to the particular course of their treatment or disease (e.g. the patient who has never had sharp debridement may never experience noncyclic acute wound pain). Another assumption is that many of our active ideas about wound pain may lack validity (e.g. diabetics do not experience wound pain due to neuropathy).

The CWPE Model can be used to guide wound pain assessment, to plan interventions related to prevention and relief of wound pain, to evaluate the efficacy of targeted interventions, or to guide research in this area. It is proposed that specific plans and targeted interventions, both pharmacologic and nonpharmacologic, be initiated based on the type of wound pain that is being experienced. Future research will confirm which interventions or groups of interventions optimize pain relief for each type of pain. For example, applying a topical anesthetic compress prior to sharp debridement may be more effective for this type of acute noncyclic pain than taking an oral pain medication. Round–the–clock medications may be most effective for continuous chronic wound pain. Applying pain–reducing dressings or selecting

---

Table 1
**Theoretical Definitions of
The Chronic Wound Pain Experience**

The Concept: The Chronic Wound Pain Experience (CWPE) is the complex, subjective phenomenon of extreme discomfort experienced by a person in response to skin and/or tissue injury. Chronic wounds include, but are not limited to, lower leg ulcers, diabetic ulcers, pressure ulcers, and open surgical wounds. Biopsychosocial assessment of the CWPE should address pain duration (e.g. periodic intermittent, persistent), pain intensity (e.g. mild, severe) and other specific descriptive characteristics (e.g. descriptors such as "throbbing," "burning," effect of ADLs and functional status.

Subconcepts: *Noncyclic acute wound pain* is single–episode acute wound pain, for example, the pain of sharp debridement or of drain removal. *Cyclic acute wound pain* is periodic acute wound pain that recurs due to repeated treatments or interventions, such as daily dressing changes or turning and repositioning. *Chronic wound pain* is the persistent pain that occurs without manipulation, such as the throbbing of an abdominal wound when a patient is just lying in bed.

© Copyright 1995 Diane Krasner

---

pressure– reducing devices may prove to reduce acute cyclic pressure ulcer pain more effectively than pharmacologic measures. Is it possible that dressing–related wound pain be reduced if able patients are allowed to change their own dressings or to call "time–outs" during dressing changes?

Modeling of the CWPE presents a conceptual road map that can guide the way for future descriptive, intervention and outcome research for patients with chronic wound pain. The need for conceptual clarity derives from the complexity of healthcare concepts as Vincent and Coler have articulated: "Classification in nursing is complex because the phenomena within the discipline are multifaceted and evolving. Given the uniqueness and complexity of human behavior, the categories in an empirical science such as nursing overlap and intertwine, unlike the traditional classification systems of mathematics in which classes are mutually exclusive."[32] As Waltz, Stickland and Lenz remind us, "Because key nursing concepts tend to be complex and relatively abstract, they must be defined and operationalized carefully, if they are to be useful

Table 2
Constitutive Patterns & Related Themes from Reflections on Patients with Pressure Ulcers Who Experience Pain

1. Nursing Expertly
   a. Reading the pain
   b. Attending to the pain
   c. Acknowledging and empathizing

2. Denying the Pain
   a. Assuming it doesn't exist
   b. Not hearing the cries
   c. Avoiding failure

3. Confronting the Challenge of Pain
   a. Coping with the frustrations
   b. Being with the patient

in building and applying knowledge."[33] It is hoped that the CWPE Model will help to clarify concepts, will inspire clinicians and researchers to explore the chronic wound pain experience more closely, and ultimately will lead to a comprehensive approach to chronic wound pain management that will optimize outcomes for patients who experience chronic wound pain.

"Using a Gentler Hand"

In a qualitative study that I conducted,[34] nurse generalists as well as advanced practice nurses who care for patients with pressure ulcers who experience pain were asked to reflect and write a story about the phenomenon. Stories from 42 participants were analyzed for the meanings derived from the nurse caregiver's reflections. A Heideggerian hermeneutical approach[35-40] was used for analysis. Text analysis included the identification of themes, common meanings and constitutive patterns which were shared and discussed with two separate qualitative research teams. Comments and insights from both groups informed and stimulated my thinking.

Three constitutive patterns and eight themes emerged from the text (Table 2). For "nursing expertly," the themes that emerged were "reading the pain," "attending to the pain," and "acknowledging and empathizing." These were the skills that nurses identified as making a difference for patients with pressure ulcer pain. Note the way one expert nurse described these skills in the following paradigm story:

"My experiences with patients with pressure ulcers always involve pain, fear and anxiety . . . My experiences have taught me this: if I can guarantee that a patient will not suffer pain with pressure ulcer care (during debridement, dressing changes, etc.), I see an immediate response of decreased anxiety and fear. But if I have inflicted pain with care, when I return to repeat that care, patients have cried and asked, "Please don't hurt me," or have exhibited signs of increased anxiety (such as sweating, bulging eyes, increased respirations, and exaggerated movement in bed). Patients who cannot verbalize their pain, show me these signs of pain, which often times, go overlooked by caregivers. My response now is – a gentler hand, a slower pace, speaking with patients and explaining every step of care, letting them know that a procedure may be uncomfortable, and offering pain medications prior to painful procedures."

For "denying the pain" the themes that were reflected in the nurses' stories were "assuming it doesn't hurt," "not hearing the cries," and "avoiding failure." While these may be effective coping strategies for healthcare providers, they leave the patient in an extremely vulnerable position. One nurse wrote:

"I've observed failure of medical and nursing staff to recognize or treat [pressure ulcer] pain. It's almost [as if there's the assumption that when] there's an absence of tissue or skin, there must be an absence of sensation in the same location. I've experienced surgeons performing debridement of nonviable tissue, which apparently is not painful, but then continue into viable tissue, without anesthesia or analgesia. They soon realize this hurts as evidenced by the patient's response, but persist as if this is acceptable or expected . . . and should not be resisted. Nurses tend not to regularly medicate pressure ulcer patients for pain as they would for other types of surgical wounds. Maybe they perceive pressure ulcers as being the patient's fault or disgusting or not a "solid" reason for pain."

For "confronting the challenge of pain," two themes emerged from the text: "coping with the frustrations" and "being with the patient." Clearly, when it comes to pressure ulcer pain, there can be a great deal of anger, helplessness, hopelessness and even pain experienced by healthcare professionals and by lay caregivers as well by patients themselves. An effective strategy for confronting the pain problem that the participants identified is being with the patient. Those participants who could just be with the patient in pain felt they had been able to answer the call to care. By being with the patient, some were even able to gain insight into the meaning that the pain experience held for the patient. For example, for one patient with a stage three pressure ulcer, the pain was a marker that she was still alive:

"She came to us on the telemetry unit, we did dressing changes, and then sent her off to surgery for skin grafts when she was strong enough. The entire time caring for this woman amazed me because she was not angry to have these wounds (which I felt were the nurses fault). She instead felt that this was just a side effect of being ill and she was happy to be alive. She was so positive and so helpful when I was changing her dressings. And after surgery she still remained so pleasant. I don't think I could have been as gracious as she was."

must do their best to address this problem. It is no longer acceptable to tell the patient in pain to "just bite the bullet." The ethical principle of nonmaleficence admonishes healthcare providers to "do no harm." With that in mind, five categories of chronic wound pain management strategies are provided for consideration. While the majority of the specific suggestions admittedly only reflect common sense, in many cases they are neither common wisdom nor common practice.

Eliminate the cause of the pain. It is often the case that the interventions chosen to treat a wound such as irrigation, adherent dressings or debridement, cause

---

Becoming more sensitive to this phenomenon and focusing on the experiences of the patients in pain (rather than just the wound) can transform our care.

Taken together these stories form a tapestry of practical insight gained through experience about patients with pressure ulcers who experience pain. Healthcare professionals possess a vast body of experiential knowledge/embodied knowing[39,41-45] related to wound pain, even though they may not always articulate or share that knowledge/knowing with others. Becoming more sensitive to this phenomenon and focusing on the experiences of the patients in pain (rather than just the wound) can transform our care. As Heidegger reminds us, we must confront the challenge of pain and suffering when our patients cry out to us:

"The point is not to listen to a series of propositions, but rather to follow the movement of showing."[45]

How can we, as a community of healthcare providers – nurses, physicians, pharmacists, physical therapists, dieticians, social workers, managers, aides and lay caregivers, expand our call to care to include pressure ulcer patients in pain? How can we work in partnership to meet the needs of pressure ulcer patients, indeed all chronic wound patients, who experience pain? How can we give voice to the silent, as well as the not–so–silent, sufferers? How can we attend to the challenge of chronic wound patients' pain in our professional practice, education and research?

Pragmatic Suggestions for Improving the Clinical Management of Chronic Wound Pain

Despite the dearth of research and information to guide practice related to chronic wound pain, clinicians who care for patients with chronic wound pain

wound pain at the same time. The AHCPR Clinical Practice Guideline #15, *Treatment of Pressure Ulcers*, states, "Manage pain by eliminating or controlling the source of pain (e.g. covering wounds, adjusting support surfaces, repositioning). Provide analgesia as needed and appropriate."[18] (p. 31). Wound pain can be controlled or eliminated by carefully choosing dressings that cover the wound bed and exposed nerve endings, that adhere as little as possible to the wound bed, and that leave minimal residue behind.[46] Avoiding cytotoxic topical agents, harsh chemicals and highly concentrated agents for wound cleansing can significantly reduce wound pain. Allowing able patients to perform their own dressing changes or to call "time–outs" can reduce the pain experienced by some patients. And whenever possible, timing the dressing change at a time of day when the patient is most prepared for it can be extremely beneficial. Give an analgesic and then schedule the dressing change when its peak effect occurs.

Wound cleansing can be used as a strategy to reduce wound pain. The build up of exudate in a wound bed can cause pressure and pain.

Removal of the exudate by gentle flushing, low pressure irrigation, or by the cautious use of whirlpool in selected patients, can bring pain relief.

Positioning patients for comfort and off their wounds can reduce pain at the wound site. If it is not possible to do so, the judicious use of support surfaces can offer pain relief to bedbound or chair-bound patients. Medicating patients before turning, repositioning, sitting or ambulation is quite logical, but it requires planning and coordination and therefore is too often omitted. Using lift sheets (to lift and move), instead of draw sheets (that drag), to move patients in bed prevents friction and shear that can cause painful injuries to the skin and deeper tissues. For many patients, splinting or immobilizing the wounded area (e.g. the use of an abdominal binder for a mid–line incision or wound) can offer significant comfort.

Protect wound margins. Eroded or denuded wound margins can contribute significantly to the pain experienced by chronic wound patients. The use of skin sealants on skin which is still intact, or ointments or skin barriers on open areas can prevent and/or minimize the pain secondary to damaged wound margins.

Select among debridement options carefully. While many factors enter into the decision about which method to select for debriding a wound containing necrotic tissue, pain is a frequently neglected consideration. The AHCPR Clinical Practice Guideline #15, *Treatment of Pressure Ulcers,* states, "Regardless of the method [of debridement] selected, the need to assess and control pain should be considered."[18] (p. 6). Many effective topical anesthetic agents are available for use prior to sharp debridement, including 2 to 4 percent xylocaine compresses (for 10 to 15 minutes, be cautions about reactions) and EMLA® for use on intact skin, not eroded, open or mucosal surfaces.[47] Using autolytic debridement when feasible and appropriate can significantly reduce the pain associated with debridement. Avoid enzymatic debridement which is associated with a high degree of pain, inflammation and possible electrolyte imbalances.

Control inflammation and edema. Inflammation and edema contribute to chronic wound pain so any measures that reduce inflammation and edema will likely also provide pain relief. These measures include thoughtful positioning (e.g. elevation of swollen legs as much as possible), appropriate selection of dressings and devices to reduce edema (e.g. compression bandaging, sequential compression pumps) and the use of systemic medications to reduce edema and inflammation.

Address the ache and the anguish. For many patients, the suffering that accompanies the chronic wound pain experience can exaccerbate the pain the person feels if it is not addressed. Whether it is holding the person's hand during care, a pat on the back or a hug, or, in selected cases, referral to a counselor, psychologist or specialized pain center, acknowledging the suffering and being with the person can make a tremendous difference in the outcome. One paradigm case stands out from my own experience. A woman in her thirties developed breakdown of her wound following a radical mastectomy. The sight of the wound and the torture three times a day of wet–to–dry dressing changes was compounding her suffering. In consulting on the case, I sought to select a dressing that would hide the wound from sight, that would not need to be changed so often, that would be less traumatic to the granulating tissue in the wound bed and that might be bulky enough to parallel her remaining breast so that she would be more "in balance" until the wound healed enough for a prosthetic device. The solution was a nonadherent impregnated gauze dressing, covered by an ABD with Montgomery straps changed daily. The dressing was effective because it not only addressed moist wound healing, but more importantly acknowledged this patient's ache and anguish.

Conclusion

Chronic wound pain, because it is so subjective and multidimensional, presents healthcare professionals and patients alike with enormous challenges. While the wound care community has tended to minimize or even ignore the problem of chronic wound pain over the years, it is now time to become sensitized to the issue. Each of us must be attuned to our patients' suffering, no matter what specialty we claim or in what setting we practice. We must listen, assess and then try pragmatic approaches to the management of chronic wound pain. It is important that we share our experiential knowledge on chronic wound pain with others so that practice, education and research related to this issue can expand and evolve.

"The real voyage of discovery consists not in seeking new landscapes but in having new eyes."
— Marcel Proust

References

1. Cavanaugh JM, Weinstein JN. Low back pain: Epidemiology, anatomy and neurophysiology. In: Wall PD, & Melzack R (eds). *Textbook of Pain.* Edinburgh, Scotland, Churchill Livingstone, 1994, p 441–455.

2. Frymoyer JW, Gordon SL (eds). *New Perspectives on Low Back Pain.* Park Ridge, IL, American Academy of Orthopaedic Surgeons, 1989.

3. Mayer TG, Mooney V, Gatchell RJ (eds). *Contemporary Conservative Care for Painful Spinal Disorders.* Philadelphia, PA, Lea & Febriger, 1991.

4. Olesen J, Tfelt–Hansen P, Welch KMA (eds). *The Headaches.* New York, NY, Raven Press, 1993.

5. Schoenen J, Maertens de Noordhout A. Headache. In: Wall PD, Melzack R (eds). *Textbook of Pain.* Edinburgh, Scotland, Churchill Livingstone, 1994, pp 495–521.

KRASNER

6. Grennan DM, Jayson MIV. Rheumatoid arthritis. In Wall PD, Melzack R (eds). *Textbook of Pain*. Edinburgh, Scotland, Churchill Livingstone, 1994, pp 394–407.

7. McCarthy C, Cushnaghan J, Dieppe P. Osteoarthritis. In: Wall PD, Melzack R (eds). *Textbook of Pain*. Edinburgh, Scotland, Churchill Livingstone, 1994, pp 387–396.

8. Choiniere M. Pain of burns. In Wall PD, Melzack R (eds). *Textbook of Pain*. Edinburgh, Scotland, Churchill Livingstone, 1994, pp 523–537.

9. Cousins M. Acute and postoperative pain. In Wall PD, Melzack R (eds). *Textbook of Pain*. Edinburgh, Scotland, Churchill Livingstone, 1994, pp 357–385.

10. Dallam L, Smyth C, Jackson BS, et al. Pressure ulcer pain: Assessment and quantification. *Journal of Wound, Ostomy Continence Nurses Society* 1995;22(5):211–218.

11. Field CK, Kerstein MD. Overview of wound healing in a moist environment. *The American Journal of Surgery* 1994;167(1A):2S–6S.

12. Franks P, Moffatt C, Connolly M, Mosanquet N, Oldroyd M, Greenhalgh RM, McCollum CN. Community leg ulcer clinics: Effect on quality of life. *Phlebology* 1994;9:83–86.

13. Hamer C, Cullum NA, Roe BH. Patients' perceptions of chronic leg ulceration. In: Proceedings of the 2nd European Conference on Advances in Wound Management. London, England, Macmillan Magazines Limited, 1992.

14. Hollinworth H. Nurses' assessment and management of pain at wound dressing changes. *Journal of Wound Care* 1995,4(2):77–83.

15. Krasner D. The chronic wound pain experience: A conceptual model. *Ostomy/Wound Management* 1995;41(3):20–27.

16. Krasner D. Managing pain from pressure ulcers. In: Pasaro CL. Pain Control [column]. *American Journal of Nursing* 1995;6:22,24.

17. Rice ASC. Pain, inflammation and wound healing. *Journal of Wound Care* 1994;3(5):246–249.

18. Bergstrom, N., Bennett, MA, Carlson, C.E., et al. (1994). *Treatment of Pressure Ulcers*. Clinical Practice Guideline, No. 15. Rockville, MD: U.S. Department of Health and Human Services, Public Health Service, Agency for Health Care Policy and Research, AHCPR Pub. No. 95–0622, December 1994. (AHCPR Clearinghouse, 1–800–358–9295, 9am–5pm EST).

19. Acute Pain Management Guideline Panel. *Acute Pain Management: Operative or Medical Procedures and Trauma*. Clinical Practice Guideline #1. AHCPR Pub. No. 92–0032. Rockville, MD: Agency for Health Care Policy and Research, Public Health Service, U.S. Department of Health and Human Services. February 1992.

20. Jacox A, Carr CB, Payne R, et al. *Management of Cancer Pain*. Clinical Practice Guideline No. 9. AHCPR Publication No. 94–0592. Rockville, MD. Agency for Health Care Policy and Research, U.S. Department of Health and Human Services, Public Health Service, March 1994.

21. McCaffery M. *Nursing Management of the Patient with Pain*. Philadelphia, PA, Lippincott, 1972.

22. Herr KA, Mobily P R. Comparison of selected pain assessment tools for use with the elderly. *Applied Nursing Research* 1993;6(1):39–46.

23. Melzack, R. The McGill pain questionnaire: Major properties and scoring methods. *Pain* 1975;1:277–299.

24. Wall PD, Melzack R. *Textbook of Pain, Third Edition*. Edinburgh, Scotland, Churchill Livingstone, 1994.

25. Corson, JA, Schneider MJ. The Dartmouth pain questionnaire: an adjunct to the McGill pain questionnaire. *Pain* 1984;19:59–69.

26. Herr, KA, Mobily PR. Pain assessment in the elderly: Clinical considerations. *Journal of Gerontological Nursing* 1991;17(4):12–19.

27. McCaffery M, Beebe A. *Pain: Clinical Manual for Nursing Practice*. St. Louis, MO, Mosby, 1989.

28. Watt–Watson JH, Donovan MI. *Pain Management: Nursing Perspective*. St. Louis, MO, Mosby, 1992.

29. National Institutes of Health. Consensus Development Conference Statement: The integrated approach to the management of pain. Bethesda, MD, National Institutes of Health 1986;6(3).

30. Krasner, D. Using a hydrogel, foam and dressing retention sheet. *Ostomy/Wound Management* 1992;38(3):28–33.

31. Ponder R, Krasner D. Gauzes and related dressings. *Ostomy/Wound Management* 1993;39(5):48–60.

32. Vincent KG, Coler MS. A unified nursing diagnostic model. *Image* 1990;22(2):93–95.

33. Waltz CF, Strickland OR, Lenz ER. Operationalizing nursing concepts. In: Waltz CF, Strickland OR, Lenz ER, (eds). *Measurement in Nursing Research, Second Edition*. Philadelphia, PA, WB Saunders, 1991, pp 27–59.

34. Krasner, D. Using a gentler hand – Reflections on patients with pressure ulcers who experience pain: A Heideggerian hermeneutical analysis. *Ostomy/Wound Management* 1996;42(3):20–29.

35. Allen D, Benner P, Diekelmann NL. Three paradigms for nursing research: Methodological implications. In: Chinn PL (ed) *Nursing Research Methodology: Issues and Implementation*. Rockville, MD, Aspen Publishers, 1986.

36. Benner P (ed). Interpretive Phenomenology: Embodiment, Caring and Ethics in Health and Illness. Thousand Oaks, CA, Sage, 1994.

37. Diekelmann NL. The emancipatory power of the narrative. In: *Curriculum Revolution: Community Building and Activism*. New York, NY, The NLN Press, 1991, pp 41–62.

38. Diekelmann NL, Allen DG. A hermeneutic analysis of the NLN criteria for the appraisal of baccalaureate programs. In: Diekelmann NL, Allen DG, Tanner C. The NLN Criteria for Appraisal of Baccalaureate Programs: A Critical Hermeneutic Analysis. (Pub. No. 15–2253). New York, NY, National League for Nursing, 1989, pp 11–31.

39. Heidegger, M. *Being and Time*. (Macquerrie J, Robinson E, Trans.). New York, NY, Harper & Row, 1962. (Original work published 1927).

40. van Manen M. Hermeneutic phenomenological reflection. In: van Manen M. *Researching Lived Experience: Human Science for an Action Sensitive Pedagogy*. New York, NY, State University of New York, 1990, pp 77–109.

41. Benner, P. Uncovering the knowledge embedded in clinical practice. *Image* 1983;15(2):36–41.

42. Benner P. *From Novice to Expert: Excellence and Power in Clinical Nursing Practice*. Menlo Park, CA: Addison Wesley, 1984.

43. Benner P, Tanner C. How expert nurses use intuition. *American Journal of Nursing* 1987;87(1):23–31.

44. Heidegger M. *Poetry, Language and Thought*. New York, NY, Harper & Row, 1971.

45. Heidegger, M. Time and being. In: Heidegger M. *On Time and Being*. New York, NY, Harper & Row, 1972.

46. Thomas, S. Pain and wound management. *Community Outlook* 1989;July: 11–15.

47. Holm J, Andren B, Grafford K. Pain control in the surgical debridement of leg ulcers by the use of a topical Lidocaine–Prilocaine cream, EMLA®. *Acta Derm Venereol (Stockh)* 1990;70:132–136.

44

Growth Factors:
A New Era in Wound Healing

Carelyn P. Fylling, RN, MSN

Fylling CP. Growth factors: A new era in wound healing. In: Krasner D, Kane D. *Chronic Wound Care, Second Edition*. Wayne, PA, Health Management Publications, Inc., 1997, pp 344–347.

The Wound Healing Evolution

Wound healing is going through an evolution. Initially, there was the passive era where health professionals would clean a wound, cover it, and hope it would heal. In the 1970's, many new wound dressings started to become available during the interactive era of wound healing. Through the years, these myriads of dressings, such as the hydrocolloids, the transparent dressings, the moisture–vapor permeable dressings, the gels, beads, pastes, foams, and the alginates, have all been designed to interact with the local wound environment to enhance wound healing. Many are designed to maintain a moist wound environment, thus making the local wound environment more conducive to wound healing. Others absorb exudate to again make the local wound environment more receptive to the wound repair process. While these products assist in creating the optimal wound environment for healing, none of them actively cause cellular growth. The newest era is the active era of wound healing in which cells are actually directed to duplicate and move into the wound space. The primary treatment used to cause this cellular growth is given through the use of growth factors.

What are Growth Factors?

Growth factors are proteins (polypeptides) which are naturally occurring in the body. The growth factors that are integral in the wound healing process are found primarily in the platelets and the macrophages. Some growth factors are mitogens (causing cellular growth) and others are chemoattractants (causing cell migration). While growth factors are known for promoting cell proliferation, many researchers are looking at these growth factors as regulatory factors, directing the unique orchestration of the wound healing process. Falanga defines the term "growth factor" as all–encompassing and includes the terms cytokines, interleukins, and colony–stimulating factors in the same category. He states that "peptides with growth–promoting activities have generally been called cytokines by cell biologists, interleukins by immunologists, and colony–stimulating factors by hematologists."[1]

As of 1993, researchers had identified epidermal growth factor (EGF), platelet derived growth factor (PDGF), insulin–like growth factors (IGF), transforming growth factors and related polypeptides (TGF–ß), and fibroblast growth factor (FGF).[2,3] It is important to distinguish these growth factor families from each other because they each have a different cellular activity with different selected cells.

All of these families of growth factors exhibit chemotactic activity *in vitro*; however, each growth factor appears to act on specific cells. TGF–ß is specific for human peripheral blood monocytes; PDGF is chemotactic for fibroblasts but not for monocytes; ßFGF and IGF–1 are chemotactic for vascular endothelial cells; and EGF stimulates chemotactic migration of epithelial cells.[3] In addition, EGF is mitogenic for epithelial tissues, fibroblasts, and endothelial cells; TGF–ß inhibits replication of keratinocytes, endothelial cells, lymphocytes, and macrophages and may inhibit or stimulate fibroblasts; IGF–1 is mitogenic for fibroblasts and endothelial cells; PDGF is mitogenic for vascular smooth muscle and fibroblasts; and FGF is mitogenic for mesenchymal and neural tissue.[2]

Falanga describes that the main overall effects of these growth factors in wound healing include the following: EGF–re–epithelialization, angiogenesis, and collagenase activity; PDGF–proliferation and chemoattraction of smooth muscle cells, fibroblasts, and other mesenchymal cells and extracellular matrix deposition; FGF–angiogenesis; TGF–ß–extracellular matrix formation, immunosuppression, and inhibition of epidermal proliferation; and IL–1–chemoattraction of keratinocytes, neutrophils, monocytes, and lymphocytes, and stimulation of collagen synthesis.[1]

Numerous review articles document the research that has been conducted to determine the roles of these growth factors.[4–13] One of the difficulties of determining how growth factors work is the fact that different effects may be observed between the *in vitro* and *in vivo* research. Falanga gives the example of TGF–ß1 which in the *in vitro* setting is a potent inhibitor of endothelial proliferation but in the *in vivo* setting results in rapid angiogenesis.[1] More research needs to be conducted to clearly identify the role of growth factors in each stage of the wound healing process in humans.

Growth Factors in Research

Because the *in vitro* studies have demonstrated that the growth factors have an integral role in cellular growth and regulation, it is theorized that these growth factors can be used to assist in wound healing. The volume of animal and human studies evaluating the use of growth factors in wound healing is increasing. The types of growth factors used in research can be categorized into two major groups: single growth factors manufactured through recombinant DNA technology and multiple growth factors secured from human platelet releasate.

Single Growth Factor Research

Acidic Fibroblast Growth Factor (aFGF). Recombinant human aFGF was applied topically to full–thickness excisional injuries in healing–impaired genetically–diabetic mice. It was found that aFGF increased wound closure in a dose dependent manner, nearly tripled the rate of healing, and increased granulation tissue formation and reepithelialization.[14]

Epidermal Growth Factor (EGF). A prospective study of recombinant EGF applied topically to human skin graft donor sites (n = 12 patients) reduced the time to complete epithelialization by 1.5 days. The concern about this study was that although it was conducted on healthy human subjects, the healing rate was not that different between the two groups.[15]

A prospective, double blind, randomized study of the use of human recombinant epidermal growth factor (h–EGF) in treating human venous ulcers (n = 35 patients) demonstrated that there was a greater reduction in ulcer size and a larger number of healed ulcers, but the results were not statistically significant.[16]

Basic Fibroblast Growth Factor (bFGF). This prospective, randomized, double blind study of the use of topical human recombinant basic fibroblast growth factor for the treatment of diabetic neurotrophic foot ulcers (n = 17 patients) found that there was no advantage over placebo. The authors stated that "because diabetes causes significant wound healing defects, we hypothesized that using a single growth factor might be insufficient to accelerate wound closure of diabetic ulcers."[17]

Platelet–Derived Growth Factor–BB. Several prospective studies have been conducted on the use of recombinant PDGF–BB to treat pressure ulcers. Robson, et al. reported that in 20 patients treated in a randomized, double–blind, placebo–controlled trial, there was a greater healing response in the 100 ug/ml PDGF–BB group, but the lower doses compared to placebo had very little effect.[18,19] Mustoe, et al. conducted a randomized, double–blind trial on 41 pressure ulcer patients.[20] They found that ulcers treated in the rPDGF–BB group were significantly smaller in volume compared with those in the placebo group. Pierce, et al. demonstrated statistically significant increased fibroblast and neovessel content in pressure ulcers treated with PDGF–BB compared to placebo.[21]

In a multi–center, prospective, randomized, double–blind, placebo controlled trial of the use of recombinant human platelet–derived growth factor (rhPDGF) to treat lower extremity diabetic ulcers (n = 118), it was found that 48 percent of the rhPDGF patients healed compared to 25 percent of the placebo group (p= 0.01).[22]

Multiple Growth Factor Research

Platelet releasate. Growth factors are stored in the α granules of the platelet.[23] When thrombin is introduced into the α granules of the platelets, growth factors are released. Because the body produces multiple growth factors that are stored in the platelets, these multiple growth factors are then released — thus, the term, platelet releasate.

Several prospective, double blind, randomized placebo controlled studies have been conducted, applying the platelet releasate topically to a non-healing wound. The first study treated 24 patients with 34 wounds of varying etiologies. Eighty one percent of the platelet releasate treated wounds achieved 100 percent epithelialization compared to 15 percent of the placebo. (p < 0.0001).[24] In following studies on diabetic ulcers (n = 13 patients), Steed documented that 71 percent of the treatment group healed compared to 17 percent of the placebo group (p < 0.05).[25] Holloway also documented that in a dose ranging study of the platelet releasate versus placebo (n = 70 patients), 63 percent of the platelet releasate wounds healed versus 29 percent of the placebo (p = 0.01) and the 1 : 100 concentration had the greatest healing rate with 80 percent healed versus 29 percent (p = 0.01).[26] In a prospective, historical controlled trial (n = 23 patients with 27 wounds), Atri found that more wounds healed in a shorter period of time when platelet releasate was used compared to comprehensive wound care alone.[27] Recent prospective studies which are being prepared for publication also documented more favorable healing with the platelet releasate than with controls. (Personal communications)

Clinical Use of Growth Factors

While it is exciting to learn about the potential of using growth factors to enhance wound repair in chronic wounds, it is important to keep them in perspective. They are not a "magic bullet." Basic research has determined that growth factors can stimulate cell growth and migration, but they do not correct the other major problems that health professionals face when trying to treat a chronic, nonhealing wound: perfusion or nutritional deficits, infection, osteomyelitis, edema, or pressure. These problems need to be treated with good quality, comprehensive wound management. Growth factor therapy can be an integral component of this care but should not be used in isolation.

Several retrospective studies have evaluated the use of a comprehensive wound management algorithm which includes the use of the platelet releasate. The algorithm includes an in–depth patient and wound assessment with the following as needed: vascular studies, revascularization, infection management, aggressive wound excision, topical platelet releasate growth factor therapy, skin grafting, the use of protection devices, nutritional management, patient education, and prevention techniques.

Utilizing this protocol, Knighton, et al. documented healing wounds that had a previous wound duration of 198 weeks in an average of 10.6 weeks.[28] Keyser demonstrated in 86 diabetic patients who had their wounds for an average of 32 weeks, that 88 percent were healed in an average of 15.8 weeks.[29] In addition, in 3 separate studies, it was documented that limbs previously recommended for amputation instead had an 83 to 93 percent limb salvage rate.[29–31]

Two cost–effectiveness studies have been conducted on outpatient comprehensive wound management programs that utilize the platelet releasate. In one study, the charges from such a program were compared to a conventional outpatient clinic. It was found that in the comprehensive wound management program there were one–third the charges, three times greater wound healing, and two–third's fewer amputations.[32] In the second study, Bentkover documented that the wound management program using the platelet releasate was 38 percent less expensive per patient healed compared to comprehensive wound care without the platelet releasate or traditional care.[33]

A large, retrospective study of 3,830 patients from 39 comprehensive wound management programs that use the platelet releasate has been conducted. The study demonstrated that more wounds healed (p = 0.00001) and there were fewer amputations (p = 0.00005) when the platelet releasate was used to treat the wounds along with the comprehensive wound management rather than comprehensive wound management alone.[34]

Growth Factor Era

The concept of using growth factors to enhance the healing of chronic, nonhealing wounds has grown tremendously in the last decade. Extensive basic research has been conducted to determine not only their role in the healing process but also how to manufacture or access the growth factors. The research has now moved beyond the animal level. Clinical studies are being conducted on difficult–to–heal chronic wounds. Efficacy has been demonstrated numerous times. While single growth factors have a role in healing, many researchers are hypothesizing that healing would be even better with multiple growth factors.[1,8,11,17] This approach would more readily mimic the body's wound repair process. Healthcare delivery studies have documented that when growth factors are used as an integral component of a comprehensive wound management program, more wounds are healed, there are fewer amputations, and it is highly cost effective. This is the era of active wound healing.

References

1. Falanga V. Growth factors and wound healing. In: Nemeth AJ. *Dermatologic Clinics*. Philadelphia, PA, W.B. Saunders, 1993, pp 667–75.

2. Bennett NT, Schultz GS. Growth factors and wound healing: Biochemical properties of growth factors and their receptors. *Am J Surg* 1993;165:728–737.

3. Bennett NT, Schultz GS. Growth factors and wound healing: Part II. Role in normal and chronic wound healing. *Am J Surg* 1993;166:74–81.

4. Davidson JM. Growth factors in wound healing. WOUNDS 1995;7(5)Suppl A:53A–64A.

5. Herndon DN, NguyenTT, Gilpin DA. Growth factors: Local and systemic. *Arch Surg* 1993;128:1227–1233.

6. Skokan SJ, Davis RH. Principles of wound healing and growth factor considerations. *J Pod Med Assn* 1993;83:223–7.

7. Lawrence WT, Diegelmann RF. Growth factors in wound healing. In: Bernstein EF. *Clinics Dermatology* 1994, pp 157–69.

8. Robinson CJ. Growth factors: therapeutic advances in wound healing. *Annals of Medicine* 1993; 25:535–538.

9. Sporn MB, Roberts AB. A major advance in the use of growth factors to enhance wound healing. *Clinical investigation* 1993;6:2565–6.

10. Steenfos HH. Growth factors and healing. *Scand J Pl Rec Surg* 1994;28:95–105.

11. Kiritsy CP, Lynch SE. Role of growth factors in cutaneous wound healing: A review. *Critical Reviews in Oral Biology and Medicine* 1993;4:729–760.

12. Martin P, Hopkinson–Woolley J, McCluskey J. Growth factors and cutaneous wound repair. *Progress in Growth Factor Research* 1992;4:25–44.

13. Pierce GF, Mustoe TA. Pharmacologic enhancement of wound healing. *Annual Review of Medicine* 1995;46:467–81.

14. Mellin TN, Cashen DE, Ronan JJ, et al. Acidic fibroblast growth factor accelerates dermal wound healing in diabetic mice. *J Invest Derm* 1995;104:850–855.

15. Brown GL, Nanney LB, Griffen J, et al. Enhancement of wound healing by topical treatment with epidermal growth factor. *N Engl J Med* 1989;321:76–79.

16. Falanga V, Eaglstein WH, Bucalo B, et al. Topical use of human recombinant epidermal growth factor (h–EGF) in venous ulcers. *J Derm Surg and Oncology* 1992;18:604–6.

17. Richard JL, Richard CP, Daures JP, et al. Effect of topical basic fibroblast growth factor on the healing of chronic diabetic neuropathic ulcer of the foot. *Diabetes Care* 1995;18(1):64–69.

18. Robson MC, Phillips LG, Thomason A, et al. Platelet–derived growth factor BB for the treatment of chronic pressure ulcers. *Lancet* 1992;339:23–25.

19. Robson MC, Phillips LG, Thomason A, et al. Recombinant human platelet–derived growth factor–BB for the treatment of chronic pressure ulcers. *Ann Pl Surg* 1992;29:193–201.

20. Mustoe TA, Cutler NR, Allman RA, et al. A phase II study to evaluate recombinant platelet–derived growth factor–BB in the treatment of stage 3 and 4 ulcers. *Arch Surg* 1994;129:213–9.

21. Pierce GF, Tarpley JE, Allman RM, et al. Tissue repair processes in healing chronic pressure ulcers treated with recombinant platelet–derived growth factor BB. *Am J Path* 1994;145:1399–410.

22. Steed DL, Diabetic Ulcer Study Group. Clinical evaluation of recombinant human platelet–derived growth factor for the treatment of lower extremity diabetic ulcers. *J Vasc Surg* 1995;21:71–81.

23. Harrison P, Cramer EM. Platelet alpha–granules. *Blood Reviews* 1993;7:52–62.

24. Knighton DR, Ciresi K, Fiegel VD, Schumerth SJ, Butler EL, Cerra FB. Stimulation of repair in chronic nonhealing cutaneous ulcers: a prospectively randomized blinded trial using platelet–derived wound healing formula. *Surg Gynecol Obstet* 1990;170:56–60.

25. Steed DL, Goslen JB, Holloway GA, Malone JM, Bunt TJ, Webster MW. CT–102 activated platelet supernatant, topical: a randomized, prospective, double blind trial in healing of chronic diabetic foot ulcers. *Diabetes Care* 1992;15:1598–1604.

26. Holloway GA, Steed DL, DeMarco MJ, Matsumoto T, Moosa H, Webster MW, Bunt TJ, Polansky M, Newman D. A randomized, controlled dose response trial of activated platelet supernatant, topical CT–102 in chronic, nonhealing, diabetic wounds. *WOUNDS* 1993;5:160–168.

27. Atri SC, Misra J, Bisht D, Misra K. Use of homologous platelet factors in achieving total healing of recalcitrant skin ulcers. *Surgery* 1990;108:508–12.

28. Knighton DR, Ciresi KF, Fiegel VD, Austin LL, Butler EL. Classification and treatment of chronic nonhealing wounds: successful treatment with autologous platelet–derived wound healing factors (PDWHF). *Ann Surg* 1986;3:322–30.

29. Keyser JE. Diabetic wound healing and limb salvage in an outpatient wound care program. *South Med Jour* 1993;86:311–317.

30. Doucette MM, Fylling CP, Knighton DR. Amputation prevention in a high–risk population through a comprehensive wound healing protocol. *Arch Phys Med Rehabil* 1989;70:780–85.

31. Knighton DR, Fylling CP, Fiegel VD, Cerra FB. Amputation prevention in an independently reviewed at–risk diabetic population using a comprehensive wound care protocol. *Amer J Surg* 1990;160:466–72.

32. Fylling CP, McKeown PC. Cost and healing efficacy of treating diabetic foot ulcers in a comprehensive wound management program with growth factor therapy. *Diabetes* 1990;39(Supplement 1):18A.

33. Bentkover JD, Champion AH. Economic evaluation of alternative methods of treatment for diabetic foot ulcer patients: cost effectiveness of platelet releasate and wound care clinics. *WOUNDS* 1993;5:207–215

34. Glover JL, Weingarten MS, Buchbinder DS, Poucher RL, Dietrick GA, Fylling CP. A four–year outcome–based review of wound healing and limb salvage in patients with chronic wounds treated in wound care centers. *Advances in Wound Care* 1997;Jan/Feb.

45

Oxygen, Oxygen Free Radicals and Reperfusion Injury

PD Coleridge Smith, DM, FRCS

Coleridge Smith PD. Oxygen, oxygen free radicals and reperfusion injury. In: Krasner D, Kane D. *Chronic Wound Care, Second Edition*. Wayne, PA, Health Management Publications, Inc., 1997, pp 348–353.

Introduction

In the human body oxygen free radicals take part in many metabolic processes and act as an element of the defense mechanism against infection. Within the mitochondria of the cell, oxidative phosphorylation and the electron transport chain supply the cell with the chemical energy required for all aspects of metabolism. A number of free radical species are generated during these processes but do not normally escape from the mitochondria to other parts of the cell. Free radicals are chemically very reactive and may cause severe damage to many chemical compounds of which cells are made, especially the lipids which comprise the cell membranes. A number of enzymes present in cells catalyze the safe breakdown of oxygen free radicals, affording protection from these compounds. These enzymes include superoxide dismutase, glutathione peroxidase and catalase. In addition tocopherol (a vitamin E component) in the lipid membranes and ascorbic acid (vitamin C) are also able to break down free radicals safely, acting as free radical scavengers.

Neutrophils generate free radicals which they use in defense against bacterial attack. When exposed to some components of bacteria or to some cytokines, the neutrophils become activated. In this condition they adhere to the endothelium, migrate into the tissues and release free radicals in their attack on invading organisms.

During ischemia, the enzyme xanthine dehydrogenase becomes converted to xanthine oxidase which catalyzes the conversion of oxygen to the superoxide anion. This free radical is very toxic to tissues and may also result in the generation of free radicals of other types. When a tissue is reperfused following a period of ischemia, the new supply of oxygen in the returning blood supply permits large amounts of the superoxide anion to be produced. This process sets in motion a chain of events that is termed "reperfusion injury." Endothelial damage occurs in the microcirculation, releasing substances that are strongly chemoattractant to neutrophils. Neutrophils adhere to the endothelium, occlude capillaries and inappropriately release free radicals. This course results in destruction of the microcirculation and is responsible for the development of the features of ischemia, including cell death. This is very much an active process and not simply a passive process dependent on the failure of delivery of oxygen to the tissues. Many complex processes are involved in ischemia–reperfusion injury and a range of drugs is available which might mitigate the worst effects of this condition. Experiments show that many of these products reduce the severity of ischemia, but it seems likely that an attack on several of these processes is required to produce a clinically useful treatment.

What are Free Radicals?

Free radicals are highly reactive molecular species which have at least one unpaired electron in the outer shell.[1] They attempt to react with other molecules to achieve an electrically more stable state in which the electron is paired with another. Further free radicals are generated when one reacts

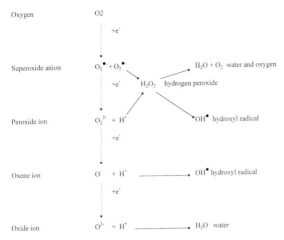

Figure 1. Formation of several species of oxygen free radicals and some of their chemical reactions to form hydroxyl radicals

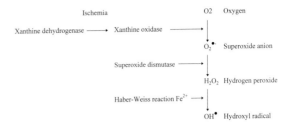

Figure 2. Production of free radicals by xanthine oxidase produced by conversion from xanthine dehydrogenase during ischemia

with a stable compound so that a chain reaction may be set up. This chain reaction ceases when two free radicals interact.

Free radicals are important to many normal functions of cells, including metabolic processes and defense against infection. Normally the free radicals are used in a well controlled manner and serve many useful functions of the human body. Free radicals are chemically very active and under some circumstances may cause harm to body tissues, resulting in cell death. Important examples of this potential are ischemia–reperfusion injury and shock. Under conditions where tissues are deprived of their blood supply and then reperfused, for example following myocardial infarction, release of free radicals from a number of sources results in the damage and death of the tissues. This pathological condition is referred to as infarction. An understanding of the complex series of processes that results in free radical release and reperfusion injury may help in the design of drugs to mitigate the worst effects of ischemia, whether it is of the extremities, the myocardium or the brain.

In biological systems the most common source of free radicals is oxygen, which has two unpaired electrons in the outer shell. A number of oxygen derived free radical species are well known (Figure 1). The reactions shown in Figure 1 illustrate that there can be rapid conversion of one type of free radical to another. Hydroxyl radicals are particularly reactive and may be important in the development of tissue injury. The lifetime of a free radical is usually very short — usually less than one second; however, this short lifespan does not prevent free radicals from causing tissue damage.

How are Free Radicals Generated in Human Cells?

The routes of normal metabolism conducted within the mitochondria during oxidative phosphorylation and the electron transfer chain involve the generation of free radicals.[2] These free radicals are usually partitioned from the rest of the cell or from other cells and do not escape to a significant degree.

Neutrophils use free radicals to attack invading bacteria. They have a specific enzyme system that enables them to generate these defense mechanisms. When neutrophils produce free radicals, a considerable metabolic surge referred to as the "respiratory burst" is required in order to generate the free radicals. These free radicals are oxidized to hydrogen peroxide by the enzyme superoxide dismutase. Hydrogen peroxide is not a free radical in itself, but can be converted to other free radicals that may cause tissue damage. For example, in the Haber–Weiss (Fenton) reaction,[3] the hydrogen peroxide reacts with the transition element iron leading to release of the hydroxyl radical.

$$[Fe^{2+} + H_2O_2 \rightarrow Fe^{3+} + OH\bullet \text{ (hydroxyl radical)}]$$

A further mechanism that results in the release of free radicals during ischemia is via a pathway involving xanthine oxidase. Under normal conditions, the enzyme xanthine dehydrogenase serves a useful function. However, when tissues are deprived of oxygen it is converted to the enzyme xanthine oxidase. This process catalyzes the conversion of oxygen to the superoxide anion, a reaction that takes place when the tissue is reperfused.[4] The superoxide anion is the source of further free radicals (Figure 2) which go on to cause more tissue damage.

How Do Free Radicals Cause Damage to the Tissues?

Free radicals have the capability of damaging a wide range of molecules which are part of the structure of cells in many tissues. When used as a

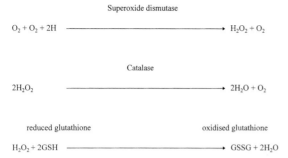

$$O_2 + O_2 + 2H \xrightarrow{\text{Superoxide dismutase}} H_2O_2 + O_2$$

$$2H_2O_2 \xrightarrow{\text{Catalase}} 2H_2O + O_2$$

$$H_2O_2 + 2GSH \xrightarrow[\text{oxidised glutathione}]{\text{reduced glutathione}} GSSG + 2H_2O$$

Figure 3. Chemical reactions of three enzymatic protectors against free radical attack: superoxide dismutase, catalase and glutathione

defense against infection they are not selective for invading bacteria. The neutrophils recognize foreign proteins and are able to release free radicals near the target organisms.

Lipids, which comprise much of the outer membranes of cells as well as the internal endoplasmic reticulum, are very susceptible to free radical injury. The mechanism of lipid damage is referred to as lipid peroxidation. It may take place in a sequential manner as interactions between free radicals and lipids result in the release of more free radicals.[5] The integrity of lipid membranes is essential for the normal functioning of cells; therefore, this mode of injury is particularly damaging. Proteins are less sensitive to free radical attack and do not have the same propensity to facilitate the chain reactions that occur during lipid peroxidation. The nucleic acid DNA is also susceptible to free radical injury, and although there are mechanisms that permit repair of DNA they may fail if damage is extensive. Carbohydrates are also readily damaged by reactions with free radicals.

How are Cells Protected from Free Radical Injury?

In general the parts of cells in which free radicals are produced during metabolic processes (the mitochondria) are constructed in such a way that the free radicals do not escape. Neutrophils release free radicals in their local vicinity, where they are often used in the defense of the body against infection. However, free radicals may reach regions in the cell where they are not required and must be disposed of safely.[6]

A number of enzyme systems specifically designed to disarm the toxicity of free radicals are present in all tissues. They are located in the cytoplasm of the cell and include superoxide dismutase, catalase and glutathione peroxidase. They all have the capability of converting free radicals to harmless

compounds themselves without being destroyed. Their reactions are shown in Figure 3. They offer limited defense against free radicals and prevent propagation of damage, which is especially important in stopping lipid peroxidation.[7]

In addition, a number of other compounds, including tocopherol, behave as non–enzymatic scavengers of free radicals. Tocopherol is a lipid soluble enzyme which is located in the lipid membranes of cells. Its main role is to prevent propagating free radical injury to lipid membranes.[8] Ascorbic acid (vitamin C), a water soluble vitamin, is also important as a scavenger of free radicals from the aqueous phase of cells.[9]

Reperfusion Injury

It has long been known that tissues temporarily deprived of their blood supply do not achieve complete restoration of blood flow when reconnected to a normal arterial supply.[10] Reperfusion injury, the reason for this enigma, has only been understood relatively recently. It occurs when the blood supply is restored to an ischemic tissue, causing further damage.[11]

Mechanisms of Reperfusion Injury

The initial phase of development of this process occurs when a tissue is rendered ischemic, allowing the breakdown of the normal mechanisms of defense against free radical injury. In particular, xanthine dehydrogenase is converted to xanthine oxidase, setting the scene for generations of free radicals. When blood flow is restored to the tissue, the renewed availability of oxygen permits the production of large amounts of free radicals. These free radicals cause damage to the endothelium by lipid peroxidation. The normal defense systems cannot cope with this level of attack and fail to prevent extensive injury. It is likely that free radicals also escape from the mitochondria to contribute to the mayhem.

A number of compounds which attract the interest of neutrophils are released by the endothelium during reperfusion. These compounds include leukotriene B_4 and thromboxane A_2. Many other inflammatory compounds are probably also released at this stage. The neutrophils are attracted and activated by these compounds, resulting in triggering of the "respiratory burst" with further release of free radicals. This process increases the damage already caused and produces further endothelial injury to the microcirculation.

The neutrophils cause occlusion of capillaries in reperfused tissues. The cytoplasm of neutrophils is very viscous compared to that of red blood cells

(RBCs). Neutrophils are also somewhat larger than RBCs and take about 1000 times longer than red cells to deform and enter a capillary.[12] When they are activated and producing free radicals, neutrophils become even more difficult to deform and adhere to the endothelium, occluding the capillaries. When required, very specific mechanisms are present to ensure that neutrophils are capable of adhering to the endothelium (Figure 4). The compounds that facilitate this adherence are located in the lipid membrane of both the neutrophils and the endothelium. Two major groups of compounds called the selectins and the integrins are responsible for this process and elsewhere are important in the adhesion of cells to one another. When activated, neutrophils are able to increase the amount of the integrin CD11b/CD18 on their surface by a considerable amount. This growth greatly increases the tendency of neutrophils to adhere to capillary endothelium. It has been shown that in ischemic reperfused tissues each occluded capillary contains on average one neutrophil irretrievably stuck in the lumen of the vessel.[13]

The endothelial lining of the capillaries plays an important role in the development of ischemia. It is responsible for the production of a wide range of vasoactive compounds. In health it produces prostaglandin which favors vasodilation and inhibits neutrophil adhesion. It also produces endothelium derived relaxing factor (EDRF) which chemically is nitric oxide.[14] This vasodilator also inhibits neutrophil adhesion.

Thromboxane A_2 (TxA_2) and leukotriene B_4 (LTB$_4$) are produced by ischemic endothelium. The TxA_2 is strongly chemoattractant to neutrophils and is released following an ischemic stimulus. LTB$_4$ is bound specifically on the surface of neutrophils and enhances expression of surface adhesion molecules, favoring the accumulation of neutrophils in ischemic tissues.[15] The platelet activating factor is another compound synthesized by the endothelium that is thought to favor white cell adhesion during reperfusion injury. Complement is a complex system of proteins that is activated in any inflammatory process. The proteins are upregulated during reperfusion injury, leading to increased capillary permeability with leakage of proteins and fluid into the tissues.

A wide range of inflammatory mediators referred to as cytokines are also involved in this complex series of events. They include the compounds interleukin–1 (IL–1), interleukin–6 (IL–6) and tumor necrosis factor α (TNFα). They cause neutrophil activation and the increased expression of endothelial adhesion molecules, favoring the adhesion of more neutrophils.[16]

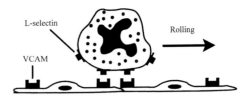

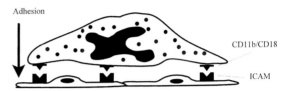

Figure 4. Mechanisms of neutrophil adhesion to vascular endothelium. Initially neutrophils roll along the endothelium in an easily reversible association mediated by L–selectin on the neutrophil surface. They may adhere firmly by a mechanism involving the integrin CD 11b/CD 18 prior to emigration into the tissues.

The number of compounds as well as the complexity and interaction of these mechanisms is very great, involving a wide range of fundamental biological processes (Figure 5). They are collectively responsible for all ischemic processes including myocardial infarction, stroke, septicemia, shock due to hypovolemia, adult respiratory distress syndrome (ARDS) and limb ischemia.

Implications of the Mechanisms Responsible for Ischemia–Reperfusion Injury

Clearly the importance of understanding the mechanisms at work in reperfusion syndrome is that some therapeutic interventions may prevent the worst features of ischemia. It has been shown in animal models and in human patients that white blood cell depletion before an ischemic insult is effective in reducing or abolishing the consequences of ischemia–reperfusion injury.[17,18] This depletion is not very practical in many situations where human subjects are being treated as patients. Pharmacological interventions have been considered as alternatives.

Free radical scavengers. Many compounds have been considered which might deactivate free radicals. Mannitol is the only compound that has been used clinically to any extent for this purpose.[19] Since free radicals are probably responsible for the initiation of the ischemia–reperfusion process, they are an attractive starting point. However, it may be difficult to find a suitable drug to address this part of the process effectively.

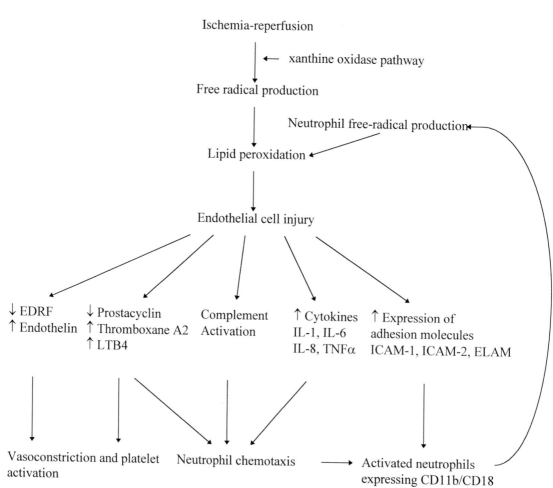

Figure 5. *Diagrammatic summary of events during ischemia–reperfusion injury. This diagram summarizes the main factors involved, but is not an exhaustive list.*

Inhibition of free radical production. The xanthine oxidase inhibitor allopurinol reduces the production of the superoxide radical from this source.[20] The Haber–Weiss reaction is dependent upon the availability of iron. This reaction can be chelated by the compound desferrioxamine, which has been shown to be useful in the mitigation of ischemia–reperfusion injury.[21]

Antioxidants. Lipid peroxidation is prevented by antioxidants, which interrupt the chain reaction that would otherwise destroy lipid membranes. Tocopherol (vitamin E) naturally prevents this process, but has also been given as a therapeutic agent. Propanolol and captopril have also been used to inhibit peroxidation.

Neutrophil inhibition. A number of the activities of neutrophils may be addressed by classes of drugs currently available or under development. The adhesion of neutrophils is greatly inhibited by the administration of monoclonal antibodies directed against the adhesion molecules which they use to attach themselves to the endothelium (CD11b/CD18). These antibodies are effective in reducing the severity of ischemia–reperfusion injury in experimental models.[22] Prostacyclin discourages neutrophil activation and has been used clinically following vascular surgery of the lower limb to reduce the ensuring reperfusion injury.

Cytokines and other inflammatory mediators. Inhibitors of cytokine activity are not widely available; however, a number of inhibitors of thromboxane production have been investigated and have a protective effect in ischemia.

Ischemia pre–conditioning and adenosine. When tissues are exposed to a series of short episodes of ischemia, their resistance to a further long exposure is greatly enhanced. The mechanisms involve the production of adenosine and heat shock proteins. The therapeutic administration of adenosine agonists experimentally mitigates ischemia, and their therapeutic use is under investigation.

Problems preventing ischemia–reperfusion injury. Despite extensive investigation, no single compound has been found that inhibits this process. So complex are the constituent processes that it seems unlikely that switching off any one of the mechanisms alone will have the desired effect. It will probably be necessary to use a combination of measures to achieve a clinically useful effect.

Role of free radical damage in the development of ulcers. Arterial ulcers are the result of severe skin ischemia and the mechanisms previously described in the ischemia–reperfusion injury section are responsible for the production of these ulcers. Neutrophil activation and release of free radicals cause the damage and lead to skin destruction.

Venous ulcers are usually the result of long term skin damage due to chronic ambulatory venous hypertension. This leads to leukocyte accumulation in the tissues of the leg, especially the skin. There is good evidence that neutrophils and monocytes initiate the damage that eventually leads to skin ulceration. In addition to free radicals, these cells replace proteolytic enzymes and inflammatory cytokines that lead to skin damage.

In patients with diabetes mellitus oxygen free radical activity is elevated and has been implicated in the etiology of vascular complications. Recent studies have shown that impaired perfusion of nerve endoneurium is a major cause of nerve fibre dysfunction in experimental diabetes. The peripheral neuropathy which results from nerve damage is one of the main causes for leg ulcers in patients with diabetes. In addition, diabetes leads to an increased susceptibility to peripheral arterial atheroma leading to stenosis and occlusion. This may lead to ulceration by causing ischemia.

Conclusions

Free radicals perform several valuable functions in health but require specific protective mechanisms to keep their toxicity in check. The protective mechanisms become deranged during ischemia and are overwhelmed after reperfusion by the extent of free radical production. This process switches on a wide range of endothelial and leukocyte mechanisms that are responsible for the production of still more free radicals and the destruction of elements of the microcirculation. They constitute the mechanisms that are responsible for the clinical manifestations of myocardial infarction, stroke, shock and peripheral ischemia. Many pharmaceutical interventions are theoretically possible and many are effective in carefully designed animal models. In human subjects the protective effect of any one of these interventions is mild. In the future it seems likely that a combination of treatments will be required to mitigate the effects of ischemia.

References

1. Halliwell B. Free radicals, reactive species and human disease: a critical evaluation with particular reference to atherosclerosis. *Br J Exp Pathol* 1989;70:737–57.
2. Boveris A. Mitochondrial production of superoxide radical and hydrogen peroxide. *Adv Exp Med Biol* 1977;78:67–82.
3. Halliwell B. Oxidants and human disease: some new concepts. *FASEB J* 1987;1:358–64.
4. Roy RS, McCord JM. Superoxide and ischaemia: conversion of xanthine dehydrogenase to xanthine oxidase. In: Greenwald RA, Cohen (eds) *Oxy Radicals and Their Scavenging Systems, Volume 2. Cellular and Medical Aspects.* New York, NY, Elsevier Science Publishing, 1993, 145–53.
5. Kellogg EW, Fridovich I. Superoxide, hydrogen peroxide and singlet oxygen in lipid peroxidation by a xanthine oxidase system. *J Biol Chem* 1975;250:8812–7.
6. Demopoulos HB. Control of free radicals in biologic systems. *Fed Proc* 1973;32:1903–8.
7. Wendel A. Glutathione peroxidase. In: Jakoby WB, Bend JR, Caldwell J (eds). *Enzymatic Basis of Detoxification.* New York, NY, Academic Press, 1980; pp 333–8.
8. di Mascio P, Murphy ME, Sies H. Anti–oxidative defense systems: the role of caretenoids, tocopherols and thiols. *Am J Clin Nutr* 1991;53: 194S–200S.
9. Stocker R, Frei B. Endogenous antioxidant defences in human blood plasma. In: Sies H (ed). Oxidative Stress: Oxidants and Antioxidants. London, UK, Academic Press, 1991, pp 213–42.
10. Quinones–Baldrich WJ, Saleh S. Acute arterial occlusion. In: Moore WS (ed). *Vascular Surgery: A Comprehensive Review.* Philadelphia, PA, WB Saunders, 1991, pp 578–97.
11. Parks DA, Granger DN. Contributions to ischaemia and reperfusion to mucosal lesion formation. *Am J Physiol* 1986;250:G749–53.
12. Braide M, Amundson B, Chien S and Bagge U. Quantitative studies of leucocytes on the vascular resistance in a skeletal muscle preparation. *Microvasc Res* 1984;27:331–352.
13. Engler RL, Dahlgren MD, Peterson MA, Dobbs A and Schmid–Schönbein GW. Accumulation of polymorphonuclear leucocytes during three hour myocardial ischemia. *Am J Physiol* 1986;251: H93–100.
14. Palmer RM, Ferrige AG, Moncada S. Nitric oxide release accounts for the biological activity of endothelium–derived relaxing factor. *Nature* 1987;327:524–6.
15. Karasawa A, Guo J, Ma X, Tsao PS, Lefer AM. Prospective actions of a leukotriene B4 antagonist in splanchnic ischaemia and reperfusion in rats. *Am J Physiol* 1991;261:G191–8.
16. Ward PA. Ischaemia, reperfusion and organ dysfunction. Biochemical and cellular events. *J Vasc Surg* 1993;18:111.
17. Romson JL, Hook BG, Kunkel SL, Abrams GD, Schorek MA, Lucchesi BR. Reduction in the extent of ischemic myocardial injury by neutrophil depletion in the dog. *Circulation* 1983;67:1016–23.
18. Chiba Y, Muraoka R, Ihaya A, Morioka K, Sasaki M, Uesaka T. Leucocyte depletion and prevention of reperfusion injury during cardiopulmonary bypass: a clinical study. *Cardiovasc Surg* 1993; 1:350–6.
19. Freeman BA, Crapo JD. Biology of disease, free radicals an d tissue injury. *Lab Invest* 1982; 47:412–26.
20. Kukreja RC, Hess ML. The oxygen free radical system: from equations through membrane protein interactions to cardiovascular injury and protection. *Cardiovas Res* 1992;26:641–55.
21. Lelli JL, Pradhan S, Mason Cobb L. Prevention of postischaemic injury in immature intestine by desferrioxamine. *J Surg Res* 1993;54:34–8.
22. Simpson PJ, Todd RF, Fantone JC, Mickelson JK, Greiffin JD, Lucchesi BR. Reduction in experimental canine reperfusion injury by monoclonal antibody (anti–Mo1, anti CD11b) that inhibits leukocyte adhesion. *J Clin Invest* 1988;81:625–9.

CHRONIC WOUND CARE, Second Edition

46

Evolution of Critical Path Methodology for Patients with Chronic Wounds

Robert W. Tallon, MD, MBA

Tallon RW. Evolution of critical path methodology for patients with chronic wounds. In: Krasner D, Kane D. *Chronic Wound Care, Second Edition*. Wayne, PA, Health Management Publications, Inc., 1997, pp 354–357.

Introduction

Rapid evolution of the United States medical services sector into an integrated managed health delivery paradigm is perceived as a threat by many wound care professionals. Will managed care recognize the unique nature of wound management or will wound care be relegated to a purely "primary care" problem? Will today's transitional healthcare environment demand the lowest cost per episode of care or will it recognize the implicit wisdom of comprehensively managing care, including disease prevention, and achieve a lower cumulative cost–of–care result?

Background

Historically, seemingly perverse incentives characterized wound care delivery. In a fee–for–service model, suppliers and providers of wound care services were reimbursed separately for the clinical diagnostic and therapeutic services ordered by the primary health professional. This payment philosophy unwittingly encouraged physicians and wound product suppliers to "provide the mostest for the longest." As long as the care provided was consistent with community practice standards and appeared medically–necessary, no prerequisite for wound healing was required for continued reimbursement. In a "pure," capitated managed care delivery system, however, physicians and plans are "at risk" for all patient–required wound care. Incentives change to motivate providers to supply the highest possible quality of health resource at the lowest possible cumulative cost. The chronic wound

in this revised health delivery scenario represents a potentially catastrophic, ongoing source of cost for the healthcare payer. In this situation, enhanced understanding of wound healing and pressure and/or leg ulcer prevention commands significantly greater importance to both health providers and durable medical equipment suppliers.

Managed care, like moist wound healing, assumes an almost sacrosanct, immutable connotation. But just as "moist wound healing" defines an optimal wound healing environment, but not a complete skin reparative solution for every patient, managed care represents merely a general philosophy of health delivery. It tells us nothing about the unique medical and social difficulties of patients for whom we care, but only assigns them to probable risk pools. Managed care tells us nothing about who delivers the care, what tools are used, how frequently the patient is seen, but only specifies how much is paid at a set monthly rate for all the medical care the patient requires.

For wound care professionals then, managed care represents an opportunity to use their clinical prowess and caring skills to most efficiently deliver the complete program of medical services patients require. To optimally function in this care delivery environment, however, it is helpful to understand the many "variants" in managed care, as well as how to best implement our clinical plans of patient management.

Managed Care

As a philosophy of healthcare delivery, managed care first emerged as prepaid health service plans in which total healthcare for plan subscribers was provided for a single, comprehensive plan premium. To achieve this financially risky assumption of total care risk, managed care plans instituted formalized mechanisms of utilization management to help control health system resource expenditures. Conversely, to maintain patient care quality in an environment that inherently valued medical resource utilization parsimony, quality assurance systems emerged as formalized management tools to guarantee a defined, minimally acceptable level of quality.

Historically, the first large managed care experiment was the Kaiser Health Plan that emerged as an aluminum company's solution to provide standardized health benefits to its employees. Later iterations arising on the West Coast, in the Southwest and in the upper Great Lakes region beginning in the late 1950s, used philosophies of preventive care, primary care–based delivery systems, health maintenance, utilization control and integrated medical delivery systems to provide a predefined "bundle" of health services to an identified pool of plan "members" among whom the risk of providing care could be spread.

For the most part, Managed Care Organizations (MCOs) in these early iterations were viewed as "second class" delivery systems, providing acceptable health services at a favorable price. Although gradually realizing steady membership growth in the 1970s and 1980s, the MCO "came of its own" as a truly powerful concept of health delivery in the 1990s. This renaissance was stimulated by the confluence of several powerful social and economic forces including the erosion of U.S. global industrial competitiveness because of ever–increasing healthcare costs; the creation of a vocal class of white–collar uninsured; the financial debacle of state Medicaid programs; and the recognition of the burgeoning use of unsubstantiated, but available, medical diagnostic and therapeutic technologies.

Should this relentless evolution of healthcare delivery to a managed care paradigm concern wound care professionals specifically and healthcare workers in general? Considered in its entirety, managed care ideally creates opportunities for wound professionals and optimizes the cumulative quality of care of wound patients. These favorable predictions are based on several key principles and incentives that are quite distinct from those encountered in fee–for–service medicine. The most vital factor is the MCO's ultimate financial responsibility for the total cost of care provided, not merely an incentive to minimize the patient's episodic health system utilization. In addition, the MCO's

responsibility spans the entire continuum of care, creating either a health delivery environment that no longer encourages "turfing" of patients from one level of care to another, alternatively, or a payment system that creates artificial reimbursement barriers to the provision of maximally–effective therapies at whatever level–of–care the patient requires as long as medically necessary. In fact, this emerging managed care scenario places health providers in positions of increased authority and responsibility. Motivated health professionals create critical paths, or rule books, themselves from which to play. The dual emergence of capitated payment models and internal stimuli to efficient resource utilization transform many of the external utilization review oversight functions, prior authorizations, and requests for medical necessity into little–missed elements of medical history.

Several key issues characterize this evolution in thinking regarding wound care delivery. They include payer and consumer requirements for clinical outcomes information; a requirement to manage patients effectively across the continuum–of–care; integration of therapeutic modalities in disease state management plans; increasing health provider collaboration; the requirement of cumulative cost–effectiveness; and the definition of scientifically–validated plans of wound management that result in significantly improved outcomes of care.

Clinical Outcomes

Since 1988 when Dr. Paul Ellwood, the "Father" of managed care, highlighted *clinical* outcomes as a significant goal of health delivery, outcomes have assumed an almost mystical quality in discussions of managed care delivery. Providers, patients, and payers frequently seem disconcerted by the presumed requirement of clinical outcomes for effective health delivery, but few actually understand what these outcomes actually are, how they are measured, and how they can be effectively integrated into the actual patient/provider health delivery interface.

First and foremost is the concept of *comprehensive* outcomes. For wound care patients, defining comprehensive outcomes is especially salient because these patients are frequently chronically–ill with multiple comorbidities. Achieving healing of a Stage 2 pressure ulcer in a patient who remains at significant risk of developing further pressure ulcers is an outcome of limited useful value. For this patient, comprehensive outcomes management involves not only healing the pressure ulcer, but also improving the patient's nutritional status, providing pressure relief, educating the caregiver, and providing a surveillance system to quickly and accurately detect evidence of future insults to the patient's skin integrity. Managed care greatly values accomplishment of these comprehensive outcomes because they go beyond episodic treatment of patient illness to an integrated process of disease state management. The embracing plan of care that spans this entire continuum of care results in the optimal cost–of–care/quality of care balance.

Support of valid, meaningful outcomes demands reliable measurement, recording, and analysis of patient–specific data. These data include not only routine patient demographics, but "sortable" records defining the site of service delivery, patient risk factors (including "pressure related" variables and those of nutrition, immune status, and coexisting disease), accurate records of the types and quantities of health resources used, and a measure of the time of professional involvement in administering the selected plan of care. These data allow the wound care professional to provide information to managed care – data from which contracting decisions can be based. Moist wound healing as a therapeutic technique may be inscrutable to the MCO. The reduced cumulative cost–of–care (facilitated by an optimized wound healing environment and decreased direct care delivery time), however, is quickly valued by even the most medically naive health system administrator. In a like manner, the ability to demonstrate reduced rates of acute care length–of–stay, a lower rehospitalization rate for wound infections, and/or a reduced required frequency of home nursing visits proves invaluable in obtaining and maintaining managed care health delivery contracts. These measurable performance criteria are critical for independent wound care speciality providers as well as for enterostomal therapy nurses, advanced practice nurses, and home care providers who arrange contracted services provided directly or as the result of an institutional affiliation with an MCO.

Disease State Management

The wound embodies the essence of an illness category that constitutes an ideal treatment setting for the implementation of disease state management (DSM) plans. One of healthcare's newest "trendy" concepts, disease specific care, emphasizes a comprehensive approach to the treatment of easily identifiable, often difficult to manage, disease processes. Wound care as a common, easily identifiable, catastrophic healthcare malady is an ideal disease category for implementation of this diagnostic and treatment methodology.

For MCOs responsible for the patient's entire course of care, disease state management proves conceptually consistent with its comprehensive care philosophy. Disease state management, as applied to wound care, involves integrated management of the patient with wounds including topical wound therapy, nutritional care, treatment of coexistent wound infection, and assuring the optimal care of any complicating comorbidity. This care delivery process demands that the wound care provider understand not only the care involved in restoring violated skin integrity, but also in principles of clinical nutrition, infectious disease, and fundamental pathophysiology as it relates to the wound healing process.

Patients managed according to this paradigm ideally benefit from a total approach to healing. For example, integrated care plans are less vulnerable to poor outcomes achieved by a program of appropriate moist wound healing in a total pathophysiologic environment characterized by a low serum albumin, poorly–controlled diabetes or coexisting immunosuppression from a cancer or steroid therapy. For the MCO whose financial and professional success is predicated on the most cost–effective "cure," failure to accomplish the goals of disease state management diminishes the organization's ultimate chance for success.

Critical Path Methodology

Quality is both a personal goal and professional obligation of the wound care provider. This pursuit of quality demands a minimization of variance in the processes of care delivery as well as an institutional requirement to optimize the cost–effectiveness of the care delivered. Use of a *critical path* (or clinical practice guidelines) can fulfill this requirement.

Critical paths are objective delineations of the recommended diagnostic and treatment guidelines for the management of the usual patient with the illness. These guidelines specifically define the expected time course of healing, the expected outcome of that care intervention, and a delineation of usual processes of care delivery. Critical paths for wound care are not meant to be immutable "cookbook" recipes for wound management, but rather to function as tools to guide the usual course of clinical management and the resulting response to that care management process for the average patient.

Key elements of the critical path include a defined plan of treatment and an expected time course of response to that treatment that allows prompt identification of patients whose actual health intervention outcomes differ from those expected for a defined patient subgroup across the continuum–of–care.

Accurate definition of a discrete patient subpopulation requires information regarding patient risk stratification. This segmentation may demand no significant difference in wound healing outcome based on any permutation or combination of wound stage, age and race. For patients identified with an elevated glucose, however, healing times may be significantly prolonged when compared to a euglycemic patient. Likewise, chronically immunosuppressed patients, either primary or secondary to medication, may require stratification to a higher risk subpopulation. This identified variable, that contributes to significant variance, would then be included as one of the critical path definition's stratification parameters.

Ultimately acquisition of a large database of wound care outcomes allows identified "variant" patients to be managed according to definable "modified" critical paths. Until that time of sufficient differentiating clinical data, however, these complicated patients can be optimally treated using the critical path as a "rough" outline guiding an individualized plan of therapy. In our former example patient with diabetes, for instance, the wound care patient is treated with a "path–specified" combination of wound debridement, surgical dressings, and support surfaces. This patient's expected time course of healing is extended, however, because of probable underlying diabetes–related delayed wound bed revascularization, disturbed leukocyte function, and/or a statistically increased incidence of infection. The defined critical path for this patient suggests the requirement for increased vigilance for evidence of wound infection and a clearly stated treatment goal of enhanced blood glucose control. In this way, clinical management according to critical path methodology, allows the clinician to comprehensively treat all disease processes contributing to delayed wound healing. This technique offers the advantages of a disease state management program for wound care.

For the average patient, the critical path might include routine elements of initial patient wound assessment, a system–defined protocol for wound healing (including suggested treatment products and dressing change intervals), an expected time course for healing, the usual site for care provision (i.e. acute care hospital, subacute center, skilled nursing facility, or home), and an appropriate recommendation for wound prevention. The definition of these elements proves invaluable to the MCO. A critical path facilitates staff compliance with a wound product formulary, which allows organizational volume and preferred contract purchasing. In addition, the critical path creates an optimal "roadmap" for the care delivery team that functions as the patient's initial contact with the health delivery system, despite that team's expertise in wound care. The ability of the critical path to facilitate the identification of therapeutic response variance permits an ideal method for assuring appropriate specialty referral or adjustment of a prescribed level–of–care. Use of the critical path also supports the MCO's quality improvement process, a byproduct of critical path implementation that is of increasing significance in an era of quality report cards, Healthplan Employer Data Information Set (HEDIS), quality comparisons, and performance–based reimbursement systems.

Lastly, the critical path provides both a risk–management and reimbursement tool, through its specification of an accepted protocol of care, response to individual patient variation.

Suggested Reading

1. Wigfeld A, Boon E. Critical care pathway development: the way forward. *British Journal of Nursing* 1996;5(12):732–735.
2. Aspling DL, Lagoe R. Benchmarking for clinical pathways in hospitals: a summary of sources. *Nursing Economics* 1996;14(2):92–97.
3. Wojner AW. Outcomes management: an interdisciplinary search for best practice. *AACN Clinical Issues* 1996;7(1):133–145.
4. Tallon R. Devising and delivering objectives for disease state management. *Nursing Management* 1995;26(12):22–24.
5. Pearson SD, Goulart–Fisher D, Lee TH. Critical pathways as a strategy for improving care: problems and potential. *Annals of Internal Medicine* 1995;123(12):941–948.
6. Tallon (ed). *Critical Concepts in Medical Practice Management*. New York, NY, McGraw–Hill, 1996.

47

Wound Care in a Quality Managed System

Jane Ellen Barr, MSN, RN, CETN

Barr JE. Wound care in a quality managed system. In: Krasner D, Kane D. *Chronic Wound Care, Second Edition*. Wayne, PA, Health Management Publications, Inc., 1997, pp 358–368.

Introduction

Quality and the road to continuous improvement are never ending. There are no short cuts to quality. Achieving quality is a deliberate and time–intensive process that often requires an individual and organizational shift in values, principles, and goals. As wound care specialists, just as we must continuously expand our wound care body of knowledge, we must learn how to be better aware of the needs and opportunities to improve our services individually and within the organizations in which we work. We must learn how to provide quality care.

This chapter on total quality management (TQM) is designed to introduce you to the principles of quality improvement. Quality will be defined. The costs of quality, various types of cost, major cost categories, and the process of estimating one's own individual cost of quality will be addressed. The concept of "customer," both internal and external, will be discussed. More significantly, the relationship between customer and suppliers will be explored. Concepts of continuous improvement, measurement, productivity, and techniques used to examine work processes will be reviewed as methods to help identify opportunities for improvement.

The Meaning of Quality

As wound care specialists, we work within the healthcare system because we care about people. The word "quality" is not just a nice idea; it is what makes us dedicated to our work, what gives us job satisfaction. Most healthcare organizations and individual practitioners are committed to quality patient care. How that commitment is translated into action varies from one organization to another and from one practitioner to another.

There are many reasons for the present focus on the concept of quality management. Escalating healthcare costs, shifts from acute to long term and home care services, and reduced payer dollars all have mandated changes in healthcare operational initiatives. The incentive for change also comes from regulatory agencies, such as JCAHO, and even from the customers themselves.

In the past when healthcare organizations focused on improving quality, they gave the responsibility for quality to one department or person, i.e., the quality assurance (QA) department. The focus was on an inspection base system where the QA staff looked at records of the work situations retrospectively to identify any errors and usually to identify those persons responsible for the errors.

In the late 1980's, healthcare executives began to incorporate TQM with newer meanings of quality into their strategic planning initiatives. Those organizations that embraced TQM concepts redefined the meaning of quality. Quality became customer oriented. Focus was placed on a balance between short and long term goals. Emphasis was placed on prevention. Patterns of problems were believed to be the result of common causes such as ineffective systems and management practices. The responsibility for quality belonged to every employee as they functioned in an environment that strived for continuous improvement. Organizational structure became fluid and integrated, allowing problem solving to involve all levels of employees in a team environment.

In healthcare today, TQM has become a management approach with a commitment to customer expectations, quality, efficiency and cost containment. Visionary leadership, commitment of top management and the entire organization, and a comprehensive database and information system have become the essential ingredients for TQM initiatives. TQM empowers employees by teaching techniques that help individuals improve and gain greater influence over their own work processes. TQM combines a way of thinking about management with a set of problem solving tools and process improvement methodologies.

The philosophy and methods of TQM are based on the work of Deming, Crosby, and Juran.[1–3] These three quality expert leaders agree that successful integration of TQM is based on several principles. The key principles include management accountability, customer orientation, teamwork, continuous improvement focused on work processes, and statistical data analysis (measurement).

Healthcare facilities and providers, while trying to thrive in the changing competitive market place, are addressing the need to redefine the meaning of quality services by incorporating these key principles into their organizations. Quality is defined as the combined efforts of the systems and the individuals within the system working collaboratively to improve patient care outcomes, while maintaining customer satisfaction, reducing costs with implementation of cost–effective operations, monitoring quality efforts, and providing opportunities for continuous improvement. Quality is becoming reality in healthcare organizations with the implementation of TQM Systems.

A quality approach draws energy from three sources: the patient/customer, the employee and the continuous improvement of work processes. Quality is redefined and achieved when there is a tight integration of these three powerful forces.

The Cost of Quality

The issue of cost is of major concern in the changing healthcare environment. Healthcare organizations have always made use of the concept of identifying the costs needed to carry out the various functions: marketing, personnel, and services. However, until the 1980s this concept had not been extended to issues of quality function, except for departmental activities of inspection. Today the concept of quality cost has emerged as a key issue in organizations. Healthcare organizations are taking a "cost of quality" approach to cost assessment.

The cost of quality includes all the costs of providing services that meet the needs of patients and other customers. Cost of quality is defined in terms of the healthcare organization's ability to successfully achieve alignment and execution.[4] Alignment, what employees do, is measured by how well the needs of the patients and other customers are met. Execution, how employees work, is measured by whether the highest return is achieved at the lowest cost.

There are two types of costs: necessary costs and avoidable costs.[3–5] Necessary costs are costs required to achieve and sustain a defined standard of work. Necessary costs include the costs of doing things right. They include prevention and inspection costs.

Avoidable costs occur whenever things are done wrong. Costs are considered avoidable costs when the system fails to do right things right. Avoidable costs include some inspection costs and failure costs.

The key to reducing cost is prevention. Prevention costs are the costs of actions intended to make sure that things will not go wrong. For example, identification of patients at high risk for pressure ulcers and the prevention of pressure ulcers have proven to be cost–effective measures.

Inspection costs are the costs of finding out if and when things are going wrong so correction and prevention can occur. A good example of an inspection cost is early identification of Stage I and II pressure ulcers through the use of prevalence and incidence studies. The next best thing to prevention is early detection and early treatment.

Despite prevention efforts, problems may still occur. Failure costs are costs incurred when a patient or another customer is or will be dissatisfied. There are internal and external failure costs. Failure of a practitioner to identify that a patient's increased pain level is causing immobility and resulting in impaired tissue integrity is an example of internal failure cost. If a specialty bed was ordered for a high risk patient, but failed to be delivered for two days, this would be an example of an external failure cost.

Practitioners can estimate their own individual cost of quality by using the quality grid.[4] The quality grid analyzes activities of the practitioner in regard to what the practitioner does, i.e. right things or wrong things, and how the practitioner does things, i.e. wrong or right. Therefore, all activities can be categorized as RTW (right things wrong), RTR (right things right), WTW (wrong things wrong), or WTR (wrong things right). The practitioner identifies all major activities that he/she does as part of the job. The activity is then categorized into the appropriate group: RTW, RTR, WTW, or WTR. The percent of time spent doing each activity is estimated. The practitioner then subtracts the percent of RTR from 100 percent to identify for the

Table 1
Example of a Quality Grid Analysis

Category	Activities	Percent Time
RTW (Right things Wrong)	Duplicated charting. Wrote policy and procedures without input from staff. Obtained wound care supplies separately throughout the day for individual patients. Spent increasing amount of time collecting wound stats from units (time consuming).	20%
RTR (Right things Right)	Assessed all patients referred for wound management using established assessment sheet. Appropriately used wound care supplies for wounds treated during various phases of healing.	65%
WTR (Wrong things Right)	Spent time answering telephones in the office when secretary stepped out. Xeroxed copies of patient education programs.	10%
WTW (Wrong things Wrong)	Spent time at alternate sites/meetings not relevant to job.	5%

100% (Total) - 65% (RTR) = 35% (Avoidable cost of quality)

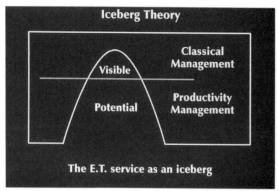

Figure 1. The iceberg theory.

practitioner the avoidable cost of quality.

A wound care specialist follows these steps: Step 1) Identify major activities; Step 2) Categorize them; Step 3) Estimate a percentage of time spent within each category; Step 4: Subtract percent RTR from 100 percent (Table 1).

After a practitioner analyzes his/her cost of quality, the iceberg theory can be utilized to facilitate more quality output from the wound care department or individual practitioner. The iceberg theory makes the assumptions that the majority of the activities carried out by the wound care practitioner, the visible part of the iceberg, would fall under the typical services expected to be provided or the minimum expectations of a department. However, beneath the visible part of the iceberg is another whole level of innovative activities that the practitioner could be involved in to increase productivity and cost of quality of services provided to customers. If a practitioner finds that 35 percent of her/his time is spent on avoidable costs of quality, correcting this problem would allow more time for innovative and more productive aspects of service (Figure 1).

One important TQM tool that helps practitioners and organizations to avoid failure costs is the use of the 1–10–100 Rule.[4] The rule states that if a problem is not fixed when it occurs, it will only become more costly to fix later in terms of both money and time. This rule of thumb recognizes that it makes a difference when a problem or error is discovered and resolved (Table 2).

It is important for all organizations and practitioners to have a good understanding of an effective cost–of–quality concept. To be cost effective, a

Table 2
The 1–10–100 Rule

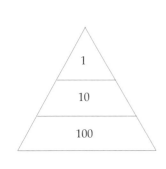

1 = Catching and fixing a problem(s) in the work area(s) (Prevention Costs)

10 = Catching and fixing a problem(s) after it has left the work area. (Inspection Costs)

100 = Repairing the damage from the problem(s) that affect patient or other external customers (Failure Costs)

cooperative organizational structure is needed to enhance output by making the most of limited resources and providing a framework for the development of measures that look at how well departments work together. Quality cost techniques provide a systematic way of measuring, reporting, and tracking the effectiveness and efficiency of all parts in the system working together at various junctures in the process. The major cost categories within a quality system are prevention, inspection (sometimes called appraisal), and internal and external failure costs.

Quality cost techniques provide a way of assessing relationships between money expended for a certain activity on both a micro–departmental and a macro–divisional level. Relationships among departments and those within departments can be evaluated. Tracking quality costs is important to demonstrate effort spent on activities in a quality system.

The Customer

The key to successful TQM implementation is managing quality customer service. A cliché often associated with TQM is "Quality begins and ends with the customer." In Japanese, the word "okyakusama" means both customer and honorable guest. Customers in today's marketplace are looking for that special treatment that is typically used to serve and honor guests.

"Customer" is an unfamiliar and sometimes uncomfortable term for healthcare providers, but it is an essential concept in improving the systems necessary for the delivery of quality healthcare. "Customer" represents the many people affected by what we do and the systems we use. No matter what our job, we provide services, materials, or information to others – our customers. A customer then is a person, a group, or an organization that uses the product, service or information that we provide.

There are both internal and external customers.[3–7] Internal customers are all employees working within an organization. Internal customers refer to persons or groups such as administration, all departments within an organization and all co–workers. External customers are those outside the organization who receive outputs from the organization. In healthcare, external customers refer to persons and groups such as the patient (the ultimate external customer), the patient's family or significant others, third party payers, HMOs, government agencies, and manufacturers who produce products needed by the organization.

All employees working in a healthcare system must see themselves as part of a structure where they are customers and suppliers to one another, linked in a chain that extends from within the organization to the ultimate customer – the patient.[3–5]

This simple structure can support complex work processes. It represents a natural flow of work across functions and between employees in an organization. In healthcare organizations, not every employee has direct contact with the patient and other external customers. However, all employees depend on other employees for the services and products they need to do their jobs. For example, the practitioner in an outpatient wound care clinic may depend on secretaries for registration, the laboratory for significant test results, or the billing department, housekeeping, medical records, dieticians, physical therapists.

Quality customer service must consist of two integral dimensions: procedural and personal dimensions.[7] The procedural dimension of service provides the mechanism by which customer needs are met. It deals with service delivery systems. A customer receives materials, information, or services from others in the organization or from an outside source. What customers receive from others is considered input. Suppliers provide material, information or service to others in the organization or to an external customer. That which is provided to others is considered output. The supplier is responsible to add value to the input.

The personal dimension, the human side of service, encompasses the attitudes, behaviors, and verbal skills that are present in every personal service interaction. Quality service standards must incorporate both the procedural and personal service dimensions.

Work can be seen as a process in which customers receive input from their suppliers, add value to that input, and then pass outputs on to their own customers. Customer needs are better satisfied if people from separate functions are all trying to meet the needs of the next internal process, rather than being primarily concerned about the welfare of their own functions. A wound care practitioner would not want the materials management department to think only of its own goals to minimize inventory and reduce costs. The practitioner would expect that supplies needed in the clinical area would be available; he/she would also understand that unnecessary supplies could not be carried in inventory.

In order to achieve customer satisfaction, it is important that the supplier's capabilities are aligned with the customer's needs. For example, if the wound care specialist of a healthcare organization makes a variety of wound care dressings available to the bedside practitioners without educating them about how to use the dressings appropriately, a misalignment can result. When customers and suppliers within an organization are not aligned, organizational goals are more difficult to meet. Customers and suppliers must work together collaboratively to achieve alignment. Alignment must occur vertically and horizontally within the organization.

Alignment should have three components: customer needs, supplier capabilities, and organizational goals. Three–way organization is achieved when supplier capabilities are matched with customer needs to reach the goals of an organization. The supplier must prevent misalignment with organizational goals. Performance gaps, which occur when the supplier capabilities lag behind the customer's requirements, or opportunity gaps, which occur when the supplier's capabilities exceed the customer's requirements, must be either prevented or utilized to expand services.

In order to be aligned with the customer's requirements, the supplier must have a customer service perspective. The customer service interaction must become the *sine quo non* of the services provided by the organization. To understand the customer, the supplier must be able to specifically define the services provided and the characteristics of the services provided and to fully realize who the customer is, what the customer wants, and how the customer perceives the service.

A service silhouette indicates how the customer perceives the service. Determinants of a service silhouette include such factors as purpose of the service, degree of necessity, magnitude of importance, view of results, relative costs and perceived risks. The supplier must aim at developing a positive service silhouette.

It is important that customers and suppliers exchange information about their requirements and provide one another with feedback as to how to meet those requirements. This exchange is best achieved by a customer feedback system. A customer feedback system must be an organized and deliberate way of finding out what customers think about the job being done. It should be planned, organized, and proactive, with the intention of optimizing customer information flow into the organization.

It also important to have an employee feedback system. An employee feedback system is an organized way of noting each employee's job performance behavior and sharing that information with the employee. It is a system whereby the management and employee mutually check on the quality level of customer service as performed by the employee. Feedback should be provided to employees by verbal recognition, posting measures of individual and group customer service productivity, and periodic performance appraisals based on measurable, observable quality customer service standards.

Continuous Improvement

Healthcare organizations can only become total quality organizations by continuously improving all the work processes to satisfy their internal and external customers. According to the theory of continuous improvement, real improvement in quality depends on understanding and revising systems or the processes that make the system work on the basis of data collected about the systems and processes themselves. Focus is on continuous improvement throughout the organization through constant effort to reduce waste, rework, and complexity.

Continuous improvement is about making refinements to processes by solving problems. Problems can be defined as sporadic and chronic.[3] A sporadic problem is a sudden, adverse change to the status quo. A chronic problem is a long standing adverse situation, which requires remedy through changing the status quo.

The distinction between sporadic and chronic problems is important in relation to continuous improvement. Sporadic problems are dramatic and must receive immediate attention. In a total quality management system, sporadic problems should be addressed by a control of quality or a process that has been established in order to meet standards. Control is largely directed at meeting goals and preventing adverse change, i.e. holding the status quo.

Chronic problems are not dramatic because they occur for a long time, are often difficult to solve, and are accepted as inevitable. Chronic problems are solved using the continuous improvement process. The danger for most organizations is that solving sporadic problems may take continuing priority over efforts to achieve the larger savings that are possible with solving chronic problems.

As wound care practitioners, we must learn how to analyze and monitor our work process so that problems can be detected before they affect the customer–supplier relationship. We need to continuously improve our processes so that they are capable of meeting competitive challenges and our customer's changing needs, both now and in the future. For example, with HMOs as one of our customers, we may need to change our processes on managing wounds in an outcome–driven, cost–effective manner in a seamless care system, as patients move through the healthcare continuum from home to acute care and back to home or long term care.

Examining the work process. Basic to the concept of continuous improvement is the ability to learn how to examine processes. A process consists of the work done to produce the service or product that the wound care practitioner delivers to his/her patients or other customers. The work process involves receiving inputs from suppliers, adding value to those inputs, and then passing them on to the patient or other customers as outputs. Work is the business of adding value to the inputs received so that they become the outputs customers need. The work process is how one goes about doing the work. It is necessary to be able to analyze work processes. Process measures help to analyze work processes over time to understand their maximum capabilities and their actual and potential flaws.

Processes that can be improved by means of systematic techniques abound in healthcare. Even individual wound care specialists create and use production processes that can be improved: the way patients are scheduled, the way patient education is provided, organization of records, billing processes, or the processes used to ensure that patients identified as high risk for pressure ulcers receive preventive measures.

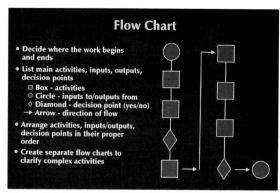

Figure 2. *Flowchart.*

Continuous improvement is an integral part of a quality organization. To implement a continuous improvement program, the work process must be able to be identified, analyzed, and monitored. Continuous improvement is seen as a cost–effective way to maintain an organization's competitive edge. When all individuals within the organization improve their work processes, the organization can better meet the needs of its patients and other customers. Key to the concept of continuous improvement is fixing problems on the spot, preventing problems from occurring, and improving abilities to meet customer requirements. Continuous improvement often means small but beneficial changes that add up.

Modern technical, theoretically grounded tools must be put to use in healthcare settings for improving processes. There are many theories and techniques by which to analyze and improve complex production processes; a few examples are the process flowchart and the control chart.

Flowcharts. Flowcharts are useful tools in continuous improvement to help analyze and improve a work process.[4,8,9] They support the principle that if you understand a process and how it works, then you will be able to identify its requirements and prevent any bottlenecks. Flowcharts graphically describe the steps of one or more work process or subprocess in the sequence in which they occur. For example, a wound care practitioner could prepare a flowchart to follow the process of a hospital outpatient visit to a clinic from the patient's time of registration to discharge. Each step in the process is denoted by a symbol indicating the nature of the action or reaction. The main elements of a simple flowchart are the circle, which indicates inputs to and outputs from; the box, indicative of activities; the diamond, which is used for decision points; and the arrow, which shows direction of flow from one activity to the next. The symbols used in the flowchart make it easy for the examiner to identify the different types of actions or transactions that occur during the process (Figure 2).

Team members should be collectively involved in flowcharting a process. They should start by defining the process under consideration. Next, they should identify the beginning and the end of the process. The team should then start to list the steps of the process in the sequence in which they occur. Certain members of the team or specific action teams should be responsible for flowcharting the technical steps in the process. Once a flowchart of the process has been produced, the team should review it and then revise it if necessary to incorporate any missing steps or correct any errors. The final version of the flowchart is then transferred to a sheet of paper, using symbols to denote the steps of the process. The flowchart is now ready to be used by the organization. Flowcharts are management tools that support the quality improvement efforts in an organization.

The following procedure is used to create a flow chart:

1. Gather a group of people who represent the various parts of the process.
2. Decide where the process begins and ends.
3. Brainstorm the main activities and decision points in the process.
4. Arrange these activities and decision points in their proper order, using arrows to show direction of flow.
5. As needed, break down the activities to show their complexity.

<u>Control charts.</u> It is very important in a quality organization to monitor work processes. It is necessary to know how well processes are performing to ensure they are capable of meeting the requirements of customers and able to correct process problems before they affect outputs and to improve processes to meet changing customer needs. Performance of processes can vary from day to day. Some minor variation is normal and results from causes easily controlled or changed. Variations that exceed normal limits are the result of specific problems or influences that should be addressed by a continuous improvement process.

Control charts are management tools that help depict how well a process is doing.[4,8,9] Control charts are designed to monitor a process over time and to study its trends and variations. They are constructed to display the stability of a process around a historical (acceptable) trend with a capability of measuring small changes in the process. A control chart helps determine whether a process is in or out of control, detects trends in a process' performance

that indicate the effect of a special cause, and evaluates the overall effect of common causes on process variation to decide whether a process should be overhauled or redesigned. A control chart is, therefore, useful in identifying opportunities to improve a process.

Control charts are basically–run charts with three additional horizontal lines. The average value is the line between the upper and lower control limits. A process is said to be in control if the trend lies within the upper and lower control limits around the average. If a trend falls outside these limits, then the process is considered to be out of control. There is an additional element to this concept. The process is considered to be out of control if at least three consecutive points on the process trend line fall below or above the average line. This concept holds true even if the process trend line continues to lie between the upper and lower control limits. An important point that needs to be mentioned is that control limits are not thresholds or standards. They are measures that describe the behavior or the nature of a process. Therefore, if a process is in control, it is not necessarily a good process; conversely, if a process is out of control, it is not necessarily a bad process.

Wound care practitioners can use control charts to monitor various processes in their practices, for example, to measure statistics such as incidence and prevalence of pressure ulcers in an organization or on specific services or units within an organization and to measure healing times of various types of wounds such as venous leg ulcers.

The procedure for using a control chart is as follows:

1. Select a variable that is a good indicator of the performance of your process, i.e. the incidence of pressure ulcers in a hospital.
2. Choose a way to measure the variable you have selected, i.e. weekly assessment and documentation of the incidence of pressure ulcers on all adult patients in the hospital by the nursing staff. Incidence is documented on weekly pressure ulcer statistics forms by nurse managers and submitted to the wound care department. Wound care practitioners then analyze the data.
3. Select time intervals at which measurements should be made, for example, data may be collected weekly but reported on control charts on a monthly basis.
4. Create a chart for the aspect of the process that is to be measured over time. Label the vertical axis with the units of measure for the variable. Label the horizontal axis with the units of time over which the variable will be measured, for example, the vertical axis for the incidence of pressure

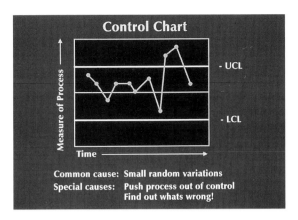

Figure 3. Control chart.

Table 3
An Example of the Why Technique

Problem:	Increased incidence of pressure ulcers on neurosurgical unit.
Why?	Increased immobility noted in patients.
Why?	Patients are complaining of increased incidence of uncontrolled pain.
Why?	Medical residency has changed. New group no longer using PCA pumps. Patients no longer receiving around the clock coverage for pain in first 48 hours after surgery.

Why did the problem actually occur and what preventive measures are needed? Poor pain management post–op caused increased immobility and therefore increased incidence of pressure ulcers. The plan is to address and correct the pain management issue.

ulcers and the horizontal axis for months as the unit of time.

5. Determine the average value for the process and the upper and lower control limits (UCL and LCL), and mark them on the chart, for example, national statistics for the incidence of pressure ulcers in acute care facilities as documented in the AHCPR guideline, *Treatment of Pressure Ulcers* are 2.7 LCL and 29.5 UCL. With the advice of statistical process control consultants, the average, UCL and LCL can be calculated based on previous performance in one's own institution. Therefore, practitioners can perform internal benchmarking while using control charts.

6. Make measurements on schedule, enter them on the chart, and monitor the chart for changes that may indicate whether the process is out of control.

By using the control chart, the wound care practitioner can monitor whether certain processes are in or out of control. Gradual trends can be identified in the process that can ultimately affect output. If a control chart is used regularly, the practitioner can be alerted to problems and opportunities for improvement (Figure 3).

Improving the work process. Continuous improvement is central to any quality organization. It can be achieved only when everyone in the healthcare organization understands the long–term advantages of a cost–of–quality approach to work processes; encourages all improvements, big and small; and focuses on prevention instead of crisis intervention. Commitment to continuous improvement results in either kaizen or breakthrough improvements, or both.[4,10,11] Kaizen refers to improvements in a series of small, gradual, ongoing changes. It is the way improvements most often occur. It also means setting

and periodically raising standards that are within reach. Breakthrough means a dramatic improvement in work processes. It can occur in technology or in the way work is organized. To make improvements, it is necessary to know how to get to the root causes of problems so that problems can eventually be prevented. Two management tools that can be utilized to get to the root causes of problems are the why technique and the cause and effect diagram.[4,8,9]

The why technuque. The why technique helps to find the root cause of a problem by moving through layers of causes to get at the preventable cause of a recurring problem. The question of why a problem exists is raised, and then by repeatedly asking why that problem exists, a final most important cause is revealed. For example, by using control charts, a wound care clinician identified that there was an increase in incidence of pressure ulcers on a neurosurgical unit for the past three months. To get to the cause of the problem, the wound care practitioner and staff members of the unit met and used the why technique. This technique, as depicted in Table 3, revealed a number of causes.

The cause and effect diagram. Sometimes called the Fishbone diagram, the cause and effect diagram

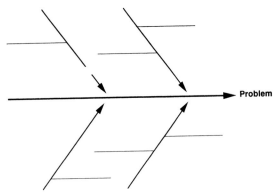

Figure 4. Schematic of a fishbone diagram.

is another tool useful in the identification of the causes and subcauses of a problem. A cause and effect diagram provides a visual representation of the relationship between an effect and its myriad of potential causes. The standard format is to have the effect stated on the right and the probable causes on the left. The lines connecting probable causes and the effect resemble a fish skeleton, hence the name "fishbone" for the process of constructing a cause and effect diagram. A cause and effect diagram displays the root cause of a problem situation in several related categories. Each category is further displayed in several subcategories, each of which either branches off into additional subcategories or displays a number of causes related to it. The use of the fishbone diagram often requires using other quality improvement tools, such as brainstorming and surveys.

Cause and effect diagrams are constructed by using several steps. Once a problem is selected for study, its causes are listed. The list is refined to reflect realistic and trackable causes meriting further study. The list of the causes is then classified into categories and subcategories, which are displayed on a diagram with arrows directed toward the main problem. Categories are either selected randomly by the team or selected from a standardized list of categories. Categories often utilized include people, materials, machines, methods/systems, measurements, policies, procedures, physical environment, and training. These categories usually apply to a wide range of problems, and using them guarantees that most of the relevant causes will be put into the diagram. Most often all the categories listed are not needed. Categories that are most meaningful to the problem being addressed need to be established (Figure 4).

To use the fishbone diagram, take the following steps:

1. Draw a fish on a sheet of paper that is large enough to allow a list of all causes by category to be documented and for all team members to read easily.

2. Enter the problem statement (25 words or less) in the head of the fish on the right side of the diagram (the effect box).

3. Generate a list of all potential causes through either brainstorming or working independently. Enter all causes onto the fish, group causes by category (see listing above for common categories).

4. Enter primary causes onto the main "bones" of the fish coming off the backbone. For each cause ask, "Why does it happen?" Answers represent sub–causes which are entered as "small bones" – branches off the major ideas.

5. Once all causes have been entered, begin a process of clarification, condensation, and evaluation of items that have been listed. Discuss entries, assure that all items listed are causes and not symptoms, and determine which causes can be addressed and which need to be referred to another body in the organization.

6. Prioritize causes and determine which are the key causes (the 20 percent that will cure 80 percent of the problem) that will become the basis for future action planning.

Measurements

In quality organizations, meeting customer requirements is the ultimate measure of quality. At every step along the fulfillment chain of service to the customer, measurements provide data that indicate how precise an organization, department, or individuals within an organization are in their managerial and operational processes. Measurements play a vital role in determining how efficient and effective an organization or individual is in serving the customer. Measurements keep organizations focused on continuous improvement according to actual results they achieve in providing services as compared to internal baseline and external benchmarks of "best practices."

Unless an organization, department, or individual makes a commitment to measure the impact of action, there will be no evidence to identify progress along the path of continuous improvement. Measurements provide critical feedback to an organization, department, or individual on how effective and efficient the organization is at meeting its goals related to such priority concerns as customer satisfaction, financial targets, market strategies, process improvements, service features, and quality and costs of poor quality.

Organizations use measurements internally to assess actual performance against established baselines of performance for individuals, departments, and teams. Baselines identify the internal view of excellence and enable companies to set targets for continuous improvement. They form the basis for assessing progress and overall performance toward the stated target or goal. Baselines respond precisely to customer requirements and set standards of excellence through the organization. As current baseline expectations are met, new expectations are created.

Benchmarking. To achieve a broader view of performance excellence, organizations benchmark.[12] Benchmarking can be defined as measuring an organization's, department's, or individual's performance against that of the best–in–class; determining how the best–in–class achieve those performance levels; and using the information as the basis for an organization, department, or individual's targets, strategies, and implementation. Benchmarking is used to understand what level of performance is really possible and why the gap exists between current performance and that optimum performance. To be effective, benchmarking must be seen as a process that requires several steps of effective planning. Benchmarking includes selecting a topic, defining what functions or processes are to be benchmarked, analyzing those functions in one's own organization, selecting appropriate organizations to benchmark, studying the organizations chosen, transforming what has been learned from benchmarking into recommended actions, integrating those actions into a planning process, and then implementing them.

Benchmarking is part of a continuous improvement process that helps to set up a standard of practice for the services provided. Searching for best standards of practice can take an organization or individual practitioners, like wound care practitioners, on a search for expertise inside and outside the healthcare arena. Benchmarking is a structured process for gaining new perspectives on the needs of patients and other customers. It helps to improve work processes by identifying, measuring, and emulating best practices both inside and outside of an organization and inside and outside of the healthcare industry. Benchmarking helps wound care practitioners to take a fresh look at standards of practice, to identify goals of excellence, to facilitate kaizen and breakthrough improvements, and to measure progress toward those improvements.

Measurements are applied to determine valued service features and process distinctions as well as deficiencies. Total quality organizations make a vigorous commitment to measurement to assess current performance, set goals for improvement, and understand what is important.

Productivity

When looking at measurements, the term "outcomes" must be addressed. In management, the term "outcome" can be considered synonymous with productivity. Organizational systems (subsystems, departments, individuals) can be described as systems consisting of three components: inputs, activities, and outputs.

Inputs include money, human resources, materials, machines, and other fixed assets, technology and information. Activities make up the design and services provided. Outputs are the results.

The organization (subsystem, departments, individuals) receives inputs and add values to get an output or result. Therefore, productivity is defined as the Output/Input ratio, the ratio of output of services produced divided by the input used to produce them.[13] If the Output/Input ratio is not a positive number, the organization (subsystem, department, individual) is in trouble.

To improve productivity means to make the Output/Input ratio bigger. The ratio can be made bigger either by increasing the output, reducing the input, or both. In a quality organization the focus to improve productivity is toward better use of the potential available through human resources. Each worker is to become his or her own industrial engineer. This process occurs by allowing and encouraging individuals to create innovative ways to improve productivity.

Productivity is improved by processes defined as reducing costs, managing growth, working smarter, paring down, and working more effectively.

Reducing costs: Output same/Input down. Without a doubt, cost reduction is the traditional and widely used approach to productivity improvement. In a QA organization, a positive approach to cost reduction involves reducing avoidable costs. For example, a wound care department, instead of stocking and utilizing multiple categories of wound dressings (or various products within the same category), analyzes the types of customers served and the types of wounds seen and streamlines products to better meet the needs of the customers. Quality organizations must be careful not to define cost reduction as "across the board cutting expenses by a given percent." Input is decreased by restructuring or re–engineering designs within the system.

Managed growth: Output up/Input up by a lesser amount. Managed growth is an approach to improvement where an investment or cost addition is made that will return more than the cost of investment, making the ratio bigger. Capital and technological improvement, systems designs, training, organizational designs, and development are among the many ways to manage growth. Initial introduction of moist wound healing products in many organizations was a technological improvement that resulted in managed growth.

Working smarter: Output up/Input same.
Working smarter is an approach to improvement where there is more output form the same input, allowing an increase in production at the same input. In a QA organization, this ratio is made bigger by reducing failure costs and some inspection costs and by improving work processes and designs.

Paring down: Output down/Input down more.
Paring down is similar to cost reduction, except that in this case production is also decreased although input is reduced by a larger amount. The ratio is still made bigger with an overall increase in productivity. This productivity improvement is frequently achieved by eliminating marginal or unproductive products, services or activities. In most organizations (subsystems, departments, individuals) there are many more opportunities than are generally realized to get rid of no–longer–productive or obsolete processes and services.

Working effectively: Output up/Input down.
Working effectively is the most effective approach to productivity improvement. Emphasis is placed on preventable costs and some inspection costs and improving the work processes.

Wound care practitioners must try to constantly improve their productivity. The payoff for relatively small increases in productivity can have a disproportionate and positive effect on the net outcomes or results, the bottom line of any organization.

Implementation

The key to becoming a quality organization is in the infiltration of the philosophy and principles of quality throughout the organization. Success in implementation lies in the development of a problem solving system, such as the use of quality teams, where emphasis is placed on problem identification and solution by all levels of employees within the organization. There are various types of quality teams, some of which include quality project teams, quality circle teams, business process quality teams, and self–managing teams. Through the actions of all the teams, quality and continuous improvement comes from the amelioration of problems by the workers within the system. All levels of employees then must be empowered with the knowledge and opportunities to become familiar with basic techniques of problem solving as well as various measurement techniques and quality strategies.

Summary

The healthcare system is changing continuously in an attempt to improve the quality of services rendered. Wound care practitioners must stay abreast of these changes, analyzing their work and work processes and implementing measures that result in continuous quality improvement in services provided for their customers. The issue of quality must take on a new meaning and must be incorporated into every aspect of wound care practice.

References

1. Aguayo R. Dr. Deming: *The American Who Taught the Japanese About Quality*. New York, NY, Fireside, Simon & Schuster, Inc., 1990.
2. Crosby PB. *Let's Talk Quality*. New York, NY, Penguin Books Inc., 1990.
3. Juran JM, Gryna FM. *Product Planning and Analysis*. New York, NY, McGraw-Hill, Inc., 1993.
4. Labovitz GH. *The Quality Advantage.* MA, Organizational Dynamics, Inc., 1991.
5. Capezio P, Morehouse D. *Taking the Mystery out of Total Quality Management*. Hawthorne, NJ, Career Press, 1993.
6. MacNeil DJ. *Customer Service Excellence*. New York, NY, Business One Irwin/Mirror Press, 1994.
7. Martin WB. *Managing Quality Customer Service*. Menlo Park, CA, Crisp Publications, Inc., 1989.
8. Al–Assaf AF, Schmele JA. *Total Quality in Healthcare*. Delray Beach, FL, St. Lucie Press, 1993.
9. Klubnik JP, Greenwood PF. *Team Based Problem Solver*. New York, NY, Irwin Professional Publishing, 1994.
10. Creech B. *The Five Pillars of TQM*. New York, NY, Truman Talley Books/Dutton, 1994.
11. Imai M. *Kaizen*. New York, NY, Random House Business Division, 1986.
12. Bernowski K. The benchmarking bandwagon. *Quality Progress.* 1991;Jan:19–24.
13. Ross JE, Ross WC. *Japanese Quality Circles & Productivity*. Reston, VA, Reston Publishing Company, Inc., 1982.

Suggested Reading

1. Blanchard K, Peale NV. *The Power of Ethical Management*. New York, NY, Fawcett Crest Books, 1988.
2. Chang RY, Niedzwiecki ME. *Continuous Improvement Tools*. Irvine, CA, Richard Chang Associates, Inc., 1993.
3. Covey SR. *The Seven Habits of Highly Effective People*. New York, NY, Fireside, Simon & Schuster, Inc., 1990.
4. Glasser W. *The Control Theory Manager*. New York, NY, Harper Collins Publishers, Inc., 1994.
5. Hammer M, Champy J. *Reengineering the Corporation*. New York, NY, Harper Collins Publishers, Inc., 1993.
6. Harper B, Harper A. *Succeeding as a Self–Directed Work Team*. New York, NY, MW Corporation, 1992.
7. Horovitz J, Cudennec–Ponn C. Putting quality service into gear. *Quality Progress.* 1991;Jan:54–58.
8. Jdner B, Gaudard MA. Variation, management, and W. Edwards Deming. *Quality Progress.* 1990;Dec:29–37.
9. Koch MW, Fairly TM. *Integrated Quality Management*. St. Louis, MO, Mosby Year Book, Inc., 1993.
10. Kriegel RJ, Patler L. *If it Ain't Broke ... Break It*. New York, NY, Waner Books, Inc., 1991.
11. Phillips DT. *Lincoln on Leadership*. New York, NY, Warner Books, Inc., 1992.
12. Rusk T, Miller DP. *The Power of Ethical Persuasion*. New York, NY, Penguin Books, 1993.
13. Sheridan JH. Are you a bad customer? *Industry Week* 1991;Aug:25–34.
14. Tracey D. *10 Steps to Empowerment: A Common–Sense Guide to Managing People*. New York, NY, Quill, 1990.
15. Walton M. *Deming Management at Work*. New York, NY, A Perigee Book, 1990.
16. Wycoff J. *Transformation Thinking*. New York, NY, Berkley Books, 1995.

48

Cost Effectiveness in Wound Care

Tania J. Phillips, MD

Phillips TJ. Cost effectiveness in wound care. In: Krasner D, Kane D. *Chronic Wound Care, Second Edition*. Wayne, PA, Health Management Publications, Inc., 1997, pp 369–372.

Introduction

Throughout the world there are increasing efforts to control healthcare costs while maintaining high quality patient care. One result of these efforts has been decreased lengths of stay in acute care facilities. The care of wounds is now often provided in the home, outpatient, or extended care setting. Without any unifying definitions or formulas for calculating the costs of wounds and measuring costs/benefits of different wound care methodologies, it is very difficult to compare cost effectiveness of different wound care treatments. This problem was addressed by the International Committee on Wound Management (ICWM) at a meeting held in Lisbon, Portugal in February 1995. This chapter will summarize background information leading up to the ICWM's consensus statement on cost effectiveness and will present the consensus statement of the ICWM.

Cost vs. Cost Effectiveness

Cost effectiveness refers to the cost of achieving a desired outcome of treatment. An extensive review of the medical literature has revealed that there is much confusion concerning the differences between "cost" and "cost effectiveness." Many of the publications reviewed which purport to measure cost effectiveness in fact only measure treatment costs without evaluating outcome. Cheaper treatments are not more effective if they cost more to achieve the same result. In the healthcare literature, cost effectiveness has been defined as cost per unit of clinical effect of a treatment.[1] Clinical effects could measure outcomes in terms of a large number of parameters, such as healing or quality of life. Studies of cost effectiveness should measure cost per unit outcome.

Costs of Wound Care

The costs of wound care can be divided into direct costs and indirect costs.

Direct costs include the costs of primary and secondary dressings used on the wound, ancillary supplies to cleanse and dress the wound, surgical and radiological interventions and investigations, treatment to manage wound complications, medications to manage wound pain, inpatient care directly related to the wound, caregiver time, travel by caregiver or patient, and disposal of wound care material or products.

Indirect costs might also be called overhead costs. Such costs might include those related to quality of life, assistance in completing activities of daily living, days lost from work, and litigation.

Outcomes

In wound care studies, outcomes are usually measured according to the goals of treatment. Many wound care studies focus on complete healing, reduction in surface area and volume, reduction in pain, debridement or reduced incidence of complications such as infection. Other parameters might include restoration of mobility, improved quality of life, and prevention of wound recurrence.

Published Cost Effectiveness Studies

Data exist regarding the annual estimated cost of chronic wound care in several countries. The annual cost of the National Health Service in the United Kingdom to care for leg ulcers ranges from £100 to 600 million pounds ($150 to 900 million dollars).[2–4] A study conducted in the United States

Table 1
Cost effectiveness of the air suspension bed (U.S. dollars)

Bed Type	Cost per 100 patients at risk	Pressure ulcers per 100 patients	Cost saved per 100 patients	Pressure ulcers prevented per 100 patients	Cost effectiveness ratio*
Standard ICU bed	125,177,12	80	–	–	–
Air Suspension bed	51,019.52	16	74,157.60	64	< 0

* Cost per pressure ulcer prevented

Adapted from: Inman KJ, et al. Clinical utility and cost effectiveness of an air suspension bed in the prevention of pressure ulcers. JAMA 1993;269:1139–1143.

reports that the cost to heal one leg ulcer ranges from $784 to $6,449.[5] For pressure ulcers, the cost in the United States to heal one wound has been reported to range from $5,000 to $40,000.[6] Pressure ulcer management costs in the Netherlands are estimated to be around 750 million guilders (approximately 420 million U.S. dollars per year).[7] Problems with many published cost effective studies include the following:

1. Cost is often confused with cost effectiveness. Studies of cost effectiveness need to address the cost per unit outcome.
2. There is no standard method of calculating wound care costs. Calculations have included various combinations of materials, labor, hospital overhead, and complications.[8–11]
3. Only a few studies have measured costs to achieve measured treatment outcomes.[12–16]
4. Outcomes are often measured or reported differently from study to study, so it is difficult to perform meta–analyses on existing research to clarify cost effectiveness of treating, debridement, pain relief, etc.

There are few cost effectiveness studies which measure the cost to achieve measured treatment outcomes. Ohlsson, et al. assessed the cost effectiveness of two treatment regimens in an outpatient population treated by visiting nurses.[16] Thirty patients with leg ulcers of venous or mixed venous–arterial etiology were randomized to treatment with saline soaked gauze or with a hydrocolloid dressing. All patients were bandaged with the same type of compression bandage. Outcome measures were healing or reduction in surface area and pain. Costs included cost of materials and supplies, nursing time, travelling time and kilometers driven. Costs for dressing materials were similar for the two groups. When the total care, including nursing time, traveling time, and kilometers driven, were analyzed the mean cost of treatment with gauze dressings was $536 (4126 Swedish kroner) and with hydrocolloid dressings $203.35 (1565 Swedish kroner). This cost difference was because the gauze group required many more dressing changes than the hydrocolloid treated group. Two patients in the gauze treatment group and seven in the hydrocolloid group healed during the study. The reduction of ulcer area was 19 percent in the gauze group and 51 percent in the hydrocolloid group. Total direct cost per percentage change in wound area per week were $28.42 for the gauze treated group and $3.97 for the hydrocolloid treated group.

Thomas examined cost effectiveness data for treatment of leg ulcers with paraffin gauze compared with alginate dressings.[2] The effectiveness parameters measured were healing rate (cm^2 per day) and time to heal in days. Included in the direct costs were cost of materials and nursing costs. Although there was a marked difference in the price of the two primary dressings [29 cents (0.18 pounds) for the paraffin gauze and $3.20 (1.95 pounds) for alginate dressings], the alginate treated group healed more quickly. Thus, the cost for complete healing of the wound in the alginate group was much lower than in the paraffin gauze treated group. The author concluded that if waste is to be avoided and products to be used cost effectively, nursing staff must carefully monitor the effectiveness of all new and expensive treatments by measuring and recording the area and volume of the wound on a regular basis.

Inman, et al. assessed the clinical utility and cost effectiveness of an air suspension bed in the prevention of pressure ulcers.[17] In this study, 100 consecutive critically ill patients at risk for the development of pressure ulcers were randomly assigned to receive treatment on either an air suspension bed or a standard intensive care unit bed with frequent turning by nurses. The outcome measures were the development of pressure ulcers by signs of severity. The costs associated with each of the two programs were calculated. In the study, the air suspension bed was associated with fewer patients developing single, multiple or severe pressure ulcers (Table 1). In patients at risk, the use of an air suspension bed in the prevention of pressure ulcers was a cost effective therapy.

It has been proposed by Detsky and Naglie[18] that new technologies be introduced when one of three conditions are met:

1. The new technology is less costly and at least as effective as the current standard.
2. The new technology is more costly and more effective than the current standard, the added benefits of the new technology being worth the added costs.
3. The new technology is less effective and less costly, the added benefits of the current standards not being worth the added costs.

The authors concluded that the air suspension bed fulfilled the first condition when applied in a critically ill patient population at risk. The air suspension bed provided increased effectiveness in the form of fewer pressure ulcers for less money than the current program of a standard ICU bed and frequent patient rotation.

Eckman, et al. examined the cost effectiveness of approaches to diagnosis and treatment of patients with type II diabetes mellitus who have foot infections and suspected osteomyelitis.[19] The prevalence of osteomyelitis, the major complications and efficacy of long term antibiotic therapy and surgery and the performance characteristics of 4 diagnostic tests (X–rays, technetium, Tc99m bone scanning, indium In 111 labeled white blood cell scanning, and magnetic resonance imaging) were examined. The interventions following hospitalization for surgical debridement and intravenous antibiotic therapy included 1) treatment for presumed soft tissue infection, 2) culture guided empiric treatment for presumed osteomyelitis, 3) Seventy–one combinations of diagnostic tests preceding antibiotic therapy for osteomyelitis, 4) Seventy–one combinations of tests preceding amputation, and 5) Immediate amputation.

The main outcome measures were quality adjusted life expectancy and average costs. The authors found that culture guided empiric treatment for osteomyelitis with 10 weeks of oral antibiotic therapy was as effective as prolonged antibiotic therapy in any patient with a positive test result. It was concluded that non–invasive testing adds significant expense to the treatment of patients with type II diabetes in whom foot osteomyelitis is suspected, and such testing results in little improvement in health outcomes. Tests which decrease diagnostic uncertainty are preferred by physicians but may expose patients to additional risk and engender unnecessary costs.[20]

Several other analyses have shown that empiric therapy within limited clinical settings produces health outcomes equivalent to more aggressive and expensive approaches. These outcomes include the empiric treatment of dyspepsia (reserving esophagogastroduodenoscopy only for patients who have an inadequate response to treatment),[21] empiric treatments of patients infected with the HIV virus who present with symptoms suggestive of pneumocystic carinii pneumonia (reserving bronchoscopy for those who do not respond within 5 days of treatment),[22] and empiric treatment of patients with idiopathic nephrotic syndrome (avoiding renal biopsy).[23]

Conclusion

In view of the paucity of studies comparing the cost effectiveness of wound care modalities, the lack of standardized methods of calculating costs of wound care, and the differences in outcomes that are measured, it is impossible to clarify cost effectiveness of healing, debridement, pain relief, etc. with regard to existing research studies.

During their February 1995 meeting, the ICWM acknowledged the need to develop measurement scales and to produce a universally acceptable method which includes only objective, measurable data.[24] Such scales should be patient centered and show wound type plus number of scores before and after treatment. Until universal, objective scales to measure cost effectiveness are available, the clinician must read published studies critically and take cost per unit outcome into account to determine if treatment measures are indeed cost effective.

Consensus Statement[2–4]

1. Diagnosis and prevention (of primary disease and recurrence) should be the first aim of all those organizing and providing wound care.
2. Patients, carers, health professionals and those who pay for care all need scientifically valid

data on the economic value of wound care therapies.

3. Economic models should take both direct and indirect cost and outcomes into account.

4. The direct costs of wound care can be identified and calculated.

5. Direct costs of care constitute a substantial and increasing proportion of total healthcare costs.

6. Indirect costs should always be taken into account and their influence on total treatment costs evaluated. This influence can vary from setting to setting.

7. Indirect costs include costs of opportunities lost for patients, carers and health professionals to perform other valuable activities.

8. In wound care, cost effectiveness can be expressed by the equation:

Cost Effectiveness = [1]direct + [2]indirect costs of achieving [3]parameters of success predetermined in a specific period of time

(1) Direct Costs: Costs of primary and secondary dressings used on wound, cost of ancillary supplies to cleanse and dress wound, cost of surgical and radiological interventions, cost of treatment to manage wound complications, cost of medications to manage wound pain, cost of in–patient care directly related to the wound, cost of caregiver time, cost of travel by caregiver or patients, cost of disposal of wound care material or products.

(2) Indirect Costs: Costs related to quality of life, related to assistance in completing activities of daily living, cost of days lost from work, costs of litigation.

(3) Parameters of Success may vary with patient and setting. Examples could include one or more of the following: complete healing, reduction in wound care, and reduction in wound surface area.

References

1. Vibbert S, Migdail KJ, Strickland D, Youngs MT (ed). *The 1995 Medical Outcomes and Guidelines Sourcebook*. Faulkner Gray, Inc., New York, NY, 1995, pp 675.
2. Thomas S. Cost effective management of leg ulcers. *Community Outlook* 1990;March:21–22.
3. Wilson E. Prevention and treatment of venous leg ulcers. *Health Trends* 1989:21–97.
4. Bosanquet N. Costs of venous ulcers: From maintenance therapy to investment programs. *Phlebology* 1992;7(Supplement):44–46.
5. Wood CR, Margolis DJ. The cost of treating venous leg ulcers to complete healing using an occlusive dressing and a compression bandage. *WOUNDS* 1992;4:138–141.
6. Makelbust J. Pressure ulcers: Etiology and prevention. *Nurs Clin North Am* 1987;22:359–377.
7. Haalboom JRE. Enkele aspecten van decubitus wondbehandling: Kunst en wetenschap. *Symp Proc; Excerpta Medica* 1990:39–42.
8. Gorse G, Messner R. Improved pressure sore healing with hydrocolloid dressings. *Arch Dermatol* 1987;123:766–771.
9. Colwell JC, Foreman MD, Trotter JP. A comparison of the efficacy and cost–effectiveness of two methods of managing pressure ulcers. *Decubitus* 1993;6:28–36.
10. Alterescu V. The financial costs of inpatient pressure ulcers to an acute care facility. *Decubitus* 1989;2:14–23.
11. Meredith K, Gray E. Dressed to heal. *Journal of District Nursing* 1988;7(3):8–10.
12. Roberts LW, McManus WF, Mason AD, Pruitt BA. DuoDerm in the management of skin graft donor sites. In: Hall CW (ed). *Surgical Research Recent Developments*. Proc Pergamon Press Inc, 1985, pp 55–58.
13. Inman KJ, Sibbald WJ, Rutledge FS, Clark BJ. Clinical utility and cost–effectiveness of an air suspension bed in the prevention of pressure ulcers. *JAMA* 1993;269:1139–1143.
14. Robinson BJ. Randomized comparative trial of DuoDerm vs Viscopaste PB7 and bandage in the management of venous leg ulceration and cost to the community. In: Ryan TJ (ed). Beyond occlusion: Wound care proceedings. *International Congress Symposium Series #136*. Royal Society of Medicine Services, London, 1988, pp 101–104.
15. Xakellis GC, Chrischilles EA. Hydrocolloid versus saline–gauze dressings in treating pressure ulcers: A cost effectiveness analysis. *Arch Phys Med Rehab* 1992;73:463–469.
16. Ohlsson P, Larsson K, Lindholm C, Möller M. A cost effectiveness study of leg ulcer treatment in primary care. *Scand J Prim Health Care* 1994;12:295–299.
17. Inman, et al. Clinical utility and cost effectiveness of an air suspension bed in the prevention of pressure ulcers. *JAMA* 1993;269:1139–1143.
18. Detsky AS, Naglie G. A clinician's guide to cost effectiveness analysis. *Annals of Internal Medicine* 1990;113:147–154.
19. Eckman MH, Greenfield S, Mackey WC, et al. Foot infections in diabetic patients: Decision and cost effective analysis. *JAMA* 1995;273:712–720.
20. Moskowitz AJ, Kuipers BJ, Kassirer JP. Dealing with uncertainty, risks and tradeoffs in clinical decisions; a cognitive science approach. *Ann Intern Med* 1988;108:435–449.
21. Kahn KL, Greenfield S. The efficacy of endoscopy in the evaluation of dyspepsia. A review of the literature and development of a sound strategy. *J Clin Gastroenterology* 1986;8:346–358.
22. Tu JV, Biem HJ, Detsky AS. Bronchoscopy versus empirical therapy in HIV patients with presumptive pneumocystic carinii pneumonia: A decision analysis. *American Review of Respiratory Diseases* 1993;148:370–377.
23. Levey AS, Lau J, Pauker SG, Kassirer JP. Idiopathic nephrotic syndrome: Puncturing the biopsy myth. *Annals of Internal Medicine* 1987;107:697–713.
24. Special Report: International Committee on Wound Management. World Council on Cost Effective Wound Care. *WOUNDS* 1995;7(3):119–120.

Acknowledgement

The author wishes to thank Laura Bolton, PhD and Lia van Rijswijk, RN, ET for invaluable help in preparation of this manuscript.

49

Controlled Clinical Evaluations vs. Case Studies: Why Wound Care Professionals Need to Know the Difference

Amy Roma, RN, CETN; Laura Bolton, PhD; and Adrienne McNally

Roma A, Bolton L, McNally A. Controlled clinical evaluations vs. case studies: Why wound care professionals need to know the difference In: Krasner D, Kane D. *Chronic Wound Care, Second Edition*. Wayne, PA, Health Management Publications, Inc., 1997, pp 373–382.

Introduction

Wound care research has made great strides in keeping pace with rapid changes in healthcare. Product availability has branched from few options to a multitude of selections now classified in product categories. Likewise, expectations regarding treatment choices have progressed from a haphazard, "it worked before" approach, to research–based decision making.[1–3] Solid rationale for established or modified treatment plans separates a knowledgeable healthcare provider from a haphazard one. (See Chapter 17, "Dressing Decisions for the 21st Century" in this source book.) Given the abundance of published literature and sales materials, all claiming product superiority, how does one discern the legitimacy of claims being made? It is the responsibility of the clinician not to accept these claims at face value, but to scrutinize the quality of information received and to use it properly.[4] Once they can identify the different kinds of research and understand what kinds of conclusions can be drawn from each, practitioners can quickly recognize the facts among the information gleaned from this vast array of literature and base care decisions solely on claims founded on scientific evidence. It is the goal of this chapter to give wound care professionals the tools to identify the various types of clinical research backing wound care product claims and to select only the legitimate conclusions derived from each as the scientific backing for their wound care decisions.

Definitions and Scope

Different types of clinical research aid healthcare decision making in various ways which are outlined in Table 1. Each type of research is valuable if the conclusions are consistent with the study design and methods. Resources abound with the "how to's" of clinical research[4,15,16] where one can learn more about the different types of research. Surveys scan current practice or opinion. Case studies provide evidence of product performance or safety for a given indication or type of wound, but do not demonstrate comparative efficacy. Controlled clinical evaluations provide evidence of comparative product efficacy or claims. Systematic reviews aid in decision making by summarizing how much or how little is known about a particular set of treatments or procedures. The strongest support for decision making is the prospective, randomized, controlled clinical evaluation in which treatments are assigned randomly to patients and measurements are made before and after treatment. If there is no scientific basis for including a particular treatment modality in one's protocol of care, one can test its comparative efficacy in achieving

Table 1
Types of Clinical Research (Examples) and Conclusions Derived from Each

Type of Study	Content	Conclusions
Survey of Clinical Practices[5,6]	Information gathered by interview or questionnaire	Frequency, prevalence, incidence or preference of a phenomenon or practice
Clinical Case Study[6-8]	Uncontrolled studies of the effect of a single treatment	Safety or performance of a clinical practice or treatment on the cases studied
Controlled Clinical Evaluation[9-11]	Controlled studies comparing treatments	Comparative safety, performance and efficacy of a clinical practice or treatment
Systematic Clinical Review[12-14]	Summary of prior research	Matches content of prior research summarized

measurable goals by conducting a controlled clinical evaluation of the treatment versus an accepted standard or control treatment.[9]

Research should also be clinically relevant if it is to support conclusions which have a bearing on healthcare practice. The more similar to one's own clinical practice a study is in setting, wound type, patient and treatment variables, the more clinically relevant it is to one's use and decision making. Though the scope of this chapter includes only clinical studies, remember that there is a wealth of preclinical research which can also aid decision making, but there is no substitute for controlled clinical evidence. *In vitro* studies are least clinically relevant since they are based on responses by cells in culture, separated from their normal environment rich in growth factors, enzymes and other naturally–occurring molecules in the body. *In vitro* studies on animals can be valuable when they parallel clinical phenomena. For example, acute animal wound healing parallels that of humans; pressure ulcer animal models attempt to simulate human pressure ulcers;[16] and ischemic ulcers can be generated in animals by prolonged ischemia.[17] However, clinical relevance should be carefully assessed before extrapolating from animal to human studies or when generalizing from one type of clinical wound to another, for example from donor sites to diabetic foot ulcers. Because of the question of clinical relevance, most of us turn to controlled clinical evaluations as a basis for treatment choices.

Conducting a controlled clinical evaluation is not forbidding. It can be fun and can open new horizons of patient care and communication with colleagues. Getting involved in some form of research helps the new researcher learn the process. However, a basic understanding of various research models is essential in establishing the foundations for clinical practice. This chapter will help the reader to discriminate between the two most common types of studies reported: uncontrolled case or product studies and controlled clinical evaluations. For the purposes of this chapter, uncontrolled studies of one or more patients will be referred to as "case studies" since comparative evaluation is not made. Controlled studies will be referred to as "clinical evaluations" since comparative product safety or efficacy is evaluated versus concurrent, historic concurrent or historic control treatments. With this basic knowledge, readers will be able to use the evidence they glean from published and unpublished professional and sales literature with a clearer understanding of exactly what it means for their practices and their patients' well being.

ROMA, ET AL.

Table 2
Product Evidence Required by the FDA

Product Classification	Product Description	Evidence Required
Class I Medial Device General controls are sufficient to ensure safety and effectiveness.	Devices that are neither life supporting or life sustaining or for a use which is of substantial importance in preventing impaired health and does not present a potential, unreasonable risk of illness or injury. These are "less risky" devices. Examples: medical adhesive tape/bandage; ostomy appliances and accessories.	Many Class I devices are exempt from pre–market notification process. Those subject to 510 (k)/Pre–Market Approval (PMA) must provide safety and, where appropriate, efficacy data. Examples of safety tests performed for a wound dressing would be cytotoxicity, hemolysis, acute systemic toxicity, dermal irritation, and sensitization.
Class II Medical Device General controls are determined to be insufficient to provide reasonable assurance of safety and effectiveness. Must comply with general controls and any applicable performance standards.	Devices not meeting Class I definitions as well as devices which may support or sustain human life. Examples: intravascular catheter; jet lavage.	Most Class II devices are subject to 510(k). Some are subject to PMA. Evidence of safety and effectiveness required.
Class III Medical Device Insufficient information exists to determine adequacy of generalcontrols, performance standards or special controls to provide reasonable assurance of safety and effectiveness.	Devices that are life sustaining or life supporting; implanted in the human body; presenting potential unreasonable risk of illness or injury. Examples: implantable pacemaker pulse generator; infant radiant warmer	Subject to PMA evidence of safety and effectiveness required.
Over the Counter (OTC) Drugs Based on prior research theFDA has agreed on safe, effective ingredient combinations, doses, labeling claims and indications.	These products are regulated by OTC monographs which dictate the "conditions under which specific active ingredients and combinations may be formulated...without prior FDA approval."[20] Example: aspirin	Safety and efficacy of OTC drugs, such as skin protectants or certain topical antimicrobial or antifungal agents is assumed, based on their manufacture to monograph specifications.
Prescription Drugs Include oral or topicalagents requiring a doctor's prescription.	These products include "substances intended for use in the diagnosis, cure, mitigation, treatment or prevention of disease in man or other animals...to effect the structure or any function of the body.[20] Example: captopril	Drugs require proof of both safety and efficacy relative to standard agents or treatments, which is submitted to the FDA in a New Drug Application (NDA) or in the case of a generic drug, an abbreviated NDA (ANDA).

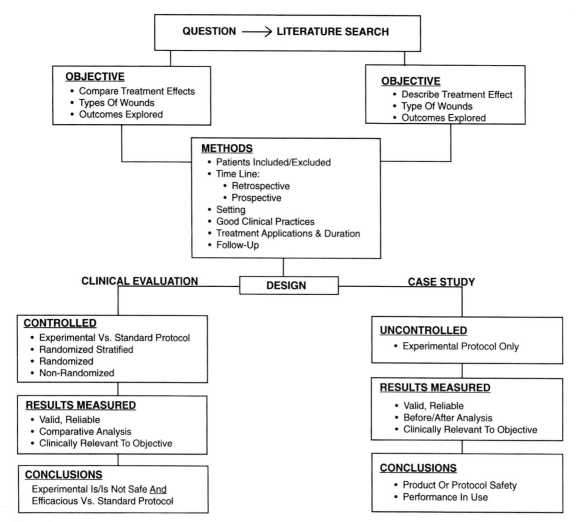

Figure 1.

Making the Most of Available Evidence

Evidence for product safety and efficacy may already have been reviewed by government authorities or by other professionals in search of answers. One may find this evidence in the product package insert, in the published literature, in posters or presentations at professional meetings or in unpublished product literature. Whatever the source, the above tools and definitions will help the clinician to draw conclusions about the clinical relevance, safety and efficacy of products, based on available literature.

Product package insert. Supporting evidence for claims, indications, warnings and contraindications have been reviewed by the Food and Drug Administration (FDA) before the agency grants clearance to market most wound care products. Different classifications of wound care products

require different supportive evidence before the product can be marketed (Table 2). Understanding these requirements for each class of product helps wound care professionals to be aware of the research base which already exists for each product, to interpret marketing claims of relative efficacy, or to confidently request evidence to support these claims.

Evidence available from industry. FDA clearance to market most wound dressings is based on substantial equivalence to another dressing previously cleared by FDA, preclinical safety studies and assurance of consistent quality, but it does not support conclusions of clinical product performance or relative clinical efficacy of the product. In some cases, studies of clinical performance characteristics may have been performed for a wound care device in order to establish "substantial equivalence" to another device, but these studies are generally not

ROMA, ET AL.

required. In general, it is not safe to assume that a wound care dressing has been tested clinically before it is marketed unless the company provides that evidence with the product literature. In the absence of published clinical evidence, wound care professionals are encouraged to contact companies marketing the devices for evidence supporting product claims.

Comparative clinical efficacy studies of most wound care devices are also not required before marketing clearance is given. For example, if manufacturer C develops an alginate dressing substantially equivalent to manufacturer B's alginate, C may produce and market its alginate in compliance with regulations without conducting a clinical study on its own alginate. C may use the "substantial equivalence" property to support clinical performance, using the same references pioneered by B to support C's claims, even if C was never used on clinical wounds. This practice benefits society by encouraging choices in each dressing category and reducing costly research. However, wound care professionals should not assume that supporting evidence exists for relative clinical performance of the two alginates. If assertions are made about comparative clinical efficacy of the two dressings, references should be provided in the associated literature. Wise professionals will review these references for accuracy or will request them from the company for verification. Evidence supporting comparative clinical claims can be provided only by a clinically relevant evaluation comparing the two dressings.

Evidence from literature and professional meetings. In addition, independent or corporate–sponsored research may provide evidence for wound care decisions beyond that evident from product package inserts and routine FDA–required data. This evidence can be found by reading or searching the wound care literature, networking with other wound care professionals, attending professional meetings and critically reading poster sessions. If the evidence is not available from any of these sources, resourceful wound care professionals can do their own research to answer questions about how wound treatments perform and which treatment modalities work best.

Building a Research Study

Specifically, research is "investigation or experimentation aimed at the discovery and interpretation of facts..."[22] An attempt to answer any question can be considered research. If a good scientific method is used to attain the answer, it will predict patient outcomes accurately and reliably. The research normally proceeds through steps similar to those involved in building a house: 1) formulate the question you want to answer (decide what kind of house you want and where); 2) develop this question into a specific objective for study (general plan); 3) write the protocol (draw the blueprint); 4) set up the study (get resources, permissions, materials, etc.) 5) conduct the study: apply treatments, observe and record effects (build the house); 6) analyze the results (certify that the structure meets codes for occupancy); 7) write up the conclusions so others can benefit. (Enjoy/assess the house).

These seven steps have been described in greater detail elsewhere.[4,16,18] They will be used here to illustrate the differences between clinical evaluations and case studies (Figure 1). The research process always begins with a basis of support, the question. The simpler the question, the better it is. The research question determines the outcome of a study in much the same way that initial choices of type and site shape a house. The site must be consistent with the anticipated structure. A literature review assesses the research environment so the researcher can "build on" secure findings of others. A researcher will need to select the questions to ask in order to determine the study methods. For example, in an environment subject to frequent flooding, it may be prudent to build the house on stilts. Knowledge regarding the use and construction of the stilts is acquired by referring to previous experience. A researcher will find this experience by searching the literature related to his/her topic. Just as the environment and past experience influence a building's structural design, a literature review helps the researcher refine the question and select the most useful methods to answer it.

With a clear question in mind, the researcher can formulate a focused research objective, specifying the type of wound, patient, setting, treatment and outcomes measured. Just as a weak foundation eventually results in instability of the structure, an unclear objective can lead to weak or uninterpretable results. A clear research objective is the foundation of the study's general plan, which is then filled in detail in the study protocol or design. The study protocol specifies the inclusion/exclusion criteria, treatments (treatment if a case study), number of patients, duration, variables measured, and anticipated analysis. Just as the blueprints of a house must be precise and clear and match the owner's vision, the study objective and protocol must clearly and accurately address the investigator's question in order to derive relevant answers at the end of the study.

When setting up the study, read product package inserts for materials carefully, making sure that the products have been cleared by the FDA for use on the type(s) and depths of wounds being studied. If performing an independent investigation on an unapproved indication, the clinician is legally responsible for adverse events.

Approvals and permissions can provide valuable tools for the success of the study, providing access to experts in study design and conduct. Facilities, whether acute, long–term, or home care, either have their own Institutional Review Board (IRB) or access to one. The IRB regulates research in order to protect human subjects, thereby assuring safety and ethical standards. It is prudent before initiating any investigation to check IRB requirements. The degree of IRB involvement in a protocol may be influenced by whether the evaluation is experimental or involves further study of an already approved indication. Experimental testing involves using a product for indications other than that for which it has already been cleared.

One additional approval to obtain is that of the patient. Guidelines regarding the necessary informed patient consent are also obtainable from the IRB. Patient informed consent is more than a formality. It is the patient's right. The right is guaranteed by the Helsinki Accord, which is a cornerstone of quality research, assuring patient understanding of and compliant participation in the study.

By informing and gaining the support of colleagues and the facility's administration, the researcher will also garner cooperation and moral support from individuals who may provide valuable assistance, feedback and tips on valid, reliable techniques for measuring or conducting the study. Additional sources of financial support and materials may include government agencies and corporations.[4] Just as a building permit assures cooperation by ascertaining conformance to local codes and standards, these approvals help to assure that the study conforms to Good Clinical Practices and the specific standards of your professional environment.

Conducting the study with integrity and diligence is another key to success. As the strength and quality of a house depend on the builders' adhering to the blueprint, so too does a well–conducted study follow its protocol as closely as possible. Anyone involved in the study requires adequate training to assure uniform treatment application, patient monitoring and measurement of outcomes. All professionals should keep the patient's welfare as the highest priority while conducting the study.

Comparing Case Studies with Clinical Evaluations

Early phases of the research process do not differ for case studies and clinical evaluations. The question sends the curious researcher to the literature to explore and learn from the experience of prior researchers. However, the objective of a case study, which explores effects of a single treatment, is clearly different from that of a clinical evaluation, which compares more than one treatment. If the objective is to describe performance, effects of a single treatment can be explored on a given wound care outcome in a case study paradigm. Case studies are time honored vehicles for informing colleagues about unusual or unexpected responses or adverse reactions to treatment modalities. For example, many journals feature special sections for case studies which spawn new research and alert professionals to new clinical findings. However, no relative safety or efficacy claims can be based on a case study.

If comparative safety or efficacy is to be determined, then two or more treatment groups can be compared in a clinical evaluation of their comparative effects on the specified outcome(s). The protocol will specify the treatments to be compared and the techniques for applying each treatment and measuring outcomes.

The study design flows from the objective. Ideally, the treatments will vary in only one parameter, and patients will be assigned in a random or other unbiased way to each treatment group. In a well designed clinical evaluation, wound and patient characteristics are measured at minimum before and after each treatment for a given duration to allow conclusions about the comparative safety and/or efficacy of the treatments applied.

The process of setting up and conducting the study is similar for clinical evaluations and case studies. Both require resources, materials and cooperation of or permission from an IRB, administration, colleagues and patients in order to succeed in meeting the objectives. Good clinical practices are essential to assure proper ethical treatment of patients, data acquisition, and analysis.

Analysis of results for a case study involves descriptive statistics before and after treatment of patient variables (e.g. age, sex, mobility, nutritional status, risk factors), wound variables (e.g. area, depth, necrosis, exudate, surrounding skin), and environmental elements (e.g. caregiver, financial constraints, footwear).

If more than one patient completes the study, paired statistics are used to compare pertinent measures before and after treatment, and optionally

ROMA, ET AL.

after a follow–up period specified in the protocol. This type of comparison gives readers a conclusion of product or protocol safety during treatment as well as durability of its effects. Clinical evaluations compare these three types of variables for the treatment groups studied, assuring similarity before the experimental and control treatments or procedures are implemented, then examining differences in the progressive treatment effects on these variables and the subsequent durability of these effects during follow–up. Comparative statistics, such as t–tests or anaylses of variance are used for the continuous, normally distributed variables, while chi–squared or other non–parametric statistics are used for discrete or skewed data. The results yield direct information about differences in effectiveness of the treatments.

Conclusions derived from a single patient case study or a multiple patient case study series report the course of events when one or more participants use a product or procedure. For example, Wilson and Dunn performed a longitudinal (over time) case study series of seven patients with systemic methicillin–resistant *S. aureus* (MRSA) infections whose leg ulcers were dressed with a hydrocolloid dressing.[7] All patients were isolated to prevent the spread of this pathogen until its presence was detected only in the wound. With the dressing isolating the wound, the patients resumed normal hospital room residence without spread of the MRSA, which eventually disappeared in all but one patient. While the study suggests safety of the product on microbially contaminated wounds, it does not extrapolate comparative efficacy of the treatment since it is not compared to an alternative treatment method. By heralding an unexpected result, the case study may set the stage for further investigations to compare this treatment modality to other management methods.

Although safety questions are essential research objectives to address, many professionals want more than assurances for safety of their wound care products. For instance, when making selections in the building scenario, two brands of window shades viewed individually may visually keep out the sun's rays. However, only by comparing them under the same sun exposure at the same time of day and using a thermometer to obtain an accurate temperature can one ascertain which window shade provides more protection against the heat. Both brands work, but which one is more effective? Wound care research answers the questions of comparative safety and efficacy, i.e. of healing, debridement or pain relief, by comparing products under similar conditions, side by side, or parallel to control treatments. The more specific the

investigation is to the condition of intended product use, the more accurate and clinically relevant the results will be. Results are only as good as the reliability (repeatability) and validity (clinical relevance) of the methods by which they are obtained and may apply only to what the original objective set out to discover.

The conclusion of a study or evaluation can only extrapolate information from the investigation that the study was designed to provide. A case study or study series describes safe usage or product performance on the patients studied. Comparative clinical evaluations allow conclusions to be made about comparative product safety and efficacy, providing a powerful basis for medical decision making. However, one must be careful to include in generalizations only the kind of population studied. For example, if an objective is stated to determine the comparative efficacy of two enzymatic debriding agents in removing necrotic tissue from pressure ulcers, the conclusion may include in generalizations only pressure ulcers, not arterial ulcers as they were not included in the evaluation. If its integrity is to be maintained, research, like building a house, must proceed in specific sequence of clearly designed steps, without leaving out a single step or exceeding its intended boundaries.

Conducting Your Own Study

With the framework of a literature search–based question and objective established, what are the details directing the outcomes? Customizing, which will differentiate case studies from product evaluations (interior design) now takes place. The following components must be included in a research design in order to obtain sound results.

Study design and methods. Inclusion criteria identifies who is being studied, for example, nursing home residents with sacral pressure ulcers. Relevance of medications, disease processes, patient status, age and sex, vary according to the objective. Narrow inclusion criteria limit the number of variables influencing the outcome, but will also limit general applicability of the results.

Exclusion criteria identify patients not studied, who cannot be included in generalizations.

The number (n) of participants contributes to the power of the study. The more participants included and the greater power, the more credible the results will be at the completion of the investigation. Obviously, the reported safety of a product after 350 applications is more convincing than a report on 25 applications. The "n" also affects the statistical significance when the results are analyzed. For a given magnitude of difference in treatment effects, the more patients in the study, the lower is the probability that the observed difference resulted from chance alone (the α probability, sometimes called "p"). The larger the "n" the more it increases the power of the study.

The setting should be relevant to the objective. For example, is the researcher comparing the practicality of two different products in the home environment? Then common sense suggests that the study should take place in the participants' homes. Otherwise, extrinsic factors (confounding variables) may influence the relevance of the results.

All research requires measures of outcomes to be reliable, valid and objective. Reliability refers to a method of data collection which achieves consistent, repeatable and accurate results or observations. If data collection is reliable, it can be replicated accurately at different times by the same observer or by another observer. An evaluation should utilize valid tools that actually measure the clinical outcome being investigated. (See Chapter 4 "Wound Assessment and Documentation" in this source book). Reliable, measurable observations make a study objective (based on observable phenomenon) as opposed to subjective (taking place within the mind). For example, if the participant's degree of risk for developing a pressure ulcer is determined solely by an unspecified criterion within the investigator's mind, it is subjective. If an objective, valid, reliable tool is used to make the observations, they are more likely to accurately match objective reality.

What data collection time line is used? A retrospective study examines specified past events during a given period of time. This process can save time and money, but inaccuracies may arise from inconsistent charting. Retrospective studies are commonly conducted by means of chart reviews. Precise records are essential for accurate data collection. In a simple illustration, a retrospective study utilizing length x width as the healing parameters must have these measurements recorded consistently at regular time frames for all wounds assessed. Prospective research, on the other hand, evaluates that which will take place. The research design applies treatments to participants who are accrued or actively enrolled in the study for a specified duration. These studies are more costly, but usually provide more accurate, reliable outcome measures and assure more consistent treatment. Treatment should be selected to reflect the study objective. For example, if the goal were to study effects of ultrasound on healing, the control may also be the "gold standard" of the treatment protocol. This standard is usually the best known or most widely used method of care. An uncontrolled or case study investigates the performance of a new product without comparing it to a standard protocol. It could also examine the use of an established procedure in a new situation. Under either circumstance, the experiment can only describe safe usage and product performance. All participants included in an uncontrolled study (product or case study) receive the same treatment protocol. No comparison against another product or procedure takes place, therefore, no conclusions regarding superior efficacy versus that of another product or procedure can be claimed. A product or case study is useful in providing professionals information regarding product use, performance and unexpected findings. Properly designed and appropriately reported, such case studies can point out techniques to avoid or highlight those which merit further research.

On the other hand, a controlled investigation or clinical evaluation utilizes comparisons and carries more power by discerning both safety and comparative efficacy of a product or procedure. Here the objective is to evaluate the experimental product or procedure against a standard control. A controlled evaluation is divided into several avenues, the selection of which are often determined by resources such as funding, time and participant availability. Experimental and control treatments may be applied to different patients, to different wounds on the same patient or, if appropriate, to different parts of the same wound. The researcher must commit to a lengthy patient accrual process to obtain a significant number of patients for a controlled study in the treatment of rare diseases, such as necrotizing fasciitis, while a controlled study of pressure ulcers in a nursing home may take less time because the latter are more abundant.

Patient or wound assignment. When using a control, the method of participation assignment must be determined. Non–randomized treatment assignment allows the investigator to determine what treatment is used on which participant. While this method does permit treatment comparison, it introduces a bias into the evaluation, thereby influencing objectivity and affecting outcomes. A less biased, more powerful assignment method is randomization. Webster defines "random" as "being or relating to a member of a set whose members have an equal probability of occurring."[22] Therefore, patients will have equal probability of being assigned to each treatment group according to a pre–selected random pattern, thus eliminating investigator bias. A stratified random pattern further defines subgroups and randomizes treatment assignment accordingly.[15] For example, two treatment groups of trochanteric pressure ulcers may each be subdivided into age–related subgroups. Treatments are then randomized within each subgroup so that half the patients over 65 are randomly

ROMA, ET AL.

assigned to receive each treatment, half the patients between 45 and 65 are similarly assigned to treatments as are half the patients younger than 45.

Evaluation of results. Unbiased evaluation of results obtained in a blinded evaluation or experiment, improves the accuracy of a study. A single–blinded evaluation is when the subjects are unaware of whether they have been assigned to the control or experimental group or procedure. In contrast, a double–blinded experiment obscures knowledge of control versus experimental assignment from both the subject and the investigator who evaluates the outcomes. This type of study significantly reduces the possibility of opportunistic biases during treatment and outcome measurement.

Analyzing and reporting results. The results should cover the outcomes cited in the study objective: no more, no less. The data reported are obtained strictly by the investigation and not surmised. Validity and reliability of outcome measures determine the quality of the results. Do the outcome measures address the original objective? Would these results have happened by chance alone? The results section should contain an appropriate analysis of all variables recorded, beginning with a section ascertaining that the treatment groups were initially similar on pertinent patient characteristics, such as wound size, duration and depth. The key tests for differences in treatment effects should reflect the original objective, be appropriate to the data, and be performed on independent subsets of data. They should be presented clearly in figures and tables which illustrate the level of statistical significance of findings. Treatment details should vary only relative to treatment specifics. When comparing two primary dressings, ideally only the dressings should differ, though this may be difficult in practice. Cleansing procedures, secondary dressings, and taping methods should be equivalent in order to isolate the specific dressing as influencing the outcome. Such procedures associated with one treatment, but not the other could cause differences in patient outcomes erroneously attributed solely to the treatments.

Forming a conclusion. Finally, the conclusion is the summation of the study. Although the conclusion is based on the investigator's interpretations of the results, it should still accurately reflect the results obtained and not include assumptions. One cannot assume in the conclusion that the results applicable to the population studied can also apply to the excluded group or other settings.[4] For example, if the effectiveness of a pressure reduction surface is established in a hospital setting, it cannot be assumed that the results apply to the home care population. Caregiver time and training level in critical areas such as repositioning or pressure relief may vary from setting to setting. Moreover, if the comparative treatments differed widely, then conclusions about why the treatment effects were different are wisely discussed as hypotheses.

Summary

Through scientific research, the wound care professional is able to make informed, knowledgeable treatment decisions. This research may be in the form of published or unpublished literature or studies conducted within one's own institution. Whatever the source, only knowledge and application of the research process can help one obtain or interpret quality information to improve patient care. To make the most of this information, a wise wound care professional will scrutinize the results as well as the conclusions that can be legitimately drawn from the context of the research design. Are the results consistent with the objective and method? Was the study sufficiently controlled to justify claims of relative efficacy and safety?

Research need not be intimidating. Become familiar with the floor plan; start at the ground and build up. Set realistic goals that will support your clinical practice. It is important to remember that research objectives will not always culminate in a final answer but may in fact lead to another question. In the context of wound and skin care, case studies may suggest safe usage of a product and descriptive functions, but only controlled clinical evaluations ideally support final decisions about the best treatments to use to achieve wound care outcomes.

References

1. Bergstrom N, Bennett MA, Carlson CE, et al. *Treatment of Pressure Ulcers.* Clinical Practice Guideline No. 15. AHCPR Publication No. 95–0652: Rockville, MD, U.S. Dept. of Health and Human Services, Agency for Health Care Policy and Research, December 1994.
2. Panel for the Prediction and Prevention of Pressure Ulcers in Adults. *Pressure Ulcers in Adults: Prediction and Prevention.* Clinical Practice Guideline No. 3. AHCPR Publication No. 92–0047: Rockville, MD, U.S. Dept. of Health and Human Services, Agency for Health Care Policy and Research, May 1992.
3. National Pressure Ulcer Advisory Panel (NPUAP). *Pressure Ulcer Research: Etiology, Assessment and Early Intervention.* NPUAP, Buffalo, NY, 1995.
4. Van Rijswijk L. Nursing research and dermatology: Where to start. *Dermatology Nursing* 1990;2(3):158–161.
5. Ballard–Krishnan S, van Rijswijk L, Polansky N. Pressure ulcers in extended care facilities: Report of a survey. *JWOCN* 1994;21(1):4–11.
6. Rowe J, Barer D. A regional specialty policy for pressure sores. *Clinical Rehabilitation* 1995;9(3):262–266.

7. Wilson P, Burroughs D, Dunn LJ. Methicillin–resistant *Staphylococcus aureus* and hydrocolloid dressings. *The Pharmaceutical Journal* 1988;243:787–788.

8. Gilchrist B, Reed C. The bacteriology of chronic venous ulcers treated with occlusive hydrocolloid dressings. *British Journal of Dermatology* 1989;121:337–344.

9. Day A. Managing sacral pressure ulcers with hydrocolloid dressings: Results of a controlled, clinical study. *Ostomy/Wound Management* 1995;41(2):52–65.

10. Arnold TE, Kerstein M. Prospective multicenter study of managing lower extremity venous ulcers. *Annals of Vascular Surgery* 1994;8(4):356–362.

11. Colwell J, Foreman MD, Trotter JP. A comparison of the efficacy and cost–effectiveness of two methods of managing pressure ulcers. *Decubitus* 1993;6(4):28–36.

12. Hutchinson JJ, McGuckin M. Occlusive dressings: A microbiologic and clinical review. *American Journal of Infection Control* 1990;18(4):257–268.

13. Bolton LL, van Rijswijk L. Wound dressings: Meeting clinical and biological needs. CE feature. *Dermatology Nursing* 1991;3:146–160.

14. Bolton LL, Fattu AJ. Topical agents and wound healing. *Clinics in Dermatology* 1994;12:95–120.

15. Bolton L. Clinical studies and product evaluations: How to maximize their value. *Ostomy/Wound Management* 1995;41(7A Suppl.):88S–95S.

16. Xakellis G, Maklebust J. Template for pressure ulcer research. *Advances in Wound Care* 1994;8:46–48.

17. Constantine B, Bolton L. A wound model for ischemic ulcers in the guinea pig. *Archives of Dermatological Research* 1986;278:429–431.

18. Salcido R, Donofrio JC, Fisher SB, LeGrand EK, Kickey K, Carney JM, Schosser R, Liang R. Histopathology of pressure ulcers as a result of sequential computer–controlled pressure sessions in a fuzzy rat model. *Advances in Wound Care* 1994;7(5):23–40.

19. The Medical Device Amendments of 1976, as Further Amended by the Safe Medical Devices Act of 1990. *International Drug & Device Regulatory Monitor*. August 1991—no. 219, Appendix B.

20. Hamer RA. Importation of drugs and medical devices in the US: An overview of FDA pre–market approval requirements. *Pharmacy International* 1986;107:214–217.

21. Day A, Dombranski B, Farkas C, Foster C, Godin J, Moody M, Morrison M, Tamer C. Managing sacral pressure ulcers with hydrocolloid dressings: Results of a controlled, clinical study. *Ostomy/Wound Management* 1995;41(2):52–65.

22. Gove PB (ed). *Webster's Seventh New Collegiate Dictionary* Springfield, MA, G & C Merriam Co., 1972.

Acknowledgment

The authors wish to acknowledge the work of Karen Edgeworth in providing graphics and other assistance with this manuscript.

50

Regulatory Issues and Reimbursement

Glenda J. Motta, RN, MPH, ET

Motta GJ. Regulatory issues and reimbursement. In: Krasner D, Kane D. *Chronic Wound Care, Second Edition*. Wayne, PA, Health Management Publications, Inc., 1997, pp 383–388.

Introduction

As healthcare professionals and clinicians, we are often uncomfortable with the business aspects of patient care. However, like it or not, healthcare is a business, resources are tight, and patients are being identified by how much revenue they generate or lose for healthcare facilities. Smart wound care clinicians are expanding their advocacy role by considering these factors when caring for their patients.[1]

Regulatory issues and reimbursement mechanisms have an enormous impact on the quality of care, the introduction of new technology, utilization of products and services, patient access to care, and the actual outcomes of care delivered. Program budgets, such as those for Medicare and Medicaid, are fixed in advance and the reimbursement or payment mechanisms often determine how funds are distributed and what products and services are covered. The key factors are 1) whether or not the product or service is a covered benefit in the particular clinical setting where provided and 2) whether the amount paid is adequate and appropriate. In order to be adequately reimbursed, clinicians must learn how to document assessments, interventions, patient compliance to treatment plan, and outcomes of wound care in a way that supports coverage and payment for products and services.

Overview of Medicare and Medicaid

Regulatory overview and administration of two major reimbursement programs, Medicare and Medicaid, are the responsibility of the Department of Health and Human Services (DHHS), acting principally through the Health Care Financing Administration (HCFA). The federal statutes set forth broad parameters for coverage, eligibility, and payment; the DHHS promulgates rules and regulations that govern the programs.

The Medicare program consists of two benefit categories: Part A, services that require hospitalization as an inpatient or that are provided by a skilled nursing facility, home health agency or hospice; and Part B, supplemental medical services that can be provided on an outpatient or ambulatory basis, such as physician office visits, outpatient hospital visits, or care in surgi–centers. Part B also covers medically necessary durable medical equipment (DME) and medical supplies, such as surgical dressings and support surfaces and pneumatic compression devices. Actual day–to–day implementation of the rules, determination of eligibility, and the payment of funds for Medicare, are handled by various insurance companies who contract with HCFA, known as fiscal intermediaries (those processing claims for Part A benefits) and carriers (those processing claims for Part B benefits). Even though Medicare benefits are the same nationwide, coverage and payment may vary by intermediary or carrier.

Each state administers its own Medicaid program which provides healthcare services for individuals who meet specific eligibility requirements. The program is administered by an agency, such as the Department of Social Services or the Department of Health. Some states contract with a fiscal agent to process and pay claims and to interact with providers. Benefits may be offered through contracts with health maintenance organizations (HMOs) or other types of prepaid, capitated, or managed care plans.

Reimbursement by Clinical Setting

There are some basic tenets which apply when working with any third–party payer (Table 1). Documentation of pertinent observations, nursing actions, and other treatment interventions is crucial to reimbursement for all payers, especially Medicare. Providing accurate, complete information on a patient admitted to a hospital, subacute care unit, skilled nursing facility, or home health agency will reinforce the determination that the admission meets third–party payer requirements. Documentation must include patient assessment, problem identification, goals of care, implementation plan, and an evaluation of the outcomes.

Acute care. Hospitals are paid a fixed amount by Medicare and Medicaid using a prospective payment system. The number of hospitals that receive a managed fee for service rather than reimbursement for charges is increasing as managed care networks expand. Wound care products are included in the fixed amount of payment. Specialty devices, such as support surfaces, which were once reimbursed by Medicare as capital equipment, are now being paid under a prospective payment system.

Subacute care. Subacute care is provided to patients who no longer satisfy the Medicare or Medicaid criteria for medically necessary acute care services, but still require medical care during a subacute phase of recovery. It is designed to meet the needs of a growing group of patients who are sufficiently stabilized and no longer require costly hospital care. Nearly all healthcare payers recognize and reimburse subacute care services. However, there is no standard payment mechanism or rate. Subacute care facilities are reimbursed on a program–specific and site–specific basis. Payment varies by payer source, based on a facility–specific contract, or may be determined on a case–by–case basis.[2] Examples of possible reimbursement arrangements are fee–for–service, discount–off charges, per diem, fixed per case rate, and capitated rate.

To substantiate the patient's need (medical necessity) for subacute care, documentation is required regarding the appropriateness of the care setting, the utilization and frequency of services provided, and resources used.

Skilled nursing facility. Skilled nursing facilities are paid a per diem by Medicare, based on their costs. However, there are limits set to encourage cost efficiency. In some states, Medicare pays under a prospective payment system, based on the assessment of characteristics and service needs of residents. Most Medicaid programs pay a fixed per diem amount and wound care supplies are often included in this allowed amount. If the patient has Part B Medicare, surgical dressings may be reimbursed under this benefit if all eligibility requirements are met.

For Part A coverage, proof that the beneficiary continues to require skilled nursing care must be clearly documented in clinicians' notes, care plans and physician orders. Documentation must prove that the care provided is skilled or rehabilitative and can only be performed by, or under, the supervision of licensed nurses or therapists. The medical record should also indicate 1) the reason why a beneficiary is certified for Medicare, (e.g., vital signs and other conditions are being monitored, complex wound treatment regimen is being provided), 2) expected outcomes, and 3) progress or decline actually observed.

Federal regulations require that all residents in nursing homes (regardless of payment source) receive the care and supplies necessary to prevent the development or worsening of pressure ulcers. Medicare guidelines state that a citation will be issued "if a resident who enters a facility without a pressure ulcer develops one, and the facility has not demonstrated that the clinical condition made this unavoidable."[3] In addition, the regulation states that providers must establish institution–wide skin care regimens that stress prevention and early intervention. Financial, civil, and criminal penalties may be imposed on a facility for the nosocomial incidence of pressure ulcers. Documentation of risk assessment, development of a comprehensive care plan that reflects measures taken to prevent ulcers, and recording outcomes is critical.

Home health agency. Medicare pays home health agencies a per visit fee based on costs, but subject to limits. Medical supplies, such as wound care products, may be billed separately if they are essential to carry out the treatment plan, documented as medically necessary, ordered by the physician, and are "non–routine" supply items.

Skilled nursing and rehabilitative services provided in the home are covered under Medicare and by many other payers. Wound care services generally fall into the categories of observation and assessment, teaching or training, and direct hands–on care.

Observation and assessment for wound care is reasonable and necessary under Medicare guidelines when the likelihood of change in a patient's condition requires skilled nursing personnel to identify and evaluate the need for either possible modification of treatment, or the initiation of additional medical procedures until the treatment regimen is stabilized.

Teaching and training activities are reasonable and necessary under Medicare to teach a beneficiary, the family, or caregivers how to manage the wound treatment regimen, reinforce teaching previously provided in an institution or in the home, provide initial instructions for wound care, or teach proper application of a specialized dressing.

The Medicare Part A Regional Home Health Intermediary Manual (HIM 11)[4] fully explains the types of wounds that usually qualify as reasonable and necessary for home healthcare (Table 2).

Medicare Part B

Claims for wound dressings, support surfaces, and pneumatic compression devices are submitted to one of four Durable Medical Equipment Regional Carriers (DMERCs), depending upon where the beneficiary lives. The DMERC defines coverage and payment for each device or medical supply. These policies define medical necessity, documentation requirements, and utilization

---

Table 2
Types of wounds for which home healthcare is deemed reasonable and necessary (Medicare Part A Regional Home Health Intermediary Manual)

- Open wounds draining purulent or colored exudate, or which have a foul odor and/or for which the beneficiary is receiving antibiotic therapy.

- Wounds with a drain or t–tube which requires shortening or movement.

- Wounds requiring irrigation or instillation of a sterile cleansing or medication solution into several layers of tissue and/or packing with sterile gauze.

- Recently debrided ulcers.

- Pressure ulcers with partial thickness tissue loss and signs of infection.

- Pressure ulcers with full thickness tissue loss that involve exposure of fat or invasion of other tissue, such as muscle or bone.

- Wounds with exposed internal vessels or a mass which may hemorrhage with dressing change.

- Open wounds or widespread skin complications following radiation therapy, immune deficiencies, or vascular insufficiencies.

- Post–operative wounds with complications or underlying disease with potential to adversely affect healing (e.g., diabetes).

- Third degree burns and second degree burns where the size of the burn or presence of complications necessitates skilled nursing care.

- Other open or complex wounds which require treatment that can only be safely and effectively provided by a licensed nurse.

---

guidelines. Payment for wound dressings, support surfaces, and pneumatic compression devices under the Part B benefit is based on a fee schedule amount. Each year, the DMERC issues a list of allowables for these products. Medicare payment for a covered item is 80 percent of the lower of either the fee schedule (allowed charge) or the actual charge/retail price.

Reimbursement for wound dressings under Medicare Part B is provided under the Surgical Dressing Benefit. Medicare defines surgical dressings as "limited to primary and secondary dressings required for the treatment of a wound caused by or treated by a surgical procedure that has been performed by a physician or other heathcare professional to the extent permissible under state law." Dressings used after any type of debridement of a non–surgically created wound are covered, as long as the debridement is reasonable and necessary.

Under Part B, wound dressings are covered for 1) wounds caused by a surgical procedure, including incisions that have dehisced and incisions allowed to heal without closure; 2) wounds debrided by any method that is reasonable and necessary, including cleaning by mechanical, chemical, or autolytic debridement, wet–to–dry dressings or enzymes; 3) sutured wounds; 4) ulcers, such as Stage III or IV pressure ulcers, diabetic ulcers, or stasis ulcers treated with debridement; 5) burns treated with debridement and/or skin grafting; and 6) catheter entry points into a blood vessel.

Wound dressings are not covered for 1) Stage I pressure ulcers; 2) radiation dermatitis; 3) cuts, abrasions, skin tears; 4) skin irritations associated with peristomal care; 5) first degree burns; and 6) any wound that does not require surgical closure or debridement.

A beneficiary may be eligible for durable medical equipment, such as support surfaces and pneumatic compression devices, under Part B if the eligibility requirements outlined in the DMERC policy are met. However, these devices are not covered if the beneficiary resides in a skilled nursing facility. Support surfaces are grouped into three categories by the DMERC policy. Each category lists the coverage and payment rules and the specific product types. Generally, the risk factors, such as immobility, impaired nutrition, incontinence, altered sensory perception, compromised circulatory status, and the existence of any pressure ulcers must be well–documented for coverage.

Although Part B does not cover compression stockings, wraps, and garments, there is coverage for a pneumatic compression device if medical necessity requirements are met. There must be significant ulceration of the lower extremity, other methods of compression must have been tried and failed, and the ulcer must have failed to heal after 6 months of continuous treatment.

Providers who treat at–risk and wound care patients (e.g. physical therapists, occupational therapists, podiatrists, physicians, outpatient clinics) bill for these services under the Part B benefit. The key to reimbursement is documentation that clearly outlines the required skills of the individual professional, the medical necessity and reasonableness of the service, and the treatment goals. For therapists it is also important to note the significant functional progress being made over time as well as the functional and safety goals being met. Reimbursement for skilled services is based on allowable costs. Support surfaces and other supplies may be submitted as therapy supply expenses. Therapy related supplies are issued incident to a skilled therapy service and are charged, identifiable to a specific patient, and ordered by a physician for a medical reason.

To support coverage for any claim, always follow the documentation requirement for that benefit as listed in the DMERC, carrier, or intermediary manual. Wound dressings, support surfaces, and pneumatic compression devices are subject to utilization limits. Criteria are often complex and confusing, so it is important to keep current with payer policies.

Wound Care Documentation Guidelines

Appropriate documentation is critical to guide treatment decisions, evaluate wound healing progress, protect against litigation, and support reimbursement claims. Documentation that is inconsistent, ambiguous, and incomplete will result in reimbursement denials. Standardized flow sheets, photography, and computerized programs should be used to ensure greater accuracy of wound assessment and documentation. Software databases, such as I–STAR™ (Individualized Support Tracking and Assessment Record) or the Wound Intelligence System, allow comprehensive data collection and analysis of patient progress. They also provide patient demographics, wound characteristics, and product utilization statistics for use in cost reporting and quality assurance monitoring.[4]

Medical Necessity Requirements

Medicare policy requires healthcare professionals to provide information to justify medical necessity for wound care. Without such documentation, payment for services and products will be denied. For more details, consult the appropriate intermediary or carrier manual for the specific care setting.

For acute, subacute care, and skilled nursing facility settings. The following are the requirements for acute, subacute care, and skilled nursing facility settings:

- location and measurement of pressure ulcers (including width, length, depth in cm) of all ulcers (on admission and daily or weekly),

- assessment of wound healing progress,
- turning and positioning and schedule,
- assessment and documentation of general skin condition,
- evaluation and documentation of nutritional intake,
- use of protective or pressure reducing devices,
- topical treatment of wounds,
- skilled nursing care provided.

For Part B. For surgical dressings, the DMERC requires that suppliers maintain current clinical information which includes at least the number of wounds, the size (including depth) of the wounds, the frequency of dressing changes, and the number of dressings per wound to support reasonableness and necessity of the type and quantity of surgical dressings provided. Document any acute problems such as increase in amount of drainage or percent of necrosis, infection, and development of additional wounds.

It is the clinician's responsibility to educate third–party payers on the cost benefits, safety and efficacy, and positive outcomes of the many treatment and management approaches for wound care.

For home health agencies. Skilled nursing care for wound treatment provided in the home must be reasonable and necessary. The following wound characteristics must be documented during the assessment and reassessment: size, depth, nature of drainage (color, odor, consistency, and quantity), condition and appearance of the surrounding skin, photographs of wound(s) at least every 4 weeks, wound measurements at least once per week and weekly wound summaries.

When assessing the wound, avoid vague terms such as "improved," "stable," or "worse." Quantifiable and measurable wound dimensions should be recorded. Medicare requires that the patient's overall condition (e.g. orientation, mobility level, continence) be noted in the treatment plan. Any effect that nutritional status or other factors have on wound healing should be included in progress notes. In general, any information that helps validate the treatment plan or the outcomes of care (positive or negative) is important.

The plan of care must contain specific instructions for the treatment of the wound. The following are outcomes and accomplishments which may be used to demonstrate efficacy of care and medical necessity for home care:
- Teaching accomplished with family/caregiver;
- Family/caregiver demonstrate understanding;
- Progress towards goal;
- Any changes in patient status or treatment plan;
- Wound documentation;
- Outcomes of care;
- Outcomes of teaching;
- Patient's level of independence in care;
- Progress toward wound healing;
- Patient or wound deterioration.

To justify support surfaces, a comprehensive pressure ulcer treatment program must be documented which includes education of the patient and caregiver on the prevention and/or management of pressure ulcers, regular assessment by a healthcare professional (usually at least weekly for a patient with a Stage III or IV ulcer), appropriate turning and positioning, appropriate wound care, management of moisture/incontinence, and nutritional assessment and intervention.

Conclusion

Reimbursement is a complex yet important area for wound care clinicians to understand. The availability of products and services to treat or manage wounds often depends on reimbursement by third–party payers. Regulatory issues and reimbursement mechanisms have an enormous impact on the quality of care, the introduction of new technology, utilization of products and services, patient access to care, and the actual outcomes of care delivered.

Every claim submitted for reimbursement is based on the premise that the care rendered or the supplies provided were medically necessary and appropriate to treat the wound. This means that facilities, practitioners, and suppliers are liable for claims filed for wound care services, products, and durable medical equipment. Some payers have initiated fraud investigations against facilities, alleging that the development of pressure ulcers indicates that the patient did not receive the care that the provider was paid to render. The clinician must document the fact that the patient actually received care, products, and services.

It is the clinician's responsibility to educate third–party payers on the cost benefits, safety and efficacy, and positive outcomes of the many treatment and management approaches for wound care. As payers continue to seek ways to reduce healthcare expenditures, coverage decisions will change. Preservation of skin integrity and prevention of ulceration is still viewed by many payers as "convenience" and not medically necessary. This view is erroneous and we must educate insurers on the cost–efficacy of maintaining skin health and intervening early when patients are at risk.

Payers cannot keep abreast of the ongoing technological advances in wound care without input from the clinical community. Manufacturers, distributors, and clinicians must assume a proactive role in determining coverage for new products as they become available. Wound care clinicians must be able to demonstrate cost efficacy of new products and positive outcomes such as decreased healing time, reduced utilization of more expensive services, and fewer patient complications.

References

1. Motta GJ. Reimbursement: Some basic facts. *Nursing Spectrum* 1992;(2):10.
2. American Health Care Association. *Subacute Care: Medical and Rehabilitation Definition and Guide to Business Development.* Washington, DC, AHCA, 1994, p 10.
3. HCFA Guidance to Surveyors. *Interpretive Guideline* S483.25.
4. Motta GJ, Whitaker KW. *Defensive Wound Management.* Mitchellville, MD, Pathways to Empowerment, 1994, p 26.

51

Wound Research

Nancy L. Parenteau, PhD; Michael L. Sabolinski, MD; Gerit Mulder, DPM, MS; and David T. Rovee, PhD

Parenteau NL, Sabolinski ML, Mulder G, Rovee DT. Wound research. In: Krasner D, Kane D. *Chronic Wound Care, Second Edition*. Wayne, PA, Health Management Publications, Inc., 1997, pp 389–395.

Introduction

The treatment of chronic wounds can be placed into two categories: 1) treatment which assists the patient's own wound healing response either by relieving the underlying cause, improving the condition of the wound, or controlling infection, all of which act to facilitate healing, and 2) treatment designed to actively manipulate the wound healing response.

Despite recent improvements in treatment,[1] the ability to positively influence the rate, frequency, and quality of healing has been limited, particularly with the sole reliance on facilitative approaches.[2]

The identification of growth factors, cell attachment factors, and extracellular matrix components which can affect cell behavior has led to the possibility of providing an active agent to the wound healing process. In addition, the relatively recent ability to cultivate skin cells and reconstitute skin tissue has led to the possibility of providing the multiple benefits of a skin graft. Growth factors, extracellular matrix/cell attachment factors, and cell therapies are now reaching the clinic on an experimental basis. Growth factors and other elements of the wound have been covered in previous chapters. This chapter will discuss current work in cell biology and cell therapy as it relates to the present and future treatment of the chronic wound.

The Cell Biology of the Wound

Since the behavior of any active therapy is dependent on cell behavior and interaction in the wound, a brief overview of some key points is warranted. The inflammatory, connective tissue, and epithelial cells of the wound communicate through the production of cytokines, such as interleukins, or growth factors. Cells also communicate with each other and the surrounding extracellular matrix through cell surface receptors called integrins and various cell–cell adhesion molecules.[3] Growth factors are often sequestered by the surrounding matrix, creating microenvironments to which the cells react and contribute. Tissue and bacterial proteases can alter the microenvironment by activating and/or releasing matrix–bound growth factors, such as transforming growth factor – beta (TGFß), and digesting the extracellular matrix.[4]

In an acute wound, the inflammatory cells such as macrophages along with neutrophils and platelets begin the cascade of events toward healing, producing growth factors and cytokines which act upon the surrounding wounded epithelium and connective tissue. Macrophages also clean the wound, engulfing bacteria and removing debris while emitting a variety of factors.[5] The wounded epithelium and connective tissue also produce cytokines such as interleukin–1 (IL–1), basic fibroblast growth factor (bFGF), platelet–derived growth factor (PDGF), and TGFß to stimulate cell proliferation and regulate matrix degradation and new matrix deposition in both an autocrine and paracrine way.

In the chronic wound, the sequence of events present in the acute wound, namely the normal inflammatory response, is not always present. The chronic wound environment can be significantly different from that of the normal healing wound and is more difficult to understand. As in the acute wound, the cellular response is dependent on the matrix of the wound, the cellular constituents of the wound, and the types and amounts of growth

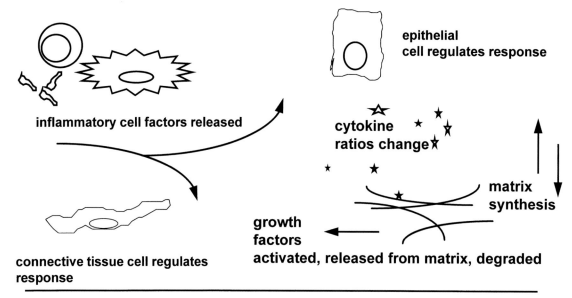

inflammatory cell factors released

epithelial cell regulates response

cytokine ratios change

matrix synthesis

growth factors activated, released from matrix, degraded

connective tissue cell regulates response

- platelets and inflammatory cells begin the process
- cytokines act in concert, activities intimately linked
- extracellular matrix orchestrates the process
- timed, balanced activity of agonist and antagonist
- coordinated mitogenic vs. synthetic response
- connective tissue and epithelial cells control their response by regulating receptor levels
- an imbalance of any of these aspects can lead to abnormal or impaired healing

Figure 1. *"Wound healing cell balance."*

factors and proteolytic enzymes present in the wound. It is the interaction of these constituents which leads to either the success or failure of the wound healing process. Assuming adequate care to relieve the underlying cause, specific wound healing needs to vary with the type of wound. For example, although wound closure by re–epithelialization remains a primary endpoint, connective tissue regeneration is particularly important in the deep pressure ulcer where substantial amounts of tissue repair may be required, while rapid epithelialization is important to minimize risk to the diabetic patient. In the venous ulcer, both stimulation of re–epithelialization and adequate dermal repair are important for persistent wound closure. The venous ulcer patient is particularly difficult to target since the cause of the compromised healing response is not entirely clear. The chronic wound is therefore a difficult and varied problem in need of active therapies which can be used to augment conventional therapy.

The non–healing wound – a puzzle of matrix, factors and cells. A key aspect in the repair and regeneration of the chronic wound is cellular ingrowth. However, many chronic wounds fail to respond beyond formation of some granulation tissue while others heal slowly even with proper dressings to control hydration of the wound and attempts to relieve the underlying cause. For example, while easing the underlying cause of the venous ulcer with compression will lead to healing over time in some patients, others, particularly those with wounds of greater duration, remain unhealed.[6] The granulation tissue matures, fibrin deposits develop and re–epithelialization does not proceed in spite of good standard care. Since the epidermis normally has a strong impetus to migrate over an open wound, why doesn't it? It appears that in these patients, the inherent wound healing ability is no longer sufficient. The cause of the deficiency is unclear. It can be due to proteolytic activity as a result of chronic contamination or inflammation,[4] a refractory cellular environment at the indolent edge, inadequate growth factor response, an imbalance of growth factors or an inadequate matrix deposition and remodeling. The cause is likely to be a combination of these elements.

Healing depends on a balance of elements. The intimate relationship between growth factors and

PARENTEAU, ET AL.

matrix is a key element in wound healing (Figure 1). Research has been done on the migration of epithelial cells on a variety of substrates *in vitro*. Fibronectin may guide cell migration during wound healing[7] although basement membrane components such as Collagen Type IV, laminin and laminin 5 (epiligrin, kalanin, nicean) may also play a role. The synthesis of metalloproteinases by the migrating epithelium also suggest that the epithelium is capable of "remodeling" the underlying matrix. Migrating keratinocytes synthesize new matrix proteins and can also change their pattern of integrin expression in response to the wound environment.[8] The stimulus or inhibition of migration and remodeling is still yet more complex since the migrating epithelium and the infiltrating fibroblasts encounter growth factors such as TGFß, bound to the matrix.[9] For example, TGFß binds tightly to both fibronectin and Type I collagen. Basic FGF binds to heparin sulfate. Therefore the cells encounter and respond to matrix and growth factors in concert. The epithelium fails to migrate from the indolent wound margins or remaining appendageal structures of a chronic venous ulcer. This failure could be due to inhibitory signals of matrix and growth factors in the wound bed or to a refractory state of the epithelium in proximity to the wound environment rendering the epithelium incapable of responding.

The Extracellular Matrix as an Active Agent in Wound Repair

Collagen substrates have been used as wound fillers to provide a scaffold for cellular ingrowth and tissue formation in burn wounds.[10] Processed native acellular dermis[11] which still contains the basement membrane, and collagen–glycosaminoglycan matrices[12] have been used to promote improved dermal healing when used in conjunction with meshed split–thickness autograft in burn wounds. However, their utility in promoting healing in the chronic wound has yet to be determined. The development of a wound filler which could act as a biological scaffold for fibroblast ingrowth may be particularly important in the treatment of deep wounds. Collagen, the primary substance of native connective tissue, should be well–suited for this application.[13] A preliminary study reported that Type I collagen sponges were able to decrease wound area in pressure ulcers by 40 percent as compared to no treatment.[14] The function of the scaffold might be further augmented by the addition of growth factors such as FGF to promote

angiogenesis and fibroblast infiltration or by the addition of fibroblasts.[15]

Methods to promote migration of connective tissue cells into the wound using cell attachment and chemotactic factors have also been studied. The arginine–glycine–aspartic acid (RGD) peptide sequence is a cell attachment peptide found in fibronectin and other matrix proteins. RGD–containing peptides promote cell attachment by binding integrin receptors present on the cell surface.[16] RGD peptide has been studied in wounds and has been found to stimulate healing by the promotion of connective tissue cell migration. RGD peptide has been shown to accelerate healing of sickle–cell leg ulcers[17] and diabetic ulcers[18] when compared to placebo controls. A related approach has involved combining a cell attachment peptide with a copper–containing compound which is chemotactic for cells.[19] However, neither treatment has yet been able to demonstrate a statistically significant difference in healing over standard (facilitative) care in controlled clinical trials.

The Use of Complex Mixtures to Augment the Healing Response

Growth factors for wound healing therapy have been covered in a previous chapter; however, it is important to review a few basic points with respect to their function. In the wound, growth factors do not act alone as they might in an *in vitro* experiment but rather in context with other factors.[20] Much of what we understand about their activity has come from *in vitro* experimentation; therefore, activities of the growth factors should be considered potential modes of action *in vivo*. Indeed, the production of transgenic mice where production of a single growth factor has been eliminated or "knocked out" has resulted more often than not in mice exhibiting a normal phenotype and normal wound healing response. This complexity and redundancy of function has made it difficult to target wound healing therapy using the addition of growth factors. The use of cocktails of multiple growth factors may partially solve this problem.

One approach has been to use complex naturally occurring mixtures of growth factors in the form of platelet extracts.[21] Platelets are recognized as major contributors to the wound healing process. Autologous platelet extracts contain PDGF, platelet–derived angiogenesis factor (PDAF), platelet–derived epidermal growth factor (PDEGF), TGFß, and platelet factor 4 (PF–4)[21]. Please refer to Chapter 44 on growth factors for more detailed information.

Cell Therapy

In a recent study comparing four types of wound contact materials combined with four layer compression for the treatment of venous ulcers, it was concluded that pinch skin grafts were the only primary wound contact material which made a difference.[22] Skin grafts can stimulate the wound healing response without having to persist as a skin graft. However, the difficulty and discomfort of creating a donor site, the pre– and post–hospitalization sometimes required, and the inability to re–apply multiple times as might be needed in large wounds of long duration, all make this a costly and less than routine option. The use of a cultured skin graft eliminates the need for a donor site and can be applied in a simple office procedure as often as might be needed, thereby reducing cost while providing similar benefits to an autologous skin graft.

cultured epithelial sheets are used together with homograft dermis.[26]

The fibroblast. Fibroblasts are a logical candidate to influence dermal healing through production of extracellualr matrix and growth factors. Fibroblasts have been shown to stimulate epithelial cell growth *in vitro* and are known to make a number of growth factors such as PDGF and FGF which could affect wound healing. However, unlike the epidermal cell, there are few published studies demonstrating the efficacy of dermal fibroblasts as wound healing agents. Improved wound strength in the healing of acute irradiated excision wounds by the application of fibroblast suspensions to the wound was demonstrated although no difference in collagen deposition was found.[27] Clinical studies have also reported improved healing of burn wounds after the application of cultured fibroblasts.[28] A product comprised of fibroblasts on

---

...the differentiated skin equivalent consists of four components which have the ability to effect healing: 1) the extracellular matrix, 2) dermal fibroblasts, 3) the epidermis and 4) a naturally occurring specialized semi–permeable membrane, the stratum corneum

---

The epidermal cell. Cell culture technology has advanced sufficiently to allow the cultivation of the epidermal keratinocyte, either autologous or allogeneic, for application to the chronic wound. Studies using autologous and allogeneic cultured epithelial sheets have shown the ability to stimulate granulation tissue formation and re–epithelialization.[23] Cultured epithelial sheets not only stimulate re–epithelialization but have been reported to stimulate the formation of underlying connective tissue as well. It has been postulated that the primary mode of action is through the production and delivery of multiple growth factors.[23] For example, cultured epithelial sheets produce TGFß and IL–1, both known to be able to affect fibroblast growth and matrix deposition. Cultured epithelial sheets have been shown to rapidly stimulate epithelial outgrowth from appendageal structures in *in vitro* explants.[24] Single center studies using cultured epithelial sheets for the treatment of venous ulcers have shown promise in the stimulation of wound healing in both venous[25] and pressure ulcers.[26] However, the efficacy of cultured epithelial sheets has yet to be directly compared to standard therapy in a randomized, controlled clinical trial. To date, they have shown the most clinical utility in the treatment of severely burned patients where autologous

a resorbable Vicryl® mesh (Dermagraft™, Advanced Tissue Sciences, La Jolla, CA) has been used under split–thickness autografts in burns but produced no significant effect on healing while the application of the mesh resulted in a slightly reduced take of the autograft.[29] The clinical utility of the fibroblast/ mesh approach for the treatment of chronic wounds is currently being examined in controlled clinical trials.

The synergy between epithelium and connective tissue. The reformation of a dermal matrix may be of particular importance in the venous ulcer where the quality of the healed wound is often minimally healed rather than ideally healed.[30] The quality and persistence of the healed wound is most likely intimately linked to the quality of dermal healing. Some researchers contend that a dermis containing the support of the fibroblasts is necessary for maintenance of the epidermal cell population.[31] However, cultured epithelial sheet grafts have appeared to persist for years in burn patients without engraftment of fibroblasts or a dermal element.[23] Cultured epithelial sheet grafts result in the formation of a "neodermis." Neodermis formation can take up to one year in burn patients. Therefore, cultured epithelial sheet grafts are now used clinically with cadaver dermis to improve take and attachment of the grafts. Neodermis formation is likely due to the effects of biologic wound closure with healthy epidermis which delivers growth factors to the underlying tissue.

The composite skin graft. Recent advances in cell culture methodology have enabled the formation of bilayered composite cultured skin grafts for clinical use.[32] The composite grafts contain both a dermal matrix with fibroblasts and an epidermis. It is now possible to provide a material possessing many properties of an autologous skin graft.[6] The cultured skin graft also has features which may increase its clinical utility over harvested human skin.

A bilayered allogeneic skin equivalent (Apligraf™, Organogenesis, Canton, MA) has now been used in controlled clinical trials for the treatment of venous ulcers[33] as well as for dermatologic surgery and burns. The skin equivalent consists of a fibroblast–populated collagen lattice overlaid with a differentiated, cornified epidermis. Because of its resemblance to skin, it contains both the advantages of a skin graft without the need for donor site harvest and the ability to reapply when and if necessary during treatment.

Keeping in mind the multiple factors influencing healing which were reviewed earlier in the chapter, the differentiated skin equivalent consists of four components which have the ability to effect healing: 1) the extracellular matrix, 2) dermal fibroblasts, 3) the epidermis and 4) a naturally occurring specialized semi–permeable membrane, the stratum corneum. These components may act alone, but more importantly, as part of a fully integrated tissue, they can act synergistically to heal a wound.[6] The goal is to re–establish new skin tissue either by stimulating the patient's own healing by secondary intention or by graft take.

The skin equivalent has been studied in a large scale randomized controlled trial on 293 venous ulcer patients. The study compared skin equivalent therapy which consisted of the cultured skin, primary non–adherent dressing, gauze and an elastic wrap to a four layer compression wrap consisting of primary non–adherent dressing, gauze, inelastic compression and an elastic wrap.[34] Preparation of the wound consisted of a standard cleaning with saline soaked gauze. No special debridement regimen, antibiotic therapy, or restricted activity was employed.

The skin equivalent was found to be more effective in achieving wound closure and in reducing time to complete healing than the four–layer compression even though the compression achieved was less–than–therapeutic.[34] According to Cox's proportional hazards regression (p < 0.0001), the skin equivalent was 60 percent more effective than standard compression in all patients, the largest difference in effectiveness, and was seen in the hardest to heal patients, those with wounds of greater than a year duration. Apligraf™ was equally effective in all treatment groups.

As expected, controlled compression therapy was most effective in small, less severe ulcers of less than 6 months to a year duration and minimally effective in patients with severe ulcers of greater than a year duration. The ability of an active therapy to heal all patients at the relatively same occurrence rate regardless of duration has also been described for RGD peptide therapy (Argidine™, Telios Pharmaceuticals, La Jolla, CA)[16] and cultured epithelial sheet grafts.[25] This ability illustrates an important difference in mode of action between facilitative and active therapies – the aim of active therapies being to directly contribute partial or complete wound healing ability to the wound. The exact mode of action of the skin equivalent may vary between individuals;[6] however, by applying a living interactive tissue, the chances of appropriate and adequate stimulation are further increased, yielding significant healing in all patients irrespective of duration and severity.

Boyce and colleagues have developed a composite culture based on a variation of the collagen–glycosaminoglycan matrix which is seeded with fibroblasts and overlaid with keratinocytes. A preliminary study on 4 patients with skin wounds of varied etiology reported stimulation of healing and graft persistence.[35]

Conclusion

To enhance healing over and above the inherent wound healing ability of the patient has been the goal of the new category of active wound healing candidates. However, large scale controlled trials against facilitative therapy alone have been met with many disappointments, particularly in the treatment of venous ulcers. Comparisons with more traditional facilitative approaches, both in efficacy and cost, have led to clinical skepticism regarding scientists' abilities to design a "breakthrough" therapy. The complexity of the wound environment may indeed require a "complex", i.e. multi–functional, solution such as a skin graft to re–establish the wound healing response. This requirement is indicated by the fact that the skin equivalent represents the first treatment to provide clinically meaningful results compared to a standard facilitative approach for the treatment of venous ulcers. Cost effectiveness using the new therapies can be obtained by significantly increasing a patient's chance of healing, reducing the time to heal, and improving the quality of healing, i.e., the therapy must not only work — it must work well. Results with skin equivalents should only improve as we learn more about how best to use them in conjunction with dressings, compression, debridement and control of contamination. The effectiveness of skin equivalents in diabetic and pressure ulcers has also yet to be determined. However, the cultured skin replacement has already shown its clinical utility in a difficult population (that of venous ulcers) and offers the chance for skin replacement in additional applications such as dermatologic surgery and burns.

References

1. Eaglstein WH , Mertz PM, Falanga V. Wound dressings: Current and future. In: Barbul A, Caldwell MD, Eaglstein WH, Hunt TK, Marshall D, Pines E, Skover G (eds). *Clinical and Experimental Approaches to Dermal and Epidermal Repair: Normal and Chronic Wounds.* New York, NY, Wiley–Liss, NY, pp. 257–265, 1991.
2. Margolis D, Cohen IK. Management of chronic venous leg ulcers: A literature–guided approach. *Clinics in Dermatol* 1994;12:19–2.
3. Mutsaers S, Laurent G. Wound healing from entropy to integrins. *The Biochemist. The Bulletin of the British Biochemical Society* 1995;17:32–38.
4. Wysocki AB, Staiano–Coico L, Grinnell F. Wound fluid from chronic leg ulcers contains elevated levels of metalloproteinases MMP–2 and MMP–9. *J Invest Dermatol* 1993;101(1):64–68.
5. Riches DW. The multiple roles of macrophages in wound healing. In: Clark RF, Henson PM. (eds) *Molecular and Cellular Biology of Wound Repair.* New York, NY, Plenum Press, 1988, pp 213–242.
6. Sabolinski ML, Alvarez O, Auletta M, Mulder G, Parenteau, NL. Cultured skin as a "smart material" for healing wounds: Experience in venous ulcers, *Biomaterials* 1996;17:311–320.
7. Clark RAF. Mechanisms of cutaneous wound repair. In: Westerhof W. (ed). *Leg Ulcers: Diagnosis and Treatment.* New York, NY, Elsevier Science Publishers, 1993, pp. 29–50, 1993.
8. Garlick JA, Taichman LB. Effect of TGF–ß1 on re–epithelialization of human keratinocytes in vitro: An organotypic model. *J Invest Dermatol* 1994;103:554–559.
9. Ruoslahti, E., and Yamaguchi Y. Proteoglycans as modulators of growth factor activities. *Cell* 1991;64:867–869.
10. Yannas IV, Burke JF, Orgill DP, Skrabut EM. Wound tissue can utilize a polymeric template to synthesize a functional extension of skin. *Science* 1982;215:174–176.
11. Livesey SA, Herndon DN, Hollyoak MA, Atkinson YH, Nag A. Transplanted accellular allograft dermal matrix. *Transplantation* 1995;60:1–9.
12. Heimbach D, Luterman A, Burke JF, et al. Artificial dermis for major burns: A multi–center randomized clinical trial. *Ann Surg* 1988;208:313–320.
13. Cavallaro JF, Kemp PD, Kraus KH. Collagen fabrics as biomaterials. *Biotechnol Bioeng* 1994;43:781–791.
14. Doillon C J, Silver FH, Olson, RM, Kamath CY, Berg, RA. Fibroblast and epidermal cell–type I collagen interactions: Cell culture and human studies. *Scanning Microsc* 1988;2:985–992.
15. Marks MG, Doillon C, Silver FH. Effects of fibroblasts and basic fibroblast growth factor on facilitation of dermal wound healing by type I collagen matrices. *J Biomed Mater Res* 1991;25(5):683–696.
16. Craig WS, Cheng S, Mullen DG, Blevitt J, Pierschbacher MD. Concept and progress in the development of RGD–containing peptide pharmaceuticals. *Biopolymers* 1995;37:157–175.
17. Wethers DL, Ramirez GM, Koshy M et al. Accelerated healing of chronic sickle–cell leg ulcers treated with RGD peptide matrix. RGD study group. *Blood* 1994;84(6):1775–1779.
18. Steed DL, Ricotta JJ, Prendergast JJ, Kaplan RJ, Webster MW, McGill JB, Schwartz SL. Promotion and acceleration of diabetic ulcer healing by arginine–glycine–aspartic acid (RGD) peptide matrix. RGD Study Group. *Diabetes Care* 1995;18:39–46.
19. Mulder GD, Patt LM, Sanders L et al. Enhanced healing of ulcers in patients with diabetes by topical treatment with glycyl–L–histidyl–L–lysine copper. *Wound Repair and Regeneration* 1995;2(4):259–269.
20. Nathan C, Sporn M. Cytokines in context. *J Cell Biol* 1991;113:981–986.
21. Knighton DR, Fiegel VD, Doucette MM, Fylling CP, Cerra FB. The use of topically applied platelet growth factors in chronic nonhealing wounds: A review. *WOUNDS* 1989;1:71–78.
22. Blair SD, Wright DD, Backhouse CM, Riddle E, McCollum CN. Sustained compression and healing of chronic ulcers. *BMJ* 1988;297(6657):1159–1161.
23. Compton C. Wound healing potential of cultured epithelium. *WOUNDS* 1993; 5:97–111.
24. Regauer S, Compton C. Cultured keratinocyte sheets enhance spontaneous re–epithelialization in a dermal explant model of partial–thickness wound healing. *J Invest Dermatol* 1990;95:341–346.
25. Limova M, Mauro T. Treatment of leg ulcers with cultured epithelial autografts. Clinical study and case reports. *Ostomy/Wound Management* 1995;41(8):48–60.
26. Phillips TJ, Kehinde O, Green H, Gilchrest BA. Treatment of skin ulcers with cultured epidermal allografts. *J Am Acad Dermatol* 1989;21:191–199.
27. Langdon R. C. , Cuono C. B. , Birchall N., Moellmann G. E., Madri J. A., McGuire J. Cryopreserved dermis is an ideal substrate for the engraftment and maturation of human epidermal keratinocyte cultures. *Mat Res Soc Symp Proc* 1989;363–371.
28. Glushchenko EV, Alekseev AA, Tumanov VP, Serov GG. [The treatment of thermal skin burns by using cultured fibroblasts]. *Arkh Patol* 1994;56(5):29–34.
29. Gorodetsky R, McBride WH, Withers HR, Miller GG. Effect of fibroblast implants on wound healing of irradiated skin: Assay of wound strength and quantitative immunohistology of collagen. *Radiat Res* 1991;125:181–186.
30. Hansbrough JF, Doré C. and Hansbrough WB. Clinical trials of a Living dermal tissue replacement placed beneath meshed, split–thickness skin grafts on excised burn wounds. *J Burn Care & Rehabilitation* 1992;13:519–528.
31. Lazarus GS, Cooper DM, Knighton DR et al. Definitions and Guidelines for Assessment of Wounds and Evaluation of Healing. *Wound Repair Regen* 1994;130:489–493.
32. Leary T, Jones PL, Appleby M, et al. Epidermal keratinocyte self–renewal is dependent upon dermal integrity. *J Invest Dermatol* 1992;99:422–430.
33. Wilkins LM, Watson SR, Prosky SJ, Meunier SF, Parenteau NL. Development of a bilayered living skin construct for clinical applications. *Biotech Bioeng* 1994;43:747–756.
34. Sabolinski M, Rovee D, Parenteau N et al. The efficacy and safety of Graftskin™ for the treatment of chronic venous ulcers. *Wound Repair and Regeneration* 1995;3(1):78.
35. Boyce ST, Glatter R, Kitsmiller J. Treatment of chronic wounds with cultured skin substitutes: A pilot study. *WOUNDS* 1995; 7:24–29.

Appendix 1
Abbreviations and their definitions

TGFß	Transforming Growth Factor–Beta
IL–1	Interleukin–1
bFGF	Basic Fibroblast Growth Factor
PDGF	Platelet–Derived Growth Factor
RGD	Arginine–Glycine–Aspartic Acid
PDAF	Platelet–Derived Angiogenesis Factor
PDEGF	Platelet–Derived Epidermal Growth Factor
EGF	Epidermal Growth Factor

52

A Profitable Partnership: The Durable Medical Equipment Industry (DME) and Healthcare Professionals

Rick Jay, BA, MBA and Jay Portnow, MD, PhD

Jay R, Portnow J. A profitable partnership: The Durable Medical Equipment Industry (DME) and healthcare professionals. In: Krasner D, Kane D. *Chronic Wound Care, Second Edition*. Wayne, PA, Health Management Publications, Inc., 1997, pp 396–402.

Introduction

The purpose of this chapter is to discuss the Durable Medical Equipment (DME) Industry, its role in providing equipment and services, the relationship between practitioners and industry, and how this relationship can be improved and enhanced to get better product, reduced costs, better funding and improved patient outcomes.

What is DME?

DME includes the equipment that healthcare professionals prescribe or recommend for their patients, including among other items, specialty beds, wheelchairs, seating systems, patient monitoring equipment, and bathing accessories. DME is usually associated with the equipment prescribed for use in the home. However, DME items are also utilized in hospitals and long term care facilities. Not included in DME are items such as pharmaceuticals and wound dressings.

The Wound Care Industry

The wound care industry primarily includes the DME equipment utilized to treat wounds (most notably specialty support surface companies such as Bio–Clinic, Cardio Systems, Hill–Rom, Invacare, KCI, Lumex, Pegasus, RIK Medical, and others); the dressings nurses utilize (from such companies as Convatec, Dow Hickam, Johnson & Johnson, Kendall, Sherwood, Smith & Nephew, and others); and supplemental wound products. Although the focus of this chapter will be on DME, this equipment is only as effective as the quality of medical care and support products that accompanies it.

Whether DME or dressings, the relationship of industry to the wound care community does not change significantly. On the industry side, the primary contacts are sales and service people. In the wound care community, there are enterostomal therapy nurses (ET nurses) who are generally the recognized "experts" in wound care. But wound care also falls into the province of most nurse managers and most general and home care nurses. General surgeons, vascular surgeons and primary care physicians are, of course, essential members of the community. Plastic surgeons are also an important part of the community as they are sometimes required to surgically intervene to help deal with the most severe wounds. When referring to practitioners, all of the above medical professionals are included.

The Role of DME in Wound Care

Pressure and shear relief mattresses, beds, and overlays can play an important role in wound treatment. That role is simple: to decrease the external forces that contribute to the occlusion of blood supply.

Support surfaces themselves do not heal wounds; blood flow does. A proper support surface primarily decreases the pressure and shear forces (and resultant issue deformation) that help cut off blood flow in the first place. Similarly, support surfaces need to be combined with quality medical care and a full wound treatment program.

Distributors. Distributors come in many shapes and sizes. They usually maintain a perpetual stock of products and are in a position to offer immediate local service on a broad variety of products from a wide variety of manufacturers. For hospitals, they have the advantage of being able to provide a daily shipment on one invoice of a large percentage of the

---

One cannot understand the respective roles of healthcare professionals and DME without first discussing the ultimate objective. This objective should be simple: to improve patient outcomes while controlling costs.

Since support surfaces are only one element in a proper wound care program, it is inappropriate for DME sales people to be recommending which patients should be on which products, unless that advice is properly integrated by the medical professional into a total wound program. On the other hand, the DME representative should be able to speak knowledgeably about the ability of his or her product to deal with all major patient issues including pressure, shear, maceration, transfers, patient sliding, patient turning, power consumption (or failure), and infection control.

How are DME Products Distributed?

Clinicians are often confused by the individuals that call on them and who they represent.

Once a manufacturer designs, tests, and produces a finished product, that manufacturer must find a way to bring that product to market, that is, get it into the hands of the user in such a way that the product is used appropriately. This task is easier said than done. Good products cannot work unless their supply chain is properly organized.

There are several methods commonly used to bring a product to market:

Going direct. This is often the most effective means. It is also the most expensive. It means that the manufacturer makes a heavy investment in local warehouses (for large products that are expensive to ship) and in a factory–trained sales organization (and service organization if needed) that represents only its products. National coverage requires a minimum of 30 to 50 sales people. However, for on–the–spot national representation, forces of 100 to 300 people are more the norm, meaning only a well–established company with over $50 million in sales can consider this route.

Using the pressure relief support surface industry as an example, the best known companies with "direct" organizations are Hill–Rom and KCI.

product needs of the hospital. Two well known companies in the field are Baxter and Owens & Minor. These companies, however, do not generally distribute higher ticket durable medical equipment products, particularly the more specialized ones such as support surfaces. They also do not perform a sales function, so the manufacturer generally needs its own sales force to educate users and prescribers. Wound dressings are often distributed through this channel.

Exclusive distributors. Another alternative is for a company to contract a series of exclusive distributors, one in each market, to distribute, service and represent its products. Dedicated representatives from the distributor are factory–trained and act like a "direct" sales force.

This method of distribution is considerably less expensive than direct distribution and can lead to considerable end user cost savings, particularly for newer, smaller companies. In the support surface industry, companies like RIK Medical and Lumex utilize this concept. KCI started this way and eventually bought out its distributors and turned them into a "direct" force.

Dealers. Dealers are generally less exclusive and carry a broader line of products, often with several competing manufacturers in each line. Conversely, one manufacturer can sell through multiple dealers in the same market. Dealers are common with home care DME products, which are often sold through virtually all home care dealers in a given city. While this is often the least costly distribution form, it also necessarily means that representatives carry multiple product lines and are not as intensively trained on any one product. In the support surface industry, Invacare utilizes this type of organization.

Mixed distribution systems. It is possible that certain companies mix their strategies. In the support surface industry, Cardio and Pegasus utilize a mix of going direct, using distributors, and using dealers, depending on the city.

CHRONIC WOUND CARE, Second Edition

Understanding Roles:
The Patient Comes First

One cannot understand the respective roles of healthcare professionals and DME without first discussing the ultimate objective. This objective should be simple: to improve patient outcomes while controlling costs. The emphasis cannot shift just to the cost side of the equation, but must balance cost with appropriate patient care.

Once people accept the above objective, it becomes apparent that the needs or desires of industry and practitioners matter only after steps are taken to insure that patient and cost requirements are simultaneously met.

Practitioners: How to Get More
From Industry

As a "for profit" industry, DME is sometimes looked at suspiciously by nurses and other healthcare professionals. This should not be the case as without profit these products would simply not exist. Furthermore, it is profit that motivates and allows companies to continually develop better and more cost effective products.

Many practitioners do not understand their power to influence their DME manufacturers and suppliers. These companies want to meet your needs. In order to facilitate this, it is important to outline what you want and expect from a product or service. Share this information with your vendors. In today's competitive environment, most companies will respond to this approach.

Tips. Treat the relationship as a partnership. It should never be adversarial. Partnerships are based on trust, mutual respect and loyalty. If your vendors cannot be trusted or respected, do not do business with them. (And be honest with them; let them know if your trust has been violated.) If they can be trusted, and they provide the best product or service for your patient, then appreciate them and commit a large portion of your business to them. Dedicated, long term customers generally get the best service and price.

Understand that your vendor's primary asset is his or her time. Respect that time, keep appointments, return phone calls and you will enjoy even better service in return.

Do not be afraid of going to the top to get what you want. When was the last time you called the president of the company? You would be amazed at the response you can get. If you do not get the answer you want from your local distributor or sales representative, then call 800 information and call the manufacturer (customer service department)

directly. Manufacturers usually know more about their products than their local office or distributor. They also appreciate hearing if their local offices or distributors are not providing you with the information you need. You can also learn a lot about a company by calling the corporate office. Are they prompt, courteous, and knowledgeable? If not, they probably do not provide their local representatives the support they need to be able to meet your long term needs.

Respect the vendor as a member of the clinical team. Ask for and expect appropriate clinical input from the vendors. For example, it is not unreasonable to expect the vendor to comment on the full range of available products, including competitors' products. A good vendor will recommend others' products to supplement or sometimes replace theirs. Be suspicious of vendors who disparage their competitors. This is usually a sign of competitive weakness on their part. It also undermines your ability to select other products when they are more appropriate. (It is a commonly accepted precept that no one product is right for all patients.)

Learn the reimbursement policies of your patient's insurer. Do not prescribe something that will not be paid for by the insurer without checking with your patient first. Products or technologies that are new to the market are most often the ones to ask the most questions about, as it usually takes insurers, including Medicare and Medicaid, two to three years to recognize and establish coding for genuinely new products.

Once you have found a vendor that meets all of the above criteria, reward the vendor with your business. The fewer vendors you use, the better the price and service you will receive and the less time you will spend doing it. Multiple sourcing is a concept that was popular in the 60's and 70's and is now being replaced with more exclusive vendor partnerships based on enhanced reliability, lower cost, and an improved understanding of each other's needs.

Industry: How to Maximize Your Return
from Practitioners

Just as practitioners sometimes misunderstand vendors, the reverse is also true. There are some cardinal rules that vendors must follow if they are to have positive long term results.

Rule 1. The outcome of the patient is more important than your sale. Never forget this motto and never represent a product to do what it cannot do. You will lose credibility, lose sales, and potentially harm the patient at the same time. This advice is more than good ethics; it is good business.

For example, a powered air overlay is generally not appropriate for a heavy patient if the head of the bed is raised, as it can lead to bottoming out at the sacrum and the development of a pressure ulcer. If a sales person knowingly or unknowingly (which is worse?) recommends such a use, and the patient is harmed, that sales person will lose many, many times the value of that one "sale."

Rule 2. Education is a better approach than selling. If you cannot educate the practitioners in a way that will help them do a better job, then do not waste their time. They are busy people. The more knowledgeable they are, the less patience they will have for ignorance.

This question should not, however, be cause for intimidation, as the right attitude and hard work will always gain the respect you need. Learn how your product meets patients' needs, improves outcomes, and reduces costs. What are the indications for its use and where should it not be used? (It is better to find out from you than from failure!)

In general, as a sales person, your knowledge in your area, though relatively narrow in overall scope, should be extremely deep, i.e. you should know more about your product and how it works than 99 percent of the clinicians you call on. The medical practitioner, on the other hand, will have a much broader medical knowledge that usually has less depth than the educated sales person's sphere of knowledge.

In general, your credibility as a sales person is your most important asset. If you do not know the answer, say so and promise to get back promptly with the proper answer. Do not ever fake it. Never compromise your credibility.

In this regard, never stop educating yourself. Attend conferences, read journals (like the medical journals and the DME Review). Ask permission to work with a healthcare professional around his or her job (and vow to yourself not to sell them anything while learning what they do). If you understand the job, you will do a much better job of meeting the practitioner's needs.

Rule 3. Service is often more important than product or price, as the latter elements are becoming available from multiple sources. How can you differentiate your value added services? (For example: what is your delivery turnaround time? Is someone on call all the time? What training accompanies the product?) Service is also the best way to get your desired price.

Rule 4. Respect the practitioners' time. They are busy people under increasing time pressures to do more with less. If you make an appointment, be early. Never take more time than the practitioner

willingly gives. If you want more time, bring knowledge to the table to make it a worthwhile expenditure of time. (Food usually helps too!)

If the practitioner asks for 60 to 90 days before evaluating your product, do not go around him or her in an effort to get it in sooner. That is a good way to lose the business forever. (Similarly, clinicians should maintain their promises to evaluate in a timely fashion!)

Rule 5. If making money is your only goal, you will not succeed. If you take care of the patients' needs first and caregiver, institutional and hospital needs second, then the profits will follow. For example, in the DME wheelchair and wheelchair seating business, there are two companies very well known for their quality, patient orientation and service — Quickie and Jay Medical. They also happen to be among the most profitable companies in their respective fields.[1]

Rule 6. Learn about the reimbursements of your products. Medicare, Medicaid, Commercial insurers, HMOs, and other payers cover products at different rates in different settings with sometimes dramatic consequences for the patient. It is important to communicate this information to practitioners so that realistic choices can be made. There is no sense in prescribing the perfect system if the patient will not be able to afford the deductibles, copays, and so on.

Rule 7. When the sale is made the work usually begins. You will need to educate everyone involved with the product (including second and third shift at the institution or with the family and homecare nurse at home.) When there is a problem (and there always will be at least one), track it to its source, (as third party information usually tells only part of the story), then solve the problem with the involvement of the appropriate medical practitioners (even if it means discontinuing the use of your own product.)

Working Together to Get Better Products and Services

There are more opportunities than ever to improve product and service delivery, particularly with the evolution of technology. There are a few keys to getting the improvements we all want:

Focus on partnerships. In a recent meeting of vice presidents of purchasing from major hospital buying groups, it was generally acknowledged that price squeezing the manufacturers, though not over, was inevitably producing diminishing results.

Instead, future focus was being placed on forming partnerships with manufacturers to reduce overall costs. One way to go about this approach is to create approved clinical pathways, and then reduce utilization by better matching products with patient needs. A 20 percent decrease in utilization will save much more money than a 5 percent reduction in cost. The era of earning more money by selling less product is rapidly coming upon manufacturers. Industry and practitioners must work cooperatively to make this concept happen without compromising patient outcomes.[2]

Similarly, products that reduce patient stays in hospitals can earn dramatic savings far beyond the cost of the product. A support surface that heals wounds faster can save over $1,000 per day. If that same product can follow the patient into the home sooner, then several more thousand dollars can be saved. These savings are huge compared to the cost of the product itself.

job? Do it by forgetting the details and looking at the bigger picture.

Study the underlying principles the product has to meet. For example, with pressure relief support surfaces, a wound professional needs to understand the underlying principles of pressure, shear, tissue deformation, and bottoming out. Once these principles are understood, it is easier to predict when a new technology might or might not work without making your patients into guinea pigs.[4]

Focus less on bells and whistles, and more on basic patient and caregiver needs. How does this new technology help meet these basic needs? Again, using support surfaces as an example, once you believe the surface meets the basic pressure and shear relief needs, you need to look at other needs

---

One thing is certain, the product you use today is not the one you will be using ten years from now!

These are two examples of where the lowest price product does not necessarily mean the lowest cost outcome. Furthermore, these two cost savings methods simply cannot happen without the intense cooperation of practitioners, purchasing, and product suppliers.

One example of developing clinical pathways to reduce costs is by developing a protocol for determining which support surface to use for which type of wound and patient. This approach is one way nurses are driving down their support surface costs, often with the cooperation of their support surface supplier. One such pathway that resulted in over $200,000 annual savings without compromising patient outcomes was documented by a group of nurses at St. Joseph's Hospital in Denver.[3]

Always strive to improve product or service. Here are some ideas on how to improve a product or service (most of these ideas need to be practiced by manufacturers, but clinicians can also play an important role):

Remember that no product or service is perfect. What are the drawbacks? How can it be improved? Through critical evaluation, improved products and superior service will evolve.

Keep an open mind to new technologies. This idea is easier said than done, especially when you believe your existing products are working. One thing is certain, the product you use today is not the one you will be using ten years from now! Better products will replace it. How do you do this without making new technology evaluation a full–time

such as patient transfers, patient sliding, patient turning, cleaning and maintenance, the ability to conduct CPR or physical therapy and the ability to utilize standard hospital sheets and underpads.

In other words, if you understand basic principles and patient needs, new technologies do not take long to figure out. Eliminate the ones that cannot answer these principles and needs; spend your time evaluating those that can.

Keep in mind that most engineers are mediocre product developers because they are more focused on their drawing boards than on patient needs. They also tend to come up with complicated solutions because the simple ones are much harder to figure out.

Get the product developers into the field to see the patient and institutional needs with their own eyes. A hands–on approach will allow for products to be developed with the patient and institution in mind.

When you do not succeed at first, try, try again. Most great products go through hundreds of evolutions, with continuing refinements every 90 days. Never stop trying to make your product or service better.

Every once in a while, forget how things are done today. Focus on the ideal product or service. What should it do? How should it accomplish its task? Only by defining a new product or level of service will it ever be developed.

When in doubt, favor the simplest solution. Technology can be wonderful and it has solved lots of difficult problems, but sometimes, it goes too far. Are the bells and whistles you are paying for really being used? How often? Do nurses and caregivers know how to use them? What happens if they are misused? What happens if the power goes out?

Most "high tech" products work wonderfully when they work. What you have to watch for is when they do not work as intended. In addition, most nurses have more alarms, computer modules, and adjustments than they want or know how to use.

As a practitioner, avoid the complicated solutions, where possible, as one huge way to save dollars. As manufacturers, focus on elegantly simple solutions that do the same job more safely and with less training time (a major cost in our system). Ironically, however, the most elegantly simple solutions are also the most difficult to come up with. (Velcro is a great example!)

Involve a team in decision making. A product has to work for everyone involved: patient, nursing, caregiver, the institution, the payor, purchasing, and house keeping. Most hospitals have new product committees to take into account the needs of everyone involved. Getting this input up front will not only result in better decisions, it will also help the program succeed because the people who have been part of the decision will help in the proper execution of that decision.

The Role of Managed Care

We all know that managed care is making cost a greater issue. In other words, every product or service needs to be questioned as to its effectiveness and its relevancy. Effectiveness has to do with design. Does the product or service do what it is supposed to do? Relevancy has to do with appropriateness. Is this product or service justifiable for the patient or situation? One of technology's primary roles will be to develop products and provide services that will be cost effective while maintaining or improving outcomes.

To be cost effective, one must question the relevancy of a product or service to a patient's needs. In the past, our healthcare system has tended to over–prescribe, so as to be on the safe side and to insure the best patient outcomes regardless of cost. With managed care, practitioners and industry need to work together to better match technology to patient needs, so as not to over–prescribe. Will an overlay do, or is a full bed system necessary? These are sometimes easy decisions to make, sometimes very difficult. More outcome studies relating to products and service will help us make better decisions in the future, so will a greater emphasis by industry to reduce utilization. (Gone are the days when product suppliers can shop the hospital floor for patients "requiring" their products.)

However, we should never allow patient outcomes to be compromised. This is where industry and practitioners must together draw a line in the sand and stand up to managed care. If you can prove you are right, managed care will follow, as they cannot afford the liability cost of providing the wrong product or service. Again, outcome studies will be key.

One area that managed care and hospital buying groups have pushed hard in order to gain price advantage is exclusive contracts. For the most part, this is a valid way to save money. With greater volume, manufacturers can reduce their prices. Furthermore, enforcement of contracts permits manufacturers to reduce their sales forces, as they do not need to defend their businesses as aggressively against competitors. This approach leads to leaner sales forces and reduced costs.* However, practitioners must still be willing to fight for specialty items that are needed by their patients, but are not covered on national contracts. These contracts invariably have provisions to allow for such purchases off contact, particularly when dealing with "new technology," so do not let purchasing or managed care say "no" without fighting for the patient.

How to Get More Funding?

Acquiring funding is a key area in which industry and practitioners must work together. As a general rule, funding sources will listen to industry only if good clinical and outcome documentation is provided. Funding sources generally listen to practitioners more, particularly when they take a stand based on proven clinical principles. So clinicians

---

* One irony of national contracts is that they often end up causing higher costs. This is because is most cases, national contracts can only be signed and supported by the largest players in a given industry. As a general rule, large companies are not innovators in the U.S. economy. It is the smaller companies that have historically pioneered most innovations. The small company with an innovative technology is increasingly shut out of this national contract system – even if the products produce better outcomes at 40 percent savings! The only way these innovative companies can succeed is if purchasers write new technology clauses into contracts or if practitioners fight for new products based on medical needs of their patients. Only by allowing innovators to gain market share in this way can they ever hope to grow and then sign the national contracts that will allow broader savings. (Ironically, the first question group purchasers ask of smaller technology companies is "which hospitals in our group are currently using your product?"! This is in spite of the fact they have signed exclusive contracts with larger competitors to shut them out of their hospitals!

must stand up for what they believe in. They must stand up for the patient. The squeaky wheel still gets the most grease. When it comes to funding, expect to get turned down the first time. Understand that you will often win on appeal. That is the way the system works. The patient is worth fighting for.

Conclusion

Durable Medical Equipment (DME) and wound dressings form the bulk of wound care products that are sold to wound care practitioners (ET nurses, nurse managers, home care nurses, and physicians and surgeons). These products are generally sold and distributed directly from manufacturers or through exclusive distributors or non–exclusive dealers.

When working together, the DME industry and medical practitioners must avoid an adversarial relationship and must agree that improving patient outcomes at reduced costs is the ultimate objective. This objective should then drive a cooperative relationship between industry and practitioners.

Medical practitioners should expect from their vendors a high degree of knowledge about their products, high integrity, and consistent follow up after the sale. In return, practitioners should value their vendors' time, involve them in clinical decisions, and be loyal to them by concentrating their business with as few suppliers as possible.

Vendors must earn their business by understanding patient and practitioner needs, understanding their products well enough to educate rather than sell, and always working for better patient outcomes.

Together, practitioners and industry must work as a partnership to improve patient outcomes by focusing on proper (and decreased) utilization of products along proven clinical pathways. Managed care will insist upon this approach, and it does not have to compromise patient care as long as clinicians fight the fight when appropriate for products that are declined, by arming themselves with conviction and well researched outcome studies.

Together, practitioners and industry should also strive for improved, yet simpler products, and they should involve a broad range of disciplines along with proper product design, choice, and implementation. They also need to work together to educate funding sources, particularly when new cost effective technologies are developed.

The model for cooperation outlined in this chapter is not theoretical. It is happening in the medical community and in general industry, whether medical or not. Huge costs savings and improved outcomes are happening in every corner of our society, medical community and industry, as parties that once considered themselves somewhat adversarial, are working together and cooperating to improve outcomes at reduced costs.

References

1. Sunrise Medical, Inc. 1995 Annual Report. 2382 Faraday Avenue, Suite 200, Carlsbad, CA 92008, (619)930–1500.
2. Orchestrating New Roles: Group Strategies for the Health Care Evolution: February 4–5, 1996, Phoenix, Arizona. Sponsored by NCI, 30211 Avenida de las Banderas, Suite 120, Rancho Santa Margarita, CA 92688, (714)589–6500.
3. Mahon D, et al. Reducing specialty bed use. *Nursing Economics* 1995;13(3).
4. Jay R. Pressure and shear: Their effects on support surface choice. *Ostomy/Wound Management* 1995;41(8):36–45.
5. Jay R. How different support surfaces address pressure and shear forces. *Durable Medical Equipment Review* 1995;2(2).

53

Opportunities for the Wound Care Clinician

Janice M. Stanfield, RN, BS, CETN

Stanfield JM. Opportunities for the wound care clinician. In: Krasner D, Kane D. *Chronic Wound Care, Second Edition*. Wayne, PA, Health Management Publications, Inc., 1997, pp 403–406.

Introduction

Healthcare is big business. It impacts us not only as providers, but also as consumers. Nursing and rehabilitative therapies are considered essential services, therefore, questions rarely arise as to their need or value. Changes are, however, occurring in the delivery of healthcare and the sophistication of diagnostic equipment, therapeutic tools and healthcare products. Healthcare providers are finding it nearly impossible to maintain current knowledge in every aspect of care. Nurses and therapists alike are following the model set by physician groups. They are defining areas of speciality and investing tremendous time and resources into intense study to become "experts" in a chosen area. Certainly the advantage to the healthcare consumer is access to a highly trained professional who can be called upon to assist when a patient or situation presents itself which warrants special intervention.

When a practitioner chooses to become specialized, he/she is limiting his/her employment opportunities to a very specific area of expertise. In addition, he/she finds the environment much more competitive with more and more specialists targeting the same markets. Although in the past, healthcare providers have been educated at some of the finest universities in the country, few healthcare educational programs include classes on business and marketing. Knowledge of marketing and business development is essential to maximizing potential opportunities.

One great change in healthcare over the past ten years is related to the management of wounds. Technological advances in wound care products and services, coupled with the changes in the delivery of healthcare, have created an environment that is complex. Certified Enterostomal Therapy Nurses (CETN), Clinical Nurse Specialists (CNS), Certified Wound Care Nurses (CWCN), Physical Therapists and some physicians have targeted wound management as their primary practice. However, as a new millennium approaches, some of these specialists are questioning the impact healthcare reform will impose upon their individual specialized practice. Others are already affected.

Administrative decisions are focusing on strict cost containment, improvement of quality care and evidence of appropriate and timely outcomes. Until now, employment opportunities have been plentiful; however, many clinicians are being thrown into dual roles (e.g., wound specialist and diabetes educator, wound specialist and discharge planner). Less fortunate specialists are finding that their positions have been completely eliminated. Clinicians are becoming more and more concerned as traditional employment opportunities are growing scarce. It is apparent that the security of one's career is based on an ability to achieve and document positive outcomes and broaden a client base. It is time to focus on the market, to investigate potential clients along with methods of marketing one's skills as leaders in the field.

Exploring Opportunities

While some wound care specialists enjoy the routine of institutional employment, others prefer the autonomy of an independent practice. One must first decide how to deliver services, (i.e., as an employee or as a contractor). Either way, the key to a secure successful practice is communicating the value of the service, i.e. marketing.

There are two basic ways to look at marketing a service. Marketing to an existing client is reinforcing value and securing a position. Marketing to a new client requires identification of a potential opportunity and then convincing the client that you are the best person to meet the challenge.

Marketing is a continuous process. The decision may be made to target one market as a primary referral source. However, it is important to keep in mind that successful specialty practice depends on diversifying or broadening a market base. An example of a broad base practice might be the hospital employed acute care based CNS, who accepts and makes home visits one day a week, is contracted through his/her hospital as part time faculty to a local nursing school or other community college and participates in product clinical trials through her hospital based outpatient clinic. Another example would be the CETN in independent practice who contracts with 5 acute care facilities, 10 home care agencies, and 2 long term care facilities for "as needed" visits. In addition, the CETN serves as a speaker on a travelling lecture circuit, reviews malpractice cases and advises attorneys and/or the court as to the validity of the pending action, participates with industry as a site investigator for clinical trial work, and advises managed care organizations as to cost effective alternative dressings. The more diverse your practice is, the more opportunity and, therefore, security will come your way.

The first step is selecting the clients you wish to service. Some target markets who have identified the need or value of wound care specialists are acute care, subacute and transitional care, rehabilitative care, long term care facilities, hospice units, home healthcare, outpatient clinics, industry, educational institutions, law firms, insurance companies, and managed care organizations.

The next step is to accumulate information. Identify individuals within the market who are responsible for making decisions about the use of ancillary services. Find out if they are currently utilizing a wound care specialist and, if so, if there are problems or concerns with respect to their existing service. Learn about the competition. If they are not currently using a specialist, do they perceive a need? What are the challenges they are facing? What are their goals?

Marketing strategies should always be directed toward assisting clients in achieving their goals in an efficient, cost effective manner. Therefore, presentations or marketing tactics must be tailored to highlight the skills you possess which will help the patient achieve his/her goals.

> *Marketing strategies should always be directed toward assisting clients in achieving their goals in an efficient, cost effective manner.*

Potential Markets

Acute Care facilities offer the most traditional roles for wound care specialists. However, with reimbursement for Medicare and many indemnity insurance programs being dictated by Diagnosis Related Groupings (DRG's), as well as the increase of capitated insurance contracts within the managed care arena, facilities are in crisis. They are being forced to weigh heavily the costs of providing services. To assure their solvency, they are not only beginning to address acute care needs, but are also setting up diagnostic and outpatient clinics, affiliated home care agencies, transitional care units, rehabilitative therapy units and outpatient surgery centers. These facilities are combining staff positions and eliminating positions which appear non-essential. Actually, for the wound care specialist, this is good news. Acute care facilities are bringing a broader market to the specialist. What are the benefits one might have to offer? A wound care specialist can become involved in staff education by preparing classes on prevention of skin problems, wound assessment, documentation, and education on the use and selection of wound care products. The specialist can assist with the management of wound care supplies and facilitation of reimbursement, assist in the consolidation of supplies in central services, serve as the liaison to associated vendors and develop and implement policies and procedures. Monitoring patient outcomes, emphasizing improvement in quality patient care, decreasing in nosocomial breakdown, and providing patient education can enhance a facility's image and decrease liability. A specialist can follow patients after discharge, thereby providing continuity of care from hospital to sub–acute, to rehabilitation, to home care.

Many specialists function as gatekeepers of specialty rental beds, saving thousands even millions of dollars related to inappropriate bed rentals.

A wound care specialist is in a unique position to establish a revenue generating center within the hospital setting. This is accomplished through the development and maintenance of a clinic where one can not only establish outpatient revenue but also be a site for clinical research and/or outpatient retail supplies.

Subacute care, transitional care, rehabilitation and long term care facilities offer similar challenges. Although these facilities have long been challenged with wound care problems related to longer acute care stays, the facilities are usually smaller; and therefore, the population which directly and clearly benefits from the employment of wound specialists is limited. Some of these facilities are monitored and controlled by state and/or federal programs and face challenges not found in acute care. Their goals may vary. Certainly, a specialist who plans on working in these environments must have a thorough understanding of state and federal regulations as well as reimbursement. As in acute care, it is the clinician who must position him/herself as a vehicle for achieving the institution's goals and saving cherished fiscal resources while improving or assuring the quality of care. Benefits similar to acute care can be offered by a wound care specialist, perhaps with the exception of an outpatient clinic or retail supply center.

Home health is one of the oldest, yet most rapidly growing, market segments. Trends toward managed care are changing their focus. Since wound specialists are expert at recommending cost effective wound management, many home care agencies have found that there is significant value to ordering a "wound specialist" consult early in the patient care regime. The clinician often cuts visit frequency, orders more cost effective treatment, and the patient experiences better outcomes. Other benefits one might offer include staff and patient education on prevention of recurring skin related problems; wound assessment, documentation and selection of appropriate wound care products; and assistance in the development of patient care plans and outcomes management. The specialist can assist with management of wound care supply reimbursement, development and implementation of policies and procedures, and can serve as a vendor liaison.

Hospital Program Evaluations are marketed by some clinicians and offer a variety of opportunities.

Some facilities prefer that an expert come in to prepare a "report card" of sorts. A clinician collects pertinent data; reviews facility contracts, DME, and disposable equipment; interviews staff and determines the assets and liabilities of each facility. The clinician then creates a document which contains a detailed picture of the facility status and recommendations for management. Sometimes it is appropriate to recommend that the clinician participate in program development by staff and patient education. One might also select and train a "skin care team" that assumes responsibilities when the clinician leaves. It is appropriate to recommend that the clinician, who is more knowledgeable with respect to wound care products, diagnostic tools, and speciality bed sales and rental, be an integral part of, if not solely responsible for, negotiation of contacts with vendors. In addition, the consultant might assist with development of standardized protocols, setting up of "outcome profiles," downsizing of central supply inventory and evaluation and recommendations to the facility with respect to documentation and liability.

The role of educator is extremely diverse. Wound care specialists are often hired to participate in travelling speaker bureaus, where 10 to 20 lectures are scheduled each year. Vendors or manufacturers, home care agencies and hospitals all have been known to hire a specialist to teach wound care, hoping to bring to a central location nurses or patients who could purchase products or services from the program sponsor. Some specialists teach programs independent of any institution or vendor and do so by utilizing their independent provider number for continuing education. A wound specialist might also work full time as faculty at an established ET or wound specialist program or serve as contract adjunct faculty, teaching community college or university level nursing education programs.

Industry is probably one of the fastest growing employment or contract markets for the wound clinician. With the sophistication of products and the huge influx of dressings on the market, industry is utilizing the wound care specialist in a variety of ways. Some of the avenues one might market include investigative product trial monitor, research associate, or clinical investigator. These options involve investigation of potential products and/or troubleshooting of current products manufactured or distributed by a company. Trial monitors and research associates are usually employed by a company; however, some are independent, contracting wound specialists. A clinical background with additional experience related to statistics is beneficial. Clinical investigators are usually practicing wound care clinicians who have a diverse practice and the ability to work with Institutional Review Boards (IRB) without creating a delay for the study sponsor. Sponsors usually prefer an investigator with a minimum of five years of patient care experience. Investigators are often called upon to publish the findings of a particular study and/or present the findings at a national conference in either oral or poster form. In addition, investigators are often used to present findings and answer questions to the sponsors sales force prior to introduction of the product onto the market.

Industry also hires clinical advisors who meet with key personnel to discuss and review the wound care market with respect to product needs and positioning. Advisors, like investigators, are usually experienced wound care specialists with a diverse practice. Since it is important for industry to consult a variety of specialists, this type of opportunity is usually limited with each company.

Another opportunity rests in consumer education and development of consumer education tools such as pamphlets and videos. Many companies seek practicing professionals to assist in the development of educational tools for consumers. Again, this opportunity is usually limited to the task at hand; however, it opens doors in many other areas.

Many companies hire wound specialists to provide other types of internal education. Classes are taught to sales associates and cover all aspects of wound management, marketing to specialist clinicians, competitor challenges, and marketing strategies with respect to competitive products.

Requests are often made of both independent clinicians and company employed wound specialists to develop papers which relate to support of their products. These papers are then submitted to journals for publication or used as selling pieces for their sales staff.

In some cases, companies actually hire wound specialists to become sales associates. Others hire or contract them for clinical sales support. These specialists are often utilized to make rounds in a facility with staff nurses and to provide education while assisting the company to position products for use in a particular facility. The opportunities in industry seem endless and are very important to the proper development and implementation of products and services in the wound care market.

Insurance companies, litigators and attorneys utilize experienced wound clinicians as expert witnesses. This type of utilization is most often fee per service, based on the hours one spends reviewing charts, flagging pertinent data, writing summaries, investigating standards of care, and locating supporting documentation. In addition, specialists are contracted to serve as expert witnesses during depositions, on court review boards and even in jury trials. Expert witnesses are usually clinicians with at least seven years experience. These opportunities can be marketed through insurance litigators and attorneys.

Conclusion

There are boundless opportunities for wound care specialists. The opportunities described above explore only some conventional and non–conventional markets for CETNs, CWCNs, physical therapists and CNSs with wound expertise. Good market research, clear demonstration of a plan to assist clients in achieving their goals, excellent client communication, and development of strategies for promoting yourself and your services are truly the key to securing your position in the field of wound management.

Suggested Reading

1. Gardenswartz L. *What it Takes*. New York, NY, Dolphin Doubleday, 1987.
2. Johnson J. Developing an effective business plan. *Nursing Economics* 1990;8:57–64.
3. Arnold N, Weir D. Retrospective analysis of healing in wounds cared for by ET nurses versus staff nurses in a home setting. *Journal of Wound Ostomy and Continence Nurses* 1994;July:156–160.
4. Taylor S. ET nurses enhance quality of care from within vendor organizations. *The Resource* 1994;1(2):1.
5. Russell Sukau B. Working our in house ET vs independent ET relationship issues. *The Resource* 1994;1(2):2.
6. Carroll L. Organizing successful seminars, how vendor reps can help. *The Resource* 1994;1(2):2.
7. Steffan J. Utilization management in managed care as an effective arena for the ET nurse, *The Resource* 1994;1(3):2–3.
8. Eichinger K. Manufacturers role in end user education. *The Resource* 1995;1(4):4–5.
9. International Association for Enterostomal Therapy. Professional Practice Manual, 1990.
10. Hale M. Pressure sores targeted for quality improvement. Innovations '93, American College of Physician Executives, pp 207–210.
11. Milazzo V. How to formulate and negotiate contracts. Medical Legal Consulting Institute, Inc. Houston Texas, 1996.
12. Milazzo V. How To become a prosperous medical legal consultant. Medical Legal Consulting Institute, Inc. Houston Texas, 1996.
13. Milazzo V. How to develop an action oriented marketing strategy for your nursing business. Medical Legal Consulting Institute, Inc. Houston Texas, 1996.
14. National Nurses in Business. How I Became a Nurse Entrepreneur: Tales from 50 Nurses in Business. National Nurses in Business, Petaloma, CA, 1991.

Conclusion

Diane Krasner, MS, RN, CETN
Dean Kane, MD, FACS

A Prescription for Advanced Wound Caring:

Assessing holistically

Developing comprehensive plans

Valuing the patient's perspective

Allowing the family to be involved

Networking on behalf of the patient

Communication with other team members

Encouraging collaboration

Developing your own expertise.

Watching for subtle wound changes

Observing the signs of progress

Undertaking treatments with care

Nourishing the patient and the wound

Demonstrating your respect for the patient and the wound.

Cultivating caring practices and comportment

Aligning care to the patient, the wound and the setting

Remaining optimistic and attentive

Inspiring excellence

Nurturing and comforting

Giving your very best.

Index

response modifiers, 184
Biology, wound, 118
Biopsy, 7–8, 49, 85, 90, 103, 325
Biotherapy, 188
Bismuth triboron phenate, 129
Blood
  capillaries, 75
  cells
  red, 350
  white, 84
  clotting, 49
  flow, 173, 322, 327
  gas, arterial, 65
  glucose, 174
  pressure
  cuffs, 321
  diastolic, 31
  stopping, 104
  supply, 114, 175
  wound, in test tube, 124
Body
  fat, 74
  water, 7
Bone
  marrow
  hypoplasia, 232
  sensitivity to radiation, 70
  scans, 173
Bony
  prominences, 236
  tissue, 40
Bowel
  disease, 335
  edema, 75
  hypo–oncotic, 75
Braden scale, 30–31
British Pharmaceutical Codex of 1923, 125
Building a Wound Care Healing Team,
Buchbinder D, Melick CF, Hilton MM, Huber
  GJ, 321–324
Burn(s)
  centers, 59
  dressings for, 129
  patients, 391
  second degree, 59
  severe, 75
  wounds, 21, 62, 191, 390, 392
Bypass, surgery, see also Surgery, 175

C

Cadaver dermis, 392
Cadexomer iodine ointment, 61
Calcium
  alginate dressings, 53
  aloe vera contains, 219
Calories, see also Nutrition, 77
Cancer(s)
  patients, 335
  skin, 3, 184, 238, 309
  squamous cell, 238
Candida albicans, 216, 271
Capillary(ies)
  blood and lymph, 75
  gauze, 7
  lymph, 75
  microscopy, 325
Carbohydrates, 67
Carbon monoxide, 65
Carcinoma, basal cell, 184, 195
Cardiff, Wales, wound healing in, 117
Cardiology, 309
Care, see also Wound care, Healthcare
  facilities, 299
  giver, 10, 210, 216
  services marketing, 404
  wound, 4–5
Case studies compared with clinical evaluations, 378
Catabolism of body protein, 67
Catheter sizes, 100
CDC, 251
Cell(s)
  balance, 395
  basal, carcinoma, 184, 195
  biology, wound, 389
  connective tissue, 390
  damage, 112
  death, 348
  destruction, 90
  epidermal, 53, 179, 391–392
  fluids, 242
  keratinized, 179
  mesanchymal, 345
  migration, 53, 390
  mitochondria, 348
  proliferation, 54
  red blood, 350
  squamous, carcinoma, 184, 195, 238
  therapy, 58

white blood, 84
Cellular
    changes in wound healing, 64
    replication, 81
Cellulitis, 88, 192
Centers for Disease Control and Prevention, 93
Cerebrovascular disease, 173
Certified Enterostomal Therapy Nurses
    (CETN), 403
Charcot deformity, 69, 172–173
Chemicals, toxic, 114
Chemotherapeutic vesicant drugs and anti-
    dotes, 190
Chemotherapy, 70, 184, 187
Chills, 192
Chloramphenicol, 232
Chlorhexidine, 129
Chloride, aloe vera contains, 219
Chloromycetin, 232
Cholesterol, aloe vera contains, 219
Chronic
    disease
    pain, 333
    venous, 20, 328, 330
    leg ulcers, 85
    wounds, see also Wounds,1–2, 4, 6–9,
    11, 20, 37, 49, 54, 59, 61, 64, 67, 70,
    84–85, 109, 111–112, 260, 269, 309, 324,
    336, 346, 354, 389–390
Chronic Wound Pain, Krasner D, 336–342
Classifications, wound, see also Wounds
    arterial ulcers, 158
    diabetic wounds, 172
    pressure ulcers, 152
Claudication, 173, 174
Claw deformity, 172, 173
Cleansers, 97, 120, 178, 214
Cleansing
    skin, 179
    wound, 97, 212, 216, 341
Clinical
    nurse specialists (CNS), 403
    research, 374
Clostridium, 8, 234
Closure, tension free, 187
Co–Factors in Impaired Wound Healing, Stotts
    NA, Wipke–Tevis D, 64–72
Cocci, aerobic gram positive, 174
Cod liver oil, 129
Cognitive ability, insufficient, 68
Colchisine, 194

Collagen
    anchoring, 238
    biosynthetic, 139
    breakdown by enzymes in wounds, 84
    expression in various wound types,
    118
    formation, 81
    hydroxyproline levels in, 65
    lysis, 64
    production, 241
    synthesis, 51, 194, 345
    type IV, 390
Collagenase, 115, 232
Colloidal oatmeal powder baths, 184
Colonization, microbe, 90
Color system of wound classification, 25, 85
Compresses, Dressings, 339
Compression
    dressings, 238
    pumps, 342
    therapy, 255, 392
Congestive heart failure, 235
Connective tissue, 195, 390, 392
Contact plate, 7
Controlled Clinical Evaluations vs. Case
    Studies: Why Wound Care
    Professionals Need to Know the
    Difference, Roma A, Bolton L, McNally
    A, 373–382
Controlled compression therapy, 392
Copper, 67, 81
Cornified epidermis, 392
Coronary artery disease, 173
Corticosteroids, 31, 184, 187
Cortisol levels, 31
Cortisone, 91
Cost
    care, 172
    containment, 217
    effectiveness, 309, 369
    prevention, 11
    reducing, 367
    wound care, 54, 354, 358–359
Cost Effectiveness in Wound Care, Phillips TJ,
    369–372
Cotton wool, 125
Cream
    general, 182
    silver sulfadiazine, 106
    topical peroxide, 266
Creatinine

Tranquilizers, 184
Transcutaneous oxygen
    analysis, 317
    measurements, 65, 160, 174
    monitoring, 327
Transfer assistance, 311
Transferrin, 76
Transient bacteremia, 176
Transitional care facilities, 304
Transparent film dressings, 41
Trauma to skin adjacent to wounds, 55
Traumatic wounds, 40, 100
Triglycerides, aloe vera contains, 219
Tubes, 202
Tulle dressings, 128
Tumors, metastatic, 184
Tunneling, 38
Turgor, tissue, 236

U

Ulcer(s) see also Wounds
    arterial, 12, 158, 237, 262, 271
    decubitus, 42, 236
    dermal, 331
    development, 353
    diabetic, 1, 59, 159, 173, 238
    ischemic, 12
    leg, 12, 18, 60, 85, 121, 331
    lower extremity, 175
    Marjolin's, 195
    medical management, 163
    neuropathic, 12, 68
    non–healing, 235
    pathogenesis, 166
    pressure, 1, 9–11, 29, 64, 67–69, 81–82,
        90, 104, 144, 159, 178, 196–198, 214,
        236, 245, 262, 284, 336–337, 340, 370,
        391
    prevention, 32, 126
    surgical management, 162
    vascular, 64
    vasculitic, 159
    venous, 1, 3, 12, 68, 159, 165, 237,
        262–263, 267–268, 331, 353, 390–391
Ulceration, 186–187
Ultrasound, 29, 251, 253, 258, 325
Ultraviolet C, 255
Undermining, 38, 44
United Kingdom wound care, 115
United States Public Health Hospital, 265

Unna boot, 170
Uremia, 70
Uric acid, aloe vera contains, 219
Urinary
    incontinence, see also Incontinence,
        178, 196–197, 248
    tract infection, 235
U,S, Preventive Services Task Force, 29

V

Vaccination scars, 195
Vaccine, influenza, 94
Vaginal dressings, 129
Validity of color system of wound classifica-
    tion, 25
Valvular insufficiency, 269
Vancomycin resistant enterococcus, 91
Vascular
    disease, 173, 175
    microcirculation system, 84
    surgery, 309
    technologists, 322
    testing, 173–174, 312
    ulcers, 64
    wounds, 40
Vascularized
    connective tissue, 195
    flaps, 236
Vasculitic ulcers, 159
Vasculitis, 2
Vasoactive drugs, 31
Venograms, 237
Venous
    doppler diagnosis, 237
    ulcers, 1–3, 12, 20, 67–68, 159, 165,
        237–238, 262, 269, 328, 330–331, 353,
        390–391, 67–68
Venous ulceration, 165
Venous Ulceration, Falanga V, 165–171
Vesicant drugs, chemotherapeutic, and recom-
    mended antidotes, 190
Vinegar, 225
Virus, cytomegalo–, hepatitis, AIDS, 176
Visceral proteins, 74
Vitamins, 67, 70, 80, 194, 246

W

Water

X

Z